The American Psychiatric Publishing

Textbook of Suicide Assessment and Management

Second Edition

The American Psychiatric Publishing

Textbook of Suicide Assessment and Management

Second Edition

Edited by

Robert I. Simon, M.D.

Robert E. Hales, M.D., M.B.A.

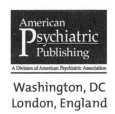

American Psychiatric Publishing
A Division of American Psychiatric Association

Washington, DC
London, England

If you would like to buy between 25 and 99 copies of this or any other American Psychiatric Publishing title, you are eligible for a 20% discount; please contact Customer Service at appi@psych.org or 800–368–5777. If you wish to buy 100 or more copies of the same title, please e-mail us at bulksales@psych.org for a price quote.

Copyright © 2012 American Psychiatric Association

ALL RIGHTS RESERVED

Manufactured in the United States of America on acid-free paper

16 15 14 13 12   5 4 3 2 1

First Edition

Typeset in Formata and Palatino

American Psychiatric Publishing
a Division of American Psychiatric Association
1000 Wilson Boulevard
Arlington, VA 22209-3901
www.appi.org

Library of Congress Cataloging-in-Publication Data
The American Psychiatric Publishing textbook of suicide assessment and management / edited by Robert I. Simon, Robert E. Hales. — 2nd ed.
    p. ; cm.
    Textbook of suicide assessment and management
    Suicide assessment and management
    Includes bibliographical references and index.
    ISBN 978-1-58562-414-0 (hardcover : alk. paper)
    I. Simon, Robert I. II. Hales, Robert E. III. American Psychiatric Publishing. IV. Title: Textbook of suicide assessment and management. V. Title: Suicide assessment and management.
    [DNLM: 1. Suicide—psychology. 2. Mental Disorders—complications. 3. Risk Assessment—methods. 4. Suicide—prevention & control. WM 165]
    616.85'8445—dc23

2012007971

British Library Cataloguing in Publication Data
A CIP record is available from the British Library.

Contents

PART I
Suicide Risk Assessment

PART II
Major Mental Disorders

PART III
Treatment

PART IV
Treatment Settings

PART V

Special Populations

PART VI

Special Topics

Contributors

Sara E. Allison, M.D.
Psychiatrist, Michael E. DeBakey Veterans Affairs Medical Center, Houston, Texas

Laura N. Antar, M.D., Ph.D.
Research Fellow, Autism and Obsessive-Compulsive Spectrum Program, Albert Einstein College of Medicine, Montefiore Medical Center, Bronx, New York

Peter Ash, M.D.
Chief, Child and Adolescent Psychiatry; Director, Psychiatry and Law Service; and Associate Professor, Department of Psychiatry and Behavioral Sciences, Emory University School of Medicine, Atlanta, Georgia

Nazanin Bahraini, Ph.D.
Clinical Research Psychologist, Department of Veterans Affairs, Mental Illness Research, Education and Clinical Center (MIRECC); Assistant Professor, Department of Psychiatry, University of Colorado Denver School of Medicine, Denver Colorado

Ross J. Baldessarini, M.D.
Professor of Psychiatry and in Neuroscience, Department of Psychiatry, Harvard Medical School; Founding Director, International Consortium for Bipolar Disorder Research and Director, Psychopharmacology Program, McLean Hospital, Belmont, Massachusetts; Senior Consulting Psychiatrist, Massachusetts General Hospital, Boston, Massachusetts

Amy Barnhorst, M.D.
Assistant Clinical Professor, Department of Psychiatry and Behavioral Sciences, University of California, Davis School of Medicine, Sacramento, California

Mark J. Bates, Ph.D.
Lieutenant Colonel (Retired), Biomedical Science Corps, U.S. Air Force; Director, Resilience and Prevention Directorate, Defense Centers of Excellence for Psychological Health and Traumatic Brain Injury (DCoE), Silver Spring, Maryland

Aaron T. Beck, M.D.
Emeritus Professor, Department of Psychiatry, Perelman School of Medicine, University of Pennsylvania

Alan L. Berman, Ph.D., A.B.P.P.
Executive Director, American Association of Suicidology, Washington, D.C.

Bruce Bongar, Ph.D., A.B.P.P., F.A.P.M.
Calvin Professor of Psychology, Pacific Graduate School of Psychology, Palo Alto; Consulting Professor of Psychiatry and Behavioral Sciences, Stanford University School of Medicine, Stanford, California

J. Michael Bostwick, M.D.
Professor of Psychiatry, Department of Psychiatry and Psychology, Mayo Clinic College of Medicine, Rochester, Minnesota

John C. Bradley, M.D.
Colonel (Retired), Medical Corps, U.S. Army; Clinical Professor of Psychiatry, Uniformed Services University of the Health Sciences; Chief of Psychiatry and Deputy Director for Mental Health, VA Boston Healthcare System, Brockton, Massachusetts

Beth S. Brodsky, Ph.D.
Associate Clinical Professor of Medical Psychology (in Psychiatry), Columbia University College of Physicians and Surgeons, New York, New York

Gregory K. Brown, Ph.D.
Research Associate Professor of Clinical Psychology in Psychiatry, Department of Psychiatry, Perelman School of Medicine, University of Pennsylvania

Frank R. Campbell, Ph.D., L.C.S.W., C.T.
Senior Consultant in Forensic Suicidology, Campbell and Associates Consulting, LLC (www.lossteam.com)

Juan J. Carballo, M.D., Ph.D.
Professor of Psychiatry, Department of Psychiatry, Fundacion Jimenez Diaz University Hospital, Autonomous University of Madrid, Madrid, Spain

Cameron S. Carter, M.D.
Professor of Psychiatry and Director, Imaging Research Center, University of California, Davis School of Medicine, Sacramento, California

Frank Chen, M.D.
Houston Adult Psychiatry, Houston, Texas

Yeates Conwell, M.D.
Professor, Department of Psychiatry, University of Rochester Medical Center, Rochester, New York

Dianne Currier, Ph.D., M.P.H.
Senior Research Fellow, Australian Longitudinal Study on Male Health, Center for Molecular, Environmental, Genetic and Analytic Epidemiology, Melbourne School of Population Health, University of Melbourne, Australia

D. Edward Deneke, M.D.
Fellow in Psychosomatic Medicine, Department of Psychiatry, University of Michigan, Ann Arbor, Michigan

Jan Fawcett, M.D.
Professor, Department of Psychiatry, University of New Mexico School of Medicine, Albuquerque, New Mexico

Glen O. Gabbard, M.D.
Professor of Psychiatry, SUNY Upstate Medical University, Syracuse, New York; Clinical Professor of Psychiatry, Baylor College of Medicine, Houston, Texas

Michael Gitlin, M.D.
Professor of Clinical Psychiatry, Geffen School of Medicine at University of California—Los Angeles, Los Angeles, California

Liza H. Gold, M.D.
Clinical Professor of Psychiatry, Georgetown University Medical Center, Washington, D.C.

Matthew N. Goldenberg, M.D.
Assistant Professor, Department of Psychiatry, Uniformed Services University of the Health Sciences, Bethesda, Maryland

Robert E. Hales, M.D., M.B.A.
Joe P. Tupin Professor and Chair, Department of Psychiatry and Behavioral Sciences, University of California–Davis School of Medicine, Sacramento, California; Medical Director, Sacramento County Mental Health Services, Sacramento, California; Editor-in-Chief, American Psychiatric Publishing

Lindsay M. Hayes, M.S.
Project Director, National Center on Institutions and Alternatives, Mansfield, Massachusetts

Marnin J. Heisel, Ph.D.
Departments of Psychiatry and Epidemiology & Biostatistics, University of Western Ontario, London, Ontario, Canada; Department of Psychiatry, University of Rochester Medical Center, Rochester, New York

Donald Hilty, M.D.
Professor of Clinical Psychiatry, Department of Psychiatry and Behavioral Sciences, University of California, Davis School of Medicine, Sacramento, California

Eric Hollander, M.D.
Clinical Professor of Psychiatry and Behavioral Sciences and Director, Autism and Obsessive-Compulsive Spectrum Program, Albert Einstein College of Medicine, Montefiore Medical Center, Bronx, New York

Marco Innamorati, Psy.D.
Professor of Psychology, Department of Neurosciences, Mental Health and Sensory Organs, Suicide Prevention Center, Department of Psychiatry, Sant'Andrea Hospital, Sapienza University of Rome, Rome, Italy

H. Florence Kim, M.D., M.A.
Houston Adult Psychiatry, Houston, Texas

Martin H. Leamon, M.D.
Health Sciences Clinical Professor of Psychiatry, Department of Psychiatry and Behavioral Sciences, University of California, Davis School of Medicine, Sacramento, California

David Lester, Ph.D.
Distinguished Professor of Psychology, The Richard Stockton College of New Jersey, Galloway, New Jersey

Carl P. Malmquist, M.D., M.S.
Professor of Forensic Psychiatry, University of Minnesota, Minneapolis, Minnesota

John T. Maltsberger, M.D.
Clinical Professor of Psychiatry, Harvard Medical School, Boston; Clinical Associate, McLean Hospital, Belmont; Boston Psychoanalytic Society and Institute, Boston, Massachusetts

J. John Mann, M.D.
Paul Janssen Professor of Translational Neuroscience and Director, Division of Molecular Imaging and Neuropathology, Department of Psychiatry, Columbia University, New York

Daryl Matthews, M.D., Ph.D.
Clinical Professor Psychiatry, John A. Burns School of Medicine, University of Hawaii at Manoa, Honolulu, Hawaii

Donald J. Meyer, M.D.
Associate Director, Forensic Psychiatry, Beth Israel Deaconess Medical Center; Member Program in Psychiatry and Law at Massachusetts Mental Health Center and Assistant Clinical Professor, Harvard Medical School, Boston, Massachusetts

Jeffrey L. Metzner, M.D.
Clinical Professor of Psychiatry, University of Colorado School of Medicine, Denver, Colorado

Paula T. Morelli, Ph.D.
Associate Professor, Myron B. Thompson School of Social Work, University of Hawaii at Manoa, Honolulu, Hawaii

Maria A. Oquendo, M.D.
Professor of Clinical Psychiatry, Columbia University College of Physicians and Surgeons; Vice Chair for Education, Director of Residency Training, and Director of the Clinical Evaluation Core of the Silvio O. Conte Center for the Neurobiology of Mental Disorders, New York State Psychiatric Institute, New York, New York

Maurizio Pompili, M.D., Ph.D.
Professor of Suicidology, Department of Neurosciences, Mental Health and Sensory Organs, Sant'Andrea Hospital, Sapienza University of Rome, Italy; Research Affiliate, International Consortium for Bipolar Disorder Research, McLean Hospital, Belmont, Massachusetts and Department of Psychiatry, Harvard Medical School, Boston, Massachusetts

Divy Ravindranath, M.D., M.S.
Clinical Assistant Professor, Department of Psychiatry, University of Michigan, Ann Arbor, Michigan

Patricia R. Recupero, J.D., M.D.
Clinical Professor of Psychiatry, Warren Alpert Medical School of Brown University; President and CEO, Butler Hospital, Providence, Rhode Island

Phillip J. Resnick, M.D.
Professor of Psychiatry and Director, Fellowship in Forensic Psychiatry, Case Western Reserve University School of Medicine, Cleveland, Ohio; Adjunct Professor, Case Western Reserve University School of Law, Cleveland, Ohio; Director of the Court Psychiatric Clinic, Cleveland, Ohio

Michelle Riba, M.D., M.S.
Clinical Professor and Associate Chair, Department of Psychiatry, University of Michigan, Ann Arbor, Michigan

M. David Rudd, Ph.D., A.B.P.P.
Dean, College of Social & Behavioral Science; Scientific Director, National Center for Veterans Studies; Professor, Department of Psychology, University of Utah, Salt Lake City, Utah

Charles L. Scott, M.D.
Chief, Division of Psychiatry and the Law, Professor of Clinical Psychiatry, Director, Forensic Psychiatry Fellowship, University of California Davis Medical Center, Sacramento, California

Andreea L. Seritan, M.D.
Associate Professor of Clinical Psychiatry and Assistant Dean, Student Wellness, University of California, Davis School of Medicine, Sacramento, California

Shawn Christopher Shea, M.D.
Director, Training Institute for Suicide Assessment and Clinical Interviewing (TISA), Stoddard, New Hampshire

Robert I. Simon, M.D.
Clinical Professor of Psychiatry and Director, Program in Psychiatry and Law, Georgetown University School of Medicine, Washington, D.C.; Chairman, Department of Psychiatry, Suburban Hospital, Johns Hopkins Medicine, Bethesda, Maryland

Barbara Stanley, Ph.D.
Lecturer in Psychiatry and Director, Suicide Intervention Center, New York State Psychiatric Institute. Columbia University College of Physicians and Surgeons, New York, New York

Joseph B. Stoklosa, M.D.
Instructor in Psychiatry, Harvard Medical School, Boston; Assistant Psychiatrist, McLean Hospital, Belmont, Massachusetts

Glenn R. Sullivan, Ph.D.
Assistant Professor, Department of Psychology and Philosophy, Virginia Military Institute, Lexington, Virginia

Michael E. Thase, M.D.
Professor, Department of Psychiatry, Perelman School of Medicine, University of Pennsylvania

Leonardo Tondo, M.D., M.Sc.
Lecturer and Research Associate, Department of Psychiatry, Harvard Medical School and International Consortium for Bipolar Disorder Research, McLean Hospital, Belmont, Massachusetts; Associate Professor (emeritus), Department of Psychology, University of Cagliari, Italy; Founding Director, Centro Lucio Bini Mood Disorders Research Center, Cagliari, Italy

Sheila Wendler, M.D.
Assistant Clinical Professor of Psychiatry, John A. Burns School of Medicine, University of Hawaii at Manoa, Honolulu, Hawaii

Jesse H. Wright, M.D., Ph.D.
Professor, Department of Psychiatry and Behavioral Sciences, University of Louisville

Glen L. Xiong, M.D.
Health Sciences Assistant Clinical Professor, Department of Psychiatry and Behavioral Sciences, University of California, Davis School of Medicine; Medical Director, Sacramento County Mental Health Treatment Center, Sacramento, California

Jong H. Yoon, M.D.
Assistant Professor of Psychiatry, University of California, Davis School of Medicine, Sacramento, California

Stuart C. Yudofsky, M.D.
D.C. and Irene Ellwood Professor and Chairman, Menninger Department of Psychiatry and Behavioral Sciences, and Drs. Beth K. and Stuart C. Yudofsky Presidential Chair of Neuropsychiatry, Baylor College of Medicine; Chairman, Department of Psychiatry, The Methodist Hospital, Houston, Texas

Disclosure of Competing Interests

The following contributors to this book have indicated a financial interest in or other affiliation with a commercial supporter, a manufacturer of a commercial product, a provider of a commercial service, a nongovernmental organization, and/or a government agency, as listed below:

Peter Ash, M.D.—Consults with attorneys and provides expert testimony in a wide variety of cases, including malpractice cases that involve child or adolescent suicides.

Michael Gitlin, M.D.—*Honoraria:* Servier; *Speaker's bureau:* AstraZeneca, Bristol-Myers Squibb, Eli Lilly; the author notes that this support presents no conflict of interest for the chapter.

Marnin J. Heisel, Ph.D.—*Research support:* Canadian Institutes of Health Research, American Foundation for Suicide Prevention, Ontario Mental Health Foundation, Ontario Ministry of Research and Innovation; *Honorarium:* Canadian Coalition for Seniors' Mental Health (for leading development of set of knowledge translation tools for late-life suicide prevention. The author notes that none of this support comprises a conflict of interest for the chapter.

Eric Hollander, M.D.—*Consultant:* Transcept

J. John Mann, M.D.—*Grants* (unrelated past grants): GlaxoSmithKline, Novartis

Maria A. Oquendo, M.D.—*Grant/research support:* American Foundation for Suicide Prevention, AstraZeneca, Bristol-Myers Squibb, Eli Lilly, Janssen, Pfizer, National Institute of Mental Health, National Institute on Alcohol Abuse and Alcoholism, Shire; *Shareholder:* Bristol-Myers Squibb (spouse is full-time employee)

Shawn Christopher Shea, M.D.—*Consultant:* Pfizer (one-time consultant on improving medication adherence; not topic of chapter)

Michael E. Thase, M.D.—The author reports no conflicts of interest related to this this chapter. However, in the spirit of full disclosure, during the past 3 years, Dr. Thase has acted as advisor/consultant for Alkermes, AstraZeneca, Bristol-Myers Squibb Company, Eli Lilly & Co., Dey Pharma, L.P., Forest Laboratories (formerly PGx Health, Inc), Gerson Lehman Group, GlaxoSmithKline, Guidepoint Global, H. Lundbeck A/S, MedAvante, Inc., Merck and Co. Inc. (formerly Schering Plough and Organon), Neuronetics, Inc., Novartis, Otsuka, Ortho-McNeil Pharmaceuticals (Johnson & Johnson), Pamlab, L.L.C., Pfizer (formerly Wyeth Ayerst Pharmaceuticals), Shire US Inc., Supernus Pharmaceuticals, Takeda, and Transcept Pharmaceuticals. During the past 3 years, he has received grant support from Agency for Healthcare Research and Quality, Eli Lilly and Company, Forest Pharmaceuticals, GlaxoSmithKline, National Institute of Mental Health, Otsuka Pharmaceuticals, and Sepracor, Inc. Prior to 2011, he served on the Speakers Bureau for AstraZeneca, Bristol-Myers Squibb Company, Eli Lilly & Co., Merck and Co. Inc., and Pfizer (formerly Wyeth Ayerst Pharmaceuticals).

Jesse H. Wright, M.D., Ph.D.—*Consultant:* Takeda Pharmaceuticals; *Stock:* Empower Interactive, Mindstreet; *Book royalties:* American Psychiatric Publishing, Guilford Press, Simon & Schuster

Glen L. Xiong, M.D.—*Research grant:* National Alliance for Research in Schizophrenia and Depression; *Consulting workgroup member:* PgxHealth

The following contributors to this book indicated that they have no competing interests or affiliations to declare:

Laura N. Antar, M.D., Ph.D.
Nazanin Bahraini, Ph.D.
Amy Barnhorst, M.D.
Mark J. Bates, Ph.D.
Aaron T. Beck, M.D.
Alan L. Berman, Ph.D., A.B.P.P.
Bruce Bongar, Ph.D., A.B.P.P., F.A.P.M.
J. Michael Bostwick, M.D.
John C. Bradley, M.D.
Beth S. Brodsky, Ph.D.
Gregory K. Brown, Ph.D.
Frank R. Campbell, Ph.D., L.C.S.W., C.T.
Juan J. Carballo, M.D., Ph.D.
Cameron S. Carter, M.D.
Frank Chen, M.D.
Yeates Conwell, M.D.
Dianne Currier, Ph.D., M.P.H.
Jan Fawcett, M.D.
Glen O. Gabbard, M.D.
Liza H. Gold, M.D.
Matthew N. Goldenberg, M.D.
Robert E. Hales, M.D., M.B.A.
Lindsay M. Hayes, M.S.
Donald Hilty, M.D.
Marco Innamorati, Psy.D.
H. Florence Kim, M.D., M.A.
Martin H. Leamon, M.D.
David Lester, Ph.D.
Carl P. Malmquist, M.D., M.S.
John T. Maltsberger, M.D.
Daryl Matthews, M.D., Ph.D.
Donald J. Meyer, M.D.
Jeffrey L. Metzner, M.D.
Paula T. Morelli, Ph.D.
Maurizio Pompili, M.D., Ph.D.
Divy Ravindranath, M.D., M.S.
Patricia R. Recupero, J.D., M.D.
Phillip J. Resnick, M.D.
Michelle Riba, M.D., M.S.
M. David Rudd, Ph.D., A.B.P.P.
Charles L. Scott, M.D.
Andreea L. Seritan, M.D.
Robert I. Simon, M.D.
Barbara Stanley, Ph.D.
Joseph B. Stoklosa, M.D.
Glenn R. Sullivan, Ph.D.
Sheila Wendler, M.D.
Jong H. Yoon, M.D.
Stuart C. Yudofsky, M.D.

Foreword

Stuart C. Yudofsky, M.D.

The "Black Wolf" of Psychiatrists

As I write this foreword, I have been practicing psychiatry for over 37 years. I care for patients on nearly every working day. Whether I am treating patients, teaching and supervising medical students and psychiatry residents, or conducting research, she is always with me. She lurks in the shadows by day, and her howlings unsettle my sleep by night. In the worst of times, her heaviness sags my back; her wet, hot breath blankets the nape of my neck; and her fangs sink deep into my being. In the best of times, she prances at my side with the pose of a harmless, domesticated pet. But she is always there. And there is just no way that I can shake her off, as she might propel crystal pellets of water following a plunge into the black swamp. I imagine her to be a ponderous, powerful, black wolf whose loyalty is inviolate. Oh how I wish she were a bit less faithful and fateful, so that I might catch a breath of peace. But this cannot be the lot of a psychiatrist—nor, do I suspect, can it be the lot of mental health professionals of other disciplines who treat patients with severe and persistent mental illnesses.

The "black wolf" of psychiatrists to which I refer is *suicide*—the littermate of depression, "the black dog" about which Sir Winston Churchill so famously spoke, as quoted by his private secretary, John Colville:

> Of course we all have moments of depression, especially after breakfast. It was then that Lord Moran [Churchill's doctor] would sometimes call to take his patient's pulse and hope to make a note of what was happening in the wide world. Churchill, not especially pleased to see any visitor at such an hour, might excuse a certain early morning surliness by saying, "I've got a black dog on my back today…" Churchill suffered from periodic bouts of acute depression, which, with the Churchillian gift for apt expression, he called "black dog." (Colville 1995)

As physicians and scientists, psychiatrists perennially glimpse and marvel at the unfathomable complexity of the human body. It matters not whether we examine the surfaces of our patients' skin with the macro lenses of our vision and touch or evaluate molecular structure of their cells with transmission electron microscopes; we can usually approach understanding the purpose of this complexity through the unifying concept of *survival*. No wonder that we find overwhelming the realization that a thought, feeling, or impulse can trump this infinite complexity that serves survival and lead to suicide.

The following case of a man who presented about 2 years ago illustrates how the black dog of suicide relentlessly stalks my everyday practice of neuropsychiatry.

The Case of Mr. Burton Harcourt

History and Presenting Illness

Congenitally congenial and characterologically gifted, Mrs. Hoffman peered into my office and whispered plaintively, "Your new patient with traumatic brain injury decided to cancel his appointment this morning; but his wife came instead. I hope that you will agree to meet with her. She seems quite distressed."

If gold and diamonds are metaphors for sinew and muscle, Mrs. Helen Harcourt could have been an Olympic weight lifter. Bejeweled and attired in opulence more appropriate for the coronation of royalty than a visit to a commoner doctor, she nonetheless appeared anxious and vulnerable. "I must apologize for my husband's not coming," she lamented. "He changed his mind at the last minute." Mrs. Harcourt acknowledged that her husband neither trusted nor liked psychiatrists: "I'm embarrassed to say that Burton believes that psychiatrists are more *troubled* than their patients—but he would use a different word."

"Would that word be *crazy*?" I speculated.

Blushing profusely, Mrs. Harcourt conceded, "Yes, that's the word. But I could not disagree with him more."

"Has he ever 'seen' a psychiatrist?" I inquired.

"No. But for many years before his skiing accident, I had asked him to go with me for couples counseling, but he always refused," she replied.

Mrs. Harcourt proceeded to disclose that she had been married for 23 years to Burton Harcourt, whom she had met when they were both students at Dartmouth College. A native of Incline Village, California, Burton was not only captain of the Dartmouth Ski team but also an outstanding student majoring in business, and president of the senior class. They married right after college and moved to New York City, where Burton worked as a securities analyst for an investment banking firm while Helen attended medical school.

"I became pregnant with my older child at the beginning my second year of medical school, and gave birth to her right before I was to begin my clinical rotations. Although I was approved to take 3 months off from school, I never went back. I had very mixed feelings about returning. On one hand, I had long been passionate about science and becoming a physician. On the other hand, I *did* want to be with our baby almost every moment. Burton made the ultimate decision, however. He told me, 'Medical school makes no sense for us; you will waste tons of time to make piddling amounts of money. Let me take care of that part.'"

For the next several years Burton spent most of his waking hours at work. Not only was he was rarely home, but he did not evidence interest in his wife or two young daughters. Upon receiving his MBA from Harvard University, Burton founded a venture capital firm that specialized in natural resource investments. With Burton as its president and CEO, the company moved to Houston, where it grew exponentially in size, profits, and influence. Shrewdly investing his personal wealth in the purchase of immense stakes in the Eagle Ford and Marcellus shale oil and gas plays in Texas, Pennsylvania, and other states, Mr. Harcourt became a billionaire by age 47. Thereafter, he devoted most of his time to traveling internationally to attend business meetings and sporting events and to take skiing, hunting, and fishing holidays with business associates and friends—rarely with his family. He even missed his older daughter's graduation from high school in order to attend a World Cup soccer match. He was perennially critical of Mrs. Harcourt's appearance and her intelligence and shy temperament.

Eighteen months prior to his scheduled meeting with me, Mr. Harcourt was seriously injured while helicopter skiing in British Columbia. Not wearing a helmet, he suffered severe brain injury when he careened, at high velocity, into an ice-hardened snowbank. After 3 weeks he emerged from coma with manifestations of prefrontal and left-brain injury, including right hemiparesis, a severe expressive aphasia, and neuropsychiatric symptoms, including impulsivity, impaired social judgment, affective lability, and depression. His intellect and cognition were spared. Over the next 18 months, he worked diligently with his team of rehabilitation professionals and made excellent progress. Nonetheless, his speech remained somewhat garbled and halting, his balance was impaired, and he ambulated slowly with a pronounced limp. Mr. Harcourt spent most of his time at home, where he would have temper tantrums—elicited by seemingly minor frustrations—in which he would scream expletives and throw and break objects. He reacted especially vehemently to Mrs. Harcourt's efforts to assist him when he lost his balance and fell. On such occasions, he would wrench away from his wife's grasp while screaming, "Stop putting me down, you fat bitch. I'm not an invalid; and you're not my mother!"

Many factors in this case raised my concerns regarding the suicidal risk of Mr. Harcourt. Among these were the damage to his left brain and prefrontal cortex, the likeli-

hood that he suffered from major depression and narcissistic personality disorder, his impulsivity, his social withdrawal, and the profound diminution in his self-esteem as a result of his physical disabilities and other losses.

I asked Mrs. Harcourt whether her husband ever exhibited self-destructive behavior or made reference to suicide or wanting to die, to which she responded, "He has never mentioned suicide directly nor overtly tried to harm himself. Nonetheless, he often says that he feels that he has nothing to look forward to and that he feels like he is a burden to everyone else. On a couple of occasions he has said, 'It's too bad that I didn't kill myself in the ski accident. Everyone would be better off.'"

Preliminary Recommendations

I recommended to Mrs. Harcourt that she begin weekly supportive treatment with me that would, initially, focus on the following:

1. Supportive psychotherapy for her situational and family related stresses
2. Neuropsychiatric education to help her understand the neurological and psychiatric bases for and implications of her husband's cognitive, behavioral, and emotional dysfunctions
3. The development of strategies to reduce her husband's neuropsychiatric symptoms and symptomatologies
4. Review of her husband's many risk factors for suicide.

   - Advising her on how to assess, on a day-to-day basis, his suicide risk.
   - Recommending how to make her home environment safer from the perspective of suicide—such as removing guns and potentially lethal medications.

- Providing a detailed *plan* of how to respond and what to do should her husband become acutely suicidal.

5. Encouragement for her to share with her husband what was relevant and constructive in our treatment sessions, and, most importantly, to invite him on a continuing basis to join her at any time to participate in our treatment.

Within 3 weeks, Mr. Harcourt joined his wife in the treatment sessions, which were then increased to twice per week. Gradually and progressively, his level of comfort with and meaningful participation in treatment increased. During the first session that he joined us in treatment, I assessed carefully his suicide risk. Essentially, what Mr. Harcourt told me was similar to what he told his wife: that while he felt pessimistic, hopeless, and "like a burden to everyone," he had no immediate plans to kill himself. He also stated, "If something were to happen and I were to die, it would be a relief." Manifestly, I was not reassured: "The black wolf of suicide" was heeling faithfully at my side—both during and outside of my initial sessions with the patient.

Diagnosis

Mr. Harcourt met the following DSM-IV-TR (American Psychiatric Association 2000) diagnoses:

- **Axis I:**
  293.83 Mood Disorder Due to Traumatic Brain Injury With Major Depressive–Like Episode
  301.1 Personality Change Due to Traumatic Brain Injury, Aggressive Type
- **Axis II:**
  301.81 Narcissistic Personality Disorder

Treatment

Mr. Harcourt's major depression responded to antidepressant treatment, as did his irritability and impulsivity to the combination of a lipid-soluble beta-blocker and an anticonvulsant. To Mrs. Harcourt's shock and his own surprise, not only did he suggest including their children in "couples therapy," but he became engaged in intensive, psychodyamically oriented psychotherapy. He gained insight into how his emotional responses to his critical, detached father and enveloping mother were directly related to his low self-esteem, constrained capacity for intimacy, poor quality of relationships, and impaired psychological adjustment to his physical limitations. The multifarious symptoms associated with all three of his diagnoses improved significantly over time, as did his suicidal ideation, enjoyment of life, and optimism.

Discussion

As enumerated and highlighted in *bold*, the case of Mr. Harcourt illuminates the following five principles about the care of patients with high suicide risk (and their families) in which traumatic brain injury (TBI) is complicated by a personality disorder.

1. *The comorbidity of personality disorders and TBI is common.* There are a number of reasons for the comorbidity of personality disorders and TBI. First, both conditions are highly prevalent. According to the Centers for Disease Control and Prevention, each year approximately 1.7 million people sustain traumatic brain injury, and the TBI results in 52,000 deaths, 275,000 hospitalizations, and 1,365,000 hospital visits (Centers for Disease Control and Prevention 2003; Orman et al. 2011). For many of the survivors of TBI, there are chronic sequelae.

The median prevalence of personality disorder from published studies of *all* personality disorders ranges from 11.55% to 12.26%, with narcissistic personality disorder making up only about 0.61% of the population (Torgersen 2005). Second, personality disorders can increase the risk for sustaining TBI, with examples including impulsivity, recklessness, irritability, and aggressiveness, leading to physical altercations for people with antisocial personality disorders. The combination of Mr. Harcourt's problems with intimacy and low self-esteem led to his not achieving mature relationship-based life satisfactions. He endeavored to compensate by calling attention to himself through participating in spectacular and dangerous sport feats, including helicopter skiing, hang gliding, and bungee jumping. The disabilities engendered from TBI further diminished his self-esteem and aggravated his impulsivity, which could easily have led to further risk of injury and, of course, suicide.

2. *TBI often intensifies the symptoms associated with personality disorders, as it does with mood and anxiety disorders, and the associated reluctance to accept help and support from family members and mental health professionals* (Yudofsky 2005). I am frequently asked by students and by family members of people with neuropsychiatric disorders whether the condition will improve personality disorder symptoms. My first response is to try to describe the unfathomable complexity of the human brain, as honed by hundreds of thousands of years of evolution, and then offer a metaphor: "If a new, flat-screen, high-definition TV were to be dropped from the roof of a 20-story building onto the cement sidewalk below, would you expect its reception to be improved?"

3. *The suddenness and multifarious deleterious consequences of TBI and many other neuropsychiatric disorders almost invariably place enormous stress on family members and caregivers of the identified patient* (Yudofsky and Hales 2012). When TBI occurs in the context of personality disorder, the familial and caregiver relationships with the patient are exceedingly complex. Interventions must be understood and carried out in the context of the nature of the pre-and post-TBI relationships, which will be significantly influenced by the identified patient's personality disorder. For example, it is especially challenging to become a caregiver for a spouse who has a long history of being selfish, demeaning, hurtful, and rejecting. The good news is that as psychiatrists, we use training and professional approaches that render us uniquely equipped among all medical disciplines to comprehend these complexities and to intervene effectively for all parties involved.

4. *Given the complexities involved in the neuropsychiatric manifestations of brain injury complicated by personality disorder, it is essential that the psychiatrist be eclectic and flexible in treatments provided.* In the case of the Mr. Harcourt, I provided psychopharmacology; individual, supportive, and insight-oriented psychotherapy for both him and his wife; neuropsychiatric counseling and education (related to brain-based aspects and implications of TBI) for him and his family; couples counseling; family counseling; and specific interventions designed to assess and address suicide risk.

5. *Psychiatric treatment of patients with TBI and a comorbid personality disorder is both essential and effective.* As described, prior to his psychiatric care, Mr. Harcourt was severely impaired by the concomitants of TBI and narcissistic personality disorder, which also adversely affected his wife and children. The identified patient and the family unit were failing. The symptoms and signs of his mood disorder and organic dyscontrol responded within 2 months to psychopharmacological treatment. Couples counseling helped Mr. and Mrs. Harcourt to reduce power struggles, to identify and agree on strategies to reduce Mr. Harcourt's risk-taking behavior and suicide risk, and to avoid the unwieldy consequences of maternal transference by curtailing Mrs. Harcourt's propensity to monitor and intervene in her husband's risk-taking behaviors, ambulatory, balance disabilities, and so forth. These interventions helped to improve their relationship to a point that it became vastly superior to what it had been before Mr. Harcourt's TBI.

Individual psychotherapy aided Mr. Harcourt in gaining insight into the role of childhood parental relationships in his low self-esteem, need for constant admiration, unrealistic goals for "complete recovery from the TBI," and relationship problems with his wife and children. Emphasis of treatment combined insight and operationalizable change in his behavioral patterns. After about 8 weeks of treatment, Mr. Harcourt no longer met the criteria for major depression, did not express feelings of hopelessness and pessimism, had increased his social interactions, and began to derive pleasure from his family and friends. He denied suicidal ideation or intent.

Finally, Mrs. Harcourt, through individual psychotherapy, came to understand the reasons for her vulnerabilities to entering and remaining in an exploitative, demeaning relationship and how to change in ways that enabled independent growth and actualization of her potential and goals. (In working with veterans with TBI, I call this not-uncommon outcome with family members "collateral benefit.") Although she had contemplated returning to medical school after her younger child entered college, she chose instead to pursue a career in science. At this time, Mrs. Harcourt reports feeling "happy and successful as a wife, mother, and graduate student in neuroscience." Interestingly, she tells me that she almost never wears jewelry these days.

The American Psychiatric Publishing Textbook of Suicide Assessment and Management, Second Edition

Although I received the galley copy of the second edition of the *Textbook of Suicide Assessment and Management,* edited by Drs. Robert I. Simon and Robert E. Hales, about 2 years into my treatment of Mr. Harcourt, I endeavored, post hoc, to sample and appraise whether this book would have been of practical use and significant benefit to me in my evaluation and treatment of Mr. Harcourt from the perspective of suicide risk and suicide mitigation.

I found the textbook to be a veritable treasure of information and guidance for the assessment and treatment of a patient at risk for suicide. The book, updated and sharpened with essential facts and references, extensively covered the areas of assessment and treatment for which I had good familiarity, such as the prevalence of suicide from the perspectives of age, diagnosis, and presenting symptoms. It filled in important gaps in my knowledge that would have improved my care of Mr. Harcourt, such as in the areas of cognitive therapy for suicide prevention and split treatment, for which there are separate chapters. The chapters on therapeutic risk management of the suicidal patient, suicide prevention by lethal means restriction, and suicide prevention programs would have importantly expanded and fortified the interventions I had employed in those realms. Additionally, during the delicate, uncertain stages of care when Mr. Harcourt was refusing treatment and I was learning from Mrs. Harcourt of his high risk factors for suicide, the chapters on patient suicide and litigation and psychiatrist reaction to patient suicide would have been enlightening, protective (of me), and reassuring.

All in all, it is my strong conviction that I, and most likely other psychiatrists, are deeply indebted to Drs. Simon and Hales and the outstanding chapter authors they have assembled for providing the best available recourse for helping to keep at bay the "black wolf" of psychiatrists.

References

American Psychiatric Association: Diagnostic and Statistical Manual of Mental Disorders. Washington, DC, American Psychiatric Association, 2000

Centers for Disease Control and Prevention: Report to Congress on Mild Traumatic Brain in the United States: Steps to Prevent a Serious Public Health Problem. Atlanta, GA, National Center for Injury Prevention and Control, September 2003. Available at: http://www.cdc.gov/ncipc/pub-res/mtbi/report.htm. Accessed December 3, 2011.

Colville J: The personality of Winston Churchill, in Winston Churchill: Resolution, Defiance, Magnanimity, Good Will. Edited by Kemper RC. Columbia, University of Missouri Press, 1995, pp 108–125

Orman JAL, Kraus JF, Zaloshnja, et al: Epidemiology, in Textbook of Traumatic Brain Injury, 2nd Edition. Edited by Silver JM, McAllister TW, Yudofsky SC. Washington, DC, American Psychiatric Publishing, 2011, pp 3–21

Torgersen S: Epidemiology, in The American Psychiatric Publishing Textbook of Personality Disorders. Edited by Oldham JM, Skodol AE, Bender DS. Washington, DC, American Psychiatric Publishing, 2005, pp 129–134

Yudofsky SC: Fatal Flaws: Navigating Destructive Relationships With People With Disorders of Personality and Character. Washington, DC, American Psychiatric Publishing, 2005, pp 87–137

Yudofsky SC, Hales RE (eds): Clinical Manual of Neuropsychiatry. Washington, DC, American Psychiatric Publishing, 2012, pp 119–163

Preface

Suicide assessment and management is a complex and challenging clinical task. The second edition of *The American Psychiatric Publishing Textbook of Suicide Assessment and Management* advances the goal of the first edition, to assist clinicians who daily undertake the assessment and management of patients at risk for suicide and often prevent their suicide. Whenever possible, core competencies are presented and discussed.

Chapters from the first edition have been extensively edited and updated. The chapters are written by recognized experts in their respective areas. To make the second edition more comprehensive, we expanded the number of chapters by approximately 20%. With the return of sizable numbers of Iraq and Afghanistan war veterans, and the significant increase in suicide among this population, a chapter on suicide in the military was essential. In addition, there has been much media attention related to suicides caused by intimidation, humiliation, and exposure of sexual acts or compromising situations. Consequently, a chapter on the role of the Internet in suicide was added. Because important neurobiological findings related to the risk and completion of suicide have been reported, we felt that an understanding of the basic biological mechanisms associated with suicide would be of interest to the clinician.

There have been a number of published studies and great interest in the use of cognitive-behavioral therapy to prevent suicide; consequently, a chapter on this topic was added. Because of managed care, insurance companies have been restricting access to psychiatrists for combined psychotherapy and pharmacotherapy, and instead authorizing pharmacological treatment by psychiatrists and psychotherapy by psychologists or social workers. "Split" treatment is becoming increasingly common, and, as in the first edition, we have included a chapter on this important topic. Psychiatrists need to know how to use this form of treatment to prevent suicide and know their responsibilities when a suicide is attempted or completed.

In the previous edition, only one chapter addressed assessment. Since we wanted the reader to know more about this important area, chapters were added on the chronological assessment of suicide events and the clinical risk assessment interview.

We felt that the first edition gave insufficient attention to prevention; consequently, an entire new section devoted to prevention was added for the new edition. This section includes chapters on suicide prevention by lethal means restrictions, suicide prevention programs, and suicide research related to prevention.

In examining the first edition, we felt that a better organizational structure of the sections and chapters was needed. To achieve this goal, we assumed the role of the clinician-reader and reorganized the sections and chapters to coincide with the natural sequence of events in evaluating and treating patients: assessment, major mental disorders, treatment, treatment settings, special populations, special topics, and prevention. Depending on where clinicians are in this series of events, they may more readily access information that they need. At the same time, we wanted the reader to obtain a more varied and sometimes new point of view from the chapter authors. As a result, 22 new chapter authors were recruited for the second edition.

For the second edition, we also added case scenario questions for self-study, along with an answer guide, so that readers can apply their knowledge of key concepts.

An understanding of suicide prevention, risk assessment, and treatment is a core competency for psychiatrists. The achievement of this competency has been made more difficult in current clinical practice because most psychiatrists no longer have the luxury of treating patients for extended periods of time and understanding them. As a result, psychiatrists must possess a reasonable working knowledge of the suicidal patient to provide competent care. This textbook is dedicated to assisting psychiatrists and other clinicians to achieve that goal.

Robert I. Simon, M.D.
Bethesda, Maryland

Robert E. Hales, M.D., M.B.A.
Sacramento, California

Acknowledgments

We would like to thank our authors for their exceptional work in writing new chapters or in updating chapters from the previous edition. The authors prepared manuscripts that are both scholarly and practical for psychiatrists and other mental health professionals who treat patients in a variety of clinical settings. We appreciate the authors' responding to our editorial suggestions in such a collegial manner and for their first-rate writing skills.

Our project administrator for this edition, as well as the first, was the indefatigable Tina Marshall. Tina possesses a winning personality along with a conscientious and persistent manner in communicating with authors on a regular basis, especially when deadlines are looming. She also keeps us on track and on schedule with all our tasks.

We would like to thank the leadership team at American Psychiatric Publishing—Rebecca Rinehart, John McDuffie, Kathy Stein, and Bob Pursell—for their support and encouragement throughout all phases of this project. The copyeditor, Jennifer Wood, and managing editor, Greg Kuny, meticulously reviewed the manuscript and worked closely with the chapter authors and us to prepare an accurate and well-edited book, and Judy Castagna very capably handled page layout and provided expert oversight for manufacturing. Finally, Tammy Cordova designed the cover and created the book design in her usual, stellar fashion.

We hope that you find the book useful in your care of patients and that you enjoy reading it as much as we did in writing and editing it.

Robert I. Simon, M.D.
Bethesda, Maryland

Robert E. Hales, M.D., M.B.A.
Sacramento, California

PART I

Suicide Risk Assessment

C H A P T E R   1

Suicide Risk Assessment

Gateway to Treatment and Management

Robert I. Simon, M.D.

Suicide risk assessment is a gateway to treatment and management. It is a core competency requirement for psychiatrists (Scheiber et al. 2003). The purpose of suicide risk assessment is to identify treatable and modifiable risks and protective factors that inform the patient's treatment and safety management requirements (Simon 2011). Patients at risk for suicide often confront the psychiatrist with life-threatening emergencies. Most clinicians rely on the clinical interview and certain valued questions and observations to assess the suicide risk (Sullivan and Bongar 2006). The psychiatrist, unlike the general physician, does not have laboratory tests and sophisticated diagnostic instruments available to assess a suicidal patient. By comparison, in evaluating an emergency cardiac patient, the clinician can order a number of diagnostic tests and procedures, such as electrocardiography, serial enzymes, imaging, and catheterization. The psychiatrist's quintessential diagnostic instrument is systematic suicide risk assess-

ment that is informed by evidence-based psychiatry.

A standard of care does not exist for prediction of suicide (Pokorny 1983, 1993). Suicide is a rare event. Efforts to predict who will die by suicide lead to a large number of false-positive and false-negative predictions. No method of suicide risk assessment can reliably identify who will die by suicide (sensitivity) and who will not (specificity). Suicide is the result of multiple factors, including diagnostic (psychiatric and medical), psychodynamic, genetic, familial, occupational, environmental, social, cultural, existential, and chance factors. Furthermore, stressful life events have a significant association with completed suicides (Heilä et al. 1999). Patients are at varying risk for suicide, and their level of risk can change rapidly. Thus, unless speaking generally, the term *patient at risk for suicide* is preferred to the generic "suicidal patient." The term *suicidality* should not be used; it is an ambiguous term that lumps together suicidal ideation, suicide attempts, suicide, and self-injurious behaviors (Meyer et al. 2010).

Standardized suicide risk prediction scales do not identify which patient will die by suicide (Busch et al. 1993). Single scores of suicide risk assessment scales and inventories should not be relied on by clinicians as the sole basis for clinical decision making. Structured or semistructured suicide scales can complement, but are not a substitute for, systematic suicide risk assessment. Malone et al. (1995) found that semistructured screening instruments improved routine clinical assessments in the documentation and detection of lifetime suicidal behavior. Oquendo et al. (2003) discussed the utility and limitations of research instruments in assessing suicide risk.

Self-administered suicide scales are overly sensitive and lack specificity. Suicide risk factors occur in many depressed patients who do not die by suicide. Although patients occasionally provide more information on a self-administered scale than in a clinical interview, patients at risk for suicide may not answer truthfully. Checklists cannot encompass all the pertinent suicide risk factors present for a given patient (Simon 2009). The plaintiff's attorney will point out the omission of pertinent suicide risk factors on the checklist used to assess the patient who later commits suicide. The standard of care does not require that specific psychological tests or checklists be used as part of the systematic assessment of suicide risk (Bongar et al. 1992).

Actuarial analysis reveals that most depressed patients do not kill themselves. For instance, the 2002 national suicide rate in the general population was 11.1 per 100,000 per year (Heron et al. 2009). The suicide rate or absolute risk of suicide for individuals with bipolar and other mood disorders was estimated to be 193 per 100,000, which repre-

sents a relative risk 18 times greater than that for the general population (Baldessarini 2003). Thus, 99,807 patients with these disorders will not die by suicide in a single year. The same actuarial analysis can be applied to other psychiatric disorders. The suicide rate for individuals with schizophrenia or alcohol or drug abuse is also 18 times the 2002 national suicide rate. On an actuarial basis alone, the vast majority of patients will not die by suicide. Actuarial analysis, however, is more useful in identifying diagnostic groups at higher risk than in trying to predict the suicide of a specific patient (Addy 1992). Actuarial analysis does not identify specific treatable risk and modifiable protective factors. The clinical challenge is to identify those patients with depression at high risk for suicide at any given time (Jacobs et al. 1999).

The standard of care does require that psychiatrists and other mental health professionals adequately assess suicide risk when it is indicated. Although open to interpretation, risk assessments that systematically evaluate both risk and protective factors should meet any reasonable definition of "adequate" (see Figure 1–1). Conceptually, suicide risk assessment is a process of analysis and synthesis that identifies, prioritizes, and integrates acute and chronic risk and protective factors. Suicide risk assessment based on current research that identifies risk and protective factors for suicide enables the clinician to make evidence-based treatment and safety management decisions (Fawcett et al. 1987; Linehan et al. 1983).

Professional organizations recognize the need for developing evidence-based and clinical consensus recommendations to be applied to the management of various diseases, including such behavioral states as suicide (Simon 2002b; Taylor 2010). The American Academy of Child and Adolescent Psychiatry published "Practice Parameter for the Assessment and Treatment of Children and Adolescents With Suicidal Behavior" (Shaffer et al. 1997).

Case Example

A 34-year-old woman is brought to an urban hospital emergency department after impulsively ingesting an unknown quantity of aspirin tablets and then slashing her arms with a knife. She is severely agitated, responding to command hallucinations to kill herself. The patient became acutely depressed and agitated following the breakup of a brief relationship, her first "serious" intimate relationship. At age 16, the patient made superficial scratches on her wrist with a razor, following a "disappointment" with a young person she idolized from afar. During the week prior to admission, she abused alcohol and methamphetamine. An admission drug screen is positive for these substances. The salicylate level is markedly elevated.

Upon admission to the psychiatric unit, the patient is placed on one-to-one safety management. Her agitation and aggressive-impulsive behaviors require placement in open-door seclusion with an attendant sitting by the door. Nursing staff protocol requires that all patients be encouraged to verbally agree with or sign a suicide prevention contract. Although the patient does not understand the purpose of the contract, she signs it. Psychiatric examination reveals a thought disorder, severe agitation, bizarre facial grimaces and mannerisms, confusion, hopelessness, command hallucinations, flat affect, insomnia, and inability to interact with the psychiatrist, unit staff, and other patients.

The psychiatrist and the psychiatric unit's social worker speak with the patient's mother and siblings at the time of admission. The psychiatrist relies on the emergency exception to consent in speaking to family members without the patient's authorization. He learns that the patient's parents were divorced when she was 7 years old. She sees her father infrequently. The patient has a close relationship with her mother, older brother, and younger sister, but feels her illness is a burden on the family. Family efforts to reassure the patient have failed.

There is no history of physical or sexual abuse. The mother reveals that her daughter was a good student, excelling in mathematics. The patient is a computer specialist, and her relationship with coworkers is good. However, she has few friends. The patient holds strong religious beliefs. She is described by her siblings as creative, artistic, and a loner. In the past, the patient has reacted to major disappointments with depression and suicidal thoughts, sometimes accompanied by "strange" facial movements and grimaces. The family history is positive for mental illness. A paternal uncle, diagnosed as a "manic-depressive," died by suicide with a shotgun 10 years ago. A reclusive maternal aunt has been diagnosed as a "chronic schizophrenic."

The patient is living at home. The psychiatrist asks about guns in the home. The patient's brother states that there is a locked-up shotgun used for skeet shooting. The brother agrees to remove the gun from the home. A follow-up call by the social worker confirms that the gun was removed from the home and secured in a safe place. The psychiatrist's systematic suicide risk assessment of the patient on admission is rated as high (see Figure 1–2).

The psychiatrist makes a diagnosis of schizophrenia, disorganized type, and substance abuse disorder (alcohol and methamphetamine). He prescribes an atypical antipsychotic medication, a benzodiazepine for control of severe agitation, and a sleep medication. The psychiatrist will consider a suicide-reduction drug, such as clozapine, if the suicidal ideation does not remit. In his initial suicide risk assessment, the psychiatrist evaluates both acute and chronic risk factors as well as current protective factors. He continues to assess the patient's acute suicide risk factors over the course of the hospitalization.

On the day after admission, the patient is less agitated. She does not require seclusion. On the third hospital day, command hallucinations are indistinct. The patient is more communicative with the hospital staff and other patients. By the fifth hospital day, the patient states the command hallucinations "have gone away." She is not agitated. Suicidal ideation continues but without intent or plan. The patient's bizarre facial grimaces and mannerisms observed on admission are no longer present. Hopelessness and confusion diminish.

The patient attends all the assigned group therapies. She benefits from individual and group supportive therapies. The patient develops a therapeutic alliance with the psychiatrist and the treatment team. Her affect, however, remains flat. Her thought processes are logical,

Systematic Suicide Risk Assessment

Assessment factors[a]	Risk	Protective
Individual		
Distinctive clinical features (prodrome)		
Religious beliefs		
Reasons for living		
Clinical		
Current attempt (lethality)		
Therapeutic alliance		
Treatment adherence		
Treatment benefit		
Suicidal ideation		
Suicide intent		
Self-injurious behaviors		
Suicide plan		
Hopelessness		
Prior attempts (lethality)		
Panic attacks		
Psychic anxiety		
Loss of pleasure and interest		
Alcohol/drug abuse		
Depressive turmoil (mixed states)		
Diminished concentration		
Global insomnia		
Psychiatric diagnoses (Axis I and Axis II)		
Symptom severity		
Comorbidity		
Recent discharge from psychiatric hospital		
Impulsivity		
Agitation (akathisia)		
Physical illness		
Family history of mental illness (suicide)		
Childhood sexual/physical abuse		
Mental competency		

FIGURE 1–1. Systematic suicide risk assessment: a conceptual model.

Source. Adapted from Simon 2011.

Interpersonal relations

Work or school

Family

Spouse or partner

Children

Situational

Living circumstances

Employment or school status

Financial status

Availability of guns

Managed care setting

Demographic

Age

Gender

Marital status

Race

Overall risk ratings[b]

[a]Rate risk and protective factors present as low (L), moderate (M), high (H), nonfactor (0), or range (e.g., L–M, M–H).
[b]Judge overall suicide risk as low, moderate, high, or a range of risk.

FIGURE 1–1. Systematic suicide risk assessments: a conceptual model *(continued)*.
Source. Adapted from Simon 2011.

---

but abstracting ability for proverbs is impaired. Mild insomnia is present. Concentration is poor. The patient willingly takes her medication, although she experiences mild to moderate side effects.

Using evidence-based studies, the psychiatrist assesses the risk factors associated with an increased risk of suicide in patients with schizophrenia. These include a previous suicide attempt (robust "predictor" of eventual completed suicide), substance abuse, depressive symptoms (especially hopelessness), male sex, early stage in illness, good premorbid history and intellectual functioning, and frequent exacerbations and remissions (Meltzer 2001). The psychiatrist has read about the International Clozaril/Leponex Suicide Prevention Trial (InterSePT), which indicated significant risk factors for suicide in patients with schizophrenia, including a diagnosis of schizoaffective disorder, current or lifetime alcohol/substance abuse or smoking, hospital-

ization in the previous 3 years to prevent a suicide attempt, and the number of lifetime suicide attempts (Meltzer et al. 2003a).

A systematic suicide risk assessment is performed on hospital day 6 (see Figure 1–3) and is compared with the admission suicide risk assessment (see Figure 1–2). Although most of the acute psychotic symptoms have improved or remitted, suicidal ideation continues. The patient's perception that she is a burden on her family has lessened with family reassurance and support. The overall risk of suicide is assessed as "moderate" on day 6. The psychiatrist determines that the patient needs an additional week of inpatient treatment. Because of the patient's overall improvement, the health care insurer authorizes coverage for 2 additional days after a doctor-to-doctor appeal. The psychiatrist's experience indicates that most patients at moderate suicide risk can be treated as outpatients, so he crafts an outpatient treatment plan based on the patient's

Admission Systematic Suicide Risk Assessment

Assessment factors[a]	Risk	Protective
Individual		
Distinctive clinical features (prodrome)	H	
Religious beliefs	O	
Reasons for living	O	
Clinical		
Current attempt (lethality)	H	
Therapeutic alliance	H	
Treatment adherence	L	
Treatment benefit	O	
Suicidal ideation (command hallucinations)	H	
Suicide intent	H	
Self-injurious behaviors	M	
Suicide plan	O	
Hopelessness	M–H	
Prior attempts (lethality)	L	
Panic attacks	O	
Psychic anxiety	O	
Loss of pleasure and interest	H	
Alcohol/drug abuse	H	
Depressive turmoil (mixed states)	O	
Diminished concentration	H	
Global insomnia	M–H	
Psychiatric diagnoses (Axis I and Axis II)	H	
Symptom severity	H	
Comorbidity	H	
Recent discharge from psychiatric hospital	O (within 3 months)	
Impulsivity/aggression	M–H	
Agitation (akathisia)	H	
Physical illness	O	
Family history of mental illness (suicide)	H	
Childhood sexual/physical abuse	O	
Mental competency	M	

FIGURE 1–2. Admission systematic suicide risk assessment: a case example.

Source. Adapted from Simon 2004.

Interpersonal relations

Work or school			L
Family		M	
Spouse or partner	H		
Children	O		
Situational			
Living circumstances		M	
Employment or school status			L
Financial status			L–M
Availability of guns	H		
Managed care setting	O		
Demographic			
Age	M		
Gender	H		
Marital status	L		
Race/ethnicity	O		
Overall risk ratings[b]	High		

ᵃRate risk and protective factors present as low (L), moderate (M), high (H), nonfactor (0), or range (e.g., L–M, M–H).
ᵇJudge overall suicide risk as low, moderate, high, or a range of risk.

FIGURE 1–2. Admission systematic suicide risk assessment: a case example *(continued)*.
Source. Adapted from Simon 2004.

clinical and safety needs. He understands that the decision to discharge a patient is the psychiatrist's responsibility. The psychiatrist's decision is not based on the insurer's denial of benefits. An insurer's denial of benefits is not considered an acceptable justification for placing the patient at increased risk for suicide.

The patient's postdischarge plan recommends once-per-week supportive psychotherapy and medication management with the psychiatrist. The patient is also referred to the hospital's partial hospitalization and substance abuse programs, which she will attend the day after discharge. The patient is eager to return to work but agrees to remain on sick leave for another 3 weeks. She recognizes the importance of adhering to the follow-up care plan. The patient plans to pursue her artistic interests. Her mother and siblings are very supportive, which is an important protective factor. The psychiatrist assesses other protective factors, including the patient's ability to form a

therapeutic alliance, adherence to treatment, treatment benefit, strong religious values, positive reasons for living, and commitment to the follow-up care plan. The psychiatrist's discharge diagnosis is schizophrenia, single episode in partial remission, and substance abuse disorder (alcohol and methamphetamine).

Standard of Care

Each state defines the legal criteria for determining the standard of care required of physicians. For example, in *Stepakoff v. Kantar* (1985), a suicide case, the standard applied by the court was the "duty to exercise that degree of skill and care ordinarily employed in similar circumstances by other psychiatrists." The duty of care established by the court was that of the "average psychiatrist." In an increasing number of states,

Discharge Systematic Suicide Risk Assessment

Assessment factors[a]	Risk	Protective
Individual		
Distinctive clinical features (prodrome)	0	
Religious beliefs		H
Reasons for living		M
Clinical		
Current attempt (lethality)	H	
Therapeutic alliance		M
Treatment adherence		H
Treatment benefit		M
Suicidal ideation (command hallucinations)	M	
Suicide intent	0	
Self-injurious behaviors	0	
Suicide plan	0	
Hopelessness	L	
Prior attempts (lethality)	L	
Panic attacks	0	
Psychic anxiety	0	
Loss of pleasure and interest	L	
Alcohol/drug abuse	M	
Depressive turmoil (mixed states)	0	
Diminished concentration	H	
Global insomnia	L	
Psychiatric diagnoses (Axis I and Axis II)	H	
Symptom severity	L–M	
Comorbidity	H	
Recent discharge from psychiatric hospital	0 (within 3 months)	
Impulsivity/aggression	L	
Agitation (akathisia)	0	
Physical illness	H	
Family history of mental illness (suicide)	H	
Childhood sexual/physical abuse	0	
Mental competency	L	

FIGURE 1–3. Discharge systematic suicide risk assessment: a case example.
Source. Adapted from Simon 2004.

Interpersonal relations

Work or school		H
Family		H
Spouse or partner	L–M	
Children	0	
Situational		
Living circumstances		M
Employment or school status		H
Financial status		M
Availability of guns		0
Managed care setting	L–M	
Demographic		
Age	M	
Gender	L	
Marital status	L	
Race/ethnicity	0	
Overall risk ratings[b]	Moderate	

[a]Rate risk and protective factors present as low (L), moderate (M), high (H), nonfactor (0), or range (e.g., L–M, M–H).
[b]Judge overall suicide risk as low, moderate, high, or a range of risk.

FIGURE 1–3. Discharge systematic risk assessment: a case example *(continued)*.
Source. Adapted from Simon 2004.

the standard of care is that of the "reasonable, prudent practitioner" (Peters 2000). The legal standard must be distinguished from the professional standard of "best practices" (Simon 2005).

In a suicide case, the courts evaluate the psychiatrist's management of the patient who attempted or completed suicide to determine whether the suicide risk assessment process was reasonable and the patient's attempt or suicide was foreseeable. An "imperfect fit," however, exists between medical and legal terminology. *Foreseeability* is a legal term of art; it is a commonsense, probabilistic concept, not a scientific construct. Foreseeability, which is defined as the reasonable anticipation that harm or injury is likely to result from certain acts or omis-

sions (Black 1999), is not the same as predicting when a patient will attempt or die by suicide. Foreseeability should not be confused with predictability, for which no professional standard exists. It also must be distinguished from preventability; a patient's suicide may be preventable in hindsight, but it was not foreseeable at the time of assessment.

Only the risk of suicide is determinable. The prediction of suicide is opaque, but there is reasonable visibility for assessing suicide risk. Contemporaneously documented systematic suicide risk assessments help provide the court with guidance. When suicide risk assessments are not performed or documented, the court is less able to evaluate the clinical complexities and ambiguities that exist in the assessment, treatment, and management of patients at risk for suicide. In malpractice litigation, the failure to perform an adequate suicide risk assessment is often alleged along with other claims of negligence. It is rarely asserted as the only complaint (Simon 2004).

Systematic Suicide Risk Assessment

Systematic suicide risk assessment identifies acute, modifiable, and treatable risk and protective factors essential to informing the psychiatrist's treatment and safety management of patients at risk for suicide (see Figure 1–1). It is easy to overlook important risk and protective factors in the absence of systematic assessment. Systematic suicide assessment helps the clinician gather important information and piece together risk factors with which to construct a clinical mosaic of the suicidal patient. Given the high stakes, getting the suicide risk assessment right is of critical importance.

Suicide risk assessment is an integral part of the psychiatric examination, yet it is rarely performed systematically, or when it is performed, it is not contemporaneously documented. Protective factors are not usually considered. It is evident from the review of quality assurance records and the forensic analysis of suicide cases in litigation that the extent of suicide risk assessment usually is no more than the statement "Patient denies HI, SI, CFS" (homicidal ideation, suicidal ideation, contracts for safety). Frequently one finds no documentation of suicide risk assessment or only the statement, "Patient denies suicidal ideation." Often, relying on a talismanic "no-harm contract" replaces performing an adequate suicide risk assessment. Laypersons could just as easily ask these same questions and obtain a no-harm contract. Moreover, there is

no evidence that suicide safety contracts decrease or prevent suicide (Stanford et al. 1994). The road to patient suicides is often strewn with broken safety contracts. In the case example, systematic suicide risk assessment supplants reliance on a suicide prevention contract.

Why do so many psychiatrists, whether they have been sued or not, fail to perform and document adequate suicide risk assessments? There is a wide variety of answers (see Table 1–1). In inpatient settings, short lengths of stay and the rapid turnover of seriously ill patients may distract the clinician from performing adequate risk assessments. Also, the focus of clinical attention rapidly shifts away from knowing the patient to pressing discharge planning.

Malone et al. (1995) found that on routine clinical assessments at admission, clinicians failed to document a history of suicidal behavior in 12 of 50 patients who were identified by research assessment as being depressed and as having attempted suicide. Fewer total suicide attempts were reported clinically than were shown by data on suicide attempts obtained by use of a comprehensive research assessment. Documentation of suicidal behavior was most accurate on hospital intake admission when a semi-structured format was used instead of discharge documentation by clinical assessment alone. Malone and colleagues suggested that use of semistructured screening instruments may improve documentation and the detection of lifetime suicidal behavior.

Approximately 25% of patients at risk for suicide do not admit having suicidal ideation to the clinician but do tell their families (Robins 1981). Hall et al. (1999) found that 69 of 100 patients had had only fleeting or no suicidal thoughts before they made a suicide attempt. None of these patients reported having had a specific plan before their impulsive suicide attempts. This was the first

TABLE 1–1. Reasons for clinician failure to perform and document adequate suicide risk assessments

Clinician does not know how to perform a systematic suicide risk assessment.

Clinician does not do suicidal risk assessments, usually delegating them to others.

Clinician performs systematic risk assessments but does not document them, (usually in a high-volume practice).

Anxiety produced by patients at substantial risk for suicide creates denial and minimization of the risk, causing failure to perform an adequate assessment.

Clinician fears that documenting the risk assessment process creates legal exposure if the assessment is wrong and the patient commits suicide.

attempt for 67% of these patients. When the patient denies suicidal ideation, additional questions should be asked (e.g., prior suicide attempts and family history of mental illness, suicide attempts, or suicide).

Patients who are determined to die by suicide regard the psychiatrist and other mental health professionals as the enemy (Resnick 2002). Therefore, just asking the patient at risk for suicide about the presence of suicidal ideation, suicide intent, and a suicide plan and receiving a denial cannot be relied upon by itself. If possible, family members or others who know the patient should be consulted. Even when the patient is telling the truth, it is unwise to equate the patient's denial of suicidal ideation with an absence of suicide risk.

The Principles of Medical Ethics With Annotations Especially Applicable to Psychiatry (American Psychiatric Association 2009) states: "Psychiatrists at times may find it necessary, in order to protect the patient or community from imminent danger, to reveal confidential information disclosed by the patient" (section 4, annotation 8). Management of patients at high risk for suicide may require breaking patient confidence and involving the family or significant others (e.g., to obtain vital information, to administer and monitor medications, to remove lethal weapons, to assist in hospitalization). Statutory waiver of confidential information is provided in some states when a patient seriously threatens self-harm (Simon and Shuman 2007). If the severely disturbed patient lacks the mental capacity to consent, a substitute health care decision-maker should be contacted. Proxy consent by next of kin is not permitted in all jurisdictions for patients with mental illnesses. If an emergency exists, the emergency exception to patient consent may be invoked (Simon and Shuman 2007). Just listening to significant others without divulging information about the patient does not violate confidentiality unless the patient withholds consent for any contact with others. It may be possible to speak with significant others once a therapeutic alliance develops and the patient consents. The Health Insurance Portability and Accountability Act of 1996 (HIPAA) permits psychiatrists and other health care providers who are treating the same patient to communicate without expressed permission from the patient (45 Code of Federal Regulations § 164.502).

Observational information obtained from the psychiatric examination may provide objective information about suicide risk factors, thus avoiding total reliance on the patient's reporting (Simon 2011). For example, slash marks on the arms or neck, burns, or other wounds may be apparent. The mental status examination may reveal diminished concentration, bizarre ideation, evidence of command hallucinations, incapacity to cooperate, restlessness, agitation, severe thought disorder, impulsivity, and alcohol or drug withdrawal symptoms. The degree of irritability can be rapidly assessed in patients with major depressive disorder and is correlated with depression severity and suicide attempts (Perlis et al. 2005).

Suicide risk assessment bears an analogy to weather forecasting (Monahan and Steadman 1996; Simon 1992). Data must be gathered in order to compose an assessment or forecast. Determining the clinician's level of confidence in the available patient data is essential for the treatment and management of suicide risk. Table 1–2 contains a suicide risk assessment approach for data gathering. The standard of care requires that the clinician gather sufficient information on which to base an adequate suicide risk assessment. The assessment approach in Table 1–2 can alert the clinician to deficiencies in the data collection.

Systematic risk assessment itself is an impetus to gather essential clinical information about the patient. It reminds the clinician to consider multiple data sources. When the clinical situation turns stormy, clinicians, like pilots, must rely on their instruments.

Suicide Risk Factors

General risk factors such as a recent suicide attempt, hopelessness, or family history of suicide apply across most clinical settings. Individual suicide risk factors are unique and specific to the patient. The stuttering patient who no longer stutters when at risk for suicide is a classic example. Suicide risk factors can be culturally determined, as is the case with shame suicides in certain Eastern cultures. Suicide risk factors occur under certain circumstances, as when an individual is jailed for the first time. Age-related contagion effect is an important sui-

TABLE 1–2. Suicide risk assessment data gathering: hospital admission

Identify distinctive individual suicide risk factors.

Identify acute suicide risk factors.

Identify protective factors.

Evaluate medical history and laboratory studies.

Obtain treatment team information.

Interview patient's significant others.

Speak with current or prior treaters.

Review patient's current and prior hospital records.

Note. Modify for outpatient use.
Source. Adapted from Simon 2002a.

cide risk factor for adolescents who have been directly exposed to a completed peer suicide. Although clinicians rely mostly on general suicide risk factors, individual, cultural, and contextual risk factors must also be considered.

There is no pathognomonic risk factor for suicide. A single suicide risk factor does not have adequate statistical power on which to base an assessment. Suicide risk assessment cannot be predicated on the basis of any one factor (Meltzer et al. 2003b); the assessment of suicide risk is multifactorial. Moreover, a number of retrospective community-based psychological autopsies and studies of psychiatric patients who completed suicide have identified general risk factors (Fawcett et al. 1993). Systematic suicide risk assessment should consider evidence-based general risk factors along with the individual patient's unique risk factors.

Short-term suicide risk factors derived from a prospective study of patients with major affective disorders were statistically significant within 1 year of assessment (Fawcett et al. 1990). These factors included panic attacks, psychic anxiety, loss of pleasure and interest, moderate alcohol abuse, depressive turmoil (mixed states), diminished concentration, and global insomnia. Short-term risk factors were predominantly severe, anxiety driven, and treatable by a variety of psychotropic drugs (Fawcett 2001). Although this is an important finding, the clinician cannot identify specifically when or if the patient will attempt suicide during the 1-year period. "Imminent" suicide, a frequently used nonclinical term, is a predictive illusion (Simon 2006). Can the clinician state what time parameters exist for predicting suicidal behaviors based upon imminence? Suicidal ideation is a key risk factor. In the National Comorbidity Survey, the transition probabilities from suicidal ideation to suicide plan and from a plan to attempt were 34% and 72%, respectively (Kessler et al. 1999).The probability of transition from suicidal ideation to an unplanned suicide attempt was 26%. In this study, approximately 90% of unplanned and 60% of planned first attempts occurred within 1 year of the onset of suicidal ideation.

Systematic suicide risk assessment should be performed when the patient reports passive suicidal ideations (e.g., "I hope God takes me" vs. "I'm going to kill myself"). Passive ideation can quickly become active. Also, the patient may be minimizing or hiding active suicidal ideation. In passive suicidal ideation, the intent is to die by indirect means. Prematurely decreasing or discontinuing precautions on a patient with passive suicidal ideation can lull the clinician into a false sense of safety. When assessing a patient's suicidal ideation, the clinician should consider specific content, intensity, duration, and prior episodes. Mann et al. (1999) found that the severity of an individual's ideation is an indicator of risk for attempting suicide. Beck et al. (1990) determined that when patients were asked about suicidal ideation at its worst point, patients with high scores were 14 times more likely to die by suicide than were patients having low scores.

Patients with major depression and generalized anxiety disorder have higher levels of suicidal ideation when compared with depressed patients with no diagnosis of generalized anxiety disorder (Zimmerman and Chelminski 2003). Comorbid anxiety and depression occur in over 50% of persons with nonbipolar major depressive disorders (Zimmerman et al. 2002). The combination of severe depression and anxiety or panic attacks can prove lethal. A patient may be able to tolerate depression. When anxiety or panic is also present, the patient's life may become unbearable, and suicide risk is dangerously elevated. Anxiety (agitation) symptoms should be treated aggressively while antidepressant medications are being given an opportunity to work. Some patients demonstrate a significant antidepressant response within the first 1–2 weeks of treatment (Posternak and Zimmerman 2005).

Time is on the side of patients at risk for suicide who are treated rapidly and effectively. Conversely, time works against patients with severe depression when treatment is delayed or ineffective. The mental disorder often progresses and becomes entrenched. Secondary effects, such as work impairment and disrupted relationships, lead to despair, demoralization, and an increased risk of suicide. Suicide-reduction medications such as lithium and clozapine should be considered for bipolar patients and schizophrenia patients, respectively (Baldessarini et al. 2006).

Long-term suicide risk factors in patients with major affective disorder are associated with suicide completion 2–10 years after assessment (Fawcett et al. 1990). Long-term suicide risk factors are derived from community-based psychological autopsies and the retrospective study of psychiatric patients who have died by suicide (Fawcett et al. 1993). Long-term suicide risk factors include suicidal ideation, suicide intent, severe hopelessness, and prior attempts. Suicide risk increases with the total number of risk factors, providing a quasi-quantitative dimension to suicide risk assessment (Murphy et al. 1992).

Patients with disorders from diagnostic groups such as major affective disorders, chronic alcoholism and substance abuse, schizophrenia, and borderline personality disorder are at increased risk for suicide (Fawcett et al. 1993). Roose et al. (1983) found that delusional depressed patients were five times more likely to die by suicide than depressed patients who were not delusional. Busch et al. (2003) also indicated that there was an association between psychosis and suicide in 54% of the 76 inpatient suicides. In the Collaborative Study of Depression (Fawcett et al. 1987), no significant difference in suicide rate was shown between depressed and delusionally depressed patients. Patients who had delusions of thought insertion, grandeur, and mind reading, however, were significantly represented in the suicide group (Fawcett et al. 1987). A number of follow-up studies have not indicated that patients with psychotic depression are more likely to die by suicide than patients with nonpsychotic depression (Coryell et al. 1996; Vythilingam et al. 2003). Research, however, indicates that suicide risk increases with the severity of psychosis (Warman et al. 2004). Electroconvulsive therapy may produce rapid reduction of suicide risk in severely depressed patients whose symptoms fail to respond to adequate drug trials.

Patients often display distinctive, individual suicide risk and preventive factor patterns. Suicide patterns may be identified from prior exacerbations of suicidal ideation, suicidal crises, or actual attempts. Understanding a patient's psychodynamics and psychological responses to past and current life stressors is important. In the case example earlier in this chapter, when the patient was depressed and at risk for suicide, she displayed bizarre facial mannerisms. Some unusual prodromal suicide risk factors can emerge when patients become suicidal, as, for example, with the stuttering patient whose speech clears, the patient who compulsively whistles, and the patient who self-inflicts facial excoriations. Many patients experience more common suicide risk patterns, such as suicidal ideation within a few hours or days following the onset of early-morning awakening. Knowing a patient's distinctive, prodromal suicide risk factors along with his or her psychodynamics is very helpful in treatment and safety management. Significant others often provide information about the patient's suicide risk prodrome. Review of prior hospitalization records may yield additional information. Strongly held values such as religious beliefs and reasons for living can be significant protective factors.

Demographic suicide risk factors include age, sex, race, and marital status, among others. The suicide rates for white males 65 years and older are elevated. White males older than 85 have the highest suicide rates. Males die by suicide at a rate three to four times greater than that of females. Females make suicide attempts at a rate three to four times greater than that of men. Divorced individuals are at significantly increased risk for suicide compared with married individuals. The suicide rate is higher among white individuals (with the exception of young adults) than among African Americans. Demographic suicide risk factors alert the clinician to perform a thorough suicide risk assessment.

A family history of mental illness, especially of suicide, is a significant risk factor. A genetic component exists in the etiology of affective disorders, schizophrenia, alcoholism and substance abuse, and Cluster B personality disorders. These psychiatric disorders are associated with most suicides (Mann and Arango 1999). Genetic and familial transmission of suicide risk is independent of the transmission of psychiatric illnesses (Brent et al. 1996). Psychiatric illnesses are a necessary but not *sufficient* cause of patient suicides. Patients with intractable, malignant psychiatric disorders that end in suicide often have strong genetic and familial components to their illnesses.

In schizophrenia, the completed lifetime suicide rate is 9%–13%. The estimated number of suicides annually in the United States among patients with schizophrenia is 3,600 (12% of total suicides). The lifetime suicide attempt rate is 20%–40%. Suicide is the leading cause of death among persons with schizophrenia who are younger than 35 years. Suicide is a risk in schizophrenia throughout the individual's life cycle (Heilä et al. 1997; Meltzer and Okaly 1995); however, suicide tends to occur in the early stages of illness and during an active phase (Meltzer 2001).

In the case example, the patient's suicide attempt was directed by command hallucinations. The earlier psychiatric literature indicated that command hallucinations accounted for relatively few suicides in patients with schizophrenia (Breier and Astrachan 1984; Roy 1982). Nonetheless, an auditory hallucination that commands suicide is an important risk factor that requires careful assessment. The patient needs to be asked: Are the auditory hallucinations that are commanding suicide acute or chronic, syntonic or dystonic, familiar or unfamiliar voices? Are you able to resist the hallucinatory commands, or have you attempted suicide in obedience to the voices?

Junginger (1990) reported that 39% of patients with command hallucinations obeyed them. Patients were more likely to comply with hallucinatory commands if they could identify the voices. Kasper et al. (1996) found that 84% of psychiatric inpatients with command hallucinations had obeyed them within the past 30 days. Resistance to command hallucinations that dictate dangerous acts appears to be greater than resistance to commands to perform nondangerous acts (Junginger 1995). This is not as true for patients who have obeyed command hallucinations dictating self-destructive behaviors. In a study of command hallucinations for suicide (Harkavy-Friedman et al. 2003), 80% of patients who attempted suicide reported having made at least one attempt in response to command hallucinations. Hellerstein et al. (1987) studied the content of command hallucinations and grouped them in the following categories: 52% involved suicide, 14% involved nonviolent acts, 12% involved nonlethal injury to self or others, 5% involved homicide, and 17% were unspecified. Thus, 69% of command hallucinations dictated violence. Patients with auditory hallucinations that command suicide should be presumptively assessed at high risk for suicide, requiring immediate psychiatric treatment and management.

Harris and Barraclough (1997) examined data from 249 reports from the medical literature regarding mortality among persons with mental disorders. They compared observed numbers of suicides in individuals with mental disorders with those expected in the general population. The standardized mortality ratio (SMR)—a measure of the relative risk of suicide for a particular disorder compared with the expected rate in the general population (SMR of 1)—was calculated for each disorder by dividing observed mortality by expected mortality. The authors concluded that "if these results can be generalized, then virtually all mental disorders have an increased risk for suicide excepting mental retardation and dementia" (p. 222).

Harris and Barraclough also calculated the SMR for all psychiatric diagnoses by the treatment setting. The SMR was 5.82 for inpatients and 18.09 for outpatients. Prior suicide attempts by any method had the highest SMR (38.36). Suicide risk was highest in the 2 years following the first attempt. The SMR for psychiatric, neurological, and medical disorders can be helpful to the psychiatrist in assessing the risk of suicide for a specific diagnosis.

Baldessarini (2003) found that the overall SMR for bipolar disorder was 21.8. The SMR was 1.4 times higher for women than for men. Most suicide acts occur within the first 5 years after the onset of illness. The SMR for bipolar II disorder was 24.1, compared with an SMR of 17.0 for bipolar I disorder and 11.8 for unipolar disorders.

The high SMR for prior suicide attempts is supported by other studies (Fawcett 2001). Between 7% and 12% of patients who have attempted suicide die by suicide within 10 years, thus making it a significant chronic risk factor for suicide. The risk of completed suicide is highest during the first year after the attempt. Suicide rehearsals, behavioral or mental, are common. Near-lethal attempts are frequently followed within days by a completed suicide. Most suicides, however, occur in patients with no history of prior attempts. The majority of patients who completed suicide did not communicate their suicide intent during their last appointment (Isometsä et al. 1995). In a retrospective study of 76 inpatient suicides, Busch et al. (2003) found that 77% of the patients denied suicidal ideation at their last recorded com-

munication. Mann et al. (1999) found that prior suicide attempts and hopelessness are the most powerful clinical "predictors" of completed suicide. The rate of suicide completion during first attempts is high, especially among males (62%; females, 38%) (Isometsä and Lönnqvist 1998). Individuals who had previously attempted suicide (82%) used at least two different methods in attempts and completed suicides. Although a suicide rehearsal is an indicator of high risk, the method of suicide attempt can change while the patient's suicide intent remains unchanged.

Research finds that high risk factors associated with attempted suicide in adults are depression, prior suicide attempt(s), hopelessness, suicidal ideation, alcohol abuse, cocaine use, and recent loss of an important relationship (Murphy et al. 1992). A suicidal patient's perception that he or she is a burden on loved ones, as in the case example earlier in this chapter, is an important suicide risk factor (Van Orden et al. 2006). In youths, the strongest factors associated with suicide attempts are depression, alcohol or other drug use disorder, and aggressive or disruptive behaviors.

Populations at Risk for Suicide

Practice parameters exist for the assessment and treatment of children and adolescents with suicidal behavior (Shaffer et al. 1997). Risk factors for adolescents include prior attempts, affective disorder, substance abuse, living alone, male sex, age 16 years or older, and a history of physical and/or sexual abuse. Adverse childhood experiences (e.g., emotional, physical, or sexual abuse) are associated with an increased risk of attempted suicide throughout the life span (Dube et al. 2001). More women than men at risk for suicide have experienced childhood abuse (Kaplan et al. 1995). Brent (2001) provides a framework for the assessment of suicide risk in the adolescent that can be used to determine immediate disposition, intensity of treatment, and level of care (see Chapter 20, "Children, Adolescents, and College Students," this volume).

In adults older than 65 years, important correlates of late-life suicide are depression, physical illnesses, functional impairment, personality traits of neuroticism, social isolation, and loss of important relationships (Conwell and Duberstein 2001). The suicide rate for men 85 years and older is substantially higher (60 per 100,000) (Loebel 2005). Affective disorder is the risk factor with the strongest correlation. Among older adults, 41% saw their primary care physician within 28 days of completing suicide (Isometsä et al. 1995). Thus, primary care is an important point of suicide prevention for elders at high risk (see Chapter 21, "The Elderly," in this volume).

Personality disorders place a patient at increased risk for suicide (Linehan et al. 2000). Patients with personality disorders are at seven times greater risk for suicide than the general population (Harris and Barraclough 1997). Among patients who complete suicide, 30%–40% have personality disorders (Bronisch 1996; Duberstein and Conwell 1997; see Chapter 11, "Personality Disorders," this volume). Cluster B personality disorders, particularly borderline and antisocial personality disorders, place patients at increased risk for suicide (Duberstein and Conwell 1997). The presence of personality disorders, when comorbid with bipolar disorder, is an independent suicide risk factor that increases lifetime risk of suicide (Garno et al. 2005). In patients with borderline personality disorder, impulsivity was associated with a high number of suicide attempts, after control for substance abuse and a lifetime diagnosis of depressive disorder (Brodsky et al. 1997). In

a longitudinal study of personality disorder, a combination of borderline personality disorder, major affective disorder, and alcoholism was found in a subgroup of completed suicides (Stone 1993).

Personality disorder, negative recent life events, and Axis I comorbidity were identified in a large sample of patients who completed suicide (Heikkinen et al. 1997). Recent stressful life events, including workplace difficulties, family problems, unemployment, and financial trouble, were highly represented among patients with personality disorders. Personality disorders and comorbidity with other disorders and conditions, such as depressive symptoms and substance abuse, are frequently found in patients who complete suicide (Isometsä et al. 1996; Suominen et al. 2000).

Gunderson and Ridolfi (2001) estimated that suicide threats and gestures occur repeatedly in 90% of patients with borderline personality disorder. The clinician, in his or her suicide risk assessment of the borderline patient, should pay special attention to comorbidity, especially mood disorder, substance abuse, prior suicide attempts or self-mutilating behaviors, impulsivity, and unpleasant recent-life events. Self-mutilating behaviors that commonly occur in borderline patients include cutting (80%), bruising (34%), burning (20%), head banging (15%), and biting (7%).

Although self-mutilation is considered to be parasuicidal behavior (without lethal intent), the risk of suicide is doubled when self-mutilation is present (Stone et al. 1987). Retrospectively, it may be difficult or impossible to distinguish a nonlethal suicide gesture from an actual suicide attempt. Weisman and Worden (1972) devised a risk-rescue rating in suicide assessment as a descriptive and quantitative method of determining the lethality of suicide attempts. *Suicide intent* is defined as the subjective expectation and desire to die by a self-destructive act. The clinician must consider intent, not just behavior. For example, a patient who takes 10 aspirin tablets in the belief that it will result in death demonstrates high intent. A patient taking 6 mg/day of a benzodiazepine who overdoses on 180 one-milligram tablets may not have intended to die by suicide and may have known that death would not likely occur. An *aborted attempt* occurs when the intent to harm is interrupted and no physical harm results. *Lethality* refers to the danger to life by a suicide method or act. O'Carroll et al. (1996) provide definitions for a variety of suicidal behaviors.

Psychiatrists have difficulty gauging the imminence of suicide. No suicide risk factors identify imminence. *Imminence* defies definition; it is not a medical or psychiatric term. Imminence is another word for prediction. When a patient points a loaded gun at his or her head or perches on a bridge, it is a high-risk psychiatric emergency. However, individuals have been "talked out" of pulling the trigger or jumping. Individuals intent on committing suicide are usually ambivalent until the last moment. Suicide risk is in constant flux. It is imperative to identify, treat, and manage the patient's acute risk factors driving a suicide crisis rather than to undertake the impossible task of trying to predict whether or when a suicide attempt may occur. "Imminent suicide" creates the illusion of short-term prediction; it has no relevance to suicide risk assessment.

Impulsivity, a trait factor or predisposition often associated with alcohol and substance abuse, is an important suicide risk factor requiring careful assessment (Moeller et al. 2001). Impulsivity also has been found in many suicide attempters with major depressive disorder, panic disorder, and aggressive behaviors linked to the serotonergic system (Pezawas et al. 2002). Simon et al. (2001), in a case-controlled study of 153 case subjects, found that 24% of the subjects had spent less than 5 minutes between the decision to attempt suicide and a near-lethal attempt.

Patients who harm themselves are more impulsive than the general population. Patients who repeatedly harm themselves have been found to be more impulsive than patients who harm themselves for the first time (Evans et al. 1996). Impulsivity can be both acute and chronic. Chronic impulsivity can become acute when heightened by life stress, loss, and anxiety. Suicide attempts or violent suicide may often result (Fawcett 2001). Mann et al. (1999) found that suicide attempters with major depressive disorder have higher levels of aggression and impulsivity than nonattempters.

Impulsivity/aggression can be assessed clinically by asking the patient questions about violent rages, assaultive behaviors, arrests, destruction of property, spending sprees, speeding tickets, sexual indiscretions, hostility, easy provocation, and other indicators of poor impulse control (McGirr et al. 2009). A history of impulsive, aggressive behaviors toward self or others is a chronic risk factor for suicide (Brent and Mann 2005).

"Shame suicides" can occur in individuals faced with intolerable humiliation (e.g., scandal, criminal charges). A shame suicide may be an impulsive act in a narcissistically vulnerable person; however, it might not be associated with a diagnosable mental disorder (Roy 1986).

A patient's suicide risk may be exacerbated by problems arising from the treater. Examples include physical or psychological impairment, patient exploitation, incompetence, indifference, negative countertransference, fatigue ("burnout"), and deficient language skills (Simon and Gutheil

2004). To perform an adequate suicide risk assessment, the clinician must be able to understand idiomatic phrases and slang expressions. In one instance, a severely depressed suicidal patient with opioid dependence told the psychiatrist that she had "gone cold turkey." The psychiatrist, who had limited English language skills, proceeded to ask the patient if she had an eating disorder.

Suicide Risk Assessment Methodology

A number of suicide risk assessment models are available to the clinician (Beck et al. 1998; Clark and Fawcett 1999; Jacobs et al. 1999; Linehan 1993; Mays 2004; Rudd et al. 2001; Shea 2004). Only a few methods can be cited here. No suicide risk assessment model has been empirically tested for reliability and validity (Busch et al. 1993). Clinicians can also develop their own systematic risk assessment methods based on their training, clinical experience, and familiarity with the evidence-based psychiatric literature. The examples of suicide risk assessment illustrated in Figures 1–1, 1–2, and 1–3 represent ways of *conceptualizing* systematic assessment. The model in Figure 1–1 is a *teaching tool* designed to encourage a systematic approach to suicide risk assessment. It should not be used as a form or protocol to be applied in a robotic fashion. The use of stand-alone suicide risk assessment forms is not recommended.

Suicide risk factors vary in number and importance according to the individual patient. The clinician's judgment is central in identifying and assigning clinical weight to risk and protective factors. A common error is to omit assessment of protective factors. It is important to assess protective factors against suicide to achieve a balanced assessment of suicide risk. As noted previously, each patient has a distinctive suicide risk factor profile that should receive a high priority for identification and assessment. Protective factors tend to be more variable. The risk factor profile or prodrome can recur during a subsequent psychiatric illness.

Malone et al. (2000) assessed inpatients with major depression for severity of depression, general psychopathology, suicide history, reasons for living, and hopelessness. The self-report Reasons for Living Inventory was used to measure beliefs that may act as preventive factors against suicide (Linehan et al. 1983). The total score for reasons for living was inversely correlated with the sum of scores for hopelessness, subjective depression, and suicidal ideation. The authors recommend including reasons for living in the clinical assessment and management of suicidal patients.

Protective factors against suicide may include family and social support, pregnancy, children at home, strong religious beliefs, and cultural sanctions against suicide (Institute of Medicine 2002). Some families, however, are not able to be supportive, for a variety of reasons. Religious affiliation was associated with less suicidal behavior in depressed patients (Dervic et al. 2004). However, severely depressed patients may feel abandoned by God or may feel that God will understand, increasing their risk for suicide. Survival and coping skills, responsibility to family, and child-related concerns are also protective factors (Linehan et al. 1983).

A therapeutic alliance between clinician and patient can be an important protective factor against suicide (Simon 1998). The therapeutic alliance is influenced by a number of factors, especially the nature and severity of the patient's illness, but can change quickly from session to session. The therapeutic alliance may not be present and protective between sessions. Clinicians have been shocked and bewildered when a patient with whom the clinician felt a strong therapeutic alliance existed attempted or died by suicide between sessions. The absence of a therapeutic alliance in a patient at risk for suicide should be considered a significant risk factor.

Protective factors, like risk factors, vary with the distinctive clinical presentation of the individual patient at suicide risk. An ebb and flow exists between suicide risk and protective factors. Protective factors are especially important for discharge planning. They are usually easier for patients to talk about than risk factors and thus tend to be overvalued by the patient or the clinician. Protective factors may not be fully effective until the patient's suicide risk is reduced. Acute high suicide risk associated with severe mental illness may nullify protective factors.

Figure 1–1 divides assessment factors into five general categories: individual, clinical, interpersonal, situational, and demographic. The practitioner ranks the risk and protective factors according to the patient's clinical presentation. Usually, acute, high-risk suicide risk factors are the focus of continuing clinical attention. *Acute* refers to the intensity (severity) and magnitude (duration) of symptoms such as early-morning awakening versus global insomnia. A high risk factor is supported by an evidence-based association with suicide.

The continuum of suicide risk is assessed on a dimensional scale of low, moderate, high, or nonfactor. A final risk rating is ultimately a reasoned clinical judgment based on the overall assessment of the risk and protective factor pattern. The overall risk assessment informs treatment, safety management, and discharge decisions. The purpose of Figure 1–1 is to provide a *conceptual model* that encourages systematic suicide

risk assessment. Assessments can be made in a time-efficient manner after thorough psychiatric examination and during continuing patient care. A concise contemporaneous note that describes the clinician's suicide risk assessment and clinical decision-making process is adequate (see Table 1–3).

TABLE 1–3. Sample suicide risk assessment note

Suicide risk factors identified and weighed (low, moderate, high)

Protective factors identified and weighed (low, moderate, high)

Overall assessment rated (low, moderate, high, or range)

Treatment and management intervention informed by the assessment

Effectiveness of interventions evaluated

Source. Adapted from Simon 2004.

For example, assessment factors can be rated as *acute* (the focus of clinical attention) or *chronic* (long-standing, usually static risk factors). After initial psychiatric examination and systematic suicide risk assessment, the clinician can evaluate the course of acute suicide risk factors that brought the patient to treatment. Modifiable and treatable suicide risk factors should be identified early and treated aggressively. For example, anxiety, depression, insomnia, and psychosis may respond rapidly to medications as well as to psychosocial interventions, while impulsivity may respond to treatment with anticonvulsants (Hollander et al. 2002) (Table 1–4). The clinician should also identify, support, and, when possible, enhance protective factors. Psychosocial interventions can help mitigate or resolve interpersonal issues at home, work, or school. At discharge, a final systematic suicide risk assessment allows comparison with the initial office visit or hospital admission assessment. The clini-

TABLE 1–4.	Modifiable and treatable suicide risk factors: some examples
Depression	Impulsivity
Anxiety	Agitation
Panic attacks	Physical illness
Psychosis	Situation (e.g., family, work)
Sleep disorders	Lethal means (e.g., guns, drugs)
Substance abuse	Drug effects (e.g., akathisia)

Source. Adapted from Simon 2004.

cian determines whether there is sufficient reduction of suicide risk to support patient discharge. The question that needs to be asked is the following: What is different?

Conclusion

Systematic suicide risk assessment encourages the gathering of relevant clinical information. Suicide risk exists along a continuum that can vary from minute to minute, hour to hour, and day to day. Thus, assessments must be performed at several clinical junctures, such as change of safety status, removal from seclusion and/or restraint, ward changes, prior to issuing passes, and at time of discharge. The suicide risk assessment process that follows the course of acute risk factors is illustrated in the case example. For outpatients, systematic suicide risk assessment is critical to clinical decision making, especially regarding voluntary or involuntary hospitalization.

Patients with Axis I psychiatric disorders such as schizophrenia, anxiety disorders, major affective disorders, and substance use disorders often present with acute (state) suicide risk factors. Patients with Axis II disorders often display chronic (trait) suicide risk factors. Exacerbation of an Axis II disorder or comorbidity with an Axis I disorder (including substance abuse) may transform a chronic suicide risk factor, such as impulsivity, into an acute risk factor. A family history of mental illness, especially when associated with suicide, is an important chronic (static) risk factor. The offspring of mood disorder patients who attempt suicide are at a significantly increased risk for completed suicide (Brent et al. 2002). In the case example, the patient's aunt was diagnosed as a "chronic schizophrenic," and a "manic-depressive" uncle completed suicide. Comorbidity significantly increases the patient's risk for suicide (Kessler et al. 1999). Suicide risk increases with the total number of risk factors, providing a quasi-quantitative dimension to suicide risk factor assessment (Murphy et al. 1992).

Systematic suicide risk assessment of the patient's risk and protective factors is a gateway to improved information gathering that informs the identification, treatment, and management of patients at risk for suicide.

Acknowledgment

This chapter was adapted with permission from Simon RI: "Suicide Risk: Assessing the Unpredictable," in *The American Psychiatric Publishing Textbook of Suicide Assessment and Management.* Edited by Simon RI, Hales RE. Washington, DC, American Psychiatric Publishing, 2006, pp. 1–12.

Key Clinical Concepts

- Fully commit time and effort to the ongoing assessment, treatment, and management of the patient at suicide risk.

- Conduct systematic suicide risk assessments to inform treatment and management of patients at risk for suicide.

- Identify treatable and modifiable suicide risk and protective factors early, and treat aggressively. Delayed or ineffective treatment can result in a psychiatric condition becoming entrenched, leading to patient demoralization, hopelessness, and adverse life consequences. Consider suicide-reduction drugs such as lithium and clozapine in bipolar patients and schizophrenic patients, respectively.

- Do not use suicide prevention contracts in place of conducting systematic suicide risk assessments.

- Suicide risk assessment is a process, not an event. Conduct suicide risk assessments at important clinical junctures (e.g., initial evaluation, discharge, changing observational levels).

- Contemporaneously document suicide risk assessments. Such documentation facilitates good clinical care and is standard practice.

References

Addy CL: Statistical concepts of prediction, in Assessment and Prediction of Suicide. Edited by Maris RW, Berman AL, Maltsberger JT, et al. New York, Guilford, 1992, pp 218–232

American Psychiatric Association: The Principles of Medical Ethics With Annotations Especially Applicable to Psychiatry. Washington, DC, American Psychiatric Association, 2009

Baldessarini RJ: Lithium: effects on depression and suicide. J Clin Psychiatry 64:7, 2003

Baldessarini RJ, Pompili M, Tondo L: Bipolar disorder, in The American Psychiatric Publishing Textbook of Suicide Assessment and Management. Edited by Simon RI, Hales RE. Washington, DC, American Psychiatric Publishing, 2006, pp 277–299

Beck AT, Brown G, Berchick RJ, et al: Relationship between hopelessness and ultimate suicide: a replication with psychiatric outpatients. Am J Psychiatry 147:190–195, 1990

Beck AT, Steer RA, Ranieri WF: Scale for suicidal ideation: psychometric properties of a self-report version. J Consult Clin Psychol 44:499–505, 1998

Black HC: Black's Law Dictionary, 7th Edition. St. Paul, MN, West Group, 1999

Bongar B, Maris RW, Bertram AL, et al: Outpatient standards of care and the suicidal patient. Suicide Life Threat Behav 22:453–478, 1992

Breier A, Astrachan BM: Characterization of schizophrenic patients who commit suicide. Am J Psychiatry 141:206–209, 1984

Brent DA: Assessment and treatment of the youthful suicidal patient. Ann N Y Acad Sci 932:106–131, 2001

Brent DA, Mann JJ: Family genetic studies, suicide and suicidal behavior. Am J Med Genet 133:13–24, 2005

Brent DA, Bridge J, Johnson BA, et al: Suicidal behavior runs in families: a controlled family study of adolescent suicide victims. Arch Gen Psychiatry 53:1145–1152, 1996

Brent DA, Oquendo M, Birmaher B, et al: Familial pathways to early onset suicide attempt. Arch Gen Psychiatry 59:801–807, 2002

Brodsky BS, Malone KM, Ellis SP, et al: Characteristics of borderline personality disorder associated with suicidal behavior. Am J Psychiatry 154:1715–1719, 1997

Bronisch T: The typology of personality disorders—diagnostic problems and their relevance for suicidal behavior. Crisis 17:55–58, 1996

Busch KA, Clark DC, Fawcett J, et al: Clinical features of inpatient suicide. Psychiatr Ann 23:256–262, 1993

Busch KA, Fawcett J, Jacobs DG: Clinical correlates of inpatient suicide. J Clin Psychiatry 64:14–19, 2003

Clark DC, Fawcett J: An empirically based model of suicide risk assessment of patients with affective disorders, in Suicide and Clinical Practice. Edited by Jacobs DJ. Washington, DC, American Psychiatric Association, 1999, pp 55–73

Conwell Y, Duberstein PR: Suicide in elders. Ann N Y Acad Sci 932:132–150, 2001

Coryell W, Leon A, Winokur G, et al: Importance of psychotic features to long-term course in major depressive disorder. Am J Psychiatry 153:483–489, 1996

Dervic K, Oquendo MA, Grunebaum MF, et al: Religious affiliation and suicide attempt. Am J Psychiatry 161:2303–2308, 2004

Dube SR, Anda RF, Felitti VJ, et al: Childhood abuse, household dysfunction, and the risk of attempted suicide throughout the life span: findings from the Adverse Childhood Experiences Study. JAMA 286:3089–3096, 2001

Duberstein P, Conwell Y: Personality disorders and completed suicide: a methodological and conceptual review. Clinical Psychology: Science and Practice 4:359–376, 1997

Evans J, Platts H, Liebenau A: Impulsiveness and deliberate self-harm: a comparison of "first-timers" and "repeaters." Acta Psychiatr Scand 93:378–380, 1996

Fawcett J: Treating impulsivity and anxiety in the suicidal patient. Ann N Y Acad Sci 932:94–105, 2001

Fawcett J, Scheftner WA, Clark DC, et al: Clinical predictors of suicide in patients with major affective disorders: a controlled prospective study. Am J Psychiatry 144:35–40, 1987

Fawcett J, Scheftner WA, Fogg L, et al: Time-related predictors of suicide in major affective disorder. Am J Psychiatry 147:1189–1194, 1990

Fawcett J, Clark DC, Busch KA: Assessing and treating the patient at suicide risk. Psychiatr Ann 23:244–255, 1993

Garno JL, Goldberg JF, Ramirez PM, et al: Bipolar disorder with comorbid cluster B personality features: impact on suicidality. J Clin Psychiatry 66:339–345, 2005

Gunderson JG, Ridolfi ME: Borderline personality disorder: suicidality and self-mutilation. Ann N Y Acad Sci 932:61–73, 2001

Hall RC, Platt DE, Hall RC: Suicide risk assessment: a review of risk factors for suicide in 100 patients who made severe suicide attempts: evaluation of suicide risk in a time of managed care. Psychosomatics 40:18–27, 1999

Harkavy-Friedman JM, Kimhy D, Nelson EA, et al: Suicide attempts in schizophrenia: the role of command auditory hallucinations for suicide. J Clin Psychiatry 64:871–874, 2003

Harris CE, Barraclough B: Suicide as an outcome for mental disorders: a meta analysis. Br J Psychiatry 170:205–228, 1997

Heikkinen ME, Henriksson MM, Erkki T, et al: Recent life events and suicide in personality disorders. J Nerv Ment Dis 185:373–381, 1997

Heilä H, Isometsä ET, Henriksson MM, et al: Suicide and schizophrenia: a nationwide psychological autopsy study on age- and sex-specific clinical characteristics of 92 suicide victims with schizophrenia. Am J Psychiatry 154:1235–1242, 1997

Heilä H, Heikkinen ME, Isometsä ET, et al: Life events and completed suicide in schizophrenia: a comparison of suicide victims with and without schizophrenia. Schizophr Bull 25:519–531, 1999

Hellerstein D, Frosch W, Koenigsbert HW: The clinical significance of command hallucinations. Am J Psychiatry 144:219–225, 1987

Heron M, Hoyert DL, Murphy SL, et al: Deaths: final data for 2006. National Vital Statistics Reports. April 17, 2009. Available at: http://www.cdc.gov/nchs/data/nvsr/nvsr57/nvsr57_14.pdf. Accessed June 20, 2011.

Hollander E, Posner N, Cherkasky S: Neuropsychiatric aspects of aggression and impulse control disorders, in The American Psychiatric Publishing Textbook of Neuropsychiatry and Behavioral Neurosciences, 4th Edition. Edited by Yudofsky SC, Hales RE. Washington, DC, American Psychiatric Publishing, 2002, pp 579–596

Institute of Medicine: Reducing Suicide: A National Imperative. Washington, DC, National Academies Press, 2002, pp 2–4

Isometsä ET, Lönnqvist JK: Suicide attempts preceding completed suicide. Br J Psychiatry 173:531–535, 1998

Isometsä ET, Heikkinen ME, Marttunen MJ, et al: The last appointment before suicide: is suicide intent communicated? Am J Psychiatry 152:919–922, 1995

Isometsä ET, Henriksson MM, Heikkinen ME, et al: Suicide among subjects with personality disorders. Am J Psychiatry 153:667–673, 1996

Jacobs DG, Brewer M, Klein-Benheim M: Suicide assessment: an overview and recommended protocol, in The Harvard Medical School Guide to Suicide Assessment and Intervention. Edited by Jacobs DJ. San Francisco, CA, Jossey-Bass, 1999, pp 3–39

Junginger J: Predicting compliance with command hallucinations. Am J Psychiatry 147:245–247, 1990

Junginger J: Command hallucinations and the prediction of dangerousness. Psychiatr Serv 46:911–914, 1995

Kaplan M, Asnis GM, Lipschitz DS, et al: Suicidal behavior and abuse in psychiatric outpatients. Compr Psychiatry 36:229–235, 1995

Kasper ME, Rogers R, Adams PA: Dangerousness and command hallucinations: an investigation of psychotic inpatients. Bull Am Acad Psychiatry Law 24:219–224, 1996

Kessler RC, Borges G, Walters EE: Prevalence of and risk factors for lifetime suicide: suicide attempts in the National Comorbidity Study. Arch Gen Psychiatry 55:617–626, 1999

Linehan MM: Cognitive Behavioral Treatment of Borderline Personality Disorder. New York, Guilford, 1993

Linehan MM, Goodstein JL, Nielsen SL, et al: Reasons for staying alive when you are thinking of killing yourself: the Reasons for Living Inventory. J Consult Clin Psychol 51:276–286, 1983

Linehan MM, Rizvi SL, Welch SS, et al: Psychiatric aspects of suicidal behaviour: personality disorders, in The International Handbook of Suicide and Attempted Suicide. Edited by Hawton K, van Heeringen K. New York, Wiley, 2000, pp 147–148

Loebel JP: Completed suicide in late life. Psychiatr Serv 56:260–262, 2005

Malone KM, Katalin S, Corbitt EM, et al: Clinical assessment versus research methods in the assessment of suicidal behavior. Am J Psychiatry 152:1601–1607, 1995

Malone KM, Oquendo MA, Hass GL, et al: Protective factors against suicidal acts in major depression: reasons for living. Am J Psychiatry 157:1084–1088, 2000

Mann JJ, Arango V: The neurobiology of suicidal behavior, in The Harvard Medical School Guide to Suicide Assessment and Intervention. Edited by Jacobs DG. San Francisco, CA, Jossey-Bass, 1999, pp 98–114

Mann JJ, Waternaux C, Haas GL, et al: Toward a clinical model of suicidal behavior in psychiatric patients. Am J Psychiatry 156:181–189, 1999

Mays D: Structured assessment methods may improve suicide prevention. Psychiatr Ann 34:367–372, 2004

McGirr A, Martin A, Séguin M, et al: Familial aggregation of suicide explained by cluster B traits: a three-group family study of suicide controlling for major depressive disorder. Am J Psychiatry 166:1124–1134, 2009

Meltzer HY: Treatment of suicidality in schizophrenia. Ann N Y Acad Sci 932:44–60, 2001

Meltzer HY, Okaly G: Reduction of suicidality during clozapine treatment of neuroleptic-resistant schizophrenia: impact of risk-benefit assessment. Am J Psychiatry 152:183–190, 1995

Meltzer HY, Alphs L, Green AI, et al: Clozapine treatment for suicidality in schizophrenia: International Suicide Prevention Trial (InterSePT). Arch Gen Psychiatry 60:82–91, 2003a

Meltzer HY, Conley RR, de Leo D, et al: Intervention strategies for suicidality. Audiograph Series. J Clin Psychiatry 6:1–18, 2003b

Meyer RE, Salzman C, Youngstrom EA, et al: Suicidality and risk of suicide—definition, drug safety concerns and a necessary target for drug development: a brief report. J Clin Psychiatry 71:1040–1046, 2010

Moeller FG, Barratt ES, Dougherty DM, et al: Psychiatric aspects of impulsivity. Am J Psychiatry 158:1783–1793, 2001

Monahan J, Steadman HJ: Violent storms and violent people: how meteorology can inform risk communication in mental health law. Am Psychol 51:931–938, 1996

Murphy GE, Wetzel RD, Robins E, et al: Multiple risk factors predict suicide in alcoholism. Arch Gen Psychiatry 49:459–462, 1992

O'Carroll PW, Berman AL, Maris RW, et al: Beyond the Tower of Babel: a nomenclature for suicidology. Suicide Life Threat Behav 26:237–252, 1996

Oquendo MA, Halberstam, Mann JJ: Risk factors for suicidal behavior: the utility and limitation of research instruments, in Standardized Evaluation in Clinical Practice. Edited by First MB. Washington, DC, American Psychiatric Publishing, 2003, pp 103–130

Perlis RH, Fraquas R, Fava M, et al: Prevalence and clinical correlates of irritability in major depressive disorder: a preliminary report from the Sequenced Treatment Alternatives to Relieve Depression study. J Clin Psychiatry 66:159–166, 2005

Peters PG Jr: The quiet demise of deference to custom: malpractice law at the millennium. Wash Lee Law Rev 57:163–205, 2000

Pezawas L, Stamenkovic M, Reinhold J, et al: A longitudinal view of triggers and thresholds of suicidal behavior in depression. J Clin Psychiatry 63:866–873, 2002

Pokorny AD: Predictions of suicide in psychiatric patients: report of a prospective study. Arch Gen Psychiatry 40:249–257, 1983

Pokorny AD: Suicide prediction revisited. Suicide Life Threat Behav 23:1–10, 1993

Posternak MA, Zimmerman M: Is there a delay in the antidepressant effect? A meta-analysis. J Clin Psychiatry 66:148–158, 2005

Resnick PJ: Recognizing that the suicidal patient views you as an adversary. Curr Psychiatr 1:8, 2002

Robins E: The Final Months: Study of the Lives of 134 Persons Who Committed Suicide. New York, Oxford University Press, 1981

Roose SP, Glassman AH, Walsh BT, et al: Depression, delusions, and suicide. Am J Psychiatry 140:1159–1162, 1983

Roy A: Suicide in chronic schizophrenia. Br J Psychiatry 141:171–177, 1982

Roy A: Suicide. Baltimore, MD, Williams & Wilkins, 1986, pp 6, 93–94

Rudd MD, Joiner T, Rajab MH: Treating Suicidal Behavior: An Effective, Time-Limited Approach. New York, Guilford, 2001

Scheiber SC, Kramer TS, Adamowski SE: Core Competencies for Psychiatric Practice: What Clinicians Need to Know (A Report of the American Board of Psychiatry and Neurology). Washington, DC, American Psychiatric Publishing, 2003

Shaffer DA, Pfeffer CR, Bernet W, et al: Practice parameter for the assessment and treatment of children and adolescents with suicidal behavior. J Am Acad Child Adolesc Psychiatry 36 (suppl), 1997

Shea SC: The delicate art of eliciting suicidal ideation. Psychiatr Ann 34:385–400, 2004

Simon RI: Clinical Psychiatry and the Law, 2nd Edition. Washington, DC, American Psychiatric Press, 1992

Simon RI: The suicidal patient, in The Mental Health Practitioner and the Law: A Comprehensive Handbook. Edited by Lifson LE, Simon RI. Cambridge, MA, Harvard University Press, 1998, pp 329–343

Simon RI: Suicide risk assessment in managed care settings. Prim Psychiatry 7:42–43, 46–49, 2002a

Simon RI: Suicide risk assessment: what is the standard of care? J Am Acad Psychiatry Law 30:340–344, 2002b

Simon RI: Assessing and Managing Suicide Risk: Guidelines for Clinically Based Risk Management. Washington, DC, American Psychiatric Publishing, 2004

Simon RI: Standard of care testimony: best practice or reasonable care? J Am Acad Psychiatry Law 33:8–11, 2005

Simon RI: Imminent suicide: the illusion of short-term prediction. Suicide Life Threat Behav 36:296–301, 2006

Simon RI: Suicide risk assessment forms: form over substance? J Am Acad Psychiatry Law 37:290–293, 2009

Simon RI: Preventing Patient Suicide: Clinical Assessment and Management. Washington, DC, American Psychiatric Publishing, 2011

Simon RI, Gutheil TG: Clinician factors associated with increased risk for patient suicide. Psychiatr Ann 330:1–4, 2004

Simon RI, Shuman DW: Clinical Manual of Psychiatry and Law. Washington, DC, American Psychiatric Publishing, 2007

Simon TR, Swann AC, Powell KE, et al: Characteristics of impulsive suicide attempts and attempters. Suicide Life Threat Behav 32(suppl):49–59, 2001

Stanford EJ, Goetz RR, Bloom JD: The no harm contract in the emergency assessment of suicide risk. J Clin Psychiatry 55:344–348, 1994

Stepakoff v Kantar, 473 N.E.2d 1131, 1134 (Mass 1985)

Stone M: Long-term outcome in personality disorders. Br J Psychiatry 162:299–313, 1993

Stone MH, Stone DK, Hurt SW: Natural history of borderline patients treated by intensive hospitalization. Psychiatr Clin North Am 10:185–206, 1987

Sullivan GR, Bongar B: Psychological testing in suicide risk management, in The American Psychiatric Publishing Textbook of Suicide Assessment and Management. Edited by Simon RI, Hales RE. Washington, DC, American Psychiatric Publishing, 2006, pp 177–196

Suominen KH, Isometsä ET, Henriksson MM, et al: Suicide attempts and personality disorder. Acta Psychiatr Scand 102:118–125, 2000

Taylor CB (ed): How to Practice Evidence-Based Psychiatry: Basic Principles. Washington, DC, American Psychiatric Publishing, 2010

Van Orden KA, Lynam ME, Hollar D, et al: Perceived burdensomeness as an indicator of suicidal symptoms. Cognit Ther Res 30:457–469, 2006

Vythilingam M, Chen J, Bremmer JD, et al: Psychotic depression and mortality. Am J Psychiatry 160:574–576, 2003

Warman DM, Forman E, Henriques GR, et al: Suicidality and psychosis: beyond depression and hopelessness. Suicide Life Threat Behav 34:77–86, 2004

Weisman AD, Worden JW: Risk-rescue rating in suicide assessment. Arch Gen Psychiatry 26:553–560, 1972

Zimmerman M, Chelminski I: Generalized anxiety disorder in patients with major depression: is DSM-IV's hierarchy correct? Am J Psychiatry 160:504–512, 2003

Zimmerman M, Chelminski I, McDermut W: Major depressive disorder and Axis I diagnostic comorbidity. J Clin Psychiatry 63:187–193, 2002

CHAPTER 2

The Interpersonal Art of Suicide Assessment

Interviewing Techniques for Uncovering Suicidal Intent, Ideation, and Actions

Shawn Christopher Shea, M.D.

The first rule of life is to reveal nothing, to be exceptionally cautious in what you say, in whatever company you may find yourself.

Elizabeth Aston, The Darcy Connection: A Novel *(2008)*

Many patients who find themselves in the company of a mental health professional unfortunately may adopt the above dictum, especially when they are asked about suicide. It is the interviewer's task to transform this potentially dangerous hesitancy. Suicide is ubiquitous. It honors no boundaries. For clinicians, exploring suicidal ideation and suicidal intent is often a daily task. Whether the patient is young or old, rich or poor, a quiet recluse or an infamous Hollywood icon, suicide is often a player—a final arbiter that, if heeded, ends the play. Many of us have been touched by suicides among our patients, friends, family members, and colleagues. Contemplation of suicide may even be a part of our own past or future history.

In this chapter, the many reasons that a patient may be hesitant to share suicidal ideation and intent are explored, such as shame ("My brother and my therapist will think less of me"), fear ("They'll remove me from the police force if they find out I've been suicidal"), or the presence of serious intent ("If I tell them about my gun, they're going to take it from me"). A flexible interviewing strategy, the Chronological Assessment of Suicide Events, or CASE Approach (Shea 2009b, 2009c, 2011c), which is designed to help patients more openly share the truth about their suicidal ideation and suicidal intent, is then described.

Before doing so, in order to better understand the focus of this chapter, it is important to review the components that constitute a suicide assessment. As delineated elsewhere (Shea 2011c), a suicide assessment is composed of three components that represent three different skill sets:

1. Gathering information related to risk factors, protective factors, and warning signs of suicide (a data-gathering process)
2. Uncovering information related to the patient's suicidal ideation, planning, behaviors, desire, and intent (a data-gathering process)
3. Arriving at a clinical formulation of risk based on these two databases (a cognitive and intuitive process)

Practical protocols for integrating these three aspects of a suicide assessment have been well delineated for adults (Bonger et al. 1998; Chiles and Strosahl 2004; Jacobs 1999; Maris et al. 2000; McKeon 2009; Rudd 2006; Shea 2011c; Simon 2004, 2011; Simon and Hales 2006) and adolescents (Berman et al. 2005). Innovative systematic protocols, such as the Collaborative Assessment and Management of Suicidality (CAMS) approach created by David Jobes (2006), have also been developed for integrating all three tasks while providing ongoing collaborative intervention, which may help lay the foundation for a more evidence-based approach for both suicide assessment and subsequent therapy. More recently, Joiner et al. (2009) delineated a promising approach based on the interpersonal theory of suicide that gracefully integrates all three components that are necessary for a suicide assessment.

In the clinical and research literature, much attention has been given to the first task (gathering risk/protective factors and warning signs) and the third task (determining a clinical formulation of risk). Significantly less attention has been given to the second task of a suicide assessment: the detailed set of interviewing skills needed to elicit effectively suicidal ideation, behaviors, planning, access to means, desire, and intent.

The CASE Approach was designed to fill this gap, and it *solely* addresses this second task. The CASE Approach complements, not replaces, the two other critical components of a sound suicide assessment protocol. The risk factors, protective factors, and warning signs must be uncovered in other sections of the interview either before or after one uses the CASE Approach.

Through the use of skilled interviewing strategies such as the CASE Approach, the resulting phenomenological picture of the patient's suicidal ideation, suicide planning, and actual suicidal intent (the second assessment task) may yield some of the most reliable data from which a clinical formulation of suicidal risk (the third assessment task) can be made. Ultimately people kill themselves not because they fit a statistical profile of risk and protective factors but because they have decided to kill themselves. When a middle-aged man whose business has collapsed pulls the trigger of a gun or a college student who has failed a semester takes a fatal step off a bridge, it is caused by phenomenological rather than statistical events. Moreover, as any clinical supervisor will testify, there is little doubt that two clinicians, after eliciting suicidal ideation from the same client, can walk away with surprisingly different information. The question is: Why?

Importance of a Comprehensive Elicitation of Suicidal Ideation: Uncovering the Patient's Real Suicidal Intent

Difficulties Encountered When Uncovering Suicidal Ideation

Not all patients at risk for suicide openly relay suicidal ideation to clinicians (Hall and Platt 1999). One could argue that many dangerous patients—those who truly want to die and see no hope for relief from their suffering—may have little incentive to do so. Even if their ambivalence about attempting suicide leads them to voluntarily call a crisis line, go to an emergency department (ED), or seek help at a campus counseling center, they may be quite cautious about revealing the full truth because a large part of them still wants to die. Such patients may be predisposed to share only some of their suicidal ideation or action taken on a particular plan, while hiding their real intent or even their method of choice (such as a gun tucked away in the back of a closet). Many reasons exist why a patient may be hesitant to openly share, including the following:

- The patient has intense suicidal ideation and is serious about completing the act, but is purposely not relaying suicidal ideation or method of choice because he or she does not want the attempt to be thwarted.
- The patient feels that suicide is a sign of weakness and is ashamed to acknowledge it.
- The patient feels that suicide is immoral or a sin.
- The patient feels that discussion of suicide is, literally, taboo.
- The patient is worried that the clinician will perceive him or her as abnormal or crazy.

- The patient fears that he or she will be locked up if suicidal ideation is shared or, during a crisis call, that the police will appear at his or her door.
- The patient fears that others will find out about his or her suicidal thoughts from a break in confidentiality, which includes fears that leaked suicidal ideation might be damaging to familial and business relationships, be damaging to career advancement or even maintaining a job (soldier, police officer, airline pilot), or be posted on the Web.
- The patient does not believe that anyone can help.
- The patient has alexithymia and has trouble describing emotional pain or material (Mays 2004).

It is sometimes easy to believe that if we ask directly about suicide, patients will answer directly—and truthfully. In many, if not most, instances they do. On the other hand, from the considerations just described, it is apparent that this is not necessarily the case.

The most dangerous patients—the patients who really intensely want to die—may be the very ones least likely to share the full truth when first asked. It is in these relatively rare yet highly lethal cases that we may have the greatest chance of actually saving a life with strategies such as the CASE Approach.

The real suicidal intent of any patient can be conceptualized by the following Equation of Suicidal Intent (Shea 2009b):

Real Suicidal Intent = Stated Intent + Reflected Intent + Withheld Intent

The Equation of Suicidal Intent postulates that the real suicidal intent of any given patient may be equal to any one of the following or a combination of the following:

- *Stated intent:* what the patient directly tells the clinician about suicidal intent
- *Reflected intent:* the amount of thinking, planning, or actions taken on suicidal ideation that may reflect the intensity of the actual suicidal intent
- *Withheld intent:* suicidal intent that is unconsciously or purposefully withheld

Thus, a patient's actual intent may be equal to his or her stated intent, reflected intent, and withheld intent; any one of these three; or any combination of the three. The more intensely a patient wants to proceed with suicide, the more likely the patient is to withhold his or her true intent. In addition, the more taboo a topic is (e.g., incest and suicide), the more one would expect a patient to withhold information. In such instances, both conscious and unconscious processes may underlie the withholding of vital information by a patient.

From a psychodynamic perspective, a curious and dangerous paradox can arise. If a patient deeply feels that suicide is a sign of weakness or a sin, unconscious defense mechanisms such as denial, repression, rationalization, and intellectualization may create the *conscious* belief in the patient that his or her suicidal intent is much less than is true. When asked directly about their suicidal intent, such patients may provide a gross underestimate of their potential lethality even though they are genuinely trying to answer the inquiry honestly. Such a patient could respond to the question "How close do you think you came to killing yourself?" with a simple "Not very," even though the night before he or she had been standing precipitously on the edge of a bridge.

Considering all of the previously mentioned factors, from unconscious to conscious, it is not surprising that from a phenomenological perspective, some patients with serious suicidal intent may relay their actual intent in stages during an interview. When evaluating such a patient, one would expect that after he or she is asked about suicide, a nuanced interpersonal dance would unfold in which the patient shares some information, reads how the clinician responds, shares some more information, reevaluates where this session is going, and so on.

Indeed, patients with serious suicidal intent who are trying to decide how much to share may consciously withhold their main method of choice (such as a gun) until they arrive at a decision during the interview that they do not want to die, at which point they may feel safe enough with the clinician to share the full truth (because they know that once they share information about the gun, a family member may be called and the gun removed). Put succinctly, there are many powerful drivers that predispose a truly dangerous patient "to reveal nothing, to be exceptionally cautious in what you say" when in the company of a clinician.

Reflected Intent: One of the Master Keys to Unlocking Real Intent

Reflected intent is the quality and quantity of the patient's suicidal thoughts and desires, suicide plans, and extent of action taken to complete the plans, which may reflect how much the patient truly wants to die by suicide. The extent, thoroughness, and time spent by the patient on suicide planning may be a better reflection of the seriousness of his or her intent and the proximity of his or her desire to act on that intent than the actual stated intent. Such reflections of intent may prove to be life-saving pieces of the suicide assessment puzzle. Recent empirical studies on the highly promising Columbia Suicide Severity Rating Scale (Posner et al. 2011) seem to lend support to the concept that reflected intent may have predictive capabilities regarding suicide risk. The work of Thomas Joiner (see Joiner 2005; Joiner et al. 2009) has provided insight into the importance of acquired capability for suicide (e.g., intensive planning, availability of methods, multiple past attempts) as a reflection of the seriousness of intent and the potential for action.

A wealth of research from an unexpected source—motivational theory—can help us better understand the importance of reflected intent. Prochaska and colleagues' (Prochaska and DiClemente 1984; Prochaska et al. 1992) transtheoretical stages of change—precontemplation, contemplation, preparation, action, and maintenance— show that when it comes to motivation to do something that is hard to do but good for oneself (e.g., substance abuse counseling), the extent of a person's goal-directed thinking and subsequent actions may be better indicators of intent to proceed than stated intent. In short, the old adage "actions speak louder than words" appears to be on the mark in predicting recovery behavior.

A patient referred to Alcoholics Anonymous (AA) may tell the referring counselor all sorts of things about his or her intent to change. Nevertheless, the amount of time the patient spends thinking about the need for change (e.g., reading literature from AA) and arranging ways to make the change (e.g., finding out where local AA meetings are) and the actions taken for change (e.g., finding someone to drive him or her to the meetings), according to Prochaska's theory, may better reflect the intent to change than the patient's verbal report.

Motivational theories are usually related to initiating difficult-to-do actions for positive change, but they may be equally effective for predicting the likelihood that a person may initiate a difficult-to-do action that is negative, such as suicide. Joiner and colleagues (2009) pointed out that suicide

can be quite a difficult act with which to proceed. Once again, the amount of time spent thinking, planning, and practicing a suicide attempt may speak louder about imminent risk than the patient's immediate words about his or her intent.

The CASE Approach— From Theory to Practice: Background

Designed specifically to address the previously discussed concerns, the CASE Approach is a flexible, practical, and easily learned interviewing strategy for eliciting suicidal ideation, planning, behavior, desire, and intent. It is not presented as the right way to elicit suicidal ideation or as a standard of care but as a reasonable way that can help clinicians develop their own way. From an understanding of the CASE approach, clinicians can directly adopt what they like, reject what they do not like, and add new ideas. Specific interviewing techniques and strategies from the CASE Approach can be used and/or adapted to any suicide assessment protocol the clinician deems useful, from a totally personalized protocol to more formal protocols such as the CAMS (Jobes 2006) and the Columbia Suicide Severity Rating Scale (Posner et al. 2011). The goal of the CASE Approach is to provide clinicians with a practical framework for exploring and better understanding how they uncover suicidal ideation no matter what suicide assessment protocol they ultimately want to use. In this way the clinician can develop an individualized approach with which he or she personally feels comfortable and competent.

First developed at the Diagnostic and Evaluation Center of the Western Psychiatric Institute and Clinic at the University of Pittsburgh in the 1980s, the CASE Approach was refined in the Department of Psychiatry at Dartmouth Medical School and in frontline community mental health center work during the 1990s. Subsequent refinements since 2000 have been implemented at the Training Institute for Suicide Assessment and Clinical Interviewing.

The CASE Approach has been extensively described in the literature (Shea 1998a, 1998b, 2001, 2002, 2004, 2009b, 2009c, 2011c). Interviewing techniques from the CASE Approach can be used in a variety of clinical arenas, as reflected by its positive reception among mental health professionals and suicidologists (Carlat 2004a, 2004b; EndingSuicide.com 2011; Joiner et al. 2009; Mays 2004; Oordt et al. 2009; Robinson 2001; see also the Web site of the University of Michigan Depression Center [www.med.umich.edu/depression/suicide_assessment/suicide_info.htm]), substance abuse counselors (Shea 2001), school and college counselors (Reed and Shea 2011), primary care clinicians (Shea 1999, 2008b), clinicians in the correctional system (Knoll 2009), legal experts (Simpson and Stacy 2004), military/Veterans Affairs mental health professionals (Shea 2008a, 2009a, 2011b), and psychiatric residency directors (Shea 2003).

The CASE Approach is a practice recommended by organizations as diverse as Magellan (Magellan Behavioral Health Care Guidelines 2002) and the government of British Columbia (Monk and Samra 2007). It is routinely taught as one of the core clinical courses provided at the annual meeting of the American Association of Suicidology (AAS) (Shea 2011a). It is also one of the techniques described in the 2-day Recognizing and Responding to Suicide Risk course sponsored by the AAS (American Association of Suicidology 2011). Didactic presentations, as well as experiential trainings resulting in both individual and group certifications in the CASE Approach, are provided by the Training Institute for Suicide Assessment and Clinical Interviewing (www.suicideassessment.com).

The Question of Validity: Its Central Role in the CASE Approach

Validity is the cornerstone of suicide assessment. Nothing more directly determines the effectiveness of the interviewer in gathering information that may forewarn of dangerousness. If the patient does not invite the clinician into the intimate details of his or her suicide planning, the best clinician in the world, armed with the best risk factor analysis available, will be limited in his or her ability to determine whether the patient is at acute, high risk.

The problem of maximizing validity was addressed in the development of the CASE Approach by returning to the core clinical interviewing literature, in which specific "validity techniques"—created to uncover sensitive and taboo material such as incest, domestic violence, substance use problems, psychological and physical abuse, and antisocial behaviors—have been described in detail (Shea 1998b). These techniques were designed by experts in various disciplines, including counseling, clinical psychology, and psychiatry. In addition to being the foundation stones for the CASE Approach, these validity techniques are useful for uncovering the numerous types of sensitive topics that may lead to suicidal thought.

Two Validity Techniques for Sensitively Raising the Topic of Suicide

Normalization

In *normalization*, described by Shea (1998b), the interviewer phrases the question so that the patient realizes that he or she is not the only person who has ever experienced the behaviors under scrutiny, as with "Sometimes when people get really angry they say things they later regret. Has that ever happened to you?" It is a simple technique in which the clinician begins the question by suggesting that he or she has heard of this behavior from other patients, metacommunicating that the patient is far from alone in having experienced the feelings or behaviors. Normalizations often, but not always, begin with phrases such as "Sometimes people who have…" The following normalization can be used to raise sensitively the topic of suicide: "Sometimes when people are in a tremendous amount of pain, they find themselves having thoughts of killing themselves. Have you been having any thoughts like that?"

Clinicians can use numerous variations of normalization to raise the topic of suicide depending on the specific situational stresses that may be prompting suicidal ideation, as with "Sometimes when people lose a spouse they loved as much as you loved Anna, they have thoughts of killing themselves. Have you been having any thoughts like that?"

Shame Attenuation

With *shame attenuation*, originally described by Shea (1998b), the client's own pain is used as the gateway to topics such as suicide (note that in the following question, there is no mention of any other people, as would be seen when using a normalization): "With all of your pain, have you been having any thoughts of killing yourself?"

Shame attenuation is very simple and somewhat less wordy than most normalizations. It can be used for raising the topic of suicide (and many other sensitive topics) with just about any patient in a wide range of situational circumstances.

If a clinician feels more comfortable substituting words such as "committing suicide" or "taking your life" for the words "killing yourself" when using normaliza-

tion or shame attenuation, he or she should feel free to do so because they are equally direct. All of these phrases are good at avoiding the confusion that can arise when clinicians raise the topic of suicide with more nebulous words such as "Have you thought of hurting yourself?" that a patient may interpret as an inquiry into nonlethal methods of self-harm (such as self-cutting or burning oneself).

My own preference is to use the words "killing yourself" because I believe that most people, when the idea first enters their mind, probably do not use relatively sophisticated phrases such as "Maybe I should take my life" or "Maybe I should commit suicide." I think it is more likely that they matter-of-factly say to themselves phrases such as "Maybe I should just kill myself." In addition, words such as *commit* often have a negative connotation in our culture, as in "*committing* a crime." As a consequence, I prefer to phrase the question with the same words that I think the patient is more likely to have used, because it may resonate more empathically in that fashion as well as avoid the potential stigmatization associated with words such as *commit*.

If the patient denies any suicidal ideation, I often inquire a second time, softening the second inquiry by asking about even subtle suicidal ideation (such as "Have you had any fleeting thoughts of killing yourself, even for a moment or two?"). Sometimes the answer is surprising, and the exchange may prompt hesitant patients to begin sharing the depth of their pain and the extent of their ideation.

Five Validity Techniques Used to Explore the Extent of Suicidal Ideation

The following five validity techniques, although not developed with suicide assessment in mind per se, form the cornerstones of the CASE Approach.

Behavioral Incident

A patient may provide distorted information for any number of reasons, including anxiety, embarrassment, keeping family secrets, cultural norms, unconscious defense mechanisms, and conscious attempts at deception. These distortions are more likely to appear if the interviewer asks a patient for opinions rather than behavioral descriptions of events. *Behavioral incidents,* originally delineated by Gerald Pascal (1983), are questions that ask for specific facts, behavioral details, or thoughts *(fact-finding behavioral incidents),* such as "How many pills did you take?," or that simply ask the patient what happened sequentially *(sequencing behavioral incidents),* such as "What did she say next?" or "What did your father do right after he hit you?" By using a series of behavioral incidents, the interviewer can sometimes help a patient enhance validity by re-creating, step by step, the unfolding of a potentially taboo topic such as a suicide attempt.

As Pascal (1983) noted, it is generally best for clinicians to make their own clinical judgments on the basis of the details of the story itself rather than relying on clients to provide "objective opinions" on matters that have strong subjective implications. The following are prototypes of typical behavioral incidents:

- Did you put the razor blade up to your wrist? (fact-finding behavioral incident)
- How many bottles of pills did you store up? (fact-finding behavioral incident)
- When you say that "you taught your son a lesson," what did you actually do? (fact-finding behavioral incident)
- What did your boyfriend say right after he hit you? (sequencing behavioral incident)

- Then what happened? (sequencing behavioral incident)

Gentle Assumption

Gentle assumption—originally defined by Pomeroy et al. (1982) for use in eliciting a valid sex history—is used when a clinician suspects that a patient may be hesitant to discuss a taboo behavior. With gentle assumption, the clinician assumes that the potentially embarrassing or incriminating behavior is occurring and frames his or her question accordingly in a gentle tone of voice. Questions about sexual history, such as "What do you experience when you masturbate?" or "How frequently do you find yourself masturbating?," have been found to be much more likely to yield valid answers than "Do you masturbate?" If the clinician is concerned that the patient may be potentially disconcerted by the assumptive nature of the question, it can be softened by adding the phrase "if at all" (e.g., "How often do you find yourself masturbating, if at all?"). If engagement has gone well and an appropriate tone of voice is used, patients are rarely bothered by gentle assumptions. The following are prototypes of gentle assumption:

- What other ways have you thought of killing yourself?
- What other street drugs have you ever tried?
- What other types of vandalism have you been involved in?

Clinical caveat: Gentle assumptions are powerfully useful at helping patients to share sensitive material, but they are also examples of leading questions. They should not be used with patients who may feel intimidated by the clinician or used with patients who are trying to provide what they think the clinician wants to hear.

For instance, gentle assumptions are inappropriate with children when uncovering abuse histories, because they could potentially lead to false reportings of abuse.

Denial of the Specific

After a patient responds with words such as "no other ways" or "none" to a gentle assumption, it is surprising how many positives will be uncovered if the patient is asked a series of questions about specific entities. This technique appears to jar the memory, and it also appears to be harder to falsely deny a specific question as opposed to a more generic question such as a gentle assumption (Shea 1998b). Examples of *denial of the specific* concerning drug use would be "Have you ever tried crystal meth?" "Have you ever smoked crack?" and "Have you ever dropped acid, even once?" The following are prototypes of denial of the specific with suicide:

- Have you thought of shooting yourself?
- Have you thought of overdosing?
- Have you thought of hanging yourself?
- Have you thought of jumping off a bridge or one of the buildings on campus?

Clinical caveat: It is important to frame each denial of the specific as a separate question, pausing between each inquiry and waiting for the patient's denial or admission before asking the next question. The clinician should avoid combining the inquiries into a single question, such as "Have you thought of shooting yourself, overdosing, or hanging yourself?" A series of items combined in this way is called a "cannon question." Such cannon questions frequently lead to invalid information because patients only hear parts of them or choose to respond to only one item in the string—often the last one. Also note that

when used to uncover suicidal ideation, denials of the specific are only utilized if the clinician suspects that the patient is *withholding a suicidal plan*, which might turn out to be the patient's method of choice.

Catch-All Question

The *catch-all question* allows an interviewer to unobtrusively see if something has been missed by literally asking if such is the case. It is useful in many situations involving sensitive material, including those areas that may generate suicidal thought:

- Are there any other things that your son is doing at school or at home that are upsetting you that we haven't talked about?
- Are there any other bad experiences you had in Iraq, perhaps even with fellow soldiers, that we haven't talked about? (may uncover sexual assault)

For suicidal ideation the catch-all question can be worded as follows: "We've been talking about different ways you've been thinking of killing yourself. Are there any ways you've thought about that we haven't talked about?" The answers are sometimes surprising.

Symptom Amplification

Symptom amplification is based on the observation that patients often minimize the frequency or amount of their disturbing behaviors, such as the amount they drink or gamble. Symptom amplification bypasses this minimizing mechanism. It sets the upper limits of the quantity in the question at such a high level that the clinician is still aware that there is a significant problem, even when the client downplays the amount (Shea 1998b).

For instance, when a clinician asks a patient who abuses hard liquor, "How much can you hold in a single night…a pint, a fifth?" and the minimizing patient responds, "Oh no, not a fifth, I don't know, maybe a pint pretty easily," the clinician is still alerted that there is a problem despite the patient's minimizations. The advantage of the technique lies in the fact that it avoids the creation of a confrontational atmosphere, even though the patient is minimizing behavior. For questions to be viewed as a symptom amplification, the interviewer must always suggest an ascending series of numbers that are set high. It is also worth repeating that symptom amplification is used in an effort to determine an actual quantity and it is *only* used if the clinician suspects that the patient is about to minimize. It would not be used with a patient who wanted to maximize, as with an adolescent who might want to give the impression that he is a "big-time drinker." The following are examples of symptom amplification:

- How many physical fights have you had in your whole life…25, 40, 50?
- How many times have you tripped on acid in your whole life…25, 40, 100 times or more?
- On the days when your thoughts of suicide are most intense, how much of the day do you spend thinking about killing yourself…10 hours a day, 14 hours a day, 18 hours a day?

Macrostructure of the CASE Approach: Avoiding Errors of Omission

Besides recovering invalid data (a problem the validity techniques attempt to address), the other major problem for the frontline clinician is missing puzzle pieces (i.e., *errors of omission*). Two questions are of immediate relevance: 1) Why do interviewers fre-

quently miss important data while eliciting suicidal ideation, and 2) Is there a way to decrease errors of omission?

The answers lie in a field of study known as *facilics* (Shea 1998b). Facilics is the study of how clinicians structure interviews, explore databases, make transitions, and use time. Over the past 20 years, facilic supervision has become a popular educational tool (Shea 1998b; Shea and Mezzich 1988; Shea et al. 1989, 2007). It is used to train psychiatric residents and graduate students across disciplines to efficiently and sensitively uncover a comprehensive database while creating a conversational feel during an initial interview (Shea and Barney 2007a).

According to facilic principles, clinicians tend to make more errors of omission as the amount and range of required data increase. Errors of omission decrease if the clinician can split a large amount of data into smaller, well-defined regions. With such well-defined and limited data regions, the interviewer can more easily recognize when a patient has wandered from the subject. The clinician is also more apt to easily track whether the desired inquiry has been completed, and does not feel as overwhelmed by the interview process.

These principles are applied to the elicitation of suicidal ideation, behavior, and intent by organizing the sprawling set of clinically relevant questions into four smaller and more manageable regions. The regions represent four contiguous time frames. In each region the clinician investigates the suicidal ideation and actions present during that specific time frame. Generally, each region is explored thoroughly before moving to the next; the clinician consciously chooses not to move with a client's tangential wandering unless there is a very good reason to do so. In the description that follows, the term *suicide events* can include any of the following: death wishes, suicidal feelings and thoughts, suicide planning, suicidal behaviors and desire, and suicidal intent.

In the CASE Approach, the interviewer sequentially explores the following four chronological regions in the order shown (see Figure 2–1):

1. Presenting suicide events (within the past 48 hours or several weeks)
2. Recent suicide events (in the preceding 2 months)
3. Past suicide events (from 2 months ago back in time)
4. Immediate suicide events (suicidal feelings, ideation, and intent that arise during the interview itself)

The sequencing of the regions was specifically designed to maximize both engagement and the validity of the obtained data. For many patients, once the topic of suicide has been raised, it seems natural to talk about the presenting ideation or attempt, if one exists, first. Following this exploration, it is easy for the interviewer to make a natural progression into recent ideation followed by past suicide events.

When performed sensitively by the interviewer, exploration of the three time frames, all of which occurred before the interview, generally improves both engagement and trust as the patient realizes that it is okay to talk about suicidal ideation. Once trust has been maximized, it is hoped that this positive alliance will increase the likelihood of the patient sharing valid information. It is then an opportune time to explore suicidal ideation and intentions *that are being experienced by the patient during the interview itself* (the region of immediate suicide events), which is a critically important area of a suicide assessment. For instance, a patient about to go on a pass from an inpatient unit may be planning to die by suicide.

During an interview directly preceding the pass, such a patient may be having suicidal thoughts such as "Don't give it away. Just look fine. Get home. Get the gun. Just get home. Get the gun." Here, the most subtle nuances of facial expression or hesitancy of speech may indicate that a dangerous suicide plan is being withheld.

Microstructure of the CASE Approach: Exploring Specific Time Frames

Step 1: Exploration of Presenting Suicide Events

Whether the patient spontaneously raises the topic of suicide or the topic is sensitively uncovered with techniques such as normalization or shame attenuation, these suicide events are viewed as *presenting events*, in the sense that the patient has been "currently" experiencing them. Such presenting suicide events may appear in the past couple of weeks or several days. If a patient presents with current suicidal behavior or with pressing suicidal ideation, it becomes critical to understand the severity. Depending on the severity of the ideation or attempt, the patient may require hospitalization, crisis intervention, and/or close follow-up.

But what specific information would give the clinician the most accurate picture of the seriousness of presenting suicidal thought or behavior? The following questions can provide a framework for eliciting the necessary information:

- How did the patient try to die by suicide? (What method was used?)
- How serious was the action taken with this method? (If the patient overdosed, what pills and how many were taken? If the patient cut himself or herself, where

was the cut, and did it require stitches and if so, how many?)

- How serious were the patient's intentions? (Did the patient tell anyone about the attempt afterward? Did the patient hint to anyone beforehand either in direct conversation or indirectly through social media such as Facebook or by texting or chatting? Did the patient make the attempt in an isolated area or in a place where he or she was likely to be found? Did the patient write a suicide note, give away prized possessions, or say goodbye to significant others in the days preceding the event? How many pills were left in the bottle?)
- How does the patient feel about the fact that the attempt was not completed? (A very good question here is "What are some of your thoughts about the fact that you are still alive now?")
- Was the attempt well planned or an impulsive act? Did the patient research suicide on the Web or in books?
- Did alcohol or drugs play a role in the attempt?
- Did interpersonal factors have a major role in the attempt? (These factors might include feelings of failure or speculation that the world would be better off without the patient, as well as anger toward others [a suicide attempt undertaken to make others feel pain or guilt, often a spouse, parent, other family member, friend, or employer].)
- Did a specific stressor or set of stressors prompt the attempt?
- At the time of the attempt, how hopeless did the patient feel?
- Why did the attempt fail? (How was the patient found and how did the patient get help?)

Answers to such questions can provide invaluable information regarding how seri-

ous the attempt was, reflecting the patient's true intent to die, no matter what the patient's stated intent might be. If no actual attempt has been made, then it is the reflected intent—the extent of suicidal desire, ideation, planning, and procurement of means—that the clinician will use in the clinical formulation of risk to determine the triage (inpatient versus outpatient) and rapidity of follow-up if outpatient care is recommended. Information uncovered in other parts of the interview regarding risk factors, protective factors, and warning signs is coupled with the preceding information to make these triage decisions.

At first glance, especially for a clinician in training, the preceding list of questions may appear intimidating to remember. Fortunately, one of the validity techniques discussed earlier—the behavioral incident—can provide the clinician with a simpler and more logical approach than memorization. The reader will recall that behavioral incidents are used when the clinician asks for a specific piece of data (e.g., "Did you put the gun up to your head?") or asks the client to continue a description of what happened sequentially (e.g., "Tell me what you did next.").

In the CASE Approach, during the exploration of the presenting events, the interviewer asks the patient to describe the suicide attempt or ideation itself from beginning to end. During this description the clinician gently but persistently uses a series of behavioral incidents, guiding the patient to create a "verbal videotape" of the attempt, step by step. Readers familiar with cognitive-behavioral therapy and dialectical behavior therapy will recognize this strategy as one of the cornerstone assessment tools—behavioral (chain) analysis. If the patient begins to skip over an important piece of the account, the clinician gently stops the patient and "rewinds the vid-

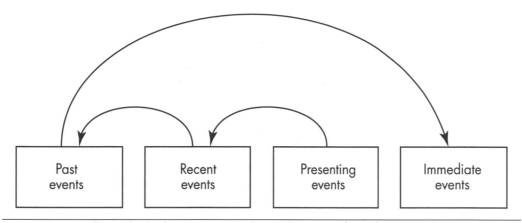

FIGURE 2–1. Chronological Assessment of Suicide Events (CASE) Approach.

eotape" by asking the patient to return to where the gap began. The clinician then uses a string of behavioral incidents from that point forward to fill in the gap until the clinician feels confident that the missing information has been provided.

This sequential use of behavioral incidents not only increases the clinician's understanding of the extent of the patient's intent and actions, but also decreases any unwarranted assumptions by the clinician that may distort the database. By creating such a verbal videotape, the clinician will frequently cover all of the previously described material in a naturally unfolding conversational mode without much need for memorization of what questions to ask when.

The serial use of behavioral incidents can be particularly powerful at uncovering the extent of action taken by the patient regarding a specific suicide plan, an area in which patients frequently minimize. For example, the series may look something like this in a patient who actually took some actions with a gun: "Do you have a gun at home?" "Have you ever gotten the gun out while you were having thoughts of killing yourself?" "When did you do this?" "Where were you sitting when you had the gun out?" "Did you load

the gun?" "What did you do next?" "Did you put the gun up to your body or head?" "Did you take the safety off or load the chamber?" "How long did you hold the gun there?" "What thoughts were going through your mind then?" "What stopped you from pulling the trigger?" "What did you do with the gun?"

In this fashion, the clinician can feel more confident at obtaining a valid picture of how close the patient actually came to committing suicide. The resulting scenario may prove to be radically different—and more suggestive of danger—from what would have been assumed if the interviewer had merely asked, "Did you come close to actually using the gun?," to which an embarrassed or cagey patient might quickly reply, "Oh no, not really." Once again, we see an example of reflected intent being potentially more accurate than the patient's stated intent.

Also note in the previous sequence the use of questions such as "When did you do this?" and "Where were you sitting when you had the gun out?" These types of questions, which are also borrowed from cognitive-behavioral therapy, are known as *anchor questions* because they anchor the patient into a specific memory as opposed to a collection of nebulous feelings. Such a refined focus will often bring forth more valid information as the episode becomes both more real and more vivid to the patient. The exploration of presenting suicide events can be summarized as follows: The clinician begins with a question such as "It sounds like last night was a very difficult time. It will help me to understand exactly what you experienced if you can sort of walk me through what happened step by step. Once you decided to kill yourself, what did you do next?" As the patient begins to describe the unfolding suicide attempt, the clinician uses one or two anchor questions to maximize validity. The interviewer then proceeds to use a series of behavioral incidents, making it easy to picture the unfolding events—the "verbal videotape." The metaphor of making a verbal videotape has been popular with trainees as well as frontline staff because the clinical task seems clear and is easily remembered, even at 3 A.M. in a busy ED.

Case Example

Frank Thompson is a good soul. He is also a tired soul. He commented to the charge nurse, "I've had a good life; I don't know, maybe it's just time to pass on." Frank has been a farmer in the rolling hills of western Pennsylvania for over five decades. His dad was a farmer. His grandfathers were both farmers. He was married to a wonderful woman, Sally, for 50 years. She died 2 years ago from brain cancer. Frank is plagued by diabetes and moderately severe heart and lung disease, having smoked far too many cigarettes for far too many years. Since Sally's death, he has developed a mild drinking problem.

Frank has 5 children and 21 grandchildren and a pack of great grandkids to boot. His children are supportive, but only one, Nick, lives nearby. It is Nick who has brought his dad to the ED. Nick heard from his dad earlier in the morning that he wasn't doing well. Nick got off work early and was caught off guard by the depressive look of his father. Later during the night, while the two of them were sitting on the front porch, his dad shared a secret that prompted Nick to get in the car and bring him down to the ED immediately. Apparently his dad had taken a handful of aspirin and some antibiotics 2 days ago.

We are picking up this reconstructed interview about 20 minutes in, when the clinician is about to enter the region of presenting events using the CASE Approach:

Patient: It's been a long haul over the past 2 years. Sometimes too long a haul, if you know what I mean. I'm way too old for all this crap.

Clinician: And it's got to be hard to do it alone.

Patient: You bet! With Sally gone, it's all so very different.

Clinician: I'm sure the pain of her loss is beyond words. With that amount of pain on board, Mr. Thompson, have you been having any thoughts of killing yourself? [shame attenuation used to gently raise the topic of suicide]

Patient: I suppose my son may have already said something to you…I took some pills…I know it was dumb, but nothing came of it anyway.

Clinician: When was that? [behavioral incident]

Patient: Couple of nights ago. But, like I said, nothing came of it. I'm not sure I need any help. I'm not going to do anything stupid; you don't have to worry about that. [Note that the clinician is not going to take the patient's "stated intent" as necessarily an accurate picture of his real intent. Instead, the clinician is going to uncover Mr. Thompson's reflected intent by weaving a verbal videotape using behavioral incidents.]

Clinician: You know what, Mr. Thompson? That may be true, but I just want to get a better feeling for what you've been going through so we can make a wise decision together. Where were you when you took the pills? [behavioral incident serving as an anchor point]

Patient: In the kitchen. I was sitting in a little kitchen nook where Sally and I used to eat lunch. I always loved that little place.

Clinician (*gently smiling*): Yeah, I bet it brings back warm memories of Sally.

Patient (*smiling back*): Yeah, it does.

Clinician: What kind of pills did you take? [behavioral incident]

Patient: Some aspirin, some penicillin.

Clinician: How much did you take of each one? [behavioral incident]

Patient: About a handful of each. [Note that there can be quite a difference in what a patient means by a "handful." It is a perfect time to clarify with a behavioral incident.]

Clinician: When you say a handful, how many of each do you mean? [behavioral incident]

Patient: About 10 of each.

Clinician: Any other pills?

Patient (*pause*): I also took about five digoxin I'm on; more than I'm supposed to, I know that. [This is a fact that the son was unaware of and had not reported to the clinician.]

Clinician: Did you have any pills left? [behavioral incident]

Patient: Not a lot. I don't keep many pills in the house, and my prescriptions have basically run out.

Clinician: Did you look for any other pills? [behavioral incident]

Patient (*pause*): Not really pills…I did go through the drawer wondering if there was any rat poison around, but I realized that was stupid, too…Trust me, suicide is not the answer. God did not put us on this earth to kill ourselves. [Unexpected information is coming to the surface. Clearly the son has not been told everything. The searching for the rat poison reflects more suicidal intent than might be expected from phrases such as "God did not put us on this earth to kill ourselves."]

Clinician: I'm glad you feel that way. And maybe we can help some too. At least I hope so.

Patient: Maybe.

Clinician: You know, right after you took the pills, what was the next thing you did? [sequencing behavioral incident]

Patient: Went to bed, just to sort of see what would happen. I was just so tired of it all.

Clinician: How did you feel about the fact that you woke up okay?

Patient: I don't know. Sort of didn't care. It's just the way it is.

Clinician: Had you been drinking at all, even a little bit? [behavioral incident]

Patient: Nope. I'm trying to lay off the stuff. It just gets me more depressed. Don't get me wrong, I'm still drinking, but not over the past couple of days. [Notice that the clinician does not pursue a complete drug and alcohol history here; this will be carefully delineated as a risk factor in a different section of the interview—the drug and alcohol history—or may have already been done.]

Clinician: I know from your son that you called him the next day. Had you tried any other ways of killing yourself before you called him?

Patient: Nope. I just thought I needed a rest of some sort, and I wanted to talk it over with Nick.

Clinician: Good. How about over the past 2 months? Have you had any other thoughts of overdosing? [behavioral incident; the clinician is gracefully moving into the region of recent suicide events with a classic bridging question]

Step 2: Exploration of Recent Suicide Events

The region of recent events may very well represent, from the perspective of motivational theory, the single richest arena for uncovering reflected intent. It is here, with a patient who strongly wants to die and is hesitant to share his or her real intent for fear of what will happen (e.g., possible hospitalization, involuntary commitment, removal of a method of choice), that a skilled interviewer may uncover suicidal ideation and suicide planning that provide a more accurate indication of the patient's real intent that is being consciously withheld.

It is also the arena when, with a patient whose unconscious defense mechanisms may be minimizing his or her conscious awareness of the intensity of his or her own suicidal intent, a more accurate picture of the patient's intent may emerge. Specifically, the patient's actions taken toward procuring a method of suicide and/or the amount of time spent preoccupied with suicide may betray the severity of the patient's real intent better than his or her stated intent would suggest.

Sometimes when the clinician raises the topic of suicide with techniques like normalization or shame attenuation, the patient's reported events do not lie within the previous 48 hours or several weeks (in essence, there are no presenting events), in which case the clinician immediately begins exploring the region of recent events. On the other hand, if the patient reports a true presenting event, after the verbal videotape is created, the clinician will need to make a bridging statement to transition into the region of recent suicide events (see Figure 2–2). Often this transition is initiated by smoothly eliciting any thoughts in the past 2 months related to the same plan that the patient discussed in the presenting events (as was done in the interview with Mr. Thompson). Once recent thoughts or actions regarding the same method, if present, have been explored, a gentle assumption is used to look for a second suicide method. My favorite gentle assumption is the simplest one: "What other ways have you thought of killing yourself?"

If a second method is uncovered, sequential behavioral incidents are used to create another verbal videotape reflecting the extent of action taken. The interviewer continues this use of gentle assumptions, with follow-up verbal videotapes as indicated with each newly uncovered method, until the patient denies any other methods when asked "What other ways have you thought of killing yourself?"

Once the use of a gentle assumption yields a blanket denial of other methods, and *if and only if* the clinician feels that the patient may be withholding other methods of suicide, the clinician uses a short series of

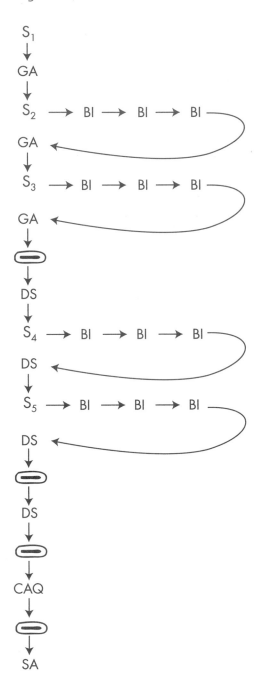

FIGURE 2–2. Prototypic exploration of the region of recent suicide events.

Should be flexibly adapted in response to client's answers and clinical presentation.

BI=behavioral incident; CAQ=catch-all question; DS=denial of the specific; GA=gentle assumption; S=suicide method; SA=symptom amplification. Solid outlined bar indicates client denial of suicidal ideation.

denials of the specific. The interviewer must use his or her clinical judgment to decide whether the use of denials of the specific is indicated. Use of this technique is not warranted if the patient has low risk factors and high protective factors and has reported minimal or no suicidal ideation up to that point in the interview. On the other hand, if the clinician's intuition suggests that this particular patient may be withholding critical information about suicidal ideation or suicide planning, then denials of the specific can be employed. This technique can be surprisingly effective at uncovering previously withheld suicidal material. The interviewer does not drive this technique into the ground with an exhaustive series of methods but simply asks for any unmentioned methods that are common to the patient's culture and that the clinician is suspicious that this specific patient might be withholding.

By way of example, if the patient has talked about overdosing, using guns, or driving a car off the road, the clinician might employ the following short list of denials of the specific, pausing after each for an answer: "Have you thought about cutting or stabbing yourself?" "Have you thought about hanging yourself?" "Have you thought about jumping off a bridge or other high place?" "Have you thought about carbon monoxide?" As before, if a new method is revealed, the clinician uncovers the extent of action taken by asking a series of behavioral incidents. It is here— with the selective and well-timed use of denials of the specific—that a highly dangerous patient who has been purposefully withholding his or her method of choice may suddenly share it, perhaps prompted by a wedge of healthy ambivalence.

Following the use of denials of the specific, the clinician can utilize the catch-all question if it is deemed to be useful ("We've been talking about different ways you've been thinking of killing yourself. Are there any ways you've thought about that we haven't talked about?"). Such an approach is generally only used if the clinician still has concerns that the client may be contemplating a serious suicide method not yet uncovered. Moreover, some hesitant, yet ambivalent, patients with dangerous intent may have continued to hide their actual method of choice, especially if it is an unusual method not covered by the clinician's denials of the specific (many unusual methods are now openly discussed on the Web). If there is enough ambivalence, the patient at this point may share his or her method of choice.

In other instances, some patients may inadvertently pause after being asked the catch-all question, revealing through nonverbal leakage that other plans may have been considered. A simple comment, said gently, can be surprisingly powerful at such moments, as with "Mr. Thompson, it looks like you may have thought of some other ways. I know it can be hard to talk about suicide, but I really want to help you. Try to share with me your thoughts even if they were fleeting in nature." The resulting information is sometimes lifesaving.

The catch-all question is useful in two other ways. Sometimes a clinician using a list of denials of the specific inadvertently forgets to mention the common method that the patient happens to be intending to use. In such cases, the method may be relayed in response to the catch-all question. The catch-all question can also prompt the patient to share that he or she has done a Web search on suicide, offering further glimpses of the patient's reflected intent.

After establishing the list of methods considered by the patient and the extent of action taken on each method, the interviewer hones in on the frequency, duration, and intensity of the suicidal ideation with a symptom amplification, such as "On your very worst days, the days when you are most thinking about killing yourself, how much time do you spend thinking about killing yourself...10 hours a day, 14 hours a day, 18 hours a day?"

The preceding strategy is easy to learn and simple to remember. It also flows imperceptibly, frequently increasing engagement, as the patient is pleasantly surprised at how easy it is to talk to the clinician about issues that were shouldered as a topic of shame. It also becomes apparent to the patient that the interviewer is quite comfortable talking about suicide and has clearly discussed it with many others. This represents yet another shame-reducing meta-communication.

Case Example (continued)

There is no better way to illustrate the power of this strategy than to see it at work with Mr. Thompson. The clinician has uncovered information suggesting that Mr. Thompson's real intent may be higher than his initially stated intent would suggest. Moreover, his list of risk factors indicates high risk, and his support system, other than his nearest son, was markedly weakened by the loss of his wife. The fact that he is wrestling with the notion that it is "wrong" to kill oneself may be creating both ambivalence (good) and a skewed self-admission—secondary to unconscious defense mechanisms—as to the depth of his suicidal desire and intent (bad).

Notice that the clinician is quite explicit with the time frame, stating the exact duration as opposed to using a vague term such as "recently." This specificity is important because it helps the patient remain focused on the desired time frame while decreasing time-wasting sidetracks.

Patient: Nope. I just thought I needed a rest of some sort, and I wanted to talk it over with Nick.

Clinician: Good. How about over the past 2 months? Have you had any other thoughts of overdosing? [behavioral incident; the clinician is gracefully moving into the region of recent suicide events with a classic bridging question]

Patient: A few times, but I never got no pills out or nothing.

Clinician: What other ways have you thought about killing yourself? [gentle assumption]

Patient: Oh, not much....I suppose I thought about hangin' myself, but that is not a good way to die. You know, it doesn't always work, at least that's what I been told.

Clinician: Have you ever gotten a rope out or something else to use to hang yourself? [behavioral incident]

Patient: No sir, I haven't.

Clinician: What other ways have you thought about killing yourself? [gentle assumption]

Patient: Well, I have gone out to the barn to see if we still had some of that pesticide I used a couple of years ago.

Clinician: And? [variant of a sequencing behavioral incident]

Patient: Oh, we did. And...and I was thinking about taking some and then burning the barn down with me inside it.

Clinician: Hmmm.

Patient: Yeah...sort of Hollywoodish (smiles) but it's no good. Way too apt to not workout right.

Clinician: How often did you go out to the barn thinking about that? [behavioral incident]

Patient: Maybe four or five times. I don't really remember exactly.

Clinician: What other ways have you thought of killing yourself? [gentle assumption]

Patient: That's about it. Nothing else, really.

The CASE Approach is doing exactly what it is supposed to be doing—getting those puzzle pieces on the table that might better reflect the severity of Mr. Thompson's suicidal intent. The resulting information is a bit surprising. The use of the gentle assumptions has resulted in a method (pesticides and burning down the barn) that quite frankly the clinician would not have thought to ask about. Gentle assumptions allow patients to provide individualized plans that might never have come to the clinician's awareness otherwise. The number of times Mr. Thompson went to the barn is also disturbing. Despite his ability to retain a sense of humor, the depth of his angst is becoming more and more apparent.

Note that Mr. Thompson has now denied any other methods when presented with a gentle assumption: "What other ways have you thought about killing yourself?" The clinician is about to use a short string of denials of the specific. His persistence is prompted by the presence of high risk factors, by the clear depth of Mr. Thompson's anguish, and by the fact that during the exploration of presenting events, and thus far in the exploration of recent events, details are being uncovered that Mr. Thompson did not share earlier. In addition, there was one other fact that seemed odd to the clinician:

Clinician: What about carbon monoxide…you know, with a car or tractor? [denial of the specific]

Patient: My old barn is so drafty, you couldn't do that if you tried. *(smiles weakly)*

Clinician: Have you thought of jumping off a building or bridge? [denial of the specific]

Patient: Nope.

Clinician: You know, Mr. Thompson, most farmers I know like to hunt or at least have a gun around to protect their animals, and sometimes when they are in a lot of pain like you've been having, they think of shooting themselves. I'm wondering if that has crossed your mind? [denial of the specific introduced with a normalization]

Patient *(long pause, looks away ever so slightly):* I suppose.

Clinician: Did you ever picture a place where you might shoot yourself? [behavioral incident]

Patient: There is a place down by Willow Creek that was the favorite place that Sally and I used to go….It's just lovely. Even in the winter it's lovely. *(sighs)* And I've often thought that if I had to go, that's where I would do it.

Clinician: Did you ever go there with a gun, thinking you might kill yourself? [behavioral incident]

Patient: Yeah…yeah, I've done that.

Clinician: Did you load the gun? [behavioral incident]

Patient: Yeah.

Clinician: What did you do next? [sequencing behavioral incident]

Patient: Put it in my mouth. I read somewhere that's how you should do it.…Someone told me once they knew a guy who did that but didn't point it upwards so the darn thing shot right out the back of his neck. *(chuckles softly)* Hard to believe. *(shakes his head)*

Clinician: Sounds like you were pretty close though.

Patient: Yeah. Yeah. I guess I was.

Clinician: Was the safety off? [behavioral incident]

Patient: Yeah. *(looks down)*

Clinician *(very gently):* You really miss her, don't you?

Patient *(bursting into tears):* Oh God, I miss her. She made my world. She was my world.

Clinician: What made you put the gun down, Mr. Thompson? [behavioral incident]

Patient: I don't really know. Maybe I thought I should be around for all my grandkids, but I just don't know anymore.

Clinician: Mr. Thompson, roughly when was this? [behavioral incident]

Patient: About 2 weeks ago.

Clinician: Right around then, when things were really tough, how much time were you spending thinking about killing yourself…70% of your waking hours, 80% of your waking hours, 90% of your waking hours? [variation of a symptom amplification]

Patient *(lifts head up and looks the clinician right in the eye):* The truth is—I couldn't get it out of my mind.

This interviewer is earning his pay. He may also be saving Mr. Thompson's life. Mr. Thompson's intent to kill himself is much higher than his originally stated intent implied. In addition, it was only through the skilled use of a denial of the specific that the patient's true method of choice emerged. With this added information reflecting the potential seriousness of Mr. Thompson's suicidal intent, hospitalization appears to be more appropriate, and there is now an opportunity to have the gun or guns removed from the farmhouse as well.

From the perspective of interviewing technique, notice that once the use of a gun was uncovered, the clinician deftly used a series of behavioral incidents to create a verbal videotape of what actually happened. Fact-finding behavioral incidents such as "Did you load the gun?" and sequencing behavioral incidents such as "What did you do next?" provided concrete information regarding the seriousness of Mr. Thompson's intent.

Also note that the string of behavioral incidents led the patient to remember and describe his inner world at the time of the gun incident. This is a rather common phenomenon. Although the behavioral incident is designed to improve the validity of hard behavioral data as the patient begins to re-imagine his experiences, the patient is often drawn into his internal cognitions and emotions at the time. This often provides a window into the the patient's soul. Within the soul, we may find strong reasons to live. As Jobes and Mann (1999) have pointed out, an understanding of a patient's reasons for living is an important aspect of suicide assessment that has traditionally not been given the attention in the literature that it warrants. On the other hand, as with Mr. Thompson, the clinician may find a shattered soul where there seem to be only good reasons to die, as reflected by his telling comment "She was my world."

Note that the interviewer saw no reason to utilize the catch-all question, because the interviewer felt comfortable that Mr. Thompson had finally shared his method of choice and was not thinking of using another unusual suicide method. This conscious decision-making highlights that the CASE Approach is not a cookbook method of exploring suicidal ideation. For instance, the extensiveness of the questioning during the region of recent events is dependent on the interviewer's ever-evolving "read" on the dangerousness of the patient. For example, if a patient has low risk factors, has high protective factors, denies any thoughts of suicide during the exploration of presenting events, and reports only one fleeting thought of shooting himself (no gun at home) during the early exploration of recent events, a clinician most likely would not use denials of the specific, the catch-all question, or symptom amplification. It would not make sense to do so, and it might even appear odd to the patient.

Step 3: Exploration of Past Suicide Events

Clinicians sometimes spend too much time on this area. Patients with complicated psychiatric histories (e.g., some people with a borderline personality disorder) may have lengthy past histories of suicidal material. One could spend an hour reviewing this material. It would be an hour poorly spent.

Under the time constraints of busy practices and managed care, initial assessments by mental health professionals usually must be completed in an hour or less and much less in an ED. In the CASE Approach, the interviewer seeks only information that could potentially change the clinical triage and follow-up of the patient. The following questions are worth investigating:

- What is the most serious past suicide attempt? (Is the current ideation focused on the same method? "Practice" can be deadly in this arena. Does the patient view the current stressors and options in the same light as during the most dangerous past attempt?)
- Are the current triggers and the patient's current psychopathological state similar to when the most serious attempts were made? (The patient may be prone to suicide following the breakup of relationships or during episodes of acute intoxication, intense anxiety, or psychosis.)
- What is the approximate number of past gestures and attempts? (Large numbers here can alert the clinician to suicide attempts made as a means of communication and/or receiving comfort, perhaps making one less concerned, or may alert the clinician that the patient has truly exhausted all hope, making one more concerned. In either case, it is important to know.)
- When was the most recent attempt outside of the 2 months explored in the region of recent events? (There could have been a significant attempt within the last 6 months that might signal the need for more immediate concern.)

Step 4: Exploration of Immediate Suicide Events

In this region the interviewer focuses on any new suicidal ideation and desire and suicidal intent that the patient may be experiencing *during the interview itself*. The interviewer also makes inquiries as to whether the patient thinks he or she is likely to have further thoughts of suicide after leaving the office, ED, or inpatient unit, or when he or she gets off the phone following a crisis call. The region of immediate events also includes appropriate safety planning. The fo-

cus of the exploration of immediate events is thus on the present and future (easily remembered as the region of Now/Next). The ultimate goal is to gather information that can help the clinician to further delineate the client's immediate suicidal intent.

Immediate desire (the intensity of the client's pain and desire to die) and the client's intent (the degree with which the client has decided to actually proceed with suicide) are clarified by discerning the relationship between the two, because they are not identical despite being intimately related. A patient could have intense pain with a strong desire to die yet have no intent, as reflected by "I could never do that to my children." Conversely, over time, a patient's pain could become so intense that it overrides his or her defenses that prevented intent, resulting in a patient who impulsively acts.

A sound starting place is the question "Right now, are you having any thoughts about wanting to kill yourself?" From this inquiry, a question such as the following can be utilized to further explore the patient's *desire* to die:

> On a scale from 0 to 10, how would you describe how bad the pain is for you in your divorce right now, ranging from a 0—'It's sort of tough, but I can handle it okay'—to a 10 '—If it doesn't let up, I don't know if I can go on.' Where would you place yourself on that scale?

Questions such as the following can then help the clinician to delineate *intent:*

- "I realize that you can't know for sure, but what is your best guess as to how likely it is that you will try to kill yourself during the next week, from highly unlikely to very likely?"
- "What keeps you from killing yourself?"

It is important to explore the patient's current level of hopelessness and to assess whether the patient is making productive plans for the future or is amenable to preparing concrete plans for dealing with current problems and stresses. Questions such as "How does the future look to you?" "Do you feel hopeful about the future?" and "What things would make you feel more or less hopeful about the future?" are useful entrance points for this exploration. If not addressed in an earlier time frame, an exploration of reasons for living can be nicely introduced here with "What things in your life make you want to go on living?"

Developing a safety plan is frequently facilitated by asking questions such as "What would you do later tonight or tomorrow if you began to have suicidal thoughts again?" From the patient's answer one can sometimes better surmise how serious the patient is about ensuring his or her safety. Such a question also provides a chance for the joint brainstorming of plans to handle the reemergence of suicidal ideation. Sound safety planning often includes a series of steps that the patient will take to transform and/or control suicidal ideation if it should arise. Such planning could begin with something as simple as taking a warm shower or listening to soothing music and end with calling a crisis line or arranging for a taxi to return to the hospital if out on a pass.

Now is a good time to address the complex issue of whether "safety contracting" as opposed to "safety planning" may be of use with any specific patient. In my opinion, each patient is unique in this regard. Safety contracting has become somewhat of a controversial topic. To understand its practical use, it is important to remember that in addition to metacommunicating care and concern on the part of the interviewer, there are two main reasons or applications for safety contracting: 1) as a method of de-

terrence and 2) as a sensitive means of suicide assessment. These applications are radically different, and their pros and cons are equally radically different. The intensity of the debate, in my opinion, is generated because most of what is "debated" deals primarily with safety contracting's application as a deterrent, which has many limitations.

For instance, safety contracting may frequently be counterproductive in patients dealing with borderline or passive-aggressive pathology. With such patients it is sometimes best to avoid the whole issue of safety contracting, because it may embroil the dyad in ineffective debates, with statements such as "I don't know what to tell you. I guess I'm safe, but on the other hand, I can't make any guarantees. Do you know anybody who can?"

If one uses safety contracting as a deterrent, it is critical to use it cautiously. It guarantees nothing and may yield a false sense of security (Miller 1999; Miller et al. 1998). Moreover, it should never be done before a sound suicide assessment has been completed (Shea 2011c). Generally speaking, I believe that safety contracting *as a deterrent* is viewed by most suicidologists as generally inferior to sound safety planning.

The power of the patient's superego and the power of the therapeutic alliance may play significant roles in whether safety contracting—employed as a deterrent—may have use with a specific patient. I am convinced that in some patients it may play a role in deterrence, as with a patient in a long-standing therapeutic alliance, with minimal characterological pathology and a powerful superego. I have had several seasoned therapists tell me after workshops that they have had patients clearly state that the safety contract functioned as a deterrent. One patient relayed on a Monday after a particularly bad weekend, "The only reason I am alive today is our contract, for I couldn't do that to you. I couldn't break my word to you."

Deterrence, however, is not the only or, in my opinion, main reason to use safety contracting. It may be more frequently useful as an exquisitely sensitive assessment tool. In this capacity it is selectively used in a small number of patients who have little or no passive-aggressive or borderline characterological pathology, in which the clinician is leaning toward nonhospitalization after completing a suicide assessment but is bothered by his or her intuition that the patient is more dangerous than he or she has stated, or analytically feels something "does not add up here." In such cases, rather than use safety *planning*, which has no interpersonal pressure to it, the clinician may opt to use safety *contracting*, in which the patient is put on the spot to make an agreement. Such an "interpersonal push" may prompt nonverbal leakage of hidden ambivalence or dangerous suicidal intent.

When contracting is used in this highly selective fashion, as the interviewer asks whether the patient can promise to contact the clinician or appropriate staff before acting on any suicidal ideation, the interviewer searches the patient's face, body, and tone of voice for any signs of hesitancy, deceit, or ambivalence. Here is the proverbial moment of truth. Nonverbal leakage of suicidal desire or intent at this juncture can be, potentially, the only indicator of the patient's true immediate risk.

Using the interpersonal process of safety contracting as an assessment tool, the clinician may completely change his or her mind about releasing a patient, based on a hesitancy to contract, avoidance of eye contact, or other signs of deceit or ambivalence displayed while the patient is reluctantly agreeing to a safety contract.

The interviewer who notices such nonverbal clues of ambivalence can simply ask,

"It looks as though this contract is hard for you to agree to. What's going on in your mind?" The answers can be benign or alarming, and the resulting piece of the puzzle—which could only be provided by the process of safety contracting—may lead to a change in disposition. This use of safety contracting as an assessment tool, based on nonverbal leakage of suicidal intent, unlike safety contracting as a deterrent (which probably has limited use in an ED), may be particularly relevant in an ED. Thus, safety contracting is complicated, and CASE-trained clinicians neither generically condemn nor condone its use, but attempt to make a wise decision based on the client's specific needs and the clinical task at hand.

For a practical review of how to effectively use safety contracting, the reader is referred to "Safety Contracting: Pros, Cons, and Documentation Issues" in *The Practical Art of Suicide Assessment* (Shea 2011c), in which one will also find references to numerous articles on the subject. Remember that safety contracting is no guarantee of safety whatsoever.

Finally, it cannot be emphasized enough that continuing concerns about the safety of the patient or the validity of the patient's self-report may require contacting collaborative sources.

Training Applications, Research Directions, and Implications for Suicide Prevention

The CASE Approach is designed to allow the clinician to enter the patient's world of suicidal preoccupation sensitively and deeply. During this delicate process, something else may be accomplished that is very important: the interviewer will help the patient to share painful information that in many instances the patient has borne alone for too long. Perhaps the thoughtfulness and thoroughness of the questioning, as illustrated with the CASE Approach, will convey that a fellow human cares. To the patient, such caring may represent the first realization of hope.

By using this strategy routinely, clinicians can become adept at it, learning how to flexibly alter it to fit the unique needs of specific clinical settings and with diverse types of patients. In most assessments, the CASE Approach can be completed within several minutes. Even with patients with more complicated conditions and factors, as might be seen in some complex ED presentations, it rarely requires more than 5–10 minutes. In patients with low risk factors and high protective factors and who answer negatively to questions in the regions of presenting suicide events, recent suicide events, and past events, the CASE Approach can be completed in three questions. With such patients, the clinician would not even enter the region of immediate suicide events.

Moreover, the CASE Approach is flexibly adapted to the psychopathology and personality traits of the individual patient. The CASE Approach is altered markedly with a patient who might want to manipulate himself or herself into a hospital or who might have borderline personality traits and may use "suicide talk" to seek comfort from caregivers. It can also be flexibly altered for use with actively psychotic patients. Note that the CASE Approach was not designed, nor is it recommended, for use with children, although future child researchers may find that some elements of the CASE Approach may prove to be useful.

Because the strategies of the CASE Approach are based on easily identifiable interviewing techniques, the skills of the trainee or staff can be easily observed, monitored over time, and objectively tested for quality assurance purposes. It is hoped that such behaviorally specific characteristics will also allow quantitative and qualitative research to be done on both the ability of the CASE Approach to be taught (and retained) and the ultimate effectiveness of the approach in procuring a comprehensive and reliable database on suicidal ideation and suicidal intent. Such research could provide the foundation for an evidence-based model for effectively eliciting suicidal ideation, similar in fashion to the way that cardiopulmonary resuscitation (CPR) was developed. As with CPR, such an evidence-based interviewing strategy could be used as the basis for certifying clinicians as having the necessary competence.

In the meantime, as we wait for the appropriate research to be undertaken, the CASE Approach allows experienced clinicians to study how they are currently eliciting suicidal ideation, as well as suggesting new ways of doing so. Returning to the Equation of Suicidal Intent, the CASE Approach provides a platform for exploring suicidal ideation and behaviors that may maximize the likelihood that 1) a patient will share what would have been withheld intent, 2) a patient will more openly share his or her reflected intent, and 3) the patient's stated intent will be as accurate as possible.

It is also hoped that the CASE Approach can play a significant role in the training of psychiatric residents and other mental health graduate students in social work, counseling, and psychology, for whom the instillation of sound suicide assessment skills is one of the most pressing of educational tasks. A training monograph on how to teach the CASE Approach to psychiatric residents and other mental health professionals, as well as an article emphasizing the importance of incorporating training in uncovering suicidal ideation in clinical interviewing courses for psychiatric residents and in other mental health disciplines, is available (Shea and Barney 2007b; Shea et al. 2007). More details on how to teach the CASE Approach and information on its effective use across disciplines and various clinical settings are available at the Web site for the Training Institute for Suicide Assessment and Clinical Interviewing (www.suicideassessment.com).

A practical example highlights the promise of the CASE Approach in yet another training arena: medical, nursing, and physician assistant student education. At least 50% of patients who kill themselves saw a primary care clinician within a month of their death (Luoma et al. 2002). A typical primary care clinician sees patients who warrant a suicide assessment on a daily basis. To prepare students for this future task, students could be asked to learn and effectively demonstrate the use of an interview strategy such as the CASE Approach for eliciting suicidal ideation. It is likely that such students would be significantly more competent in eliciting suicidal ideation, and more apt to do so, than the typical graduate of today.

In the final analysis, language can indeed be misleading, and during a suicide assessment miscommunication is not only problematic but also sometimes lethal. The Victorian writer Oscar Wilde once wisely commented, "My reality is constantly blurred by the mists of words." The CASE Approach is an attempt to cut through some of the mists created by language to the truth regarding a patient's intent to die by suicide. If we are lucky, when the mists recede it is hope that remains.

Key Clinical Concepts

- Remember that patients who have the most serious suicidal intent may be the most likely to withhold it.

- When formulating risk, keep in mind that the actual suicidal intent of the patient may be a combination of what the patient tells the interviewer is his or her intent, what plans and actions may reflect the patient's actual intent, and what intent the patient consciously or unconsciously withholds.

- Motivational theory suggests that in some instances *reflected intent*— amount of ideation, extent of planning, and actions taken on planning— may be a more accurate indicator of actual intent than what a patient states is his or her intent.

- Becoming familiar with a flexible interviewing strategy for uncovering suicidal ideation, planning, and intent (such as the CASE Approach) allows you to adapt your questioning to the unique needs of the patient and the clinical circumstance.

- Remember that each of the following validity techniques—normalization, shame attenuation, the behavioral incident, gentle assumption, denial of the specific, the catch-all question, and symptom amplification— can provide you with specific tools designed to meet specific challenges in eliciting suicidal ideation and intent.

References

American Association of Suicidology: Recognizing and responding to suicide risk (two-day course). 2011. Available at: http://www.suicidology.org/web/guest/education-and-training/rrsr. Accessed September 7, 2011.

Aston E: The Darcy Connection: A Novel. Austin, TX, Touchstone Publishing, 2008

Berman AL, Jobes DA, Silverman MM: Adolescent Suicide: Assessment and Intervention. Washington, DC, American Psychological Association, 2005

Bongar B, Berman AL, Maris RW, et al: Risk Management With Suicidal Patients. New York, Guilford, 1998

Carlat D: The Psychiatric Interview, 2nd Edition. Philadelphia, PA, Lippincott Williams & Wilkins, 2004a

Carlat D: Q&A regarding the chronological assessment of suicide events (CASE Approach). Carlat Report On Psychiatric Treatment 2, 2004b

Chiles JA, Strosahl KD: Clinical Manual for Assessment and Treatment of Suicidal Patients. Washington, DC, American Psychiatric Publishing, 2004

EndingSuicide.com: Education on ending suicide. 2011. Available at: http://www.larasig.com/suicide. Accessed September 9, 2011.

Hall RC, Platt DE: Suicide risk assessment: a review of risk factors for suicide in 100 patients who made severe suicide attempts: evaluation of suicide risk in a time of managed care. Psychosomatics 40:18–27, 1999

Jacobs DG: The Harvard Medical School Guide to Suicide Assessment and Intervention. San Francisco, CA, Jossey-Bass, 1999

Jobes DA: Managing Suicidal Risk: A Collaborative Approach. New York, Guilford, 2006

Jobes DA, Mann RE: Reasons for living versus reasons for dying: examining the internal debate of suicide. Suicide Life Threat Behav 29:97–104, 1999

Joiner TE Jr: Why People Die by Suicide. Cambridge, MA, Harvard University Press, 2005

Joiner TE Jr, Van Orden KA, Witte TK, et al: The Interpersonal Theory of Suicide: Guidance for Working With Suicidal Clients. Washington, DC, American Psychological Association, 2009

Knoll J: Correctional suicide risk assessment and prevention. Correctional Mental Health Report: Practice, Administration, Law 10:65–80, 2009

Luoma JB, Martin CE, Pearson JL: Contact with mental health and primary care providers before suicide: a review of the evidence. Am J Psychiatry 159:909–916, 2002

Magellan Behavioral Health Care Guidelines: CASE Approach Recommended to Participating Clinicians. Columbia, MD, Magellan Behavioral Health, 2002

Maris RW, Berman AL, Silverman MM: Comprehensive Textbook of Suicidology. New York, Guilford, 2000

Mays D: Structured assessment methods may improve suicide prevention. Psychiatr Ann 34:367–372, 2004

McKeon R: Advances in Psychotherapy: Evidence Based Practice, Vol 14: Suicidal Behavior. Cambridge, MA, Hogrefe, 2009

Miller MC: Suicide-prevention contracts: advantages, disadvantages, and an alternative approach, in The Harvard Medical School Guide to Suicide Assessment and Intervention. Edited by Jacobs DG. San Francisco, CA, Jossey-Bass, 1999, pp 463–481

Miller MC, Jacobs DG, Gutheil TG: Talisman or taboo: controversy of the suicide prevention contract. Harv Rev Psychiatry 6:78–87, 1998

Monk L, Samra J: Working with the client who is suicidal: a tool for adult mental health and addiction services. The British Columbia Ministry of Health and the Centre for Applied Research in Mental Health and Addiction. 2007. Available at: http://www.comh.ca/publications/resources/pub_wwcwis/WWCWIS.pdf. Accessed September 9, 2011.

Oordt MS, Jobes DA, Fonseca VP, et al: Training mental health professionals to assess and manage suicidal behavior: can provider confidence and practice behaviors be altered? Suicide Life Threat Behav 39:21–32, 2009

Pascal GR: The Practical Art of Diagnostic Interviewing. Homewood, IL, Dow Jones-Irwin, 1983

Pomeroy WB, Flax CC, Wheeler CC: Taking a Sex History: Interviewing and Recording. New York, Free Press, 1982

Posner K, Brown GK, Stanley B, et al: The Columbia-Suicide Severity Rating Scale: initial validity and internal consistency findings from three multisite studies with adolescents and adults. Am J Psychiatry 168:1266–1277, 2011

Prochaska J, DiClemente C: The Transtheoretical Approach: Crossing Traditional Boundaries of Therapy. Homewood, IL, Dow Jones-Irwin, 1984

Prochaska JO, Norcross J, DiClemente C: Changing for Good. New York, William Morrow, 1992

Reed MH, Shea SC: Suicide assessment in college students: innovations in uncovering suicidal ideation and intent, in Understanding and Preventing College Student Suicide. Edited by Lamis DA, Lester D. Springfield, IL, Charles C Thomas, 2011

Robinson DJ: Brain Calipers: Descriptive Psychopathology and the Psychiatric Mental Status Examination, 2nd Edition. Port Huron, MI, Rapid Psychler Press, 2001

Rudd MD: The Assessment and Management of Suicidality (Practitioner's Resource). Sarasota, FL, The Professional Resource Exchange, 2006

Shea SC: The Chronological Assessment of Suicide Events: a practical interviewing strategy for eliciting suicidal ideation. J Clin Psychiatry 59 (suppl 20):58–72, 1998a

Shea SC: Psychiatric Interviewing: The Art of Understanding, 2nd Edition. Philadelphia, PA, WB Saunders, 1998b, pp 463–495

Shea SC: Tips for uncovering suicidal ideation in the primary care setting, in Hidden Diagnosis: Uncovering Anxiety and Depressive Disorders (4-part CD-ROM series, version 2.0). Rancho Mirage, CA, Annenberg Center for Health Sciences, Eisenhower Medical Center/GlaxoSmithKline, 1999

Shea SC: Practical tips for eliciting suicidal ideation for the substance abuse professional. Counselor: The Magazine for Addiction Professionals 2:14–24, 2001

Shea SC: The Chronological Assessment of Suicide Events (the CASE Approach): an introduction for the front-line clinician. NewsLink (Newsletter of the American Association of Suicidology) 29:12–13, 2002

Shea SC: The Chronological Assessment of Suicide Events: an innovative method for training residents to competently elicit suicidal ideation. Presented at the annual meeting of the American Association of Directors of Psychiatric Residency Training, San Juan, PR, 2003

Shea SC: The delicate art of eliciting suicidal ideation. Psychiatr Ann 34:385–400, 2004

Shea SC: Innovations in uncovering suicidal ideation with vets and soldiers: the Chronological Assessment of Suicide Events (CASE Approach). Presented at the Eastern VISN of Nebraska, Veterans Administration, Omaha, NE, 2008a

Shea SC: Uncovering suicidal ideation in a primary care setting with vets and soldiers: the Chronological Assessment of Suicide Events (CASE Approach). Presented for the Primary Care Department, Tripler Army Base, Honolulu, HI, 2008b

Shea SC: Innovations in uncovering suicidal ideation with vets and soldiers: the Chronological Assessment of Suicide Events (CASE Approach). Presented at the Department of Defense/Veterans Administration Annual Suicide Prevention Conference, San Antonio, TX, 2009a

Shea SC: Suicide assessment: part 1—uncovering suicidal intent, a sophisticated art. Psychiatric Times. 2009b. Available at: http://www.psychiatrictimes.com/print/article/10168/1491291?printable=true. Accessed September 10, 2011.

Shea SC: Suicide assessment: part 2—uncovering suicidal intent, using the Chronological Assessment of Suicidal Events (CASE Approach). Psychiatric Times. 2009c. Available at: http://www.psychiatrictimes.com/depression/content/article/10168/1501845?pageNumber=17. Accessed September 10, 2011.

Shea SC: Innovations in eliciting suicidal ideation: the Chronological Assessment of Suicide Events (CASE Approach). Presented at annual meetings of the American Association of Suicidology from 1999 through 2011a

Shea SC: Experiential, full-day role-playing workshop on the Chronological Assessment of Suicide Events with veterans. Presented at VA Northern Indiana Health Care System, Fort Wayne, IN, 2011b

Shea SC: The Practical Art of Suicide Assessment: A Guide for Mental Health Professionals and Substance Abuse Counselors. Stoddard, NH, Mental Health Presses, 2011c

Shea SC, Barney C: Facilic supervision and schematics: the art of training psychiatric residents and other mental health professionals how to structure clinical interviews sensitively. Psychiatr Clin North Am 30:e51–e96, 2007a

Shea SC, Barney C: Macrotraining: a "how-to" primer for using serial role-playing to train complex clinical interviewing tasks such as suicide assessment. Psychiatr Clin North Am 30:e1–e29, 2007b

Shea SC, Mezzich JE: Contemporary psychiatric interviewing: new directions for training. Psychiatry: Interpersonal and Biological Processes 51(4):385–397, 1988

Shea SC, Mezzich JE, Bohon S, et al: A comprehensive and individualized psychiatric interviewing training program. Acad Psychiatry 13(2):61–72, 1989

Shea SC, Green R, Barney C, et al: Designing clinical interviewing training courses for psychiatric residents: a practical primer for interviewing mentors. Psychiatr Clin North Am 30:283–314, 2007

Simon RI: Assessing and Managing Suicide Risk: Guidelines for Clinically Based Risk Management. Washington, DC, American Psychiatric Publishing, 2004

Simon RI: Preventing Patient Suicide: Clinical Assessment and Management. Washington, DC, American Psychiatric Publishing, 2011

Simon RI, Hales RE: The American Psychiatric Publishing Textbook of Suicide Assessment and Management. Washington, DC, American Psychiatric Publishing, 2006

Simpson S, Stacy M: Avoiding the malpractice snare: documenting suicide risk assessment. J Psychiatr Pract 10:185–189, 2004

Acknowledgment

Portions of this chapter were adapted, with the permission of UBM Medica, from several articles in *Psychiatric Times* (Shea 2009b, 2009c).

CHAPTER 3

The Clinical Risk Assessment Interview

M. David Rudd, Ph.D., A.B.P.P.

The Therapeutic Relationship as a Foundation for Risk Assessment

The focus of this chapter is on the clinical interview for suicide risk assessment, but I would be remiss not to briefly mention the importance of the therapeutic relationship. To conduct a thorough, incisive, and accurate clinical interview targeting suicide risk, establishing a strong and caring relationship with the suicidal patient is essential. Therapeutic technique and clinical interventions can be of limited value when a meaningful relationship has not been established with the patient. Interestingly enough, a meaningful relationship can be established even in the face of significant time constraints and in settings as dissimilar as the emergency department, inpatient milieu, and private clinic office. Bongar (1992) emphasized that the quality of the therapeutic relationship is one of the most important factors in assessing risk and managing suicidal patients, while others have stressed that a solid therapeutic rela-

tionship is essential to successful assessment and management of suicide risk and suicidal behavior, both acute and chronic in nature (see, e.g., Michel and Jobes 2010; Shneidman 1981, 1984).

Among the variables most frequently cited as important in establishing a good relationship are *comfort* and *trust*. Motto (1979) identified a number of clinician behaviors that facilitate a stable attachment and positive alliance with the patient. He identified availability and access as crucial (i.e., making oneself available during an emergency, returning phone calls, and scheduling more frequent appointments when necessary). Shneidman (1981, 1984) even suggested that it is sometimes necessary for the clinician to "foster dependency" in order to ensure a strong initial attachment, noting that such dependency is often the natural consequence of a caring, compassionate, consistent, and predictable interpersonal style with suicidal patients. Linehan (1993) emphasized the need to differentiate the relationship during the initial evaluation process from that during short- and long-term therapy. Although considerable overlap exists, there are certainly unique elements to each. In terms of the initial suicide risk assessment interview, emotional reactions by the clinician need to be recognized and monitored and effectively managed. In a now classic contribution, Maltsberger and Buie (1974, 1989) referred to "countertransference hate" as arguably the most problematic reaction, not dissimilar to what Linehan (1993) refers to as "therapy interfering behaviors," with both being characterized by a range of negative emotions and disruptive behaviors (e.g., exhibiting fear, malice, aversion, hate, anxiety, or worry; ending sessions early; taking phone calls during session; being late for appointments; and rescheduling or canceling appointments). The ability to quickly identify and effectively respond to negative emotions and disruptive behaviors is an indispensable skill for clinicians wanting to effectively engage, assess, and manage suicidal patients, something that should be stressed from the very beginning of clinical supervision and training in a practitioner's career.

Suicidal patients withdraw prematurely from and obfuscate evaluations and treatment not because of improvement in their acute symptoms but because of severe psychopathology (Axis I and II), related interpersonal dysfunction, and identifiable skill deficits (Rudd et al. 1995). The intimate nature of the interpersonal contact in an assessment interview is often overwhelming to suicidal patients, accentuating their inability to effectively regulate emotion, poor interpersonal skills, and limited tolerance for intimacy even in a clinical context. It is important for clinicians to remember the following when attempting to establish and maintain a relationship with an acutely suicidal patient:

- The patient is likely at his or her worst since he or she is actively suicidal and

highly symptomatic, with symptoms creating difficulty across a number of functional domains (e.g., concentration, communication, and emotion regulation) and making the clinical interview a genuine challenge. The clinician can do several things to help diffuse the patient's anxiety and apprehension, including providing a simple explanation of the disruptive role of acute symptoms and offering reassurance that he or she will work in collaborative fashion with the patient to achieve an accurate understanding of current risk. Providing an explanation of why the patient is struggling to express himself or herself can be remarkably comforting during a period of acute crisis, enhancing a sense of personal control, safety, and hope. Reassurance in this context can take many forms, but here are a few examples of what the clinician can say:

> Sometimes it's difficult to concentrate and describe how you feel when you are so upset. Why don't you take a minute to organize your thoughts? Is there anything I can do to help you feel more comfortable and make it easier for you to talk? If you need to just take a few minutes to catch your breath, you can do that. I can slow down if needed; just let me know. Sometimes it's easier to talk after you've had a few minutes to relax. I realize what a difficult time this is for you and that it might be not be easy to talk. It's important that you feel comfortable so we can fully and accurately understand the extent of the problems you've been struggling with, so please let me know if there's anything in particular I can do to help you feel at ease.

- The clinician should recognize the important role played by shame and guilt in suicidal patients, particularly during an initial assessment where the patient is not familiar with the clinician. Given disproportionately high rates of abuse (physical, sexual, and emotional), patients struggling with suicidal crises are characterized by high rates of shame and guilt (Rudd et al. 2004). Unchecked shame and guilt can quickly derail an assessment, resulting in the patient's simply disengaging or providing limited or misleading reports. Awareness, careful monitoring, and, occasionally, a strategic intervention are crucial to establishing a good relationship when shame is prominent. If necessary, helping the patient understand the developmental context for shame (e.g., the relationship between shame and prior abuse) can prove highly effective at diffusing any escalation.

- Given the crisis nature of the interaction, the clinician needs to anticipate the possibility that the patient will be provocative, challenging, and potentially hostile. For patients with chronic suicidal problems, provocative and undercontrolled behavior is more often than not the routine. When facing provocation, the clinician needs to acknowledge the patient's upset in the context of the current crisis and redirect the patient to the task at hand (i.e., the need to complete the assessment leading to an immediate clinical disposition), emphasizing the collaborative nature of the evaluation process. For example:

> I can understand why you'd be so upset. You've had some very painful things happen in the last several weeks. We can take a few minutes and talk more about some of those things if you'd like, but in the next 5 or 10 minutes I'm going to need to ask you some

questions and get some information so that we can make a decision about how to respond today and over the next several days. We will come back to some of the things that have happened to you after we make a decision about what is best to do right now.

- The clinician should recognize that in completing the initial assessment process the groundwork is being laid for ongoing care, regardless of the eventual provider. Evaluations and assessments are psychotherapeutic exchanges, even if it is a brief assessment in the emergency department. This initial contact and evaluation can have considerable influence on whether or not a patient decides to continue in care. The initial evaluation can provide a foundation of hope for subsequent interactions.

- Trust and comfort are facilitated by the use of clear, unambiguous language, along with good eye contact when asking difficult questions. Using the terms "thinking of killing yourself" and "thoughts of suicide" provide little, if any, room for misinterpretation. For example:

> You said you've been having thoughts of killing yourself. What exactly have you been thinking? When did you first have thoughts of suicide?

- It can be comforting for some patients if the clinician provides developmental and historical context for their interpersonal distress. It is perhaps easiest and most effective to do this with patients who have significant abuse histories. For example, providing a simple explanation that the lack of trust and consistency in early foundational relationships (e.g., with their mother or father) has impact on how they approach all relationships (i.e., with caution and apprehension), particularly those that provoke anxiety and are somewhat threatening. It is important to help the patient understand that in the context of his or her developmental history, anxiety and apprehension are understandable. Normalization can be a powerful clinical intervention, facilitating trust and comfort in fairly dramatic fashion with an acutely distressed and suicidal patient. Simple models of understanding also help build hope, an important goal in any clinical intervention targeting suicide risk.

- Helping a patient recognize and respond to his or her own ambivalence can provide comfort. Hopeless and acutely distressed patients often do not recognize that they are ambivalent about dying, hence, the need to identify both reasons for living and reasons for dying in the assessment process (discussed in more detail below). Taking a minute to help patients explore (and write down on a coping card) reasons for living (toward the end of the initial interview) can be a powerful and enduring intervention for patients who struggle to identify any reason for hope.

Conducting a clinical interview for suicide risk assessment can be a challenge. The failure to establish a good relationship, even if the interaction faces severe time constraints (e.g., in the emergency department), adds unnecessary complications. Attention to the issues summarized above will hopefully ease the challenge and improve the patient's comfort and trust, with the outcome a more accurate and clinically meaningful assessment and eventual disposition. It is important to remember that during suicidal crises, simple and subtle things can help build hope, arguably the primary goal of any intervention.

Assessing Suicidal Thinking and Behaviors: Understanding Intent and Gauging Risk

The core of the clinical interview for suicide risk is a careful and thorough assessment of suicidal thinking and behavior, with a particular focus on an accurate understanding of suicidal intent. Accordingly, the bulk of this chapter concentrates on a thorough assessment and understanding of suicidal thinking and related behaviors, and how these elements help the clinician formulate a more precise understanding of the patient's suicidal intent and overall risk, both acute and chronic in nature.

Figure 3–1 provides a flowchart of six identifiable steps, with questions that need to be asked of the suicidal patient in order to clarify the nature and severity of his or her suicidal thinking and behavior and ultimately to gauge intent. Some of these ideas were originally presented by Rudd (2006), but they have since been modified and extended, based on subsequent empirical findings. The flowchart is structured in hierarchical fashion, with the goal of reducing anxiety, apprehension, and associated resistance by transitioning from past episodes back to the current crisis after the initial screening question(s). As illustrated, the guiding question is *Have you had thoughts about suicide, thoughts of killing yourself?* For some patients this is simply the presenting problem. For others, it may take time and effort to reveal suicidal risk (addressed in more detail later).

As mentioned earlier, it is important to use unambiguous language. Three constructs are important to remember: suicidal thoughts, morbid ruminations, and self-harm. Far too few clinicians differentiate between active suicidal thoughts, morbid ruminations, and self-harm. Although there is certainly overlap across the three constructs, morbid ruminations (thoughts about death, dying, and not wanting to be alive but *without* active thoughts of killing oneself), suicidal thoughts (thoughts of killing oneself), and self-harm (underlying motivation is emotion regulation or for a reason other than death) are distinct and convey remarkably different levels of risk. Suicidal thinking is differentiated by an active desire to kill oneself (see, e.g., Rudd 2006). Some have referred to morbid ruminations as passive suicidal thoughts, noting their routine occurrence in cases of clinical depression (Maris et al. 1992). It is important for clinicians to carefully differentiate these three constructs, providing definitions for patients when needed. Clarification early in the assessment process eases and improves subsequent efforts to monitor clinical status. It can be argued that precise definitions can serve as a clinical intervention, allowing the patient a heightened sense of control in efforts to self-monitor and effectively regulate affective states (see, e.g., Rudd et al. 2004). It is not unusual for suicidal patients, particularly those with chronic suicidal behavior (Nock 2009), to also engage in repetitive self-harm. Although these episodes can co-occur, differentiating them is important for an accurate understanding of current risk.

Many, if not the majority of, seriously depressed patients will report morbid ruminations. The clinician can work to normalize the thoughts within the context of an active depressive problem, an intervention that often helps reduce anxiety, agitation, and associated acute dysphoria, particularly for adolescents and the elderly. For example, the following statement can be used to normalize morbid thoughts within the context of a depressive episode: *It's not unusual for someone that is depressed to feel hopeless and have thoughts about death or dy-*ing. When making the distinction between morbid and suicidal thoughts, the clinician still needs to complete a detailed exploration of the patient's suicidal history, even when the patient does not endorse active suicidal thoughts. If the patient does not have an extensive history, it should only take a few minutes. As Figure 3–1 illustrates, morbid ruminations convey lower risk. However, patients can quickly transition from morbid to suicidal thoughts, something that is not uncommon for those with a history of previous attempts. The clinician can help the patient understand the difference, using the transition from morbid to suicidal thinking as an easily recognized warning sign that needs to be openly shared and can be integrated into a subsequent safety plan (Wenzel et al. 2008).

When the clinician is documenting suicidal thoughts, direct and spontaneous quotes from the patient are recommended. For example: *Can you tell me exactly what you've been thinking? What are the thoughts that go through your head?* Taking direct quotes at the beginning of the interview, without providing prompts, provides a metric to assess the specificity of the patient's thinking, a useful marker of intent. Intent has both subjective (a patient's stated intent) and objective (the patient's demonstrated intent) elements (Rudd 2006). The specificity of suicidal thinking is one marker of intent, with greater detail and specificity suggesting greater intent. Specificity is captured in the how, when, where, and why of the suicidal crisis. Greater specificity often translates to longer duration of the thoughts and associated behavior (e.g., preparation and rehearsal). Additional markers of objective intent include the following:

- Preparation behavior (e.g., writing a letter(s), redoing one's will or insurance, accessing a method, researching methods on the Internet)

No—Indicate in the chart that the patient did not manifest acute suicidal thoughts. Provide a specific quote of the morbid thoughts: *I've been thinking a lot about what it'd be like for my family if I were gone.* Again, differentiate the terms for the patient, noting that suicidal means that the patient is thinking of killing himself/herself. If the patient is NOT having active suicidal thoughts, it's still important to assess his or her suicidal history for an accurate understanding. Identify the emergence of suicidal thinking as a "warning sign" and integrate into a safety plan.

Step 1:
Is the patient having suicidal thoughts?
Have you been thinking about killing yourself? Have you thought about suicide? Differentiate between suicidal thoughts (wanting to kill oneself), self-harm (emotion regulation as the primary goal), and morbid ruminations (thoughts of death, dying, or wanting to be dead, but not active thoughts of killing oneself). Define the terms for the patient. Document carefully in the chart using direct quotes from the patient.

Yes—*Can you tell me exactly what you've been thinking?* Get a direct quote from the patient without providing prompts. This provides a means to assess the specificity of the patient's thinking, one marker of intent. Explore each individual method separately. Always question for "multiple methods."

Step 2:
Reduce resistance and anxiety surrounding suicidal thinking by exploring patient's suicide history before examining the current episode in detail. This will reduce anxiety and resistance by helping the patient become more comfortable with the general topic of suicide. *Before we go into detail about what's going on now, can you tell me about the first time you ever thought about or attempted suicide? Tell me about what was going on at the time. What was the outcome? Were you injured? Did you get medical care? How did you end up at the hospital? Why did you want to die? Did you think [method] would kill you? How did you feel about surviving? Did you learn anything from the previous attempt? How many suicide attempts have you made? Have you thought about suicide in the past year or the past month?* For those with multiple attempts, target only two previous attempts, the "first" and "worst," with the patient subjectively defining "worst."

Step 3:
Transition back to the current suicidal crisis. *O.K., we've talked about some of the previous crises;* let's talk in more detail about what brought you here today. **Assess specificity of thinking, including frequency, intensity, and duration (and access). You can use the acronym F-I-D.** *How have you been thinking about killing yourself? Have you decided when and where? How often do you have the thoughts: daily, more than once a day, weekly, monthly? Can you tell me how intense or severe the thoughts are for you? How long do the thoughts last: a few seconds, minutes, or longer? How much time do you spend thinking about suicide in an average day/week/month? Do you have access to [method] or have you taken steps to get access? Have you thought about any other method of suicide?* It's important to ask the multiple method question until the patient says no.

FIGURE 3–1. A hierarchical approach to identifying and exploring suicidal thoughts.

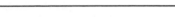

Step 4:
Assess subjective intent, including reasons for dying. *What are your reasons for dying? Why do you want to kill yourself? Do you have any intention of acting on your thoughts? Can you rate your intent on a scale of 1 to 10, with 1 being "no intent at all" and 10 being "certain that you'll act on your thoughts as quickly as you can"?*

Step 5:
Assess objective intent. *Have you taken steps to act on your suicidal thoughts? Have you done anything in preparation for your death (e.g., life insurance, letters to loved ones, research on the Internet)? Have you in any way rehearsed your suicide? In other words, have you gotten your [method] out and gone through the steps of what you'd do to kill yourself?*

Step 6:
Assess protective factors, including reasons for living. *What are your reasons for living? What keeps you going in difficult times like this?*

FIGURE 3–1. A hierarchical approach to identifying and exploring suicidal thoughts (*continued*).
Source. Adapted and expanded from Rudd 2006.

- Rehearsal behavior (actually getting one's method out and "practicing" or preparing for suicide)
- Stated reasons for living and reasons for dying (the simple numeric difference conveys evidence of intent)
- Perceived lethality of previous suicide attempts (*Did you think [method] would kill you?*)
- Any efforts to prevent discovery or rescue in previous suicide attempts
- Emotional reactions to previous attempts (*How did you feel about surviving? Did you learn anything about yourself from the attempt?*)

As noted above, the imbalance between identified reasons for living and reasons for dying provides a useful metric by which to measure manifest intent and ambivalence (e.g., 10 reasons for dying and 2 reasons for living; intent is disproportionately weighted toward death). As Joiner (2005) has discussed, the patient's capacity for suicide builds with exposure, including self-harm, multiple attempts, and preparation and rehearsal behaviors.

It is important for the clinician to recognize that mounting evidence of objective intent often means that the patient has progressed from "thinking" about suicide to actively implementing a suicide plan— clear evidence not only of greater intent but also of heightened risk. It is also important for the clinician to recognize that the patient's emotional reactions to previous attempts can help identify the persistence of what I have called "residual" intent (e.g., answers such as *"I learned that next time I need to use a gun"*) (Rudd 2006).

As demonstrated in Figure 3–1, a hierarchical approach can help reduce anxiety and resistance prior to exploring the details of the current suicidal crisis. When a patient endorses active suicidal thoughts, resistance can be reduced by briefly exploring the patient's history of suicidal behavior before examining the current crisis in detail and depth. For example: *Before we go into detail about what's going on now, can you tell me about the first time you ever thought about or attempted suicide?* If the patient endorses previous suicidal crises, it is important to eventually explore each event in detail. Thoughtful examination of all past suicide attempts will likely take multiple sessions if the patient has an extensive history. Current risk, however, can be understood with good accuracy by exploring the "first" and "worst" of the attempts (Joiner et al. 2003), with the patient identifying "worst" subjectively. Rudd (2006) has recommended the use of an "extended evaluation" for patients with chronic suicidal problems. An extended evaluation may require three to five sessions before the clinician makes a collaborative decision with the patient about providing ongoing care and treatment.

I would encourage clinicians, when examining specific suicide attempts, to consider the contextual factors (the acronym P-M-O-R is helpful for recall; see Table 3–1). Perhaps most important, the answers to the questions provided in Table 3–1 help the clinician assess both subjective and objective markers of intent, enabling the clinician to explore the convergence of data. Although there is no precise formula for compiling the various markers of objective intent, more often than not there is reasonable convergence. The patient's answers also provide a means to assess the similarity across more than one reported suicidal crisis. Recognizing the evolution and trajectory of intent for a patient is important. If there

is a trend of escalating lethality, it will be apparent across episodes. As mentioned earlier, time constraints are usually paramount in initial evaluations. Accordingly, it is incumbent on the clinician to accurately gauge time and defer detailed exploration of some previous crises or suicide attempts to later sessions if necessary. As mentioned above, sometimes it will be necessary to complete an "extended evaluation" of three to five sessions in order to fully understand a patient's suicidal history. If the clinician does not have time for such an extensive evaluation, it is important to make note of that in the chart, deferring the historical review to the next clinician, but clearly indicating that such an extensive review has not yet been accomplished.

As indicated in Figure 3–1, after exploration of a patient's suicide history (either in full or abbreviated fashion) is accomplished, the clinician can transition back to the current crisis. This can be done in any number of ways, but here is an example of a sequential transition (previous to current episode):

- *Can you tell me about the first time you ever thought about suicide [or attempted suicide]?*
- *Have you thought about or attempted suicide in the past year?*
- *Have you thought about or attempted suicide in the past few months?*
- *Now let's talk in more detail about the suicidal thoughts [or attempt] that brought you here today.*

Once the clinician transitions to the current episode, he or she needs to assess the *specificity* of the patient's thinking. This includes the frequency, intensity, and duration of thoughts, along with questions about when and where and about access to the stated method(s). As was mentioned earlier

TABLE 3–1. Contextual factors of past attempts

Precipitant?

What triggered the crisis, according to the patient?	*What triggered your thinking about attempting suicide? What was going on in your life at the time you made the suicide attempt?*

Motivation for the attempt?

Did the patient want to die?	*What were your reasons for dying? Did you want to die when you [method]?*
What did the patient actually do?	*Please tell me exactly what you did.*
What was the patient's perception of lethality?	*Did you think [method] would kill you?*

Outcome?

Was there any associated injury? If so, was medical care required? If required, did the patient follow through and get recommended medical care?	*Were you injured by the suicide attempt? Did you receive medical care? Why did you choose not to get medical care when it was recommended?*
How did the patient end up accessing care? Was care seeking initiated by the patient? Was it by random chance?	*How did you get to the hospital? Did you call someone?*
Did the patient take active steps to prevent discovery or rescue?	*Did you take steps to try to prevent discovery or rescue when you made the suicide attempt? Did you time the attempt or otherwise make it difficult for someone to find you?*

Reaction?

What was the patient's emotional reaction to surviving the suicide attempt?	*How do you feel about surviving? Did you learn anything helpful about yourself [or others] from the previous attempt?*

in this chapter, do not initially provide the patient options to choose from when questioning about method. One indicator of intent is the specificity of the patient's thinking. Early prompts can undermine an accurate assessment. They can also lead to a unilateral and unbalanced exchange that can undermine the development of a solid therapeutic relationship. Using the patient's own words (i.e., quoting them directly about suicidal thoughts) conveys that you will be, and are, listening.

It is also important, as noted below, to emphasize the need to question about multiple methods. The clinician needs to continue to ask the patient about possible methods and access until patient says no other methods have been considered. Patients will sometimes withhold their accessible method until questioned more thoroughly. Asking about multiple methods communicates not only that the clinician cares about the patient but also that he or she is going to be thorough, specific, and detailed in the evaluation process. This is yet another example of how detailed inquiry helps build trust and a stronger therapeutic alliance. Specific details about a patient's suicidal thinking can be captured with the following questions:

- *How are you thinking about killing yourself?*
- *Do you have access to [method]?*
- *Have you made arrangements or planned to get access to [method]?*

- *Have you thought about any other way to kill yourself?* [Ask this question until the patient says that no other methods have been considered.]
- *How often do you think about killing yourself? Once a day, more than once a day, once a week, monthly?*
- *You said you think about suicide every day. How many times a day?*
- *When you have these thoughts, how long do they last? A few seconds, minutes, or longer?*
- *On average, how much time [every day, week, or month] do you spend thinking about suicide?*
- *What exactly do you think about [or do] for that [period of time]?*
- *When you have these thoughts, how intense or severe are they? Can you rate them on a scale of 1 to 10, with 1 being "not severe at all" and 10 being "so severe that I will act on them."*
- *Have you thought about* when *you would kill yourself?*
- *Have you thought about* where *you would kill yourself?*
- *Have you thought about taking steps or timing your attempt to prevent anyone from finding or stopping you?*
- *Have you prepared for your death?*
- *Have you rehearsed or practiced your suicide?*
- *Do you have any intention of acting on your thoughts? Can you rate your intent on a scale of 1 to 10, with 1 being "no intent at all" and 10 being "certain that I'll act on them as quickly as I can"?*

Assessing suicidal thinking in such great detail provides a means not only to assess initial risk but also to track progress across sessions. It is entirely possible for a patient to improve and evidence little acute or chronic risk despite continuing to think about suicide with some regularity. With chronic suicidality in particular, simple notations in the chart about the presence or absence of suicidal thoughts are misleading. It may well be that a patient has been experiencing suicidal thoughts for decades. In these cases, the simple presence or absence of suicidal thinking is not a particularly good indicator of escalating risk. Some patients may think about suicide for the rest of their lives, given a history of multiple attempts and the web of associated memories. Fleeting, nonspecific suicidal thoughts with no associated intent (subjective or objective) are not unexpected and are not evidence of risk escalation beyond the individual's chronic baseline level. It is important to recognize that a patient could continue to think about suicide daily but actually be making considerable progress and evidence no significant risk if the duration (and associated specificity) of the thoughts is reduced from, say, several hours a day to less than a few minutes. Reduced duration frequently translates to reduced specificity, less severity, and lower intent, along with lower risk. This frequently parallels a drop in other associated symptoms as well. It is also important to recognize that frequency, specificity, intent, and intensity are often interrelated. Simply tracking the daily, weekly, or monthly time allocated to suicidal thinking can be incredibly useful for the practicing clinician. As with any repetitive thought, the acronym F-I-D (frequency-intensity-duration) can prove useful.

The presence or absence of protective factors is critical to a clear understanding of a patient's suicidal intent and associated risk estimate. Most important among protective factors are social support and an active treatment relationship (Rudd et al. 2004). Protective factors can be captured with the following questions:

- *Even though you've had a very difficult time, something has kept you going. What are your reasons for living?*

- *Are you hopeful about the future? Can you rate your hopefulness on a scale of 1 to 10 (with 1 being hopeless and 10 being hopeful for the future)?*
- *What would need to happen to help you be more hopeful about the future?*
- *In the past, what has kept you going in difficult times like this?*
- *Whom do you rely on during difficult times?*
- *Has treatment been effective for you in the past?*

It is important for all clinicians to recognize that a detailed and specific evaluation of suicidal thinking does not result in increased dysphoria; rather, it can actually reduce acute risk (Gould et al. 2005). Such detailed questioning helps set the tone and expectations for all subsequent clinical interactions with the patient. It provides an implicit sanction, approval, and reinforcement for the patient being honest and specific with the clinician. Detailed questioning is an intervention that facilitates a good therapeutic alliance. Most important, though, such an approach provides the details necessary to make accurate risk assessment decisions. An accurate understanding of suicide risk starts with a thorough and detailed understanding of the patient's suicidal thinking.

Assessing Related Risk Factors

The detailed assessment of suicidal thinking needs to be supplemented with an assessment of additional risk factors, all embedded within a common framework for clinical decision making. It is expected that a complete and comprehensive intake history, diagnostic interview, and mental status exam will always be conducted as a part of psychiatric and psychological evaluations. The focus of this chapter is on the elements that are unique to a suicide risk assessment.

In addition to a detailed and thorough assessment of suicidal thinking, there are a number of empirically supported domains essential to accurately assessing suicide risk (Rudd et al. 2004). As detailed in Table 3–2, the domains I recommend are identifiable precipitant(s), the patient's current symptomatic presentation, presence of hopelessness, nature of suicidal thinking, previous suicidal behavior, impulsivity and self-control, and protective factors. Although by no means exhaustive, these recommended domains are those that have good empirical support. In addition to recognizing the importance of these particular domains, I would encourage all clinicians to be keenly aware of the emerging evidence regarding suicide warning signs (Rudd et al. 2006), with acute symptoms anxiety, sleep disturbance, and perceived burdensomeness being of particular concern.

Perhaps the easiest approach to assessing each of the specific domains is to move in hierarchical fashion from the precipitating event, to the patient's current symptom presentation, to hopelessness, then to active suicidal thinking and intent. The approach for a detailed assessment of suicidal thinking and intent was covered earlier. The clinician can transition from the patient's symptoms to the issue of hopelessness and suicidality, normalizing the experience within the context of the psychiatric illness. As mentioned earlier in the discussion about assessing suicidal thinking, sequential transitions help reduce anxiety and apprehension during the whole of the interview. For example, when a patient is clinically depressed and anxious, the clinician can say, *It's not unusual for someone who's been depressed and anxious to feel hopeless. Do you feel hopeless?* If hopelessness is endorsed, the clinician can transition to morbid thoughts and eventually suicidal thinking, providing

TABLE 3–2. Additional domains of risk assessment

I. Predisposition to suicidal behavior

Previous history of psychiatric diagnoses (increased risk with recurrent disorders, comorbidity, and chronicity), including major depressive disorder, bipolar disorder, schizophrenia, substance abuse, and personality disorders such as borderline personality disorder

Previous history of suicidal behavior (increased risk with previous attempts, high lethality, and chronic disturbance) (Those having made multiple attempts [i.e., two or more] are considered at chronic risk.)

Recent discharge from inpatient psychiatric treatment (increased risk within first year of release) (Risk is highest during the first month after discharge.)

Same-sex sexual orientation (increased risk among homosexual men)

Male gender

History of abuse (sexual, physical, or emotional)

II. Identifiable precipitants or stressors (most can be conceptualized as losses)

Significant loss (e.g., financial, interpersonal relationship[s], professional, identity)

Acute or chronic health problems (loss of independence, autonomy, or function)

Relationship instability (loss of meaningful relationships and related support and resources)

III. Symptomatic presentation (have patient rate severity on 1–10 scale)

Depressive symptoms (e.g., anhedonia, low self-esteem, sadness, dyssomnia, fatigue [increased risk when combined with anxiety and substance abuse])

Bipolar disorder (increased risk early in disorder's course)

Anxiety (increased risk with trait anxiety and acute agitation)

Schizophrenia (increased risk following active phases)

Borderline and antisocial personality features

IV. Presence of hopelessness (have patient rate severity on 1–10 scale)

Severity of hopelessness

Duration of hopelessness

V. Nature of suicidal thinking

Current ideation frequency, intensity, and duration

Presence of suicidal plan (increased risk with specificity)

Availability of means (multiple methods)

Lethality of means (including both medical and perceived lethality)

Active suicidal behaviors

Suicidal intent (subjective and objective markers)

VI. Previous suicidal behavior

Frequency and context of previous suicidal behaviors

Perceived lethality and outcome

Opportunity for rescue and help seeking

Preparatory behaviors (including rehearsal)

VII. Impulsivity and self-control (have patient rate on 1–10 scale)

Subjective self-control

Objective control (e.g., substance abuse, impulsive behaviors, aggression)

TABLE 3–2.   Additional domains of risk assessment *(continued)*

VIII. Protective factors

Presence of social support (Support needs to be both present and accessible. Make sure that relationships are healthy.)

Problem-solving skills and history of coping skills

Active participation in treatment

Presence of hopefulness

Children present in the home

Pregnancy

Religious commitment

Life satisfaction. (Have the patient rate life satisfaction on a scale of 1–10. Life satisfaction should correspond with the patient's stated reasons for living and dying.)

Intact reality testing

Fear of social disapproval

Fear of suicide or death (This suggests that the patient has not yet habituated to the idea of death, a very good sign.)

---

the opportunity for a thorough exploration. At each step along the way, the clinician can normalize the patient's symptoms in the context of the identified disorder. This strategic clinical intervention serves to reduce anxiety and any related resistance.

What follows is an example of a hierarchical approach to the interview as a whole (Figure 3–2):

- **Precipitant:** *Is there anything in particular that happened that triggered thoughts about suicide?* Every patient has a "story," and providing an opportunity for its exploration is essential to an effective assessment process. Some patients, particularly those struggling with chronic suicidality, may have trouble identifying an external precipitant. The clinician needs to recognize the importance of both "internal" and "external" triggers, educating the patient that internal processes (e.g., a feeling, a thought, a physical sensation) can trigger an episode of suicidality.
- **Symptomatic presentation:** *Tell me about how you've been feeling lately. It sounds like you've been feeling depressed. Have you been feeling anxious, nervous, or panicky? Have*

you been down, low, or blue lately? Have you had trouble sleeping [additional symptoms of depression and anxiety]? Table 3–1 provides a list of the most prominent symptoms associated with heightened suicide risk.

- **Hopelessness:** *It's not unusual for someone who's been feeling depressed to feel hopeless, like things won't change or get any better. Do you ever feel that way?*
- **Morbid ruminations:** *It's not unusual when you're feeling depressed and hopeless to have thoughts about death and dying. Do you ever think about death or dying?*
- **Suicidal thinking:** *It's not unusual when feeling depressed, hopeless and having thoughts about death and dying to have thoughts about suicide. Have you ever thought about suicide?*

In the vast majority of cases, hierarchical questioning is unnecessary, since suicidality is raised immediately by the patient or is the presenting problem. In some cases, though, a more gentle and hierarchical approach is useful. I have found this to be particularly true with adolescents and the elderly, both populations that present unique

Precipitant: *Is there anything in particular that happened that triggered thoughts about suicide?*

Symptomatic presentation: *Tell me about how you've been feeling lately. It sounds like you've been feeling depressed. Have you been feeling anxious, nervous, or panicky? Have you been down, low, or blue lately? Have you had trouble sleeping [additional symptoms of depression and anxiety]?*

Hopelessness: *It's not unusual for someone who's been feeling depressed to feel hopeless, like things won't change or get any better. Do you ever feel that way?*

Morbid ruminations: *It's not unusual when you're feeling depressed and hopeless to have thoughts about death and dying. Do you ever think about death or dying?*

Suicidal thinking: *It's not unusual when feeling depressed, hopeless, and having thoughts about death and dying to have thoughts about suicide. Have you ever thought about suicide?*

FIGURE 3–2. Hierarchical approach to the interview as a whole: an example.

challenges. A gradual and progressive approach to the interview reduces anxiety and associated resistance, along with facilitating the therapeutic relationships, all of which are geared toward a more accurate risk assessment.

Consistent with the construct of chronic risk, some of the latest findings indicate that those recently discharged from an inpatient unit (e.g., following suicide attempts) are at markedly greater risk in the first weeks and months following discharge, with a gradual lowering of risk over the course of the first year (Goldston et al. 1999). In short, the general idea is that a patient's acute symptoms remit during the brief inpatient stay but chronic suicide risk persists, as evidenced by subsequent attempts following discharge. This chronic risk can be exacerbated following discharge by a new precipitant or stressor, triggering a new suicidal crisis. Monitoring patients closely following discharge is important. Patients need more intensive follow-up and contact immediately following discharge. Research also has emphasized the importance of sexual orientation as a predisposing factor. Russell and Joyner (2001) consistently found elevated suicide risk among gay, lesbian, bisexual, and transgender individuals, with homosexual men being at highest risk.

Most identifiable precipitants and stressors can be conceptualized as losses—that is, interpersonal loss, financial loss, or identity loss. Also of importance, the clinician needs to weigh acute and chronic health problems, along with acute family disruption. Medical illnesses have been associated with increased suicide risk. The risk is heightened when the medical illness occurs in the context of psychiatric disorder(s). In many respects, serious medical illness translates to loss of autonomy and independence. All too often this loss of autonomy is both physical and financial.

Assessment and monitoring of symptomatic presentation are particularly important. The focus here is on nonpsychotic states. The decision making for suicidal patients who are acutely psychotic is straightforward; they need to be in the hospital. Naturally, the clinician needs to assess both Axis I and II diagnoses, with an eye toward comorbidity. Separate from establishing a diagnosis, it is important for the clinician to assess and monitor identifiable symptom clusters, including depression, anxiety, agitation, anger, and any associated sense of urgency. This can be done in a straightforward and simple fashion by having the patient rate his or her symptoms on a 1 to 10 scale. For example, *You said you've been feeling depressed [or other symptom]. Can you rate how you're feeling now on a scale of 1 to 10, with 1 being the best you've ever felt and 10 being so depressed you're thinking about suicide?* The numerical ratings serve multiple purposes, including improving clarity in communication between patient and clinician, tracking symptom recovery over time, and providing the patient with a sense of control by quantifying his or her emotional experience.

As indicated in Table 3–2, hopelessness is treated as a separate domain, because of its significance in assessing suicide risk. It is not just the presence or absence of hopelessness that is important, but also its duration and severity. As evidenced in the hierarchical question sequence described earlier, hopelessness can be assessed with a few simple questions. As with the other symptoms, I would suggest the use of a simple rating scale to track the severity of reported hopelessness over time. For example: *Can you rate your hopelessness on a scale of 1 to 10, with 1 being very hopeful and optimistic about the future and 10 being so hopeless that you see suicide as the only option?* Clearly, patients who report enduring hopelessness are more likely to be multiple attempters and represent chronic risk.

The assessment of impulsivity is very similar to intent in that the clinician needs to consider both subjective and objective elements. More specifically, the clinician needs to consider not just what the patient says (i.e., subjective self-control) but also what the patient does (i.e., objective self-control). Objective markers of impulsivity include substance abuse, aggression, acute interpersonal withdrawal, and sexual promiscuity. Much as in the assessment of subjective intent, the clinician can simply ask the patient, *Do you feel in control right now?* Additional questions include the following:

- *Do you consider yourself an impulsive person? Why or why not?*
- *When have you felt out of control in the past?*
- *What did you do that you thought was out of control?*
- *What did you do to help yourself feel more in control?*
- *When you're feeling out of control, how long does it usually take for you to recover?*

As with the distinction between subjective and objective markers of intent, the clinician needs to reconcile discrepancies between what the patient reports about himself or herself and what is being observed. For example: *You said you felt in control, but your behavior over the past week suggests anything but being in control. You were intoxicated several times and drove wildly and did other things that put you at risk. Can you explain this to me?*

The final domain to assess is protective factors. As might be expected, social support is a central concern. Social support needs to be both available and accessible. Simple questions, like the following, can help assess the availability of support:

- *Do you have access to family and friends whom you can talk to and whom you know will be supportive?*
- *What usually happens when you ask for support [from family or friends]?*
- *Whom can you turn to in times of crisis?*

- *Are there people you need to avoid when you're feeling like this?*

The availability of support needs to be coupled with the other variables listed in Table 3–2, including in particular a strong therapeutic relationship. As discussed earlier in this chapter, assessment of the patient's reasons for living is tremendously helpful in identifying not only intent but also hopefulness. The clinician should also consider and query about close relationships like those with a spouse, partner, friends, and children. Similarly, expressed hopefulness about treatment, previous treatment success, religious commitment, and fear of death or dying are critical to consider. Patients who express a fear of dying or self-injury have yet to habituate to the idea of suicide; this is a very good factor to emerge in the assessment process.

Key Clinical Concepts

- A comprehensive assessment, including a full differential diagnosis, intake history, and mental status examination, should be completed for every patient when suicidality is an issue.

- Identified targeted domains, including precipitant(s), suicidal thinking and past behavior (to include an assessment of subjective and objective markers of intent), symptom presentation, hopelessness, impulsivity, and self-control, and protective factors, should always be covered in the assessment.

- A detailed assessment of suicidal thinking, including a thorough understanding of both subjective and objective markers of intent, is essential.

- Simple 1–10 patient ratings are remarkably useful to gauge the patient's current symptom severity and intent and to monitor fluctuations over time, including improvement and resolution of a suicidal crisis.

- Simple and strategic clinical interventions during the assessment interview can reduce the patient's anxiety, apprehension, and resistance.

- A hierarchical approach to questioning is a useful guiding framework for interviewing suicidal patients.

- It is important to recognize emerging suicide warning signs as part of the assessment process.

References

Bongar B (ed): Suicide: Guidelines for Assessment, Management, and Treatment. New York, Oxford University Press, 1992

Goldston DB, Daniel SS, Reboussin DM, et al: Suicide attempts among formerly hospitalized adolescents: a prospective naturalistic study of risk during the first 5 years after discharge. J Am Acad Child Adolesc Psychiatry 38:660–671, 1999

Gould MS, Marrocco FA, Kleinman M, et al: Evaluating iatrogenic risk of youth suicide screening programs. JAMA 293:1635–1643, 2005

Joiner TE: Why People Die by Suicide. Cambridge, MA, Harvard University Press, 2005

Joiner TE, Steer RA, Brown G, et al: Worst point suicidal plans: a dimension of suicidality predictive of past suicide attempts and eventual death by suicide. Behav Res Ther 41:1469–1480, 2003

Linehan MM: Cognitive-Behavioral Treatment of Borderline Personality Disorder. New York, Guilford, 1993

Maltsberger JT, Buie DH: Countertransference hate in the treatment of suicidal patients. Arch Gen Psychiatry 30:625–633, 1974

Maltsberger JT, Buie DH: Common errors in the management of suicidal patients, in Suicide: Understanding and Responding: Harvard Medical School Perspectives. Edited by Jacobs D, Brown HN. Madison, CT, International Universities Press, 1989

Maris RW, Berman AL, Maltsberger JT, et al: Assessment and Prediction of Suicide. New York, Guilford, 1992

Michel K, Jobes DA (eds): Building a Therapeutic Relationship With the Suicidal Patient. Washington, DC, American Psychological Association, 2010

Motto J: The psychopathology of suicide: a clinical approach. Am J Psychiatry 136:516–520, 1979

Nock MK: Understanding Nonsuicidal Self-Injury: Origins, Assessment, and Treatment. Washington, DC, American Psychological Association, 2009

Rudd MD: The Assessment and Management of Suicidality. Sarasota, FL, Professional Resource Exchange, 2006

Rudd M, Joiner T, Rajab H: Help negation after acute suicidal crisis. J Consult Clin Psychol 63:499–503, 1995

Rudd MD, Joiner TE, Rajab H: Treating Suicidal Behavior. New York, Guilford, 2004

Rudd MD, Berman L, Joiner TE, et al: Warning signs for suicide: theory, research, and clinical application. Suicide Life Threat Behav 36:255–262, 2006

Russell ST, Joyner K: Adolescent sexual orientation and suicide risk: evidence from a national study. Am J Publ Health 91:1276–1281, 2001

Shneidman E: Psychotherapy with suicidal patients. Suicide Life Threat Behav 11:341–348, 1981

Shneidman E: Aphorisms of suicide and some implications for psychotherapy. Am J Psychother 38:319–328, 1984

Wenzel A, Brown C, Beck AT: Cognitive Therapy for Suicidal Patients: Scientific and Clinical Applications. Washington, DC, American Psychological Association, 2008

CHAPTER 4

Cultural Competence in Suicide Risk Assessment

Sheila Wendler, M.D.

Daryl Matthews, M.D., Ph.D.

Paula T. Morelli, Ph.D.

> Culture is characterized by the way of life of a group of people, the configuration of the more or less stereotyped patterns of learned behavior which are handed down from one generation to the next through the means of language and imitation.
>
> *Victor Barnouw (1963)*

The word *culture* refers to the unique behavior patterns and lifestyle shared by a group of people that distinguish it from other groups. A culture is characterized by a set of views, beliefs, values, and attitudes. Culture shapes people's behavior, but at the same time it is molded by the ideas and behavior of the members of the culture. Thus, culture and people influence each other reciprocally and interactionally. The individual may be aware of these influences, or the influences may be operating at a subconscious level (Tseng et al. 2001).

Cultural competence is the ability to work successfully in a multicultural, multiethnic society. It does not consist in developing a large fund of knowledge about a particular culture or cultures. Rather, it involves being

- Sensitive to the operation of culture in human behavior, including suicidal behavior.
- Willing to get cultural consultation when necessary.
- Empathic to the emotional issues posed by cultural factors.
- Willing to view the clinician-patient interaction in a cultural context.
- Willing to use cultural factors in developing treatment plans and approaches.

Cultural variables do not operate alone; they operate in a rich interaction with other variables: biological, psychological, and social. Terminology in this area is confusing as well, because terms go in and out of fashion and varying lay meanings are applied to them.

Race usually refers to a biological group that may or may not coincide with a culture system shared by the group. Although it may be possible to define races by biological factors (Tseng and Streltzer 1997), ethnic groups are generally a social phenomenon. The term *ethnicity* refers to social groups that distinguish themselves from other groups by a common history, normative system, and group identity. *Culture* refers to behavior patterns and value systems of a social group, whereas *ethnicity* refers to a group of people sharing a common culture (Tseng and Streltzer 1997).

Suicide is a complex phenomenon that is greatly influenced by social, psychological, and cultural factors. Yet studies that investigate whether what are usually considered risk factors for suicide differ by these variables and that adjust for confounding variables are rare (Kung et al. 1998). Culture affects suicide rates or risk of suicide both directly and indirectly through interactions with variables of other types. Just as it has been learned that there are psychological factors that enhance risk (e.g., "hopelessness"), so there are cultural factors enhancing risk (e.g., "lack of acculturation"). However, rarely does cultural research relate to an altogether relevant clinical population, and rarely are more than two cultures compared; when they are, it is often on measures vastly different from similar studies of other cultural groups. Because of the international character of some of this research, there exists much nonstandardization of definitions, methods, and instruments.

There is marked international variation in suicidal behavior, some of which is based on cultural factors. Variations also in part reflect culturally based international differences in the reporting of suicide. This in turn impedes the understanding of cultural factors in suicidal behavior. Negative cultural attitudes about suicide may lead to the suppression of information about suicidal behaviors. Rates of attempted suicides are more seriously underestimated than suicide rates. This is because the latter generally require medical-legal attention, so figures are closer to reality, whereas figures for the former depend on the extent to which those who attempted suicide are referred for medical attention. In societies in which suicide is highly stigmatized, such as India, where, until recently, suicidal behavior was regarded as "a punishable legal offense" (Latha et al. 1996), suicide attempts tend to be concealed by the community (Tseng et al. 2001).

Because empirical evidence showing the differential effects of the various risk factors across cultures, races, or ethnicities is generally not available, the detection of cultural influences in suicide assessment will depend on cultural sensitivity and cultural empathy. There are no algorithms permitting the inclusion of culture in suicide risk assessment.

The literature reveals a few cross-cultural consistencies about suicidal behavior. For example, it appears generally true across cultures that women attempt suicide more often than men but that men are more likely to complete suicide. Men tend to use more violent methods. Additionally, suicide is associated with mental illness across a great range of international studies. Mental illness—particularly mood disorders—appears to be the most common risk factor cross-culturally. The comorbidity of a major mental illness and a personality disorder and/or an addictive disorder increases the suicide risk among the younger population.

Otherwise, suicide appears to be strongly culturally shaped. In 2009, the World Health Organization documented suicide rates for women ranging from 0.1 per 100,000 in Iran to 16.8 per 100,000 in Sri Lanka, and for men ranging from 0.1 per 100,000 in Egypt to 63.3 per 100,000 in Belarus. This wide range in suicide rates indicates that significant cultural and other social factors are at work. Many cultural differences in suicide rates operate through intervening variables. Key intervening variables between culture and suicide include the following:

- Degree of acculturation
- Differences in cultural attitudes toward suicide
- Variations in the prevalence of risk factors such as unemployment, poverty, and alcohol and drug abuse
- Differences in religious views of suicide
- Differences in the lethality of the methods used for suicide in that culture
- Genetic differences in susceptibility to depressive disorders
- International differences in detecting and reporting suicide
- Issues in the therapeutic alliance between individuals of different cultures

Immigration and Acculturation

Much of our information on culture and suicide comes from research conducted on national population groups—for example, on Poles in Poland and Brazilians in São Paulo. The relevance of risk factors of migrant Poles or Brazilians or their descendant groups is altogether unclear. National information should merely sensitize the clinician to the presence of a potential cultural issue.

Suicide rates generally are found to change within the same ethnic groups after migration to other cultures. For example, the suicidal behavior of Japanese who migrate to Hawaii changed in frequency and method after three or four generations, compared with that of Japanese nationals in Japan (Tseng and Kok 1992). Immigration and adjustment to a new society are stressful life events. Suicide rates are frequently higher among immigrants compared with the native born. Poles, Russians, French people, Germans, and South Africans who immigrated to Britain showed higher rates compared with British-born people and those born in their country of origin (Johansson et al. 1997).

Anthropologists have identified acculturation as an important sociocultural factor related to mental health among natives or immigrants in multicultural societies (Liu and Cheng 1998; Mavreas and Bebbington 1990; Neff and Hoppe 1992; Rogler et al. 1991). The concept of acculturation was originally developed to describe the sociocultural changes that occurred in precontact societies when they came in contact with Western cultures (Linton 1940; Redfield et al. 1936). Sociocultural changes in this situation are more or less one-sided, with the less developed societies being assimilated into the more developed societies. Some studies show that less assimilation into the dominant culture increases the risk for suicide. Natives who are less assimilated into the dominant society may be less prepared to handle the stress of an imposed new lifestyle and are at greater risk for suicide (Lee et al. 2002).

Lee et al. (2002) found that less assimilation into the host Chinese society was associated with an increased risk for suicide among native Taiwanese, particularly in males. A similar observation was reported with depression as an outcome among Greek Cypriot immigrants in the United Kingdom (Mavreas and Bebbington 1990).

Analogously, researchers have generally found high suicide rates among aboriginal or indigenous groups compared with their nonnative counterparts. Groups studied include Maori populations in New Zealand (Skegg et al. 1995), native Australians (Clayer and Czechowicz 1991), Alaska Natives (Kettl and Bixler 1991), native Hawaiians (Andrade et al. 2006; Else and Andrade 2008), Native Americans (Alcántara and Gone 2008), and native Canadians (Malchy et al. 1997). Several authors have proposed that social disruption due to rapid social, economic, and cultural changes is responsible for high suicide rates among native groups in Australia, Alaska, and Canada (Clayer and Czechowicz 1991; Kettl and Bixler 1991; Malchy et al. 1997). The concept of *anomie* proposed by Durkheim in 1897 to describe the phenomenon of a lack of social norms due to weakened social and cultural affiliation has been postulated to be an important contributor to the high suicide rates among natives in Australia, Alaska, and Manitoba (Clayer and Czechowicz 1991; Durkheim 1897/1951; Kettl and Bixler 1991; Malchy et al. 1997; Thorslund 1990). Canadian aboriginal youth have one of the highest suicide rates in the world. Youths ages 10–29 years living on reservations have a five to six times higher probability of dying from suicide than their peers in the general population (Berry 1985; Kirmayer et al. 1994).

Two types of hypotheses are generally proposed to explain the effect of acculturation on suicide. One emphasizes cultural confusion or identifies difficulty between the original and the dominant new culture, leading to social disintegration; the other involves social disadvantage compared with mainstream society. The former is based on a global and populational perspective and therefore is usually applied to describe the differences between natives and nonnatives. The latter emphasizes heterogeneity in the same population and is often used to explain individual variability. Both condi-

tions place natives at greater risk for mental disorders (Lee et al. 2002).

Somewhat paradoxically, increasing assimilation into the larger culture may also increase vulnerability to suicide. Assimilation may remove the protection formerly afforded by membership in the minority subculture (Seiden 1981; Shaffer et al. 1994), increase social disruption and concomitant feelings of normlessness (Davenport and Davenport 1987; Earls et al. 1991; Trovato 1986), and result in a state of marginality in which the individual feels isolated because he or she is unaccepted by either group (Range et al. 1997). This sense of isolation may result from inability to acquire the skills (including language skills), values, and traditions of either culture. This applies to many native youth, who may not have had a deep education in their tradition, yet are cut off from mainstream society by poverty, isolation, and educational barriers. Berry (1985) states that among native youth in northern Ontario, suicide "is related to the situation of being caught between two cultures, and being unable to find satisfaction in either" (quoted in Kirmayer et al. 1994, p. 30). This may be true of many cultural groups in the United States and Canada with high suicide rates. There may be an "inverted U" relationship between traditionalism and suicide, in which both very traditional and highly assimilated individuals or communities are protected from suicide, whereas those in the intermediate state experience greater conflict and confusion about identity, resulting in increased risk for suicide (Berry 1985, 1993, Group for the Advancement of Psychiatry 1989).

Therapeutic Alliance

One of the major challenges of developing cultural competence is improving one's skills in establishing and maintaining a therapeutic alliance with individuals from backgrounds greatly dissimilar to one's own. As Tseng and Streltzer (2004) pointed out, the sphere of interpersonal relations is closely governed by cultural norms, and the clinician-patient relationship is powerfully regulated in this way.

The quality of the therapeutic alliance is a major factor in assessing and responding to suicidality (Simon 2004). In a culturally competent suicide risk assessment, the clinician takes into account both difficulties that may arise in the development of an effective therapeutic alliance and those that may prevent an adequate assessment of its nature and strength.

Barriers to effective therapeutic communication between cultures relevant to suicide risk assessment include the following:

- Western views of therapy as a collaborative effort versus Eastern views of the therapist as a learned teacher (Bernstein 2001).
- Male views, within paternalistic cultures, that revealing weakness to females is shameful. (This has been described in both Latin and Arabic cultures; see Comas-Diaz 1988; Javier and Yussef 1995; Mass and Al-Krenawi 1994.)
- Cultural views that may generally favor nondisclosure to therapists. (For example, an Arabic proverb teaches that "complaining to anyone other than God is a disgrace" [Dwairy and Van Sickle 1996], whereas many Asian cultures view patient disclosure as a betrayal of family secrets [Uba 1994].)
- Cultural practices that may favor a passive patient role, including avoiding questioning or confronting an authority figure. (These traits have largely been described in Asian cultural groups [Eungprabhanth 1975; Uba 1994; Wong and

Piran 1995]. Eye contact may be avoided as a demonstration of respect rather than anger, withdrawal, or something else. Complaints about the treatment process or the therapist may be suppressed, and patients may avoid taking medications, producing adverse effects, rather than describe such effects to the health care provider. Studies also indicate that culturally appropriate interventions [Walker et al. 2008] and worldview matching in the case of Asians [Kim et al. 2005] result in stronger therapeutic alliances.)

Attitudes toward the communication of suicidal ideas vary across cultures. People in some cultures consider suicidal ideas disgraceful and unsuitable for revelation to others, including general medical or mental health professionals. In contrast, people in other cultures may feel quite comfortable disclosing thoughts of suicide. Tseng (2001) noted, "In some societies, people have even learned that expressing suicidal ideas is a powerful way of getting professional attention and care, even if, in reality, they are not seriously occupied with 'depressive thoughts'" (p. 294).

Religion

Case Example 1

Father Sean is a 53-year-old Irish-American Catholic priest who as a teenager developed juvenile-onset diabetes mellitus (type 1 diabetes) and has had many medical sequelae. He spent many years as rector of a small parish in suburban Minneapolis. Because of the decline in the number of individuals entering the priesthood, Father Sean was assigned additional pastoral duties in a neighboring parish. As the months passed, Father Sean became increasingly depressed. His sister encouraged him to obtain counseling through his diocese, but Father Sean demurred and remained without care. When his sister noticed his weight loss and withdrawal, she became insistent that he get help, and he finally agreed to see a private psychiatrist for an evaluation.

When the doctor asks Father Sean if he is considering suicide, the priest reacts strongly and says, "Absolutely not; it is a mortal sin. And it would destroy my sister if I were to kill myself." The psychiatrist knows that aging males with serious medical problems are at serious risk of suicide, and she wonders how much of a protective effect his religious convictions provide.

Evidence for the protective effect against suicide of social factors includes the often reported link between religion and lower suicide rates (Payne et al. 1991; Stack 1983). Since the initial publication of Durkheim's *Suicide* in 1897 (with first English translation appearing in 1951), it has been claimed that religion affects the suicide rate, with higher rates found among Protestants as compared with Catholics and Jews. However, in a study of U.S. suicide rates, Stack and Lester (1991) found no effect by religious affiliation, but more frequent church attendance was associated with a lower rate of suicide. This effect of religiosity was independent of education, sex, age, and marital status. Similarly, a high proportion in a community of individuals without religious affiliation was found to be associated with an increased risk of suicide (Hasselback et al. 1991). A study of Inuit youth found that regular church attendance was associated with less likelihood of suicide attempts (Malus et al. 1994).

Quality of family life and religiosity are highly correlated (Stack 1992). The impact of religion on suicide rates may be understood not solely in terms of specific beliefs about suicide, death, suffering, and the afterlife but also by the extent to which religious affiliations and practices organize social support networks (Pescosolido and Georgianna 1989). Religiosity may reduce the suicide rate through its effects on strengthening

social ties through adherence to rules and customs; such support networks have a protective effect on suicide risk.

Durkheim (1897/1951) believed that integration into collective society leads members to focus on the needs and goals of the group, diverting their attention from their own concerns, including suicidal thinking. Stack (1983, 1992) has argued that religion provides protective power through members' commitment to a few core lifesaving beliefs. Stack and others have provided empirical support for the religious commitment theory using church attendance, religious affiliation, and the number of religious books produced nationally as measures of commitment (Hasselback et al. 1991; Stack 1992, 2000; Stack and Lester 1991). Stack (1992) noted, however, that familial integration may reinforce or coincide with church attendance and therefore is itself a potent predictor of suicide risk. The religiously unaffiliated tend to identify fewer reasons for living and have weaker moral objections to suicide (Stack 1992).

Eastern religions, in which traditions of reincarnation and circularity are prominent, generally do not vigorously condemn suicide. However, depending on context, culture, and individual and regional perspectives, there are multiple ways suicide may be interpreted in Buddhism, Confucianism, Hinduism, or Taoism. In Buddhist teachings, for example, death is considered a part of life. The act of suicide would short-circuit preparation for entrance into the larger cycle and is considered a disruptive, selfish act as well as an affront to ancestors (Leong et al. 2008). A study by Braun and Nichols (1997) found that Buddhist and other spiritual leaders from Hawaii representing Chinese, Japanese, Filipino, and Vietnamese communities all viewed suicide negatively.

The monotheistic religions of the West (Judaism, Christianity, and Islam) are essentially linear and function on the presumption of eternal redemption or damnation based on the actions of a single lifetime. Suicide has generally been seen as a moral crime in these societies (Ladrido-Ignacio and Gensayaok 1992).

Marital Status, Support, and Interpersonal and Economic Factors

The prevalence of completed suicide, in most societies, is higher among men; an exception for this seems to be mainland China, where the suicide rate is considerably higher for females. Rates are particularly high among young females in rural areas, where the role of women is less favorable than that of men due to the former's lower social status and the highly restrictive environment in which they live (Tseng 2001; Tseng and Streltzer 1997). Suicide in the general population in Western societies is more frequent among both men and women who are single, separated, divorced, or widowed compared with those who are married (Trovato 1991). Those who are married with children have still lower rates. There are some cross-cultural data as well: among native Canadians, an analysis of data covering three decades (1951–1981) supported the hypothesis that a change from single or widowed to married status reduces suicide risk for men significantly more than for women (Trovato 1991). In the case of a transition from divorced to married status, both sexes benefited equally in terms of reduction in suicide potential (Kirmayer et al. 1994).

The quality of an individual's social network is a strong predictor of the risk for suicide attempts (Grossi and Violato 1992; Hart and Williams 1987; Magne-Ingvar et al. 1992; Wasserman 1992). Interpersonal conflicts—usually family or marital discord, a breakup of a significant relationship, or loss of personal resources—are the most common precipitants of suicide attempts (Weissman 1974). Several Western studies confirm that the most common immediate precipitants of youth suicide are acute romantic, academic, and vocational failures (Hawton 1986; Shaffer et al. 1988; Tallis 2000).

Because personal loss is well known to be a factor in many suicides, a culturally competent suicide assessment will take into account that social groups may differ in what constitutes a sufficiently grave loss. Suicide often derives from family conflict in societies in which family relationships are highly valued and there is a strong emphasis on hierarchy within the family system, characteristics common to many Asian cultures. In a Filipino study, 79.3% of suicides were attributed to family-related stress (Ladrido-Ignacio and Gensaya 1992); similar findings have emerged for Chinese and Indian populations (Ganapathi and Rao 1966; Zhang 1996).

In many Western societies, when faced with overwhelming financial debt, people are given the more or less socially acceptable opportunity to declare bankruptcy as a solution. Tseng (2001), however, points out that in other, highly interpersonally oriented cultures such as Japan, it is considered disgraceful to claim bankruptcy, an act that shames the family for many generations. In such cultures, financial catastrophe may be more likely to result in suicide (Takahashi et al. 1998; Yoshimatsu 1992). Poverty and debt as motivation for suicide are relatively rare in economically developed societies; however, financial difficulty as a motive for suicide is still relatively common in undeveloped or developing societies (Tseng et al. 2001). Unemployment as a risk factor for suicide must be examined in the context of the economic history and values of specific cultures. In cultures in which unemployment is viewed by society as a community problem rather than an individual problem, unemployment is not as strongly related to suicide risk as it is in cultures in which unemployment is linked to individual self-esteem (Kirmayer et al. 1994).

Male-female relationship problems are common reasons for suicide in societies in which romance is highly valued and the man-woman relationship is a predominant axis in interpersonal relations (Tseng et al. 2001). A failure in such relationships is associated with suicide in Western cultures.

Youth and Old Age

Regardless of place or time, there does not appear to be an exception to the observation that suicide attempts—and to a lesser extent completed suicides—tend to occur among the young (those between the ages of 20 and 30 years, with the peak from ages 20 to 24). There is substantial evidence that in the West this trend is exaggerated for disadvantaged minority populations. For example, this is true of the Alaskan and Canadian aboriginal population (Kirmayer et al. 1994), among Native American groups in the United States (Group for the Advancement of Psychiatry 1989; Kettl and Bixler 1991), and among African American youth (Garlow et al. 2005).

Although the suicide rate for African American adolescents is still lower than for white adolescents, this gap has narrowed (Gould and Kramer 2001; Greening and Stoppelbein 2002). Psychiatric disturbances, stressful life events, and poor parent-child relationships seem to account for a significant proportion of the variance in suicidal ideation and attempts among Af-

rican American youth (Greening and Stoppelbein 2002; Harris and Molock 2000; Joe and Kaplan 2001; King et al. 1990; Summerville et al. 1996). Gutierrez et al. (2001) suggested that Hispanic youth should be targeted for suicide prevention efforts, based on the higher prevalence of suicidal ideation and other risk factors for suicidal behavior, such as substance abuse, acculturative stress, and lower socioeconomic status, and on the high rates of suicide they identified in this study.

The high suicide rate among young men in Micronesia partially reflects their role confusion in a largely matriarchal society. With the change of the economy in Micronesia from agrarian to cash-based and the subsequent increase in unemployment, young male contributions to family subsistence declined, leading to the loss of a major male societal task. As the population urbanized, young people's access to extended family and a large social network began to suffer, and adolescent males found themselves in an increasingly unsupportive and unstructured environment (Tseng and Streltzer 1997).

Over the last 45 years, suicide rates have increased 60% globally. Traditionally, the rate was highest among elderly men, but it is now rivaled by the increasing rate among young people in a third of countries, both developing and developed (World Health Organization 2009). In the United States, the Suicide Prevention Resource Center (2005) reported that from 1999 through 2005, the highest rate of suicide was among those 70 years and older, 2.1 times the rate for those 15–19 years of age. In most Latin countries, as well as in some Asian nations (e.g., Hong Kong), social changes and the collapse of traditional family structures may have contributed to increases in suicide rates in older age. In Asia, for example, industrialization and Westernization have transformed traditional family life into nuclear family arrangements, which may produce in the elderly, once supported by the extended family, a state of social isolation (De Leo and Spathonis 2004).

Because the use of religion and spirituality as coping strategies tends to increase with age (Koenig et al. 1988), this may be a protective factor for the group. In contrast to such attitudes, the data are clear that most older adults who die by suicide were in some form of psychological distress and that major depression is the specific form of psychopathology most linked to elder suicide (Duberstein and Conwell 2000). In the older age groups, somatic illness and stressful life events are also common risk factors (Kung et al. 1998).

Ethnicity

Among racial groups, whites die by suicide twice as frequently as African Americans, although sharp increases have been reported in the suicide rate among young African American men (Kung et al. 1998; Suicide Prevention Resource Center 2005). In the multiethnic society of Hawaii, the rate of suicide varies considerably among different ethnic groups. This variation is reflected more sharply in the male population. From 1978 through 1982, the rate per 100,000 population was relatively higher among the Hawaiians (29.2) and Korean Americans (24.4) and relatively lower among the Filipino Americans (8.7) and the Chinese Americans (7.1), with whites (18.5) and Japanese Americans (11.7) in between (Tseng et al. 1992). These findings suggest greater differences than similarities among different ethnic-cultural groups, even though they shared the same geographical and social environment over a period of time (Tseng 2001).

Interactions between a minority group and the larger society of which it is a part also influence suicidality, often in complex ways. For instance, African American young adults may be more suicidal than older African Americans because they encounter intense discrimination at a time when they have not yet developed coping skills that have enabled their elders to survive (Seiden 1981). Attention should be paid, in considering suicide rates among various ethnic groups, to differences not only between individual ethnic groups but also between ethnic subgroups. For instance, Native Americans have an exceptionally high suicide rate. However, members of the Apache tribe have much higher rates than members of the Navajo and Pueblo tribes (Earls et al. 1991; Young 1991). Variations among tribes in the cultural acceptability of self-destructive behavior may explain some of the inter-tribal difference in suicide rates (Range et al. 1997; Young 1991).

The presence or absence of support networks in the community available to various ethnic groups also affects suicide rates; ethnic groups may differ, for example, in having viable social roles for the elderly. The elevated suicide rate in one study of elderly Chinese Americans may have been due to the social isolation among that cohort. In contrast, Native and African American groups may provide more satisfactory social roles for the elderly (Seiden 1981). The suicide rate among young Indian women is particularly higher than that among older Indian women (Banerjee et al. 1990). This finding has been explained by the relatively lower status of young women in traditional Hindu Indian culture and difficulties associated with the cultural practice of arranged marriage to a man of the parents' choice (Maniam 1988).

Cultural Attitudes Toward Suicide

Native American cultures have no strong sanctions against suicide, and some have actually favored altruistic suicidal acts (Davenport and Davenport 1987). Altruistic suicide is characterized by insufficient individualism, and its primary attributes are duty, moral obligations, and self-sacrifice for a higher cause, as illustrated in the Japanese kamikaze missions during World War II (Maris et al. 2000). Another example of altruistic suicide is presented in the following case example:

Case Example 2

Ernenek is an elderly Yuit Eskimo who lives in Seattle with his wife, Umiak; his adult son, Papik, and his wife; and a 6-month-old grandson, Amuzian. Papik is a computer programmer who was educated in the United States. As his parents aged, Papik arranged to bring them to his home. Ernenek's age and his years of hard outdoor work in the Arctic environment have taken their toll; Ernenek has no teeth, has difficulty walking and seeing, and is unable to work or even to help the family with any household work. Amuzian developed health problems, and Papik had to take time off work to help care for him. As a result, the family developed financial difficulties.

Ernenek considers himself useless and is particularly unhappy that he cannot even help care for his grandson. To spare the family the cost and effort of caring for him as well as Amuzian, he asks Umiak and Papik to shoot him. An intense, emotional discussion ensues; in Yuit culture this request is not unreasonable, but Papik refuses, in part because he has adopted mainstream U.S. societal views about suicide. The family agrees to go to the emergency department and discuss the situation with the psychiatrist there before taking any action.

In this culture, suicide is a social process; the decision to die and the carrying out of the necessary actions are done as a group, usually including the suicidal person's relatives and friends. In this nomadic hunting and gathering society, becoming old, sick, and dependent might mean placing the well-being and even survival of the family at risk. It is a common practice in this society for the individual contemplating suicide to request help from a family member in carrying out the plan. This request traditionally must be denied initially. However, if the request is repeated at least three times, it must be honored by the family. Suicide, when carried out in consideration of the welfare of the family and others in the group, is considered by the Yuit to be an act of respect, courage, and wisdom (Maris et al. 2000).

Hispanic Americans often have strong antisuicide attitudes deriving from the Roman Catholic Church, although this prohibition may not apply to some Hispanics (e.g., young Puerto Rican men) (Queralt 1993). Similarly, women from groups with strong religious prohibitions against suicide (e.g., Islamic cultures) have lower suicide rates than women from groups who have no strong prohibitions, such as Buddhists and Confucians (Kok 1988).

In Pakistan, suicidal behavior is socioculturally considered to be gravely wrong. By contrast, in some Asian cultures suicide is often considered to be altruistic. In Japan, people believe that if a person is willing to take his own life, he should be excused from any prior misbehavior or debt. Most European countries formally decriminalized suicide in the eighteenth and nineteenth centuries, although it remained a crime in England and Wales until 1961 and in Ireland until 1993 (Jamison 1999), and it continues to be recognized as a crime in several U.S. jurisdictions (Simon at al. 2005). Given the complexity of the risk factors and the increasingly multicultural nature of American society, identifying and clarifying the factors associated with suicide among cultural groups while adjusting for confounding factors could provide a valuable focus for further research (Kung et al. 1998).

Key Clinical Concepts[1]

- Develop general cultural competence in psychiatric evaluation.

- Become familiar with any special traditional suicidal behaviors that may exist in a cultural group.

- Explore the meaning of suicide from the patient's cultural point of view. Is it an act of sacrifice, a social statement, or an attempt to end personal suffering? It is important to avoid the projection of one's own value system onto the patient and to recognize that a seemingly trivial stressor, such as an argument with a parent, can have culturally magnified consequences.

- Be aware of the cultural context of help-seeking behavior and the varying expectations of the patient toward the clinician. Some people behave deferentially, others look to the evaluator for advice and guidance, and others need a safe place to express emotions. Avoid the assumption that the patient wants what the clinician would want in similar circumstance.

- Distinguish between suicidal behavior that is culturally sanctioned and that which is pathological. Treatable illness is strongly associated with suicide in all cultures, and even in societies that are tolerant of suicide there will always be individuals who, if prevented from killing themselves, will eventually be grateful for the intervention.

References

Alcántara C, Gone JP: Suicide in Native American communities: a transactional-ecological formulation of the problem, in Suicide Among Racial and Ethnic Groups: Theory, Research, and Practice. Edited by Leong FTL, Leach MM. New York, Routledge, 2008, pp 173–199

Andrade NN, Hishinuma ES, McDermott JF Jr, et al: The National Center on Indigenous Hawaiian Behavioral Health study of prevalence of psychiatric disorders in Native Hawaiian adolescents. J Am Acad Child Adolesc Psychiatry 45:26–36, 2006

Banerjee G, Nandi S, Sarkar S, et al: The vulnerability of Indian woman to suicide: a field study. Indian J Psychiatry 32:305–308, 1990

Barnouw V: Culture and Personality. Homewood, IL, Dorsey Press, 1963

Bernstein DM: Therapist-patient relations and ethnic transference, in Culture and Psychotherapy: A Guide to Clinical Practice. Edited by Tseng W-S, Streltzer J. Washington, DC, American Psychiatric Press, 2001, pp 103–121

Berry JW: Acculturation among circumpolar people: implications for health status. Arctic Med Res 40:21–27, 1985

Berry JW: Psychological and social health of Aboriginal people in Canada. Paper presented at the Workshop on Children's Mental Health and Wellness in First Nations Communities, Victoria, BC, Canada, 1993

---

[1]These key clinical concepts for the culturally competent management of suicidal patients are adapted from the work of Wen-Shing Tseng, M.D., of the University of Hawaii, who has spent 30 years instilling cultural competence in his students and residents.

Braun KL, Nichols R: Death and dying in four Asian American cultures: a descriptive study. Death Stud 21:327–359, 1997

Clayer JR, Czechowicz AS: Suicide by Aboriginal people in Australia: comparison with suicidal deaths in the total rural and urban population. Med J Aust 154:683–685, 1991

Comas-Diaz L: Cross-cultural mental health treatment, in Clinical Guidelines in Cross Cultural Mental Health. Edited by Comas-Diaz L, Griffith EEH. New York, Wiley, 1988, pp 335–361

Davenport JA, Davenport J: Native American suicide: a Durkheimian analysis. Soc Casework 68:533–539, 1987

De Leo D, Spathonis K: Culture and suicide in late life. Psychiatric Times 20:3, 2004

Duberstein PR, Conwell Y: Suicide, in Psychopathology in Later Adulthood. Edited by Whitbourne SK. New York, Wiley, 2000, pp 245–275

Durkheim E: Suicide: A Study in Sociology (1897). Translated by Spaulding JA, Simpson G. New York, Free Press, 1951

Dwairy M, Van Sickle T: Western psychotherapy in traditional Arabic societies. Clin Psychol Rev 16:231–249, 1996

Earls F, Escobar JI, Manson SM: Suicide in minority groups: epidemiological and cultural perspectives, in Suicide Over the Life Cycle. Edited by Blumenthal SJ, Kupfer DJ. Washington, DC, American Psychiatric Press, 1991, pp 571–589

Else IRN, Andrade NN: Examining suicide and suicide-related behaviors among indigenous Pacific Islanders in the United States: a historical perspective, in Suicide Among Racial and Ethnic Minority Groups: Theory, Research, and Practice. Edited by Leong FTL, Leach MM. New York, Routledge, 2008, pp 143–172

Eungprabhanth V: Suicide in Thailand. Forensic Sci 5:46–51, 1975

Ganapathi MN, Rao AV: A study of suicide in Madurai. J Indian Med Assoc 46:18–23, 1966

Garlow SJ, Purselle D, Heninger M: Ethnic differences in patterns of suicide across the life cycle. Am J Psychiatry 162:319–323, 2005

Gould MS, Kramer RA: Youth suicide prevention. Suicide Life Threat Behav 31:6–31, 2001

Greening L, Stoppelbein L: Religiosity, attributional style, and social support as psychosocial buffers for African American and white adolescents' perceived risk for suicide. Suicide Life Threat Behav 32:404–417, 2002

Grossi V, Violato C: Attempted suicide among adolescents: a stepwise discriminant analysis. Can J Behav Sci 24:410–412, 1992

Group for the Advancement of Psychiatry, Committee on Cultural Psychiatry: Suicide and Ethnicity in the United States. New York, Brunner/Mazel, 1989

Gutierrez P, Rodriguez PJ, Garcia P: Suicide risk factors for young adults: testing a model across ethnicities. Death Stud 25:319–340, 2001

Harris TL, Molock SD: Cultural orientation, family cohesion and family support in suicide ideation and depression among African American college students. Suicide Life Threat Behav 30:341–353, 2000

Hart EE, Williams CL: Suicidal behaviour and interpersonal network. Crisis 8:112–124, 1987

Hasselback P, Lee KI, Mao Y, et al: The relationship of suicide rates to sociodemographic factors in Canadian census divisions. Can J Psychiatry 36:655–659, 1991

Hawton K: Suicide and Attempted Suicide Among Children and Adolescents. Newbury Park, CA, Sage, 1986

Jamison KR: Night Falls Fast: Understanding Suicide. New York, Knopf, 1999

Javier R, Yussef M: A Latino perspective on the role of ethnicity in the development of moral values: implications for psychoanalytic theory and practice. J Am Acad Psychoanal 23:79–97, 1995

Joe S, Kaplan M: Suicide among African American men. Suicide Life Threat Behav 31:106–131, 2001

Johansson LM, Johansson SE, Bergman B, et al: Suicide, ethnicity and psychiatric in-patient care: a case-control study. Arch Suicide Res 3:253–269, 1997

Kettl PA, Bixler EO: Suicide in Alaska Natives, 1979–1984. Psychiatry 54:55–63, 1991

Kim BS, Ng GF, Ahn AJ: Effects of client expectation for counseling success, client-counselor worldview match, and client adherence to Asian and European American cultural values on counseling process with Asian Americans. J Couns Psychol 52:67–76, 2005

King CA, Raskin A, Gdowski CL, et al: Psychosocial factors associated with urban adolescent female suicide attempts. J Am Acad Child Adolesc Psychiatry 29:289–294, 1990

Kirmayer LJ, Malus M, Delage M, et al: Characteristics of Completed Suicides Among the Inuit of East Coast of Hudson Bay, 1982 to 1991: Chart Review Study (Culture and Mental Health Research Unit Report No 4). Montreal, Quebec, Canada, Institute of Community and Family Psychiatry, Sir Mortimer B. Davis– Jewish General Hospital, 1994

Koenig H, George L, Siegler I: The use of religion and other emotion-regulating coping strategies among older adults. Gerontologist 28:303–310, 1998

Kok LP: Race, religion and female suicide attempters in Singapore. Soc Psychiatry Psychiatr Epidemiol 23:236–239, 1988

Kung HC, Liu X, Juon HS: Risk factors for suicide in Caucasians and in African-Americans: a matched case-control study. Soc Psychiatry Psychiatr Epidemiol 33:155–161, 1998

Ladrido-Ignacio L, Gensaya JP: Suicidal behavior in Manila, Philippines, in Suicidal Behavior in the Asia-Pacific Region. Edited by Kok LP, Tseng W-S. Singapore, Singapore University, 1992, pp 112–126

Latha KS, Bhat SM, D'Souza P: Suicide attempters in a general hospital unit in India: their socio-demographic and clinical profile— emphasis on cross-cultural aspects. Acta Psychiatr Scand 94:26–30, 1996

Lee CS, Chang JC, Cheng ATA: Acculturation and suicide: a case-control psychological autopsy study. Psychol Med 32:133–144, 2002

Leong FTL, Leach MM, Gupta A: Suicide among American Asians, in Suicide Among Racial and Ethnic Minority Groups: Theory, Research, and Practice. Edited by Leong FTL, Leach MM. New York, Routledge, 2008, pp 117–141

Linton R: Acculturation in Seven American Indian Tribes. New York, Appleton-Century Company, 1940

Liu SI, Cheng ATA: Alcohol use disorders among the Yami aborigines in Taiwan: an inter-ethnic comparison. Br J Psychiatry 172:168–174, 1998

Magne-Ingvar U, Ojehagen A, Träskman-Bendz L: The social network of people who attempt suicide. Acta Psychiatr Scand 86:153–158, 1992

Malchy B, Enns MW, Young TK, et al: Suicide among Manitoba's aboriginal people, 1988 to 1994. CMAJ 156:1133–1138, 1997

Malus M, Kirmayer LJ, Boothroyd L: Risk factors of suicide among Inuit youth: a community survey (Culture and Mental Health Research Unit Report No 3). Montreal, Quebec, Canada, Institute of Community and Family Psychiatry, Sir Mortimer B. Davis–Jewish General Hospital, 1994

Maniam T: Suicide and parasuicide in hill resort in Malaysia. Br J Psychiatry 153:222–225, 1988

Maris RW, Berman AL, Silverman MM (eds): Comprehensive Textbook of Suicidology. New York, Guilford, 2000, pp 170–191

Mass M, Al-Krenawi A: When a man encounters a woman, Satan is also present: clinical relationships in Bedouin society. Am J Orthopsychiatry 64:357–367, 1994

Mavreas V, Bebbington P: Acculturation and psychiatric disorder: a study of Greek Cypriot immigrants. Psychol Med 20:941–951, 1990

Neff JA, Hoppe SK: Acculturation and drinking patterns among U.S. Anglos, blacks, and Mexican Americans. Alcohol Alcohol 27:293–308, 1992

Payne IR, Bergin AE, Bielema KA, et al: Review of religion and mental health: prevention and enhancement of psychosocial functioning. Prev Hum Serv 9:11–40, 1991

Pescosolido B, Georgianna S: Durkheim, suicide and religion: toward a network theory of suicide. Am Sociol Rev 54:33–48, 1989

Queralt M: Risk factors associated with completed suicide in Latino adolescents. Adolescence 28:831–850, 1993

Range LM, MacIntyre DI, Rutherford D, et al: Suicide in special populations and circumstances: a review. Aggress Violent Behav 2:53–63, 1997

Redfield R, Linton R, Herskovits MJ: Memorandum for the study of acculturation. Am Anthropol 38:149–152, 1936

Rogler LH, Cortes DE, Malgady RG: Acculturation and mental health status among Hispanics: convergence and new directions for research. Am Psychol 46:585–597, 1991

Seiden RH: Mellowing with age: factors influencing the nonwhite suicide rate. Int J Aging Hum Dev 13:265–284, 1981

Shaffer D, Garland A, Gould M, et al: Preventing teenage suicide: a critical review. J Am Acad Child Adolesc Psychiatry 27:675–687, 1988

Shaffer D, Gould M, Hicks RC: Worsening suicide rate in black teenagers. Am J Psychiatry 151:1810–1812, 1994

Simon RI: Assessing and Managing Suicide Risk: Guidelines for Clinically Based Risk Management. Washington, DC, American Psychiatric Publishing, 2004

Simon RI, Levenson JL, Shuman DW: On Sound and Unsound Mind: The Role of Suicide in Tort and Insurance Litigation. J Am Acad Psychiatry Law 33:176–182, 2005

Skegg K, Cox B, Broughton J: Suicide among New Zealand Maori: is history repeating itself? Acta Psychiatr Scand 92:453–459, 1995

Stack S: The effects of religious commitment on suicide: a cross-national analysis. J Health Soc Behav 24:362–374, 1983

Stack S: Marriage, family, religion and suicide, in Assessment and Prediction of Suicide. Edited by Marris RW, Berman AL, Maltsberger JT, et al. New York, Guilford, 1992, pp 540–552

Stack S: Suicide: a 15-year review of the sociological literature, Part II: modernization and social integration perspectives. Suicide Life Threat Behav 30:163–176, 2000

Stack S, Lester D: The effect of religion on suicide. Soc Psychiatry Psychiatr Epidemiol 26:168–170, 1991

Suicide Prevention Resource Center: Suicide among black Americans. 2005. Available at: http://www.sprc.org/library/black.am.facts.pdf. Accessed June 20, 2011.

Summerville MB, Kaslow NJ, Doepke KJ: Psychopathology and cognitive and family functioning in suicidal African American adolescents. Curr Dir Psychol Sci 5:7–11, 1996

Takahashi Y, Hirasawa H, Koyama K, et al: Suicide in Japan: present state and future directions for prevention. Transcult Psychiatry 35:271–289, 1998

Tallis F: Love Sick: Love as Mental Illness. New York, Thunder's Mouth Press, 2000

Thorslund J: Inuit suicides in Greenland. Artic Med Res 49:25–33, 1990

Trovato F: Interprovincial migration and suicide in Canada, 1971–1978. Int J Soc Psychiatry 32:14–21, 1986

Trovato F: Sex, marital status and suicide in Canada: 1951–1981. Sociol Perspect 34:427–445, 1991

Tseng W-S: Handbook of Cultural Psychiatry. San Diego, CA, Academic Press, 2001

Tseng W-S, Kok LP: Comparison of reports from Asia and the Pacific, in Suicidal Behavior in the Asia-Pacific Region. Edited by Kok LP, Tseng W-S. Singapore, Singapore University, 1992, pp 249–265

Tseng W-S, Streltzer J (eds): Culture and Psychopathology. New York, Brunner/Mazel, 1997

Tseng W-S, Streltzer J (eds): Cultural Competence in Clinical Psychiatry. Washington, DC, American Psychiatric Publishing, 2004

Tseng W-S, Hsu J, Omori A, et al: Suicidal behavior in Hawaii, in Suicidal Behavior in the Asia-Pacific Region. Edited by Kok LP, Tseng W-S. Singapore, Singapore University, 1992, pp 238–248

Tseng W-S, Ebata K, Kim KI, et al: Mental health in Asia: social improvement and challenges. Int J Soc Psychiatry 4:8–23, 2001

Uba L: Asian Americans: Personality Patterns, Identity and Mental Health. New York, Guilford, 1994

Walker RL, Townley GE, Asiamah DD: Suicide prevention in U.S. ethnic minority populations, in Suicide Among Racial and Ethnic Minority Groups: Theory, Research, and Practice. Edited by Leong FTL, Leach MM. New York, Routledge, 2008, pp 203–227

Wasserman IM: Economy, work, occupation and suicide, in Assessment and Prediction of Suicide. Edited by Maris RW, Berman AL, Maltsberger JT, et al. New York, Guilford, 1992, pp 520–539

Weissman MM: The epidemiology of suicide attempts, 1960 to 1971. Arch Gen Psychiatry 30:737–746, 1974

Wong OC, Piran N: Western biases and assumptions as impediments in counseling traditional Chinese clients. Canadian Journal of Counseling 29:107–119, 1995

World Health Organization: Suicide rates per 100,000 by country, year, and sex. 2009. Available at: http://www.who.int/mental_health/prevention/suicide_rates. Accessed June 20, 2011.

Yoshimatsu K: Suicidal behavior in Japan, in Suicidal Behavior in the Asia-Pacific Region. Edited by Kok LP, Tseng W-S. Singapore, Singapore University, 1992, pp 15–40

Young TJ: Suicide and homicide among Native Americans: anomie or social learning? Psychol Rep 68:1137–1138, 1991

Zhang J: Suicide in Beijing, China, 1992–1993. Suicide Life Threat Behav 26:175–180, 1996

CHAPTER 5

Psychological Testing in Suicide Risk Management

Glenn R. Sullivan, Ph.D.

Bruce Bongar, Ph.D., A.B.P.P., F.A.P.M.

The ultimate challenge and responsibility of suicide risk assessment is the elimination of false negatives—that is, the misclassification of suicidal people as nonsuicidal. This process is fraught with both personal and professional anxiety on the part of the mental health professional. The use of psychological testing is a common approach to managing this anxiety. In this chapter, we review some of the most commonly used psychological tests, suicide scales, and risk estimators and offer suggestions regarding their role in suicide risk assessment.

Most clinicians rely primarily on the clinical interview and certain valued questions and observations to assess suicide risk. Traditional psychological tests, such as the Minnesota Multiphasic Personality Inventory–2 (MMPI-2; Greene 2000), Rorschach Inkblot Test (Exner 2003), and Beck Depression Inventory (BDI; Beck et al. 1996), are used by less than half of psychologists, psychiatrists, and clinical social workers who evaluate suicidal adults and adolescents

(Jobes et al. 1995). Suicide assessment instruments such as the Beck Hopelessness Scale (BHS; Beck and Steer 1988) and the Beck Suicide Intent Scale (Beck et al. 1974) are considered by practitioners to be somewhat more useful in the evaluation of suicide risk than traditional psychological tests, but only a minority of practitioners routinely use them (Jobes et al. 1995).

Suicide is too complex a behavior to be adequately captured by a single sign or score (Eyman and Eyman 1991). Assessment of a patient's risk for suicide should never be based solely on the results of psychological testing. A complete evaluation of risk factors, such as the patient's psychiatric diagnosis, previous suicide attempts, substance abuse, family history of suicide, social isolation, physical illness, perceived burden to others, and availability of lethal means (especially firearms), should be considered in conjunction with psychological assessment results (Maris et al. 1992). Demographic risk factors, including gender, age, race/ethnicity, and religious beliefs, must also be considered when assessing a patient's suicide potential.

Since Pokorny published his work on suicide prediction in 1983, it has become increasingly clear that the critical issue for clinicians and researchers is not the *prediction* of suicide but rather the assessment of suicide *risk* (Pokorny 1983). For a variety of reasons, the low base rates of completed suicide in both clinical and general populations make it statistically impossible to develop a test or scale that can accurately predict whether a given individual will die by suicide over the long term. Despite this difficulty, the ability to predict suicide is perceived by the courts and public to be a prime competency of mental health practitioners and perhaps their most salient duty. Within that context, psychological tests and scales can be employed effectively to assist in the identification of individuals at increased risk for self-harm.

Table 5–1 briefly describes the tests and scales discussed in this chapter.

Minnesota Multiphasic Personality Inventory–2

The MMPI-2 is the most widely used instrument for assessing psychopathology in clinical practice (Greene 2000). Inconsistent findings of retrospective comparisons of suicide attempters and nonattempting comparison groups have led some researchers to conclude that despite considerable research effort, no item, scale, or profile configuration on the original MMPI consistently differentiated suicidal and nonsuicidal patients. Initial hopes that the restandardized MMPI-2 would provide more valid indicators of suicidality have yet to be realized. Nevertheless, when used properly, the MMPI-2 can be an important tool in the as-

sessment of suicide risk, if not the prediction of actual completed or attempted suicide.

The 567-item MMPI-2 represents a significant time investment for both administration (90% of patients complete the test in 90 minutes or less; Greene 2000) and interpretation (which should be performed by a qualified clinical psychologist). However, this method can provide important data about a patient's subjective experience that are usually not collected in a standard clinical interview. Psychological tests such as the MMPI-2 should be viewed as providing the clinician with hypotheses that can be verified with other methods (Osborne 1985). These other methods could include other psychological tests, suicide scales and risk estimators, and a comprehensive clinical interview and history (Hendren 1990).

Clinical Scales

The MMPI-2 (and the earlier version of the test, the MMPI) is composed of 10 basic clinical scales that measure a broad band of psychopathology. The two highest elevations on these clinical scales determine a patient's MMPI-2 code type. Elevations in scores on scale 2 (Depression) of the MMPI were frequently associated with a preoccupation with death and suicide (Dahlstrom et al. 1972). Clopton (1974) noted that "the one standard MMPI scale found most frequently to differentiate suicidal and nonsuicidal groups is scale 2" (p. 129). Agreeing with that assertion, Meyer (1993) stated that the prototypical pattern for suicidal individuals is the 2–7/7–2 code type (Depression and Psychasthenia). People with this code type are described as anxious, tense, and depressed. Suicidal ideation and attempts are "fairly likely" among persons with the 2–7/7–2 code type (Greene 2000).

It should give clinicians pause that the 2–7/7–2 code type is the third most fre-

TABLE 5–1. Brief descriptions of tests/scales discussed

Test/Scale	Description	Administered by
Minnesota Multiphasic Personality Inventory–2	567 true/false items yielding scores on 10 clinical scales (e.g., Psychopathic Deviancy, Depression, Paranoia), 14 content scales (e.g., Anger, Low Self-Esteem, Family Problems), and validity scales that detect attempts to overreport or underreport psychopathology. Most patients complete in 90 minutes or less.	Clinical psychologist only
Rorschach Inkblot Test	10 stimulus cards presented to patients whose verbatim responses are recorded by administrator. Well-established ability to detect psychotic processes. Suicide Constellation scale has potential for predicting future suicidal behavior. Administration takes about 45 minutes, and scoring/interpretation takes about 90 minutes.	Clinical psychologist only
Beck Depression Inventory—Revised (BDI-II)	21-item self-report inventory completed by patient in about 5 minutes. Each item has four rating options used to describe how the patient has been feeling or behaving over the past 2 weeks. Can be used to track depressive symptom severity over course of treatment.	Any trained mental health professional
Beck Hopelessness Scale (BHS)	20-item true/false self-report inventory completed by patient in about 5 minutes. BHS scores are more strongly related to suicidal behavior than BDI-II scores, but it is recommended that both be used in combination.	Any trained mental health professional
Scale for Suicide Ideation	19-item rating scale completed by a trained clinician. Measures suicidal desire (active and passive) and suicide preparation.	Any trained mental health professional
Firestone Assessment for Self-Destructive Thoughts	84-item self-report inventory that measures intensity and scope of self-destructive thoughts. Potential use involves identifying and targeting maladaptive cognitions for more effective cognitive therapy.	Clinical psychologist only
Linehan Reasons for Living Inventory (LRFL)	Various versions of the LRFL are available in the public domain (e.g., 48-item, 72-item, college student). Can be completed by patient in about 10 minutes. Takes a positive approach that focuses on reasons for not killing oneself rather than on the intensity of one's suicidal thoughts.	Any trained mental health professional
Risk Estimator for Suicide	An empirically derived, 15-item scale based on patient psychosocial variables that provides a risk rating for suicidal behavior within the next 2 years. Predictive validity not well established.	Any trained mental health professional

quently observed code type in the Caldwell clinical data set, an aggregation of more than 50,000 MMPI patient profiles (Greene 2000). Over 21% of men and nearly 20% of women with that code type endorse at least one of the "I mean business" items that directly assess suicidal intent on the MMPI-2 (Sepaher et al. 1999). The clinical presentation of these patients centers on anxious depression. They are hyperresponsible, worried, tense, and guilt-ridden; they feel inadequate, lack self-confidence, have problems with work effectiveness, and have disturbed sleep. In other words, they seem to be similar in many respects to the "typical" patient treated with antidepressants or anxiolytics by general practitioners.

Meyer (1993) pointed out that the likelihood of suicidal ideation resulting in an attempt increases as scores on scales 4 (Psychopathic Deviancy), 8 (Schizophrenia), and 9 (Hypomania) rise. The increased elevations on these scales reflect greater impulsivity and/or resentment (scale 4), heightened alienation from self and others (scale 8), and increased energy to carry out a suicide attempt (scale 9). Based on data from Sepaher et al. (1999), and drawing from a wide range of MMPI-2 sources, Table 5–2 presents suicide-relevant patient descriptions for 14 MMPI-2 code types. Taken together, these 14 elevated-risk code types represent nearly 41% of the patients in a very large clinical MMPI-2 data set.

Content Scales and Critical Items

The results of a survey of specialists who use the MMPI-2 to assess suicide risk revealed that among the Validity scales, high F (a measure of distress) and high L (a potential sign of overcontrol or denial) scores were both considered important variables to examine (Glassmire et al. 1999). However, K scores were rated as important to exam-

ine regardless of whether they were high (suggestive of overcontrol or denial) or low (indicating poor coping resources). The clinical scales most frequently cited by these experts as important in evaluating suicide risk were scale 2 (Depression), followed by scale 4 (Psychopathic Deviancy) and finally scale 8 (Schizophrenia). Examination of the 14 elevated-risk code types described in Table 5–2 confirms the experts' consensus, because only two of those code types do not include scale 2, 4, or 8 (2–3/3–2 and 3–6/6–3).

Extreme elevation of any clinical scale or the elevation of multiple scales also warrants careful review. The MMPI-2 content scales most often cited by experts were DEP (Depression), followed by ANG (Anger) and MAC-R (MacAndrews Alcoholism). The Content Component scale DEP4 (Suicidal Ideation) was also cited by these experts as useful.

The MMPI-2's five-item DEP4 (Suicidal Ideation) Content Component scale is regarded by many clinicians as highly useful when assessing suicide risk. However, there is a need for empirical studies of the association between this MMPI-2 scale and actual patient suicidal behaviors. The DEP4 scale is thought to assess "a pessimism about the future that is so dire as to support a wish to die and thoughts of suicide" (Greene 2000, p. 190). In addition to three of the six MMPI-2 suicide content items (303, 506, and 520), the DEP4 scale contains item 454 (pertaining to hopelessness about the future) and item 546 (pertaining to morbid thoughts about death and dying). We strongly caution clinicians to remember that a raw score of zero on DEP4 or a negative finding on any other suicide scale or indicator does *not* indicate the absence of suicide risk. For some patients, refusal to acknowledge suicidal ideation or intent on psychological testing may represent not an absence of suicidal intent, but rather a particularly strong determination to die.

The MMPI-2's Koss-Butcher Critical Item Set—Revised lists 22 items that are related specifically to depressed suicidal ideation. However, Butcher (1989) noted that these critical items are not "designed to operate as scales. They are used to highlight item content that might be particularly significant in the individual's case. As sources of clinical hypotheses, the critical items might be used to key the clinician into problem areas or concerns the patient may have" (p. 17).

Six items on the MMPI-2 directly inquire about suicidal ideation or behavior. These items address impulses to self-harm (item 150), recent suicidal ideation (506 and 520), desire for death (303), history of concealed past attempts (524), and current deliberate self-harm (530). Sepaher et al. (1999) found endorsement base rates of approximately 20% or more for two of the most direct MMPI-2 suicide items (506 and 520) among nine different well-defined MMPI-2 code types. These researchers dubbed these two items the "I mean business" items because patient endorsement directly communicates current suicidal intent. In their study, none of the patients who verbally endorsed the interview question "Are you currently suicidal?" failed to endorse item 506, and only 1% of those patients failed to endorse item 520.

Kaplan et al. (1994) found that many patients tend to disclose more information regarding recent suicidal ideation on self-report forms than they do in clinical face-to-face interviews. Glassmire et al. (2001) found that psychotherapy outpatients who failed to endorse suicidal ideation or behaviors during direct clinical inquiry often endorsed suicide-related items on the MMPI-2. This suggests that certain MMPI-2 items have greater sensitivity for the de-

tection of suicide potential than even direct verbal inquiry.

These findings have important risk management implications because they suggest that—at a minimum—clinicians should always review the six MMPI-2 suicide items, particularly items 506 and 520, even when clients do not report depressed mood, current suicidal ideation, or past suicidal behavior. We feel that these findings also suggest that comprehensive suicide risk management should involve multimethod assessment that includes more than a clinical interview. It may be easier for suicidal patients to endorse their self-destructive thoughts within the "confessional" of a paper-and-pencil test than before the potentially judgmental eyes of a clinician.

Rorschach Inkblot Test

Historically, the Rorschach technique was the most commonly used method for estimating the risk of suicide, although use of the instrument has declined steadily in recent years because of the low reimbursement rates for psychological testing under managed care, controversy over the test's psychometric attributes (e.g., Wood et al. 1996), and reduced opportunities for obtaining Rorschach training in clinical psychology doctoral programs.

The Rorschach may still be a potent tool for assessing suicide risk, if it is used correctly. Among the recent changes to the Rorschach Comprehensive System (Exner 2003) is the inclusion of a Suicide Constellation (S-CON) among the Rorschach special indices. The S-CON consists of 12 variables and highlights certain features that are common in the Rorschach protocols of individuals who completed suicide within 60 days of test administration. A total of 101 individual protocols now compose the S-CON data set, an increase from the original

TABLE 5–2. Suicide-relevant patient descriptions for 14 MMPI-2 code types

Code type/ Prevalence	Patient description	Endorsement of items 506 and 520
6–8/8–6 5.48%	Serious psychopathology; paranoid schizophrenia is a diagnosis traditionally associated with this code type. Likely history of prior psychiatric hospitalizations. Poor reality contact; perceived as strange, distrustful. May be preoccupied with self-protection.	47% men 46% women
2–8/8–2 3.05%	Depression that is perhaps psychotic or near-psychotic in severity. Social withdrawal, agitation, and difficulty concentrating. Impulse control deteriorating and losing the will to live.	35% men 41% women
7–8/8–7 3.59%	Acute psychic turmoil. Difficulty concentrating, tense, agitated. Insomnia and potential for impulsive suicidal behavior or self-mutilation. They feel fundamentally defective. Alcohol abuse is likely.	32% men 27% women
3–8/8–3 1.25%	Code type suggests use of hysterical defenses to ward off underlying psychotic processes. They desperately need affection but drive others away with their strange and immature approaches. Dissociative episodes or even brief episodes of acute psychosis may be observed, especially when patient is feeling threatened.	28% men 29% women
1–8/8–1 1.44%	Somatic delusions or varied somatic complaints or preoccupations that serve to ward off psychotic episodes. Socially and sexually maladjusted. Emotional constriction and flatness alternates with spells of explosive anger when feeling "cornered."	24% men 27% women
4–8/8–4 1.97%	Likely either psychotic or severe personality disorder (e.g., borderline). Alienated from others, unpredictable, hostile. Impulsive acting out, self-destructive behavior, and substance abuse are all associated with this code type. Possible history of sexual abuse. Intense anger and a sense of being irredeemably "damaged."	23% men 30% women
2–7/7–2 5.49%	Anxious and depressed. Apprehensive, tense, and intensely self-reproaching. They engage in ruthless self-examination of their flaws and deficiencies. They take on too much because they can't say no, and then they feel as if they have let everyone down.	22% men 19% women
2–6/6–2 3.14%	"Martyred depression." They blame their current problems on other people's poor treatment of them. They accumulate and catalog their resentments. They feel trapped and reject others before they can be rejected.	20% men 23% women
2–4/4–2 2.43%	Depressed, angry, and frustrated. Perhaps an impulsive, alcohol-abusing, hostile thug who is depressed because he is being constrained within the correctional system. For individuals with this code type, substance abuse is very likely, and suicide might be envisioned as a way to "settle a score."	16% men 21% women

TABLE 5–2. Suicide-relevant patient descriptions for 14 MMPI-2 code types *(continued)*

Code type/ Prevalence	Patient description	Endorsement of items 506 and 520
6–7/7–6 1.40%	Hypersensitive to actual or perceived criticism or judgment. Thin-skinned and resentful. They feel wronged by others and may launch preemptive attacks, criticizing others before they can be criticized themselves. Severely strained interpersonal relations.	20% men 16% women
8–0/0–8 0.27%	Socially isolated and anhedonic. Absorbed in personal fantasies. Often silent, as if drawn into a defensive cocoon. They feel misunderstood and are often confused by their own thoughts and feelings.	23% men 11% women
3–6/6–3 2.08%	On the surface, they are exquisitely appropriate in word, deed, and appearance. They seek approval, fear criticism, and harbor intense resentments that episodically erupt when their rigid self-control breaks down. They can be morally rigid and defensive.	16% men 16% women
8–9/9–8 1.20%	Insomnia, flight of ideas, distractibility, and agitation. Severe sense of inferiority, of being "broken." They fear intimacy. Religious delusions or paranoid ideation may be present.	14% men 18% women
2–3/3–2 8.07%	This profile could represent a "smiling depression" made possible by hysterical defenses. They might complain of fatigue, somatic problems, inefficiency at work, and being unappreciated. However, they have great difficulty expressing any underlying anger or depression.	15% men 16% women

Note. MMPI-2=Minnesota Multiphasic Personality Inventory–2. MMPI items 506 and 520 directly inquire about recent suicidal ideation.
Source. Adapted from Sepaher et al. 1999 and various MMPI-2 interpretive manuals, including Greene 2000; Friedman et al. 2001; and Graham 2005. Prevalence rates from Caldwell clinical data set (N=50,966), as reported in Greene 2000.

59 individuals whose protocols were first used to develop the index in the 1970s.

Exner (2000) stated that proper interpretation of the Rorschach protocol of any person age 15 or older must begin with the scoring and review of the S-CON index. The endorsement of 8 of the 12 variables of the S-CON can serve as a red flag to warn a psychologist that commonalities exist between the patient being tested and the 101 suicide completers. Exner (2000) cautioned strongly that a score of less than 8 does not ensure that an individual will not attempt or complete suicide. In fact, the suicide sample was found to contain approximately 20%–25% false-negative records. Hence, an endorsement of 7, or even 6, S-CON variables should prompt the clinician to carefully rescore the protocol and to attend to the possibility of self-destructive preoccupation. Many of the items in the original adult S-CON contained variables that were developmentally normal for children and adolescents. To date, efforts to develop a child/adolescent version of S-CON have been disappointing.

Fowler et al. (2001) found that S-CON scores of 7 or greater predicted near-lethal suicide attempts in a highly disturbed inpatient population, with an impressive 81%

accuracy. In addition, S-CON scores differentiated near-lethal attempters from parasuicidal patients (e.g., superficial wristcutters). S-CON scores in this study were independent of demographic or diagnostic variables and were not mere artifacts of impulsivity or psychotic disturbance. Further, Fowler et al. presented data that show a superior overall classification rate for the S-CON (0.86) compared with paper-and-pencil instruments such as the BHS (0.51).

A detailed discussion of the conceptual foundations of the Rorschach variables that are indicative of potential suicide risk is beyond the scope of this chapter (for review, see Exner 2003; Eyman and Eyman 1991; Meyer 1993). Lundbäck et al. (2006) presented data that trace the association between Rorschach S-CON scores and cerebrospinal fluid (CSF) 5-hydroxyindoleacetic acid (5-HIAA) levels in 38 hospitalized suicide attempters. These authors contended that Vista responses (a key component of the S-CON) "play an important role for the correlation" between S-CON scores and CSF 5-HIAA levels ($r=-0.517$, $P=0.033$). Vista responses to Rorschach stimuli involve dimension or depth (e.g., "It looks like staring down a well—it's so black. Must be deep. Nasty slime on the walls. Good luck climbing out of that one."). Vista responses are commonly interpreted as reflecting painful self-examination (e.g., "I am looking inside myself and I am shamed or disgusted by what I see."). Based on their findings, Lundbäck et al. (2006) proposed that a biologically based vulnerability to shame may increase suicide risk.

Whenever overt (e.g., "It looks like a man hanging from a bridge") or covert (e.g., "A broken-down wreck of something") suicidal content is provided during the administration of a Rorschach test (or any other projective test), it should be viewed as a possible indication of self-destructive intent. In these cases, it should be assumed that the patient has used the Rorschach administration to communicate suicidal intent or feelings (Neuringer 1974).

At this point, it is appropriate to comment on the production of false positives when using psychological testing in the assessment of suicide risk. Historically, much concern has been expressed about the importance of minimizing the number of false-positive identifications (i.e., the percentage of nonsuicidal patients misclassified as suicidal). In our opinion, it is possible for this concern to be overstated. Realistically, the negative consequences are limited for a patient who completes a psychological test or screen in a manner similar to that of suicidal patients but who is not actually suicidal. It is highly unlikely that an unjustified involuntary hospitalization or inappropriate psychopharmacological intervention would result solely from a score on a suicide risk scale. If done frankly and within the context of the clinician's concern for the patient's safety, the communication of positive test findings should not damage the therapeutic alliance.

A conservative stance on the matter of false positives acknowledges that the purpose of testing is the assessment of risk, not the prediction of suicide, and that *all* patients who seek the services of mental health professionals are, in varying degrees, at elevated risk for suicide. As a rule, it is better to overreact (in the direction of providing additional patient care) and be proved wrong than to underreact and be proved wrong (in the form of a patient's suicidal behavior).

Other Measures

There continues to be enormous interest in the development of suicide risk scales and estimators. Contemporary efforts at scale construction began in 1963 when the Los Angeles Suicide Prevention Center developed a special scale for assessing callers to their center (Farberow et al. 1968). Although scales that employ demographic and clinical characteristics of patients have been widely used by suicide prevention and crisis centers, such instruments remain primarily useful "as research tools rather than aids for the front-line clinician" (Motto 1989, p. 133).

Motto (1989) noted that methodological and practical problems have plagued the development of scales of suicide risk

> to the point of discouraging even devoted and experienced workers in the field of suicide prevention....These obstacles have been small samples, limited data, a low base rate, nongeneralizability of critical stressors, the individual uniqueness of suicidal persons, unknown and uncontrollable variables that contribute to outcome, ambiguity of outcome (e.g., "suicidal behavior"), and problems of demonstrating reliability and especially validity. (p. 133)

Nevertheless, an abundance of suicide assessment measures are available to clinicians. None of these, however (with the possible exception of the BDI), has attained common and widespread use.

One probable explanation for the lack of impact of such scales, collectively or individually, is that in their development, "little attention was paid to providing clinicians with a simple, brief procedure that could be quickly translated into a clear indication of suicide risk" (Motto 1989, p. 134). However, there have recently been many attempts to construct clinically useful screening instruments for use by the clinician. One review included more than 35 suicide assessments (Rogers and Oney 2005). The following examples are meant to be representative of this approach to the assessment of suicide

rather than an exhaustive listing of all available instruments.

Beck Depression Inventory and Beck Hopelessness Scale

The revised Beck Depression Inventory (BDI-II; Beck et al. 1996) consists of 21 items designed to assess the severity of depression in adolescents and adults. Each item is rated on a three-point scale, so total scores can range from 0 (no reported symptoms of depression) to 63 (extreme symptom endorsement). Scores from 0 to 13 indicate minimal depression; 14–19, mild depression; 20–28, moderate depression; and 29–63, severe depression. The BDI-II is a clear and concise instrument that enables patients to self-report depressive symptoms in less than 10 minutes. The BDI-II supplants the original BDI, which over the past 30 years became one of the most widely accepted and used instruments for assessing depression.

In addition to the overall level of depression, it is important to attend to specific item content, particularly the item that directly assesses suicidal ideation (item 9). Beck et al. (1985) also emphasized the importance of the BDI's Pessimism item (item 2) in the prediction of eventual suicide. In fact, on the BDI, pessimism is a more powerful predictor of suicidal behavior than suicidal ideation. The possible mediating effect of pessimism/hopelessness on suicidality contributed to the development of the BHS, a set of 20 true-or-false items that measure three major aspects of hopelessness: feelings about the future, loss of motivation, and expectations. Beck et al. (1985) reported that BHS scores of 9 or more were predictive of eventual suicide in 10 out of 11 depressed suicide ideators who were followed for 5–10 years after discharge from the hospital. In a subsequent study of outpatients (Beck et al.

1990), a BHS cutoff score of 9 or above identified 16 of the 17 eventual suicides (94.2%). The outpatients in the high-risk group identified by this cutoff score were 11 times more likely to die by suicide than the rest of the outpatients. These findings strongly suggest that hopelessness is an even stronger predictor of suicidal intention than severity of depressive symptoms.

Beck and Steer (1988) provided a vivid case example that demonstrates the complexities involved in using the BHS and BDI as predictors of suicide during therapy. At the time of his evaluation, the patient presented with severe depression and hopelessness but denied suicidal ideation. Over the course of three subsequent sessions, the tests were readministered; his BHS score held steady (at 20) but his BDI score dropped from 45 on intake to 35 and then rose only to 37 by the third session. The case of this patient, who killed himself 3 days prior to the next scheduled appointment, demonstrates that "in the presence of a high BHS and dropping BDI, a psychotherapist should be alert to the possibility of a suicide attempt" (Beck and Steer 1988, p. 22).

Direct verbal inquiry about specific responses to BHS items is recommended, because clinical exploration of these responses may allow the patient to acknowledge suicidal intent, may erode pervasive hopelessness, and may foster therapeutic collaboration (Beck and Steer 1988). Young et al. (1996) reported that stable levels of hopelessness over time could be more predictive of suicide attempts in patients with remitted depression than a high level of current hopelessness at any one point in time.

Beck's Scale for Suicide Ideation

Beck and colleagues also developed an important and widely adopted scale specifi-cally developed for the measurement of suicidal ideation and intent: the Scale for Suicide Ideation (SSI; Beck et al. 1979). The SSI is a 19-item rating scale that a trained clinician can use to measure the intensity of a patient's current suicidal ideation. Each item presents three options graded on a three-point scale ranging from 0 (low suicidal intensity) to 2 (high suicidal intensity). The ratings for the 19 items are summed to yield a total score ranging from 0 to 38.

Factor analysis has revealed three factors measured by the SSI: 1) active suicidal desire (e.g., attitudes toward living or dying), 2) suicide preparation (e.g., acquisition of lethal means, writing of a suicide note), and 3) passive suicidal desire (e.g., concealment of plans, avoidance of help) (Reinecke and Franklin-Scott 2005). Patients who scored 3 or higher on the SSI have been found to be seven times more likely to kill themselves than those who scored less than 3 (Brown et al. 2000). Rather than employing cutoff scores, however, it is recommended that any positive response to an SSI item be immediately followed by thorough clinical inquiry. The SSI is not intended to replace the clinical interview; it is intended to provide clinicians with a rapid and reliable instrument for multimethod assessment of suicide ideation.

The SSI has been shown to discriminate between depressed outpatients and hospitalized patients at risk for suicide (Beck et al. 1979). "Worst-point" suicidal ideation (i.e., reports of the most intense suicidal ideation that a patient has ever felt during his or her lifetime) has been found to be better predictor of eventual suicide than either current suicidal ideation or hopelessness (Beck et al. 1999). A self-report version of the SSI is also available (SSI-SR; Beck et al. 1988). Again, we see the interesting phenomenon that self-reported SSI scores tend to be higher than clinician-rated SSI scores (Beck et al. 1988). Evidently, patients are more willing to confess suicidal thoughts to paper-and-pencil instruments than to clinicians.

Firestone Assessment for Self-Destructive Thoughts

The conceptual foundation for the Firestone Assessment for Self-Destructive Thoughts (FAST; Firestone and Seiden 1990) is that suicide and self-destructive behavior are influenced by an inner "voice" (e.g., a negative thought process). The voice process represents a pattern of thoughts, attitudes, and beliefs that are antithetical to the self and hostile toward others. The voice ranges along a continuum of intensity, from self-defeating (e.g., "You're stupid," "You don't deserve good things to happen to you") to self-annihilating (e.g., "People would be better off without you," "It's the only way to end the pain").

The FAST is an 84-item self-report questionnaire that is designed to be used as a screening instrument. It can also be used to track changes in self-destructive thinking over time. The patient reports the frequency of negative thoughts on a five-point Likert-type scale (0="never"; 4 = "almost always"). (A Likert-type scale is a rating scale designed to measure user attitudes or reactions by quantifying subjective information.) The FAST helps clinicians identify the self-destructive thoughts that drive a patient's self-destructive behaviors and facilitates directed interventions toward those areas (Firestone and Seiden 1990). Knowledge of where a patient's score falls on the continuum can also assist clinicians in identifying patients who are at increased risk for suicide.

As would be expected, FAST scores correlate significantly with BDI scores (r=0.73)

and BHS scores (r=0.63) (Firestone and Firestone 1998). To date, we are unaware of any predictive validity studies involving the FAST. This theory-based measure is intriguing in its potential for identifying specific maladaptive cognitions related to suicidal ideation, thereby enhancing cognitive treatment interventions. However, treatment outcome studies using the FAST have yet to be published.

Linehan Reasons for Living Inventory

The Linehan Reasons for Living Inventory (LRFL; Linehan et al. 1983) assesses the strength of an individual's commitment not to die. The 48-item self-report measure takes about 10 minutes to administer; a 72-item version is also available. Internal consistency is high, and test-retest reliability over 3 weeks is moderately high. The LRFL has been noted to be sensitive to reductions in depression, hopelessness, and suicidal ideation in female patients receiving treatment for borderline personality disorder (Linehan et al. 1991).

Conceptually, the basis for the LRFL is that the lack of positive reasons to live is as strong a contributor to suicide as the wish to die. Patients are asked to rate a series of reasons for *not* killing themselves, using a six-point Likert-type scale (1="not at all important"; 6="extremely important"). Subscales include Responsibility to Family (e.g., "My family depends on me and needs me"), Fear of Suicide (e.g., "I am afraid of the unknown"), and Moral Objections (e.g., "I believe only God has the right to end life"). The LRFL is a useful method of monitoring chronic suicidality in high-risk patients and measuring the effectiveness of suicide-focused treatment interventions.

No evidence exists to support the widely held notion that asking a person about suicide increases that person's suicide risk. It is perhaps shocking that 25% of physicians in general practice (and 20% of their patients) endorse the belief that screening for suicidal ideation could *induce* a person to self-harm (Bajaj et al. 2008). However, it could be that asking a person about his or her reasons *not* to die by suicide might reduce that person's suicide risk. In clinical practice, we have observed suicidal patients use this measure to identify (and through therapy, enhance) personal strengths and reasons for living that had been otherwise inaccessible to them.

Risk Estimator for Suicide

Motto et al. (1985) developed an empirical suicide risk scale for adults hospitalized due to a depressive or suicidal state. Their study of 2,753 suicidal patients prospectively examined 101 psychosocial variables. After a 2-year follow-up, 136 (4.94%) of the participants had died by suicide. The authors used rigorous statistical analysis, including a validation procedure, to identify 15 variables as significant predictors of suicidal outcome. Their findings were translated into a paper-and-pencil scale that gives an estimated risk of suicide within 2 years. Motto (1989) noted that instruments such as these could provide a valuable supplement to clinical judgment as well as the kind of quantitative expression of suicide risk that represents to many clinicians an opportunity to fine-tune their clinical judgment.

However, Clark et al. (1987) undertook a field test of Motto et al.'s (1985) Risk Estimator for Suicide that "raised questions" about the instrument, although without invalidating the scale. They selected a subset of psychiatric patients with major or chronic affective disorders that corresponded to Motto's sample. The subjects in the sample

exhibited distinctly lower suicide rates over a 2-year follow-up (2.4%) than the sample reported by Motto (4.9%). The study by Clark et al. (1987) highlights the critical need to understand the limitations of all such scales, particularly

> the likelihood that suicide scales derived by multivariate analysis of a large number of clinical, psychosocial, and demographic variables may tend to be arbitrary and sample specific. Our impression is that empirically derived scales based on a single cross-sectional assessment are always difficult to validate. Repeated assessments over time on a broad array of clinical features may be necessary to develop an adequate and replicable prediction system. (p. 926)

Clark et al. (1987) recommended the use of serial assessments that monitor changing clinical symptoms and life stressors and consider the patient's long-standing character structure.

Consultative Suicide Risk Assessment

Yufit (1988) proposed that the assessment of suicidal behavior is best conducted through the use of a Suicide Assessment Team. Such a team would comprise a multidisciplinary staff of psychologists, social workers, nurses, and psychology graduate students specially trained in the use of a focused screening interview format and other assessment techniques for the identification and evaluation of suicide potential. (We further suggest the inclusion of psychiatrists on such a team whenever possible.) The Suicide Assessment Team is intended to serve as consultants to inpatient psychiatric treatment teams and to conduct three levels of suicide assessment: a focused interview (Level I), specialized rating scales (Level II), and an extended psychological assessment (Level III), including the interviews and ratings described earlier as well as special psychological assessment techniques, termed the *Suicide Assessment Battery*. Proposed Level II rating scales include the BDI, the Risk-Rescue Rating Scale, and the Los Angeles Suicide Prevention Center Assessment of Suicide Potential. Some of the 13 recommended components of the Suicide Assessment Battery include the Suicide Assessment Checklist, Coping Abilities Questionnaire, Time Questionnaire, Sentence Completion Test, Draw-a-Person-in-the-Rain test, Thematic Apperception Test, Rorschach Inkblot Test, Experience Inventory, Autobiography, and Erikson Questionnaire. Yufit (1988) concluded that

> even in a psychiatric hospital setting, where psychiatric sophistication may be considered deep, there is a need for more *comprehensive* evaluation procedures of the complex behavior of suicide. At this stage of development, these techniques are not necessarily conclusive, nor are they often objective, but they very often do serve as important *guidelines* to assist in the identification and the assessment of the components of suicide potential. They should supplement clinical judgment, not substitute for it. (p. 33)

In short, instruments such as those included in the Suicide Assessment Battery may allow clinicians to supplement their own clinical judgment with a systematized approach to collecting assessment information. Such instruments also have the potential to provide treatment providers with actionable insights into the suicidal patient's long-term character structure and current psychological processes.

Comprehensive Suicide Assessment Teams are rarely used today and may be economically infeasible in the best of cir-

cumstances. However, consultation with a clinical psychologist skilled in the assessment of both suicide risk and personality is an underutilized resource available to many psychiatrists and other health care providers. In the following case example, we briefly outline a consultative partnership that informed the treatment of a suicidal patient.

Case Example

Dr. O is a psychiatrist in private practice in a Midwestern state. A new patient is referred to him by a primary care physician. Kurt is a 38-year-old married white male who returned from a combat tour in Afghanistan 18 months prior to intake. The patient reports insomnia, fatigue, diarrhea, back pain, occasional blurred vision, and chronic headaches. He also reports that he "can't remember anything—my wife tells me to go to the store to get X, Y, and Z for the kids, and I come back with X, but not Y and not Z. Sometimes by the time I get to the store, I can't for the life of me remember why I'm there." The patient was treated with stimulant medication for attention-deficit/hyperactivity disorder (ADHD) from age 11 to 17 years ("I stopped because I heard that you couldn't enlist if you were taking any medicines."). He reports having been in close proximity (i.e., within 100 yards) to "at least" four roadside bomb blasts while in Afghanistan. He says that he "had my bell rung" on several occasions but he does not recall ever having lost consciousness, nor does he recall having experienced any proximate postconcussional symptoms. A magnetic resonance imaging scan done 6 months prior to intake at the local Veterans Affairs medical center was inconclusive. During the clinical interview, Kurt denies any current or past suicidal ideation or attempts.

After starting Kurt on duloxetine and trazodone, Dr. O refers the patient to a clinical psychologist, Dr. W, for evaluation of the memory complaints and ADHD. Testing takes place in Dr. W's office and requires a total of 6 hours over 2 days, including a 1-hour feedback session. Kurt's performance on the Wechsler Memory Scales is in the low average range, with no significant deterioration of newly learned material after a 20-minute delay. His Wechsler Adult Intelligence Scale (WAIS-IV) performance is in the high average range (Full Scale IQ=118), but with a relative deficit in Processing Speed (PSI=97). His lowest WAIS-IV score is on a subtest that required him to scan a field of similar colored shapes and select only those that were of a specified shape and color (Cancellation=5).

Kurt's MMPI-2 profile reveals a high-point code type of 8–9(2). The elevations of his clinical and other MMPI-2 scale scores suggest severe alienation from others, serious questions about his identity, and fears that he is "losing my mind." In addition, the profile suggests severe agitation, tension, somatic symptoms (e.g., heart pounding and shortness of breath), and sleep disturbance, including "nightmares every few nights." Kurt's score on the MMPI-2 Posttraumatic Stress–Keane (PK) scale is T90 (four standard deviations above the mean for nonpatients). He endorsed four of the six items on the MMPI-2 Suicide Potential scale (Glassmire et al. 2001).

Kurt's responses to the Rorschach Inkblot Test are notable for morbid content, particularly involving body disintegration: "It looks like a pile of guts"; "There's a brain over there, and another one there—blown out of their skulls, I guess"; "I don't know why but I want to say it looks like a sucking chest wound—like you are staring deep down into somebody's chest and you can see the…the…, what's the word . . . viscera. The viscera thumping away down in there." Kurt's S-CON score is 6. His test scores suggest that he is currently experiencing a great deal of stress, to the point where he might occasionally lose contact with consensual reality.

On the LRFL, Kurt endorsed only four items as reasons why he would not kill himself: "I have a responsibility and commitment to my family"; "It would not be fair to leave the children for others to take care of"; "The effect on my children could be harmful"; and "It would hurt my family too much and I would not want them to suffer." On inquiry, he revealed that he had decided within the past few months that he would kill himself soon after his children graduated from high school but that he would hold off until that time. He had already planned the circumstances of his demise, which involved shooting himself with a particular firearm (his deceased father's sidearm from his service in Vietnam), in a particular location (on his small fishing boat in the middle of a local lake), and at a particular day and time ("Monday morning, after graduation—real early, I'd set off before dawn: I don't sleep anyway"). His youngest child recently started the ninth grade.

During the feedback session, Dr. W suggests that Kurt's test results paint a picture of someone who has been through an unusually shocking—even horrifying—experience. Dr. W says that many people with similar testing profiles often feel terribly different from other people, like there is no way that other people could understand them, and that if others did understand how they were feeling, it would only result in hatred, rejection, or disgust. He suggests that often the best way to reconnect with other people is by talking first with a professional experienced in the treatment of combat veterans. Dr. W reinforces Kurt's beliefs about the harmful impact his suicide would have on his children and wife.

After receiving the report of Dr. W, Dr. O switches Kurt from trazodone to gabapentin, which has shown some efficacy for trauma-related nightmares and is also less lethal in overdose (Hamner et al. 2001). He also adds quetiapine both at night and during the day to reduce agitation. Perhaps most importantly, he refers Kurt to a psychotherapist colleague who is experienced in treating combat trauma. Kurt's wife receives psychoeducation regarding posttraumatic stress disorder and suicide, and the couple decides to place their personal firearms in the hands of a relative for the duration of treatment. After 24 weeks of twice-weekly psychotherapy and continued pharmacotherapy, Kurt demonstrates improved ability to confront and process his war experiences, improved sleep quality and decreased nightmare frequency, improved mood, decreased somatic symptoms, decreased frequency and intensity of headaches, and, as measured by the BHS, steadily increasing hopefulness.

Clinical Inquiry

We agree with Motto (1989) that the most straightforward way to determine the probability of suicide, although not strictly a "test," is to ask the patient directly. This approach should emphasize matter-of-factness, clarity, and freedom from implied criticism. A typical sequence might be to ask the following questions:

1. Do you ever have periods of feeling sad or depressed about how your life is going?
2. How long do such periods last? How frequent are they? How bad do they get? Does the depression produce crying or interfere with daily activities, sleep, concentration, sex drive, or appetite?
3. Do you ever feel hopeless, discouraged, or self-critical? Do these feelings ever get so intense that life doesn't seem worthwhile? (In a study of subintentioned death by Pompili et al. [2006], the item "Have you ever felt tired of living or thought that life was not worth living?" was endorsed by 53.3% of hospitalized drivers involved in single-car accidents, versus 23.3% of the control subjects.)
4. How often do thoughts of suicide come to mind? How persistent are such thoughts? How strong have they been? Does it require much effort to resist them? Have you had any impulses to carry them out?
5. Have you made any plans to end your life? How would you go about doing it? Have you taken any initial steps, such as hoarding medications or buying a gun?
6. Are there any firearms in your home? If you wanted to, how quickly could you get hold of a gun? Where would you get it? Are you satisfied that this situation is safe for you? If not, how can it be made safer?
7. Can you manage these feelings if they come back? If you can't, is there a support system for you to turn to in helping to manage these feelings? What is your plan for getting through the next down period? Whom should you tell when you have these feelings?

Motto (1989) pointed out that the above brief inquiry, when carried out in an empathic and understanding way, will provide the clinician with a preliminary estimate of risk. The approach rests on the premise that "going directly to the heart of the issue is a practical and effective clinical tool, and patients and collaterals will usually provide valid information if an attitude of caring concern is communicated to them." As always, however, the clinician should remember that the absence of reported suicidal thoughts or behaviors does not rule out the presence of suicide risk.

Key Clinical Concepts

- Use reliable and valid suicide risk assessment instruments to supplement clinical judgment. Obtain consultation from qualified practitioners who are trained in the appropriate use of these instruments.

- Routinely use suicide scales and consultative psychological testing because

  - Patients often disclose more information regarding suicidal thoughts and behaviors on self-report measures than during clinical interviews.

  - Suicidal ideation and elevated suicide risk are often present in patients whose initial presentation may not trigger a detailed suicide inquiry.

➤ Tests and scales contribute to a multimethod assessment that challenges the biases and blind spots of clinical judgment.

➤ Psychological testing can inform the psychodiagnostic process. Accurate psychiatric diagnosis is perhaps the most important signal to alert clinicians to suicidal behavior over the life cycle.

➤ Psychological testing can inform treatment planning. Assessment results can suggest, for example, whether a patient is suitable for group psychotherapy or whether an underlying psychotic process is present. Measures such as the Minnesota Multiphasic Personality Inventory–2 (MMPI-2) provide a rational, empirical method of identifying and rank-ordering a patient's subjective complaints.

■ Review the patient's responses on any test or scale that has been administered, preferably before the patient leaves the clinician's office. It is negligent, for example, for a testing consultant to obtain a Rorschach protocol and not score the Suicide Constellation (S-CON). Investigate red flag items (e.g., the MMPI-2 suicide items) thoroughly and document the ensuing follow-up inquiry. Review omitted items on suicide measures with the patient and explore the reasons for the omissions.

■ Document suicide risk assessment, even in cases when the risk is deemed minimal. The importance of thorough documentation cannot be overstated. Suicide risk assessment is a clinical procedure that should always be carefully documented in a timely manner. Psychological tests, when administered, should be properly scored and interpreted, and documentation added to the patient's chart.

■ Perform clinical inquiries regarding suicide throughout the course of treatment. Instruments such as the revised Beck Depression Inventory (BDI-II) or the Linehan Reasons for Living Inventory can be used not only at intake but also as a means of measuring patient progress at various time intervals.

References

Bajaj P, Borreani E, Ghosh P, et al: Screening for suicidal thoughts in primary care: the views of patients and general practitioners. Ment Health Fam Med 5:229–235, 2008

Beck AT, Steer RA: Manual for the Beck Hopelessness Scale. San Antonio, TX, The Psychological Corporation, 1988

Beck AT, Schuyler D, Herman I: Development of suicidal intent scales, in The Prediction of Suicide. Edited by Beck AT, Resnik HLP, Lettieri DJ. Bowie, MD, Charles Press, 1974, pp 45–56

Beck AT, Kovacs M, Weissman A: Assessment of suicidal intention: the Scale for Suicide Ideation. J Consult Clin Psychol 47:343–352, 1979

Beck AT, Steer RA, Kovacs M, et al: Hopelessness and eventual suicide: a 10-year prospective study of patients hospitalized with suicidal ideation. Am J Psychiatry 142:559–563, 1985

Beck AT, Steer RA, Ranieri W: Scale for Suicide Ideation: psychometric properties of a self-report version. J Consult Clin Psychol 44:499–505, 1988

Beck AT, Brown GK, Berchick RJ, et al: Relationship between hopelessness and ultimate suicide: a replication with psychiatric outpatients. Am J Psychiatry 147:190–195, 1990

Beck AT, Brown GK, Steer RA: Beck Depression Inventory II Manual. San Antonio, TX, The Psychological Corporation, 1996

Beck AT, Brown GK, Steer RA: Suicide ideation at its worst point: a predictor of eventual suicide in psychiatric outpatients. Suicide Life Threat Behav 29:1–9, 1999

Brown GK, Beck AT, Steer RA, et al: Risk factors for suicide in psychiatric outpatients: a 20-year prospective study. J Consult Clin Psychol 68:371–377, 2000

Butcher JN: The Minnesota Report: Adult Clinical System MMPI-2. Minneapolis, University of Minnesota Press, 1989

Clark DC, Young MA, Scheftner WA, et al: A field test of Motto's Risk Estimator for Suicide. Am J Psychiatry 144:923–926, 1987

Clopton JR: Suicidal risk via the Minnesota Multiphasic Personality Inventory (MMPI), in Psychological Assessment of Suicide Risk. Edited by Neuringer C. Springfield, IL, Charles C Thomas, 1974, pp 118–133

Dahlstrom WG, Welsh GS, Dahlstrom LE: An MMPI Handbook, Vol I. Minneapolis, University of Minnesota Press, 1972

Exner JE: A Primer for Rorschach Interpretation. Asheville, NC, Rorschach Workshops, 2000

Exner JE: The Rorschach: A Comprehensive System, Vol I: Basic Foundations, 4th Edition. New York, Wiley, 2003

Eyman JR, Eyman SK: Personality assessment in suicide prediction. Suicide Life Threat Behav 21:37–55, 1991

Farberow NL, Helig S, Litman R: Techniques in Crisis Intervention: A Training Manual. Los Angeles, CA, Suicide Prevention Center, 1968

Firestone RW, Firestone L: Voices in suicide: the relationship between self-destructive thought processes, maladaptive behavior, and self-destructive manifestations. Death Stud 22:411–443, 1998

Firestone RW, Seiden RH: Suicide and the continuum of self-destructive behavior. J Am Coll Health 38:207–213, 1990

Fowler JC, Piers C, Hilsenroth MJ, et al: The Rorschach Suicide Constellation: assessing various degrees of lethality. J Pers Assess 76:333–351, 2001

Friedman AF, Lewak R, Nichols DS, et al: Psychological assessment with the MMPI-2. Mahwah, NJ, Erlbaum, 2001

Glassmire DM, Stolberg RA, Ricci CM, et al: The utility of MMPI-2 suicide items for assessing suicide history. Paper presented at the 34th Annual Symposium on Recent Developments in the Use of the MMPI-2/MMPI-A Workshop and Symposia, Huntington Beach, CA, April 1999

Glassmire DM, Stolberg RA, Greene RL, et al: The utility of MMPI-2 suicide items for assessing suicidal potential: development of a Suicidal Potential Scale. Assessment 8:281–290, 2001

Graham JR: MMPI-2: Assessing Personality and Psychopathology, 4th Edition. New York, Oxford University Press, 2005

Greene RL: The MMPI-2: An Interpretive Manual. Boston, MA, Allyn & Bacon, 2000

Hamner MB, Brodrick PS, Labbate LA: Gabapentin in PTSD: a retrospective, clinical series of adjunctive therapy. Ann Clin Psychiatry 13:141–146, 2001

Hendren RL: Assessment and interviewing strategies for suicidal patients over the life cycle, in Suicide Over the Life Cycle: Risk Factors, Assessment, and Treatment of Suicidal Patients. Edited by Blumenthal SJ, Kupfer DJ. Washington, DC, American Psychiatric Press, 1990, pp 235–252

Jobes DA, Eyman JR, Yufit RI: How clinicians assess suicide risk in adolescents and adults. Crisis Intervention and Time-Limited Treatment 2:1–12, 1995

Kaplan ML, Asnis GM, Sanderson WC, et al: Suicide assessment: clinical interview vs. self-report. J Clin Psychol 50:294–298, 1994

Linehan MM, Goodstein JL, Nielsen SL, et al: Reasons for staying alive when you are thinking of killing yourself: the Reasons for Living Inventory. J Consult Clin Psychol 51:276–286, 1983

Linehan MM, Armstrong HE, Suarez A, et al: Cognitive-behavioral treatment of chronically parasuicidal borderline patients. Arch Gen Psychiatry 48:1060–1064, 1991

Lundbäck E, Forslund K, Rylander G, et al: CSF 5-HIAA and the Rorschach test in patients who have attempted suicide. Arch Suicide Res 10:339–345, 2006

Maris RW, Berman AL, Maltsberger JT, et al (eds): Assessment and Prediction of Suicide. New York, Guilford, 1992

Meyer RG: The Clinician's Handbook: Integrated Diagnostics, Assessment, and Intervention in Adult and Adolescent Psychopathology, 3rd Edition. Boston, MA, Allyn & Bacon, 1993

Motto JA: Problems in suicide risk assessment, in Suicide: Understanding and Responding: Harvard Medical School Perspectives. Edited by Jacobs DG, Brown HN. Madison, CT, International Universities Press, 1989, pp 129–142

Motto JA, Heilbron DC, Juster RP: Development of a clinical instrument to estimate suicide risk. Am J Psychiatry 142:680–686, 1985

Neuringer C: Rorschach inkblot test assessment of suicidal risk, in Psychological Assessment of Suicide Risk. Edited by Neuringer C. Springfield, IL, Charles C Thomas, 1974, pp 74–94

Osborne D: The MMPI in psychiatric practice. Psychiatr Ann 15:542–545, 1985

Pokorny AD: Prediction of suicide in psychiatric patients: report of a prospective study. Arch Gen Psychiatry 40:249–257, 1983

Pompili M, Girardi P, Tatarelli G, et al: Suicidal intent in single-car accidents: review and new preliminary findings. Crisis 27:92–99, 2006

Reinecke MA, Franklin-Scott RL: Assessment of suicide: Beck's scales for assessing mood and suicidality, in Assessment, Treatment, and Prevention of Suicidal Behavior. Edited by Yufit RI, Lester D. New York, Wiley, 2005, pp 29–61

Rogers JR, Oney KM: Clinical use of suicide assessment scales: enhancing reliability and validity through the therapeutic relationship, in Assessment, Treatment, and Prevention of Suicidal Behavior. Edited by Yufit RI, Lester D. New York, Wiley, 2005, pp 7–27

Sepaher I, Bongar B, Greene RL: Codetype base rates for the "I Mean Business" suicide items on the MMPI-2. J Clin Psychol 55:1167–1173, 1999

Wood JM, Nezworski MT, Stejskal WJ: The comprehensive system for the Rorschach: a critical examination. Psychol Sci 7:3–10, 1996

Young MA, Fogg LF, Scheftner W, et al: Stable trait components of hopelessness: baseline and sensitivity to depression. J Abnorm Psychol 105:155–165, 1996

Yufit RI: Manual of Procedures: Assessing Suicide Potential: Suicide Assessment Team. Unpublished manual, 1988

PART II

Major Mental Disorders

C H A P T E R 6

Depressive Disorders

Jan Fawcett, M.D.

In this chapter, I review the evidence supporting suicide risk assessment and prevention in depression. At present, there is no evidence that suicide can be predicted in an individual, and the evidence supporting the effectiveness of treatment in preventing suicide is limited. Suicide is the worst outcome in the treatment of depressive disorders and has been shown to be unpredictable in an individual case (Farbarow and MacKinnon 1975; Luoma et al. 2002; Pokorny 1983, 1993). Despite these limitations, it remains a standard of care in psychiatry and mental health treatment that a suicide risk assessment be performed at clinically appropriate times in the course of treatment and that every effort be made to prevent suicide in the patients we treat. The fact that treatment alone is not enough to prevent suicide is illustrated by the finding that in 50%–70% of cases of suicide, the individual was in treatment with a psychiatrist or, in the case of the higher figure, a psychiatrist or primary care physician (Baraclough et al. 1974; Robins 1981). Furthermore, a review of 30 studies found that 30% of suicides occur in patients receiving some form of mental health treatment (Luoma et al. 2002).

Assessment of Suicide Risk

Acute and Chronic Risk Factors: Severe Psychic Anxiety and Impulsivity

Despite the finding that suicide is currently unpredictable in the individual, there is evidence for the presence of chronic and acute suicide risk factors (Fawcett et al. 1990) (Table 6–1) and evidence that pharmacological treatment sustained for a minimum of 6 months can prevent suicide in a significant proportion of patients (Angst et al. 2005). This is important to note because suicide and suicide attempts have not declined despite the introduction of new pharmacological treatments (Kessler et al. 2005), even though suicidal ideation is decreased with selective serotonin reuptake inhibitor (SSRI) medication treatment, and suicide attempts have been found to decrease with dialectical behavior therapy (Beasley et al. 2007; Linehan et al. 2008; Tollefson et al. 1993). Also, meta-analyses show that short-term treatment (8- to 12-week U.S. Food and Drug Administration registration studies) with second-generation antidepressants is no more effective at preventing suicide than placebo treatment (Khan et al. 2003).

TABLE 6–1. Suicide risk factors

Any history of suicide attempt

Tendency to lose temper or to become aggressive with little provocation

Family history of suicide attempts or suicide

Living alone, chronic severe pain, or recent (past 3 months) loss

Recent psychiatric admission/discharge or first diagnosis of major depressive disorder, bipolar disorder, or schizophrenia

Recent increase in alcohol abuse or worsening of depressive symptoms

Current (past week) preoccupation with or plans for suicide

Current psychomotor agitation, marked anxiety, or hopelessness

Recent or current real or anticipated loss, major stress, or significant medical diagnosis (e.g., cancer, dementia)

In 1990, a prospective study of suicide in 954 patients with major mood disorders demonstrated that clinical risk factors for short-term or acute risk (from weeks up to 1 year in this study) differed from long-term risk factors (from 1 year to 10 years of follow-up) (Fawcett et al. 1990). In this study, the severity of risk symptoms was compared between the minority of patients who died by suicide and the majority of the sample who survived. A research interview using trained professional raters who had established acceptable reliability with one another across six academic research sites found significantly more severe psychic anxiety (as measured by the Schedule for Affective Disorders and Schizophrenia— Change Version), more severe insomnia, panic attacks, and recent onset of moderate alcohol abuse in the baseline clinical evaluation of 13 suicides that occurred over the first year of follow-up (Endicott and Spitzer 1978). Standard risk factors such as recent or past suicide attempts, severity of hopelessness, and severity of suicidal ideation

did not differ in the suicide group from the patients who survived. After 2–10 years of follow-up, these standard risk factors were significantly increased in the 21 additional cases of suicide that occurred. This study raised the concept of acute versus chronic risk factors for suicide, with each having different effects. As far as this author could tell from a literature search, no study based on clinical research findings had separated risk factors into acute versus chronic risk types (referring to the time until occurrence or imminence of suicide), an approach made possible in the 1990 study by its prospective design.

A more recent epidemiological study by Nock et al. (2009) of suicide attempts in 108,000 subjects interviewed in 21 countries found that suicidal ideation was related to depression but did not predict suicide attempt. This study found that conditions that resulted in comorbid anxiety and increased impulsivity in depressed patients (e.g., bipolar disorder, borderline or antisocial personality disorder, substance abuse), in addition to depressed mood with suicidal ideation, led to suicide attempts. Although this study did not address the temporal sequence of symptoms leading up to suicide—as did the study by Hall et al. (1999), which found that 90% of hospitalized suicide attempters had reported high psychic anxiety 1 month before their attempt—it raised the question of whether an increase of anxiety or impulsivity resulting from either stressful events or a worsening of depressive illness may constitute acute clinical risk factors for suicide.

A rather unusual epidemiological health study in Norway (Stordal et al. 2008) was based on the self-report Hospital Anxiety and Depression Scale, which was filled out monthly (except for the month of July) from 1969 through 1994 by more than 60,000 subjects. Data were obtained from more than

6,000 male and 3,000 female suicide completers. In this study, suicide peaked in the months that both depression and anxiety were reported to be at their highest level simultaneously ($r=0.72$, $P=0.001$). Again, in this study, the suicides peaked in the summer and fall, when anxiety, which tended to remain elevated, was matched by an increase in depression. Unlike some earlier studies, anxiety levels remained high in the subjects who completed suicide, whereas depression fluctuated based on the self-ratings, with suicide peaking at periods when depression severity ratings, as well as anxiety levels, were increased.

Since the prospective study of suicide that found that severe psychic anxiety, global insomnia, severe panic attacks, and recent onset of alcohol abuse were associated acutely in time with suicide, other studies have appeared that support the association of anxiety and suicide attempts or completion. A chart study of 76 patients who died by suicide in a hospital or within 3 days of discharge found that the chart notes of 79% of the patients documented the presence of severe anxiety/agitation for at least 3 days in the week before their suicide (Busch et al. 2003). Seventy-six percent of this group denied suicidal ideation as their last recorded response to nursing queries before their suicide, and 28% had made "no-suicide contracts" or "no self-harm contracts" as recorded in the clinical record by staff.

A number of epidemiological studies have found the presence of anxiety disorders to be associated with suicide attempts (Boden et al. 2007; Bolton et al. 2010; Sareen et al. 2005a, 2005b), and one study found that increased rates of suicide attempts were associated with increased numbers of comorbid anxiety disorder diagnoses (Wunderlich et al. 1998). Other studies of suicidal behavior in both unipolar major depression and bipolar depression found

that both were associated with comorbid anxiety disorders (N.M. Simon 2009; N.M. Simon et al. 2007). G.E. Simon et al. (2007), in a study of two large managed care databases of patients diagnosed with bipolar depression, found that a comorbid anxiety diagnosis of generalized anxiety disorder (GAD) or panic disorder predicted an increased odds of both suicide (odds ratio [OR]=1.7) and suicide attempts (OR=1.4), whereas comorbid substance abuse predicted only an increased odds of suicide attempts (OR=2.2) but not suicide.

Another large study, by Pfeiffer et al. (2009), points to the association of severity of anxiety with depression. In this study of 887,000 depressed veterans, suicide occurred at significantly elevated rates in individuals with comorbid GAD, anxiety disorder not otherwise specified, and panic disorder, but not in those with other anxiety disorders (OR=1.23–1.27). The finding that pointed to anxiety severity was that patients receiving antianxiety treatment (benzodiazepines and/or buspirone) during the daytime were found to have significantly elevated odds of suicide (OR=1.7). Additionally, the small group of patients who received high-dose anxiolytic medications (benzodiazepines and buspirone) was found to have a higher odds of suicide (OR=2.2). Although these data argue for a severity dimension of anxiety being associated with suicide, they also raise questions about the effectiveness of these anxiolytic treatments.

The data reviewed above argue for an association of severe anxiety and depression with suicide, a possible association of severity of anxiety with suicide, and a possible time-related association of the occurrence of severe anxiety symptoms with suicide in patients with mood disorder. They also point to a time-related, acute risk factor, in contrast to a history of a prior medically serious suicide attempt, which has been found to correlate most highly with subsequent suicide but specifies only a general time of risk. (The risk is elevated over a 5-year period following a medically serious suicide attempt, with the highest risk in the first 12 months; the rate of suicide over this 5-year period was found to be 6.67% [Beautrais 2003].)

Coryell and Young (2005) found that a prior suicide attempt, as well as evidence of a preparation (or rehearsal) for suicide, as measured by the Suicide Tendencies Scale, was associated with a significant risk of suicide over a 10-year follow-up period.

Angry impulsivity has been found to be a trait related to suicide and suicidal behavior, irrespective of diagnosis. Brent (2010) found this trait to be transmitted intergenerationally in families, unrelated to specific diagnoses, and enhanced by child abuse, which is also transmitted across generations. Swann et al. (2005) showed that impulsivity is related to suicidal behavior in bipolar patients. Taylor et al. (2008) reported findings showing an association between increased anxiety and increased impulsivity in bipolar patients.

Relation of Risk Assessment to Treatment and Management

Another important reason for detecting severe anxiety and increased impulsivity in patients with mood disorders is the possibility that treatment with second-generation, or even some older, antipsychotic medications may reduce these symptoms and possibly reduce suicidal behavior, although no studies have confirmed this effect (Baker et al. 2003; Hirschfeld et al. 2006; Houston et al. 2006).

What other acute indicators of suicide risk might be found? Recent literature has indicated an elevated risk of suicide after the diagnosis of cancer (Ann et al. 2010).

Studies have shown an elevated risk of suicide within 1 year after the diagnosis of prostate cancer (Feng et al. 2010). This is interesting because prostate cancer is highly treatable, and the suicides are occurring especially within a year of diagnosis, which is generally too early for the development of a terminal state. Is it possible that these deaths are occurring in patients with undiagnosed depression associated with anxiety associated with the diagnosis of cancer? If a screen for depression and anxious symptoms were performed, could some of these deaths be prevented?

A recent study found that the majority of suicide attempts occurred within 5 minutes of decision making; more severe attempts took a longer time to occur from the time they were first thought of, suggesting that more lethal attempts require more time to plan and consider (Deisenhammer et al. 2009). This finding suggests that prevention of suicide may require that we understand the preconditions driving a suicidal impulse in patients. Studies of implicit cognition suggest that suicidal behavior may be predictable over 6 months by implicit associations, the first behavioral marker for suicidal behavior (Nock et al. 2010). This may be one fruitful way to proceed to understand the formation of the impulse to die by suicide.

This leads to the question of whether a given patient may under certain conditions enter a "presuicidal state" that could be recognized and tapped into by the right questions at the right time by the therapist. Could we imagine and construct certain scenarios that might lead the patient into a state that we could tap into if we recognized the state and asked the right questions? A patient may be struggling with depression that has been unresponsive to a series of treatments—both pharmacological and psychotherapeutic. Or the patient may be facing a relapse of depression that initially improved with treatment, underlining the fear that the disease is unmanageable. The patient may have lost an important relationship, a job or career, or a large sum of money, or may have been diagnosed with cancer or some other medical condition, such as multiple sclerosis, that to him or her predicts personal disaster and suffering. We can imagine many scenarios. Would it be unexpected, especially in the presence of clinical depression with its inherent pessimism or hopelessness, that the thought of suicide would cross the person's mind? Experience reviewing suicide cases suggests to this author that the occurrence of a major loss may be the most important of acute suicide risk factors in the patient made vulnerable by depression and severe anxiety.

Timing of Suicide Assessments

It is not always clear just when in the course of treatment suicidal assessments should be done. Although these assessments are probably not necessary in every patient contact, particularly when the patient is doing well, in the presence of a life reversal or a clinical recurrence of symptoms such as those outlined above as well as a sudden worsening of symptoms in what seemed to be a trajectory of progress, a suicide risk assessment is called for. Also, the high risk of suicide occurring within 1 year of hospital discharge, with the risk at its highest immediately after discharge, supports a case for close follow-up and frequent suicide risk assessments during this time (Goldacre et al. 1993; Kan et al. 2007).

Suicide Assessment and DSM-5

A process for the development of a new psychiatric diagnostic system, DSM-5, is currently under way, with a publication target date of May 2013. The Suicide Subworkgroup of the Mood Disorders Work Group, a subgroup of the 13 work groups working on this project, has initiated proposals for increasing attention to the assessment of suicide risk as well as proposals to better record the presence of significant suicidal or self-harmful behavior. These proposals include a guide to risk factors for suicide supported in the literature for the assessment of concern regarding suicide risk in the treatment planning for a patient (see Table 6–2). The guide is based on a review of literature that has generated risk factors shown to be correlated with suicide, leading the clinician to add his or her own experience and clinical judgment while deciding on a 5-point assessment of concern ranging from 0, no concern, to 4, very high concern, which would imply that the main goal of treatment planning is aimed at preventing suicide in the patient. This "dimensional" assessment would be recorded evidence that the clinician gave the assessment of suicide risk careful concern, even if the clinician proved to be incorrect in his or her assessment. It would attempt to prompt a more thoughtful assessment than is conveyed by the common "no suicidal ideation or plan" often seen recorded in clinical notes. This assessment is intended to be used across diagnoses, because although suicide may be more common in mood disorders, it can occur across the diagnostic spectrum, especially in eating disorders, schizophrenia, borderline and antisocial personality disorders, and alcohol and opiate dependency disorders, as well as anxiety disorders.

There has been a proposal to add a dimension of anxiety severity to the diagnosis of mood disorders, because the presence of severe anxiety has been shown to lead to poor treatment response and outcome

---

TABLE 6–2. DSM-5 proposed risk factors for suicide

Long-term factors
1. Any history of suicide attempt
2. Any history of mental illness
3. Any history of physical or sexual abuse
4. Long-standing tendency to lose temper or become aggressive with little provocation
5. Chronic severe pain

Recent events (within 3 months)
1. Recent significant loss
2. Recent psychiatric admission or discharge
3. Recent first psychiatric diagnosis
4. Recent worsening of depressive symptoms or increase in alcohol abuse

Current (within last week)
1. Current preoccupation with plans for suicide
2. Current psychomotor agitation or marked anxiety
3. Current prominent feelings of hopelessness
4. Current living alone

Clinician's Severity of Concern Scale
0: Lowest concern (no prior or current concern about suicidal behavior)
1: Some concern (prior history of suicidal ideation or behavior, but preventing suicidal behavior is not a focus of current management)
2: Moderate concern (preventing suicidal behavior is part of the current clinical management of the patient)
3: High concern (preventing suicidal behavior is one of the main goals in the current management of the patient)
4: Imminent concern (preventing suicidal behavior is the most important goal in the current clinical management of the patient)

---

across two major studies (Coryell et al. 2009; Fava et al. 2006) and because there is evidence of a relationship of suicide risk and severity of anxiety in mood disorders (Faw-cett et al. 1990; Pfeiffer et al. 2009). The clinician utilizing a short five-item scale (Table 6–3) would then make an estimate of the anxiety severity accompanying the diagnosis of a mood disorder.

Other proposals to increase the clinician's focus on suicide prevention include that of a suicidal behavior disorder diagnosis, based on a history of a suicide attempt (with intent to die) in the past 12 months that could be made as a comorbid diagnosis across all diagnoses; and the proposal of a nonsuicidal self-injury diagnosis meant to capture people (usually of younger age) who repeatedly cut or injure themselves, not in an attempt to die but for relief of their psychic turmoil. The purpose of this latter diagnosis, paired with suicidal behavior disorder, is to separate patients who injure themselves in an attempt to die from those who have no such intent but injure themselves repeatedly to attain relief from feelings of psychic pain or turmoil.

It is important to note that these proposals must first pass scrutiny by the scientific review committee, must be found useful in the ongoing clinical field trials, and must receive the endorsement of the DSM-5 task force before being included in DSM-5.

Need for More Effective Acute Risk Assessment

What can we do to be more successful at assessing acute suicide risk in the patient who systematically plans to die by suicide but who does not communicate the state that has led him or her to this point? This is perhaps the most difficult question we face in our efforts to prevent suicide. For example, should we ask, now that something has occurred (e.g., the patient has just received a diagnosis of cancer), "What are your thoughts about your future? How will you approach life given this new turn

TABLE 6–3. Clinician's Anxiety Scale

Anxious symptoms

1. Describes (irrational worries)
2. Feeling uneasy
3. Feeling nervous
4. Motor tension
5. Feels something awful may happen

Clinical Severity Rating Scale

0: None
1: Mildly anxious
2: Moderate anxiety: 2 symptoms
3: Severely anxious: 3–5 symptoms
4: Severely anxious with psychomotor agitation

of events?" Should we be more proactive, more probing in this situation? Could we uncover a suicide plan in people who do not manifest anxiety or hopelessness but who make a calculation that life is too painful to be worth living?

We know that suicide is more common in people living alone, in people who have suffered a major loss, in people who have significant chronic pain, and especially in people who have made previous attempts. Instead of asking about suicidal thoughts or plans, should we be more challenging and ask the patient if the current turn of events has led to thoughts that suicide would be a more positive alternative? Could we uncover more planning for suicide in our patients? In a classic report, Isometsä et al. (1995) found that of 100 patients who died by suicide on the day they saw a therapist, only 20% had admitted to suicidal thoughts.

A Missed Planned Suicide

I continue to replay in my mind the case of a young and very talented man who suffered from bipolar mixed states and who, despite hospitalization and electroconvulsive therapy (ECT) that was continued

weekly after his discharge, hanged himself in his apartment with elaborate climbing lines he had installed over days—within hours of his last appointment with me. I had previously hospitalized the patient, walking him to the inpatient unit from my office after he admitted to me that he had bought a shotgun, loaded it, and held it to his chest. He seemed to improve with ECT in the hospital, was discharged, and returned to work. He still had a "dead" look in his eyes but claimed to feel better and joked with me about a work assignment that would finally utilize the specific skills he had studied in obtaining his college degree. He was planning on leaving to travel to do this assignment, which he seemed to look forward to, in 1 week.

It turned out after his death that he had not told me about a divorce, despite my asking about his marriage, as well as a recent breakup with a woman he had been seeing most recently. He had told her that he could not tell me about his divorce because it could affect his green card status—implying that this information would be divulged and he would be deported. Was he paranoid, or was this just an excuse?

The patient had admitted to some chronic suicidal ideation but denied any plan and showed no signs of distress. However, despite his obvious improvement with ECT, the patient still had "dead eyes"—with no expression or life in them.

I wonder whether I could have asked some question that could have penetrated his determined plan to kill himself. After all, if he had irrevocably planned the suicide, why would he bother to visit me? According to the notes he left, I did not ask the "right" question, we planned his next appointment, and he left my office knowing he was going to hang himself in his apartment, that night, after eating the meals he had planned for the past 3 nights and installing an elaborate system of climbing lines to guarantee the "success" of his self-hanging.

What is the magic question I could have asked that might have made him open up and given me a chance to guide him in another direction? In this case, based on his notes, he was following a careful 4-day plan to suicide. It could be that in other cases, patients have not fully planned the suicide but are in a presuicidal state that could be discerned with the proper questions.

In this case, the patient told me about his plan the first time, and I had him hospitalized, not involuntarily. He had walked with me to the admitting area in another building. In the final case, he indicated nothing—he decided he did not want my disruption—but he still attended his appointment. He always had chronic risk factors: chronic suicidal ideation, impulsivity related to bipolar disorder, living alone. He did not tell me about his lost relationships but had recently been discharged from the hospital (he was still receiving outpatient ECT on a weekly basis) and was functioning at work as far as I knew. He seemed to look forward to his new work travel assignment. I have seen several cases of death by suicide in individuals who were looking forward to a future event. This case illustrates the difficulties in gathering acute suicide risk information.

We do not have data that allow us to weigh the relative significance of either chronic or acute risk factors for suicide. Whereas factors such as previous suicidal behavior seem to be the best actuarial predictor, acute distress and a recent loss that is overwhelming from the patient's perspective, when present, seem, to this author, to be the most important acute predictors thus far. Isometsä has observed that in his reported series of 5,000 suicides, males completed suicide on their first attempt in 62% of cases, and females completed suicide on their first attempt in 38% of cases (Isometsä and Lönnqvist 1998). This finding warns us that although common, prior suicidal behavior is not by any means a requirement for the presence of acute suicide risk.

Management of Patients Deemed at High Risk for Suicide

A common situation in practice is to find a patient who clearly has acute high risk factors for suicide, who will not agree to hospitalization, and who cannot be involuntarily committed for various reasons. The management of such a patient requires persistence in staying in close touch with the patient and the patient's significant others. A patient manifesting severe anxiety, agitation, or heightened impulsivity can be treated by the constant use of effective anti-anxiety treatment. Second-generation antipsychotics may be useful in the treatment of anxiety and even depression, especially the more sedative ones such as quetiapine and olanzapine. This class of medications recently has shown a capacity for antidepressant effects, either alone or in combination with antidepressant medications (Baker et al. 2003; Hirschfeld et al. 2006; Houston et al. 2006; Vieta et al. 2007).

With this wide spectrum of action, sedative second-generation antipsychotics are particularly useful in treating severe anxiety and agitated states that present in mood disorders, schizophrenic disorders, personality disorders, and even severe anxiety disorders such as posttraumatic stress disorder. These medications require careful medical monitoring of blood sugar and serum lipids when used long term (i.e., longer than 3 months). Studies have documented the effect of quetiapine in significantly reducing anxiety in bipolar I and II depressed patients (Baker et al. 2003) and olanzapine in reducing suicidal ideation when administered as an augmentation to other mood stabilizers in patients with bipolar mixed states (Houston et al. 2006).

Benzodiazepines, especially longer-acting compounds such as clonazepam, may be helpful, but care must be taken because evidence suggests that these compounds, especially if short acting, may lead to disinhibition, with possible rebound anxiety recurring when the medication effect begins to wear off, and may increase suicidal behavior (Cowdry and Gardner 1988; Youssef and Rich 2008). It is important to inquire about the availability of handguns or other lethal means and to try to ensure that the patient no longer has access to them. Although it is true that there are always means of suicide available, a patient's admitting to the presence of a particular means of suicide may be presumptive evidence for the clinician if the patient has been thinking about employing those means.

There are a considerable number of studies showing that lithium carbonate reduces suicide and suicide attempts. Studies have found that lithium reduced these events in approximately 80% of patients with both bipolar and unipolar depression when compared with patients not treated with lithium, after 18 months of follow-up (Baldessarini et al. 2006; Müller-Oerlinghausen et al. 2005; Tondo and Baldessarini 2009). Although clinicians often worry about the danger of overdoses with lithium or problems with side effects, data continue to show a consistent reduction in suicides. One study (Müller-Oerlinghausen et al. 2005) even showed a reduction of suicidal behavior in bipolar patients who had not achieved a full response to lithium therapy, suggesting that the antisuicide effect may

be independent of the effect on other symptoms of bipolar disorder. There also are studies suggesting that lithium may reduce aggression and impulsivity (Sheard et al. 1976). From these reviews of clinical studies, it appears that like antidepressants, lithium may require up to 6 months of regular use in order to be fully effective in this role. Lithium would therefore be less likely to be of help in the treatment of the acute risk symptoms mentioned previously.

Case Example

I teach psychiatric residents who are managing outpatients that in the presence of concerns about a possible suicide, a direct inquiry about access to firearms should be made and recorded. A young patient with schizophrenia and depression, with the delusion that administering the antibiotic bacitracin to a skin abrasion had caused him progressive hearing loss, was seen by a resident under my supervision. He refused SSRI antidepressants on the grounds that they would further hasten his deafness. The patient admitted to normal audiology testing but was unshaken in his delusion. He denied having suicidal ideation or a suicide plan, and the resident dutifully noted in her suicide assessment that the patient denied access to guns. The patient was severely depressed and hopeless about his "progressive hearing loss." He appeared to be quite anxious but denied this when asked. He was encouraged to take mirtazapine for his depression and anxiety, and his risperidone dosage was increased, and he was told that mirtazapine was not an SSRI. He reluctantly agreed but expressed doubts that anything could help because he felt doomed to total hearing loss.

Three weeks later, the treating resident received a call from the patient's family stating that the patient had shot himself in the head and asking the resident to meet with them. The resident was understandably shocked and fearful about this meeting. I accompanied her to this meeting. The family brought in two bottles of concomitant prescriptions by two different general physicians of the benzodiazepine lorazepam, each for a dose of 1 mg four times daily. It appeared that the patient had been taking both prescriptions. As we reviewed his chart with the parents at their request, we came to the last note, where the suicide assessment stated, "Patient denies access to firearms." The parents were very impressed by this and said, "Doctor, we can see that you did everything possible for our son. Thank you for your efforts and for this meeting." At this point they seemed satisfied, had no further questions, and left.

Because suicide is a relatively infrequent event, practitioners can ignore procedures to conscientiously do careful suicide risk assessments and often get by without a suicide occurring. Not placing enough emphasis on careful suicide risk assessments is tantamount to speeding. It often goes undetected, but the more often we speed, the greater the probability that we will be stopped by an officer and ticketed.

As with many important pursuits, the effort to prevent suicide as well as our knowledge in this area will always be lacking. We can only try to improve. I remember treating a suicidal patient with treatment-refractory depression who finally attained a full recovery. It was only then that the patient told me: "I had planned to commit suicide but put it off for a while because you made me curious. You were so insistent that if I didn't give up I would eventually get better that I assumed either you were lying to me or you were delusional, because you seemed to believe it. I decided to stay around long enough to find out which it was—now I'm better, just like you said."

As difficult as it is, as imperfect as our best efforts may be—a life is at stake. We need to do our best for our patients—learning from the patients we lose as well as continuing research to improve our detection of acute risk factors.

Key Clinical Concepts

- There is a significant incidence of suicide among patients under care.
- Suicide assessments should be repeated depending on the patient's clinical course and the occurrence of major stressful life events.
- Both chronic and acute suicide risk factors should be included in a suicide assessment.
- Severe anxiety, agitation, and increased impulsivity are important acute risk factors, especially in the presence of a major loss or life stress.
- Although positive suicidal ideation and especially suicide planning are important acute risk factors, the denial of these elements does not alone provide reassurance that risk is not present, and such denial must be considered in the context of a full clinical evaluation.
- Available information from concerned others should be taken into account in a suicide assessment.
- Appropriate pharmacological and psychotherapeutic treatment can reduce both chronic and acute suicide risk factors.
- Management of a patient with high acute suicide risk who for various reasons cannot be hospitalized requires adequate pharmacologic treatment with very close follow-up with the patient and concerned significant others.

- Although careful suicide risk assessment and management are a standard of care, suicide is not predictable in an individual. It is important for the clinician to document a suicide assessment and the means taken to prevent suicide, because although suicide may be preventable, some patients may be lost despite every possible clinical effort.

References

Angst J, Angst F, Gerber-Werder R, et al: Suicide in 406 mood-disorder patients with and without long-term medication: a 40 to 44 years' follow-up. Arch Suicide Res 9:279–300, 2005

Ann E, Shin DW, Cho SI, et al: Suicide rates and risk factors among Korean cancer patients, 1993–2005. Cancer Epidemiol Biomarkers Prev 19:2097–2105, 2010

Baker RW, Tohen M, Fawcett J, et al: Acute dysphoric mania: treatment response to olanzapine versus placebo. J Clin Psychopharmacol 23:132–137, 2003

Baldessarini RJ, Tondo L, Davis P, et al: Decreased risk of suicides and attempts during long-term lithium: a meta-analytic review. Bipolar Disord 8:625–639, 2006

Baraclough B, Bunch J, Nelson B, et al: A hundred cases of suicide. Br J Psychiatry 125:355–373, 1974

Beasley CM Jr, Ball SG, Nilsson ME, et al: Fluoxetine and adult suicidality revisited: an updated meta-analysis using expanded data sources from placebo-controlled trials. J Clin Psychopharmacol 27:682–686, 2007

Beautrais A: Subsequent mortality in medically serious suicide attempts: a 5 year follow-up. Aust N Z J Psychiatry 37:595–599, 2003

Boden JM, Fergusson DM, Horwood LJ: Anxiety disorders and suicidal behaviours in adolescence and young adulthood: findings from a longitudinal study. Psychol Med 37:431–440, 2007

Bolton JM, Pagura J, Enns MW, et al: A population-based longitudinal study of risk factors for suicide attempts in major depressive disorder. J Psychiatr Res 44:817–826, 2010

Brent D: What family studies teach us about suicidal behavior: implications for research, treatment and prevention. Eur Psychiatry 25:260–263, 2010

Busch KA, Fawcett J, Jacobs D: Clinical correlates of inpatient suicide. J Clin Psychiatry 64:14–19, 2003

Coryell W, Young EA: Clinical predictors of suicide in primary major depressive disorder. J Clin Psychiatry 66:412–417, 2005

Coryell W, Solomon DA, Fiedorowicz JG, et al: Anxiety and outcome in bipolar disorder. Am J Psychiatry 166:1238–1243, 2009

Cowdry RW, Gardner DL: Pharmacotherapy of borderline personality disorder: alprazolam, carbamazepine, trifluoperazine and tranylcypromine. Arch Gen Psychiatry 45:111–119, 1988

Deisenhammer EA, Ing CM, Strauss R, et al: The duration of the suicidal process: how much time is left for intervention between consideration and accomplishment of a suicide attempt? J Clin Psychiatry 70:19–24, 2009

Endicott J, Spitzer RL: A diagnostic interview: the Schedule for Affective Disorders and Schizophrenia. Arch Gen Psychiatry 35:837–844, 1978

Farbarow NL, MacKinnon D: Prediction of suicide: a replication study. J Pers Assess 39:497–501, 1975

Fava M, Rush AJ, Alpert JE, et al: What clinical and symptom features and comorbid disorders characterize outpatients with anxious major depressive disorder: a replication and extension. Can J Psychiatry 51:823–835, 2006

Fawcett J, Scheftner WA, Fogg L, et al: Time-related predictors of suicide in major affective disorder. Am J Psychiatry 147:1189–1194, 1990

Feng F, Keating NL, Mucci LA, et al: Immediate risk of suicide and cardiovascular death after a prostate cancer diagnosis: cohort study in the United States. J Natl Cancer Inst 102:307–314, 2010

Goldacre M, Seagroat V, Hawton K: Suicide after discharge from psychiatric inpatient care. Lancet 342:283–286, 1993

Hall RC, Platt DE, Hall RC: Suicide risk assessment: a review of risk factors for suicide in 100 outpatients who made severe suicide attempts. Psychosomatics 40:18–27, 1999

Hirschfeld RM, Weisler RH, Raines SR, et al: Quetiapine in the treatment of anxiety in patients with bipolar I or II depression: a secondary analysis from a randomized, double-blind, placebo-controlled study. J Clin Psychiatry 67:355–362, 2006

Houston JP, Ahl J, Meyers AL, et al: Reduced suicidal ideation in bipolar I disorder mixed-episode patients in a placebo-controlled trial of olanzapine combined with lithium or divalproex. J Clin Psychiatry 67:1246–1252, 2006

Isometsä ET, Lönnqvist JK: Suicide attempts preceding completed suicide. Br J Psychiatry 173:531–535, 1998

Isometsä ET, Heikkinen ME, Marttunen MJ, et al: The last appointment before suicide: is suicide intent communicated? Am J Psychiatry 152:919–922, 1995

Kan CK, Ho TP, Dong JY, et al: Risk factors for suicide in the immediate post-discharge period. Soc Psychiatry Psychiatr Epidemiol 42:208–214, 2007

Kessler RC, Berglund P, Borges G: Trends in suicide ideation, plans, gestures and attempts in the United States, 1990–1992 to 2001–2003. JAMA 293:2487–2495, 2005

Khan A, Khan S, Kolts R, et al: Suicide rates in clinical trials of SSRIs, other antidepressants, and placebo: analysis of FDA reports. Am J Psychiatry 160:790–792, 2003

Linehan MM, McDavid JD, Brown MZ, et al: Olanzapine plus dialectical behavior therapy for women with high irritability who meet criteria for borderline personality disorder: a double-blind, placebo-controlled pilot study. J Clin Psychiatry 69:999–1005, 2008

Luoma JB, Martin CE, Oearson JL: Contact with mental health and primary care providers before suicide: a review of the evidence. Am J Psychiatry 159:908–916, 2002

Müller-Oerlinghausen B, Felber W, Berghöfer A, et al: The impact of lithium long-term medication on suicidal behavior and mortality of bipolar patients. Arch Suicide Res 9:307–319, 2005

Nock MK, Hwang I, Sampson N, et al: Cross-national analysis of the associations among mental disorders and suicidal behavior: findings from the WHO World Mental Health Surveys. PLoS Med 6:1–17, 2009

Nock MK, Park JM, Finn CT, et al: Measuring the suicidal mind: implicit cognition predicts suicidal behavior. Psychol Sci 21:511–517, 2010

Pfeiffer PN, Ganoczy D, Ilgen M, et al: Comorbid anxiety as a suicide risk factor among depressed veterans. Depress Anxiety 26:752–757, 2009

Pokorny AD: Prediction of suicide in psychiatric patients: report of a prospective study. Arch Gen Psychiatry 40:249–257, 1983

Pokorny AD: Suicide prediction revisited. Suicide Life Threat Behav 23:1–10, 1993

Robins E: The Final Months. New York, Oxford University Press, 1981, p 47

Sareen J, Cox BJ, Afifi TO, et al: Anxiety disorders and risk for suicidal ideation and suicide attempts: a population-based longitudinal study of adults. Arch Gen Psychiatry 62:1249–1257, 2005a

Sareen J, Houlahan T, Cox BJ, et al: Anxiety disorders associated with suicidal ideation and suicide attempts in the National Comorbidity Survey. J Nerv Ment Dis 193:450–454, 2005b

Sheard MH, Marini JL, Bridges CL, et al: The effect of lithium on impulsive-aggressive behavior in man. Am J Psychiatry 133:1409–1413, 1976

Simon GE, Hunkeler E, Fireman B, et al: Risk of suicide attempt and suicide death in patients treated for bipolar disorder. Bipolar Disord 9:526–530, 2007

Simon NM: Generalized anxiety disorder and psychiatric comorbidities such as depression, bipolar disorder, and substance abuse. J Clin Psychiatry 70 (suppl 2):10–14, 2009

Simon NM, Zalta AK, Otto MW, et al: The association of co-morbid anxiety disorders with suicide attempts and suicidal ideation in outpatients with bipolar disorder. J Psychiatr Res 41:255–264, 2007

Stordal E, Morken G, Mykietun A, et al: Monthly variation in rates of comorbid depression and anxiety in the general population at 63–65 degrees north: the HUNT study. J Affect Disord 106:273–278, 2008

Swann AC, Dougherty DM, Pazzagalia PJ, et al: Increased impulsivity associated with severity of suicide attempt history in patients with bipolar disorder. Am J Psychiatry 162:1680–1687, 2005

Taylor CT, Hirschfeld-Becker DR, Ostacher MJ, et al: Anxiety is associated with impulsivity in bipolar disorder. J Anxiety Disord 22:868–876, 2008

Tollefson GD, Fawcett J, Winokur G: Evaluation of suicidality during pharmacologic treatment of mood and nonmood disorders. Ann Clin Psychiatry 5:209–224, 1993

Tondo L, Baldessarini RJ: Long-term lithium treatment in the prevention of suicidal behavior in bipolar disorder patients. Epidemiol Psichiatr Soc 18:179–183, 2009

Vieta E, Calabrese JR, Goikolea JM, et al: Quetiapine monotherapy in the treatment of patients with bipolar I or II depression and a rapid-cycling disease course: a randomized, double-blind, placebo-controlled study. Bipolar Disord 9:413–425, 2007

Wunderlich U, Bronisch T, Wittchen HU: Comorbidity patterns in adolescents and young adults with suicide attempts. Eur Arch Psychiatry Clin Neurosci 248:87–95, 1998

Youssef NA, Rich CL: Does acute treatment with sedative/hypnotics for anxiety in depressed patients affect suicide risk? A literature review. Ann Clin Psychiatry 20:157–169, 2008

C H A P T E R   7

Anxiety Disorders

Laura N. Antar, M.D., Ph.D.

Eric Hollander, M.D.

It may seem counterintuitive at first that an anxious patient would consider suicide. However, a major survey found that over 70% of individuals with a lifetime history of suicide attempt had an anxiety disorder (Nepon et al. 2010). The presence of an anxiety disorder was significantly associated with having made a suicide attempt (odds ratio [OR]=1.70, 95% confidence interval [CI]=1.40–2.08), even after adjustment for social and demographic factors and Axis I and Axis II disorders (Nepon et al. 2010). Given that 18.1% of U.S. adults have a 12-month prevalence for any anxiety disorder and 4.1% have severe anxiety (Kessler et al. 2005a, 2005b), there is potential for considerable health risk.

Suicide assessment and management of this at-risk population are neither insignificant nor straightforward. Some research groups distinguish between anxiety disorders that predict suicidal ideation—social anxiety disorder (SAD), posttraumatic stress disorder (PTSD), generalized anxiety disorder (GAD), and panic disorder—from those that predict suicide attempts—SAD, PTSD, and GAD (Cougle et al. 2009). Other groups report that all anxiety disorders predict both suicidal ideation and behavior and thus expand both lists to include SAD, simple phobia, GAD, panic disorder, agoraphobia, and obsessive-compulsive disorder (OCD) (Bolton et al. 2008; Sareen et al. 2005). An examination of data from the World Health Organization (WHO) World Mental Health Surveys, derived from 108,664 respondents from 21 countries, found that all mental disorders were predictive of suicide in both developed and developing countries but that the strongest predictors of suicide differed between these groups of countries. In developed countries the strongest predictor of suicide was presence of mood disorders, whereas in developing countries the strongest predictor was presence of disorders of impulse control, substance abuse, or PTSD (Nock et al. 2009). As expected, respondents with both a mood disorder and anxiety had a higher probability of suicide attempt compared with respondents with a mood disorder alone (Nock et al. 2009; Pfeiffer et al. 2009; Sareen et al. 2005).

It remains unknown if treatment of anxiety disorders actually reduces suicide risk (Sareen et al. 2005). Among depressed veterans who also had anxiety, the odds of completed suicide were actually greater for patients who were administered anxiolytic medication (Pfeiffer 2009). However, successful treatment of psychiatric illness in general leads to a decrease in the suicide rate, and so treatment is thought to be protective (Tidemalm et al. 2008).

It is postulated that the increased awareness of the link between suicide and anxiety may be due to increased recognition and diagnosis of anxiety disorders. This growing recognition of these disorders represents an opportunity for early treatment intervention, in hopes of diminishing the suicide rate, although it remains to be proven that mortality is diminished through treatment.

In this chapter, we discuss suicide risk in relation to panic disorder, GAD, SAD, OCD, and PTSD. An illustrative case example is provided for each disorder. We conclude the chapter with a discussion of assessment and management.

Panic Disorder

The issue of whether panic disorder causes increased suicidality has been controversial for decades. However, most recent studies have determined that panic disorder, in the absence of other comorbidities, does increase the risk for suicide (Nepon et al. 2010; Norton et al. 2008; Sareen et al. 2005), although there are notable qualifiers (Cougle et al. 2009). Panic disorder, like many other psychiatric disorders, is often accompanied by numerous comorbidities that exacerbate the patient's suffering and further increase the risk of suicide. Data indicate, for example, that although panic and depression carry their own suicide risk, together they may act synergistically to con-

TABLE 7–1. Factors that increase suicidal ideation in panic disorder

Younger age
Early onset of illness
Low socioeconomic status
Current alcohol use
More severe panic symptoms
Perceived less social support
Perceived more severe adverse side effects of
  medication

Source. Adapted from Huang et al. 2010.

fer additional risk (Norton et al. 2008) (Table 7–1). Other comorbidities that increase the risk for suicide in patients with panic disorder include personality disorders (especially Cluster B [dramatic-emotional] and Cluster C [anxious-fearful]), eating disorders, and substance abuse, and severity of panic symptoms and sex of the individual are also factors (Friedman et al. 1999; Nepon et al. 2010; Warshaw et al. 2000) (Table 7–2). The implications of this and other findings are that patients with panic disorder must be screened for comorbid disorders and also for the severity of the panic and comorbidity.

TABLE 7–2. Comorbid disorders that increase the risk for suicide attempts

Mood disorders
Personality disorders
Eating disorders
Substance use

Source. Adapted from Cougle et al. 2009; Friedman et al. 1999; Nepon et al. 2010; Warshaw et al. 2000.

It is unclear at this time exactly which elements of panic disorder itself lead to suicidality, although factors leading to suicidal ideation, such as overall anxiety, anticipatory anxiety, avoidance of bodily sensations, vigilance to bodily changes, and fear of going crazy, have begun to be elucidated (Schmidt et al. 2001) (Table 7–3). It remains uncertain to what degree other impairments—social, occupational, or functional—lead to suicidal behavior; the role of hopelessness about recovery has not been clearly quantified (Norton et al. 2008). However, the landmark study in the *New England Journal of Medicine* that found a 47% rate of suicidal ideation and a 20% rate of suicide attempts in adults with a lifetime diagnosis of panic disorder (Weissman et al. 1989) is important to consider when seeing a patient with panic disorder in the office, whether or not the numbers are confounded by other comorbidities, as the following case example illustrates.

Case Example 1

Kate was a 28-year-old single woman who lived with her parents. She had had panic attacks from the time she was 16, when a date had to bring her to the hospital because she thought she was having a heart attack. She became afraid that panic attacks would occur while she was out. Within 2 years the panic disorder episodes escalated, intruding when she was alone or with friends and occasionally waking her from sleep. The attacks were always accompanied by shortness of breath, shaking, and the feeling that she was having a heart attack. Just after attacks, she had flashing thoughts about it possibly being less painful if she were dead. She struggled not to call 911 during attacks because she was embarrassed to be sent home with "nothing wrong." She felt she was going crazy. When she went away to college, she found that drinking diminished her attacks.

Kate saw the college therapist because it was getting hard to leave her dorm to attend class. He sent her to a doctor who prescribed alprazolam, which helped instantly. She took alprazolam to ward off attacks, during attacks, and then to feel better after attacks. She often felt sedated and began to fail her courses because she was still unable to go to class or complete assignments. She left school to go back and live with her parents.

TABLE 7–3. Panic-specific variables that predict suicidal ideation (but not suicide attempt)

Increased severity of anxiety
Anticipatory anxiety
Avoidance of bodily sensations
Vigilance to bodily changes
Fear of going crazy

Source. Adapted from Schmidt et al. 2001.

At home, Kate started dating a young man who understood her and made her feel safe. He and her parents encouraged her to see a psychiatrist, who weaned her off alprazolam and simultaneously prescribed a selective serotonin reuptake inhibitor (SSRI). He also referred her for cognitive-behavioral therapy (CBT). Kate soon enrolled in a community college. With her therapist and boyfriend, who she hoped would become her husband, she could "face the world." When the boyfriend discussed that he needed more space, Kate entirely severed the relationship. She stopped therapy and medications, and quit school. Within weeks, the panic attacks returned with a vengeance. She tried drinking, but alcohol did not ward off panic, and she felt defenseless. She feared she would never get well enough to leave her parents' house and cursed her former boyfriend, while feeling unlovable as a cripple. She got the alprazolam she had been taking and swallowed all of the tablets with a beer. She instantly regretted her action and told her parents. They rushed her to the emergency department, where she was stabilized and admitted to a psychiatric hospital.

Kate has many of the conflicts and comorbidities that other sufferers of panic disorder endure. Since the 1989 Weissman et al. study, there has been much debate about whether comorbidity is really the only contributor to the ideation and risk of suicide in individuals with panic disorder. To examine the effect of panic and suicide on a large scale, Nepon et al. (2010) used data from Wave 2 of the National Epidemiologic Survey on Alcohol and Related Conditions (NESARC-II), which is a longitudinal epidemiologic survey of the civilian, noninstitutionalized adult population of the United States. The first part, Wave 1, was conducted from 2001 to 2002, and Wave 2 followed up from 2004 to 2005. The group examined the role of anxiety disorders, including panic, in the 34,653 respondents in Wave 2. As noted earlier in this chapter, Nepon et al. found that 70% of the people who had made a suicide attempt had an anxiety disorder. After adjusting for sociodemographic factors, mood disorders, substance abuse, and schizophrenia or a psychotic illness, the researchers found that all anxiety disorders, except agoraphobia without panic disorder, continued to be significantly associated with suicide attempts. After adjustment for any personality disorder, however, only panic disorder and PTSD were still significantly associated with lifetime suicide attempts. Cougle et al. (2009) used data from Part I and Part II of the National Comorbidity Survey Replication (NCS-R) (N=4,131) to examine lifetime diagnostic histories, including suicidal ideation, and demographic information that was collected through surveys and structured interviews. They reported slightly different findings: that GAD, PTSD, SAD, and panic disorder were all predictors of suicidal thoughts. In contrast, attempts were only associated with GAD, PTSD and SAD, which contradicts the notion that panic disorder is related to suicide attempts. In patients with panic disorder, with or without agoraphobia, the prevalence of lifetime suicidal ideation was 39.4%, and the prevalence of lifetime suicide attempts was 17.3% (P<0.01). Cougle et al.'s multivariate logistic regression analysis of suicidal ideation and suicide attempts for men and woman with panic disorder showed significant results only for suicidal ideation in women (P<0.01) and for suicide attempts in men (P<0.05). They cautioned that the numbers for men were small

and therefore that those findings may not be predictive of reality (Cougle et al. 2009).

Although there are still discrepancies in the literature about suicide risk for pure panic disorder versus comorbid panic disorder, all studies taken together suggest that suicide attempts in individuals with panic disorder are strongly associated with comorbid disorders, including mood disorders, personality disorders, and substance use disorders. Most new data also indicate some association between pure panic disorder and suicidality.

In caring for Kate, it was important to keep in mind that her disease had become traumatic for her—she feared the next panic attack, and her function had declined so that she was unable to leave her house. She also exhibited Cluster A and B traits combined with polysubstance abuse. By the time Kate was discharged from the hospital, she had recommitted to CBT, had a better knowledge of her disease, had begun to do interoceptive therapy, and had begun taking medication. She saw her therapist frequently to address her panic disorder, substance abuse disorder, and personality disorder.

Generalized Anxiety Disorder

GAD is one of the most common anxiety disorders, with a level of impairment equal to that of major depressive disorder (MDD) (Katzman 2009). In most recent studies, GAD has been associated with both suicidal ideation and suicide attempt (Katzman 2009; Ma et al. 2009; Pfeiffer et al. 2009; Sareen et al. 2005), especially in women (Cougle et al. 2009), but not all studies concur (Nepon et al. 2010). GAD has a 12-month prevalence that ranges from 2% to 5%, and in most cases of GAD there is concurrent MDD (Stein 2004). In the Sequenced Treatment Alternatives to Relieve Depression

(STAR*D) trial, patients with anxious major depression were more likely to be at risk for suicide than were those with nonanxious depression, and they often had comorbid GAD (Fava et al. 2004).

The lifetime prevalence of GAD is estimated at 5%, and GAD rates are notably high in middle-aged women, with a 10% lifetime prevalence. The risk of suicide increases as a function of age, rising steadily from adolescence through young adulthood, and this increase may be due to the associated impairment that is the result of the disease (Goldston et al. 2009; Wittchen et al. 2001). GAD is a recurring and pernicious disorder. Because patients with GAD attend primary care settings at a rate of about 8%, there is an opportunity to evaluate and treat these patients and to work to alleviate morbidity and mortality with early and regular intervention and monitoring (Wittchen and Hoyer 2001).

The following case example helps illustrate the progression and degree of debility the illness can elicit in both patient and family.

Case Example 2

Tina was a 45-year-old mother of two teenage girls and a former graphic designer who was faced with divorce from her husband after she discovered his long-term affair with another woman. Although she was angry and humiliated, she was not sure she wanted a divorce. Tina had been anxious as far back as she could recall. In elementary school, she worried about her grades and would get headaches before tests. She worried people would not come to her birthday parties or that she would never find the man she wanted to marry. Although she was good at oil painting, she was too anxious to show her work to her teachers or take the art lessons that her parents offered to pay for. She also worried that when her parents fought, they would get a divorce and that her mother, who was a homemaker, would not be able to support the family if her father left.

She reluctantly went away to college, rather than staying at home, because her closest friend was going, and she compromised her dream of being a studio artist by majoring in graphic design, which had a better chance for employment after college. She saw the college counselor a couple of times for her anxiety, referred by the student health service, where she had gone for recurrent headaches. It helped for her to discuss some of her anxious feelings, and she especially liked the applied relaxation therapy the therapist taught her. In her fourth year, she met her future husband, who was an advertising major and who always seemed to know what he wanted and how to get it.

Tina experienced postpartum depression that progressed to major depression with both of her pregnancies. Each time, in addition to her depressive symptoms, she felt overwhelmed and unprepared for motherhood and was plagued by feelings of inadequacy and impending doom. She was treated with CBT and venlafaxine for several months; she felt both of these modalities provided her with significant relief. One month after the depressive symptoms had passed, she stopped the medication because of sexual side-effects. Because she was busy with her daughters, she didn't finish her course of CBT either. When her oldest child was three, Tina gave up her job to care for her children, because she had been unable to concentrate at work, fearing something would happen when she left them with the nanny. At that time, Tina also began to have many digestive complaints and was placed on a special diet after her gastroenterologist diagnosed her with possible celiac sprue, or gluten-sensitive enteropathy.

It became increasingly difficult for Tina to go to advertising dinners with her husband, because she always worried that she came off poorly. She began having a couple of drinks at home before a party in order to calm her nerves. At the party, she would always nurse a drink, and once she even stumbled and fell after too much wine and had to be brought home early by her husband. The notion of hosting a party made her worry weeks in advance so that no one in the family could relax. She began to feel like a burden to her husband, and she feared he would leave her for another, more capable woman. She felt humiliated that what she feared would happen to her mother was now what she feared would happen to her: that her husband would leave her and she would be unable to support herself or her family. Sometimes she confided her troubles to friends, but she was also afraid she was becoming a burden to them. To make things worse, she began to develop a horrible fear of driving on the highway, especially because she thought her vision was getting a little blurry. This was affecting her now teenage daughters' ability to go to parties. Her mind began to drift to worries that her blurry vision was a brain tumor, and she requested a magnetic resonance imaging (MRI) scan from her doctor. In the waiting room, sitting next to her very frustrated husband, she began to fantasize how the family would do better with another wife and mother.

When she became cognizant of her husband's long-term affair, she meekly confronted him. He apologized for the betrayal and told her he would leave the house and the children to her, and of course pay child support, which he thought was the right thing to do. She saw no way for herself to be able to provide what the children needed, even if she were financially secure, and considered taking a full bottle of Tylenol with wine. Her husband, realizing her danger, took her to see her primary doctor, who referred her to a psychiatrist.

It is important to note that GAD is the anxiety disorder most known to have comorbidities: up to 80% of patients with GAD have another psychiatric disorder (Ma et al. 2009). The presence of comorbidity foretells a less favorable response to both psychotherapeutic and pharmacological treatments. However, patients who are treated for a primary disorder often experience relief from their GAD symptoms (Noyes 2001).

As is suggested in our clinical example, it is often difficult to entirely distinguish GAD from other disorders—including MDD and panic disorder or other anxiety disorders—but treatment is important, because the disease is debilitating and potentially life-threatening (Table 7–4).

Social Anxiety Disorder

Social anxiety disorder is common and occurs by age 13 in 50% and by age 23 in 90% of individuals who develop the disorder (Stein 2006). Comorbid disorders are common in SAD (69% lifetime comorbidity; Schneier et al. 1992), and the SAD often predates, by many years, comorbid disorders that are known predictors of suicide. In the NCS-R, the lifetime prevalence of SAD was 12.1%, with only depression, alcohol abuse, and specific phobia having higher rates (Kessler et al. 2005a). Even when mild cases were excluded, it was found that 4.5% of the population had SAD of moderate to serious severity that impaired functioning and caused work disability (Stein 2006). Studies of more than 13,000 adults in the Epidemiologic Catchment Area (ECA) study found that SAD was associated with increased risk for suicidal ideation but not with higher rates of suicide attempt (Cox et al. 1994; Schneier et al. 1992). In contrast, recent analysis from the NCS-R, in which a similar number of people were surveyed as in the ECA study, has shown, through multivariate analyses covaried for demographic variables and for comorbidity, that women with SAD are at increased risk for both suicidal ideation and suicide attempt (Cougle et al. 2009).

TABLE 7–4. Significant comorbid disorders and imitators of generalized anxiety disorder

Major depressive disorder
Panic disorder
Social phobia
Agoraphobia
Bipolar disorder
Alcohol abuse or dependence

It has been known for decades that SAD increases the general risk of suicide (15.7%) when the SAD is accompanied by a comorbid disorder (Sareen et al. 2005; Schneider et al. 2006). SAD, especially in the generalized form, which involves anxiety in several social situations, has been found to be comorbid with depression and with other anxiety disorders. SAD is associated with an increased risk of depression, and the comorbid depression is often more difficult to treat, prolonging the disorder and increasing the risk of suicide (Stein 2006). Of special note, Perroud et al. (2007) found that SAD was the only anxiety disorder found more commonly in bipolar patients with a lifetime history of suicide attempt than in bipolar patients who had never made a suicide attempt. This finding suggested a potential subtype of bipolar disorder. Unlike many patients with other anxiety disorders, SAD patients do not present to mental health professionals with great frequency. This represents a missed opportunity to diagnose and treat SAD and to see prodromal symptoms of other burgeoning disorders. The following case example demonstrates the long and complicated course of SAD in a patient with early SAD and later comorbidity that led to significant suffering, affecting her self-image, her social life, and her job.

Case Example 3

Sarah was a 39-year-old single woman living alone and employed as a software designer for a Fortune 500 company. She had been a shy child, terrified of speaking up in class since elementary school. Although she always had one or two good friends, she felt unable to approach her peers in the hall or lunchroom and had chills and heard blood rush in her ears when she tried to participate in class. She felt socially awkward and isolated, never attended parties, and never seemed to show interest in her classmates.

When she was a teenager, boys rarely asked her out; she was regarded as being too bright, aloof, and boring. Despite her performance anxiety, she excelled in school and played piano beautifully for her family, although she never gave a public recital. Teachers commented that her potential was clear but that her timidity hindered her from living up to it. Her outgoing mother concurred and tried to push Sarah to "just get out there."

Sarah attended college, where she did well academically despite remaining socially isolated and longing for social contact. She subsequently was hired by a Fortune 500 company to write some individualized programs and, because of her creativity and ingenuity, was hired as permanent staff. She was lauded for her skill and tireless dedication but failed to progress to team manager because she could not lead groups of engineers and always had others give team presentations to their superiors.

As she grew older, she gave up hope of establishing meaningful, romantic relationships. Some affairs had ended painfully, because her partners felt that they could not get to know her. When she was 39 years old, Sarah fell in love with Jerry, an engineer at the firm, with whom she had been thrown together for long hours to work on a special project. They developed a warm friendship as they worked, and she slowly shared personal information. She felt optimistic that something might come of their relationship. She loved children and fantasized that she might marry and have children. Her mother gently pressured her for grandchildren, and Sarah called her to say this could still happen.

Several months into their acquaintance, Jerry dated another engineer and confided his feelings for this woman to Sarah. She lost all hope, not only with him but with any man. She lost sleep and appetite because she felt doomed that she would live a life of trepidation and seclusion. She began to feel more strongly that her life was not worth living. She pondered ways to kill herself that would seem an accident to spare her family humiliation. After much rumination, she revealed her thoughts to her only close friend, who urged her to seek psychiatric help. Sarah responded to a trial of CBT and an SSRI.

This case example depicts the acute pain and loss of potential that accompany SAD, which can lead patients with SAD to desperate measures. There is a chronic course to the disease and a privacy about the the patient that makes it difficult to bring him or her onto the physician's "radar." The greater the number of anxieties, the worse the outcome.

Neuroimaging studies have yielded results, showing that norepinephrine, dopamine, and serotonin are the primary neurotransmitters in SAD. Functional MRI studies demonstrate a role of the amygdala and insula in the neurophysiology of this disorder. CBT has been found useful in treating SAD, and it is not surprising that SSRIs are first-line pharmacotherapies. Serotonin-norepinephrine reuptake inhibitors, monoamine oxidase inhibitors, and benzodiazepines (Fink et al. 2009) have also been found to be beneficial.

Obsessive-Compulsive Disorder

OCD, in both its simple and comorbid forms, has been shown to be associated with increased rates of suicidal ideation and suicide attempt (Hollander et al. 1996). In an early National Institute of Mental Health ECA study, the lifetime rate of OCD was 1.9%–3.3% without exclusions for comorbidity, and 1.2%–2.4% with comorbid exclusions. This distinction is important because individuals with OCD with comorbid disorders were found to have significantly higher rates of suicide attempts (15.0%; 40/266) compared with those with other psychiatric disorders (7.0%; 283/4,020; OR=2.2; 95% CI=1.5–3.2; Hollander et al. 1996). Adults with uncomplicated OCD had significantly higher suicide attempt rates (3.6%; 5/140) compared with those with no psychiatric complaint (0.9%; 128/13,899; OR=3.2, CI=1.3–8.1; Hollander et al. 1996). The Brazilian Research Consortium on Obsessive-Compulsive Spectrum Disorders

found, in a sample of 582 outpatients with primary OCD, that 36% of OCD patients had lifetime suicidal thoughts, whereas 20% had suicidal ideation with a plan, and the suicide attempt rate was 13% (Torres et al. 2011). Factors that distinguished patients who had OCD with accompanying suicidal ideation included past history of MDD, hopelessness, and previous suicide attempts, as reported in another study of 100 patients with OCD in India (Kamath et al. 2007). Patients who had attempted suicide were notable for association with "worst-ever" suicidal ideation. Comorbidity significantly increased prevalence of suicidal ideation in that study, in which 47%–69% of patients with OCD and comorbid MDD and 80% of patients with concurrent OCD and schizophrenia had suicidal thoughts (Kamath et al. 2007). Although adult populations with OCD show a clear increased risk of suicide, a study of a clinic-based sample of 1,979 children and adolescents failed to show any increase in suicidality in this age range (Strauss et al. 2000). Also, no increase in suicide risk was found in an inpatient population of adolescents with OCD (Apter et al. 2003). These findings suggest that a chronic and deteriorating course may lead patients with OCD to desperate thoughts and acts of suicide in later life.

The heightened risk of suicide in adult individuals with OCD has been associated with aggressive obsessions and self-mutilation, both of which encompass violence toward oneself (Rasmussen and Tsuang 1986). Additionally, certain kinds of obsessions and compulsions are associated with higher suicide risk: religious and sexual obsessions, repeating and reassurance-seeking compulsions (Kamath et al. 2007; Torres et al. 2011), and symmetry/ordering obsessions have been independently associated with suicidal behaviors (Alonso et al. 2010). Univariate analysis showed severity of OCD was also correlated with suicide attempt (Balci and Sevincok 2010; Kamath et al. 2007). However, poor-insight OCD, which has been associated with MDD and suicidal ideation in prior studies, bore no association to suicide risk in a study by Kamath et al. (2007).

It has been reported that suicidality in individuals with OCD may be predicted by elevated scores on certain inventories. For example, suicidality was significantly associated with a Yale-Brown Obsessive Compulsive Scale score of greater than 16 and past suicidal ideation was associated with a Beck Depression Inventory score of greater than 19 in a sample of 50 outpatients in Brazil, 14% of whom displayed suicidality (Torres et al. 2007). This finding suggests that assessment scales may be reliable tools to help evaluate suicide risk in OCD patients. Because severity of disease in adults is correlated with suicidality, it is important to understand how patients experience their OCD in humanistic terms, not just in terms of rating scale scores. In a survey of 701 patients with OCD, it was found that their symptoms hindered career aspirations (66%), affected marital relationships (64%), lessened academic achievements (60%), caused loss of intimate relationships (43%), and caused loss of work (22%) (Hollander et al. 1996–1997). These statistics are borne out in the following case example.

Case Example 4

Stan was a 54-year-old man who lived with his brother in a one-bedroom apartment. Stan developed OCD symptoms at the age of 7, with symmetry and counting rituals that severely interfered with his home and school performance. To leave the house, he had to kiss his mother's cheek 100 times and have her turn the lock 25 times because he felt that otherwise something bad might happen to her. At school, he had to push his little toes against his shoes as he walked or, he feared, he would lose these

unnecessary digits. Stan's classmates noticed that he walked strangely and teased him.

In high school, Stan developed intrusive, disturbing sexual obsessions. He saw a psychiatrist, and with CBT and a high dose of an SSRI he was able to get his symptoms under moderate control. He completed a local 4-year college in 7 years. His symptoms continued to make him feel uncomfortable and appear too bizarre to make friends. Stan's brother, a manager at a retail store, got him a job in the stockroom. Stan was reliable and meticulous, but slow. He never advanced and struggled just to keep up.

Adding an atypical antipsychotic and a benzodiazepine to his SSRI in his mid-30s brought about some relief, but when his parents retired to Florida and Stan moved in with his brother, who tried to get him dates, his OCD worsened. On dates, Stan compulsively rearranged the flatware in an attempt to distract himself from unwanted sexual thoughts. His daily repetition and counting was taking up to 6 hours, and his sexual thoughts were humiliating. Stan began to question if his life was worth living. He expressed his hopelessness to his psychiatrist but kept from him his suicidal thoughts.

One night, after his brother told him he was going to marry a woman from work, he realized he could not cope on his own and did not want to intrude on his brother's happiness. Over the next week, he formulated a meticulous suicide plan. When his brother was out visiting his girlfriend, he performed his nighttime counting ritual, wrote a note asking his brother's forgiveness, dressed in his best suit, swallowed 90 of his pills, took the elevator to the roof of his apartment building, and jumped to his death.

Stan had several of the risk factors for suicidality that are found in patients with OCD (Table 7–5). He had repeating compulsions, reassurance-seeking compulsions, and sexual obsessions. He also had a comorbid MDD. The severity of his treatment-refractory symptoms was also a risk factor. Stan had been in therapy and been receiving proper care for his condition for years, which emphasizes the continuing need for research into more effective treatments for OCD. In fact, many patients with OCD are resistant to treatment, and even treatment responders still have considerable OCD symptoms. The high comorbidity that occurs in OCD (Table 7–6) and the meticulous planning that can occur with this disorder are associated with suicide attempts. Suicide attempts can also be associated with discontinuation or withdrawal symptoms in these patients.

Posttraumatic Stress Disorder

Although there is clear evidence that patients with PTSD have an elevated risk of suicide, it remains unproven if the association is due to comorbidity or PTSD alone (Krysinska and Lester 2010; Oquendo et al. 2005; Sareen et al. 2007). Nock et al. (2010) used multivariate analysis of data from the NCS-R (*N*=9,282) to examine this question, investigating individual factors that lead to actual suicide attempts rather than just suicidal ideation. They found, after eliminating comorbidities, that even though depression above all other Axis I psychiatric disorders predicts suicidal ideation, it does not predict attempt. Rather, the disorders that lead to suicide attempt are related to either anxiety/agitation (e.g., PTSD) or poor impulse control (i.e., bipolar disorder, conduct disorder, substance abuse). Nock et al. (2010) emphasized that suicide risk is elevated by one of two factors: increased wish for death and decreased impulse control.

In the United States, lifetime prevalence rates for PTSD are between 1.3% and 7.8%, but individuals at high risk for PTSD who have a history of trauma, such as Vietnam veterans, show rates between 15% and 17% (Krysinska and Lester 2010). In male veterans with PTSD, suicidal thoughts were reported in 70% and suicide attempts were reported in up to 25% (Butterfield et al. 2005). Among high-risk groups internationally, 31% of female rape survivors of the war in Croatia and Bosnia had PTSD, and

TABLE 7–5. Obsessions and compulsions associated with increased suicidality

Religious obsessions
Sexual obsessions
Symmetry obsessions
Ordering obsessions
Repeating compulsions
Reassurance-seeking compulsions

another study showed that 52% of Israeli battered women had PTSD. Swedish refugees with a history of torture and imprisonment showed a staggering (but not surprising) 83% prevalence of PTSD (for review, see Krysinska and Lester 2010). As mentioned above, information from the WHO World Mental Health Surveys revealed that in developed countries, mood disorders tended to predict suicidal behavior, whereas in developing countries, impulse-control disorders, substance use disorders, and PTSD were most predictive of suicidal behavior (Nock et al. 2009).

Data from patients with histories of physical or sexual assault or who have been abused by their partners indicate that PTSD is related to higher rates of suicidal behavior. The diagnosis of PTSD in battered women was shown to be important, because suicide risk was more severe in battered women with PTSD than in battered women without PTSD (Panagioti et al. 2011; Sharhabani-Arzy et al. 2003). Among civilians with chronic PTSD, suicidal ideation was reported in 38%, and suicide attempts were reported in 10% of the sample (Tarrier and Gregg 2004). Adolescents and children also have higher rates of suicidality when they carry the diagnosis of PTSD (De Bellis et al. 1999; Mazza 2000). Factors that influence suicidality in adolescents with PTSD include mood disorders, traumatic grief, childhood abuse, family or peer sui-

TABLE 7–6. Comorbidities leading to increase in suicidality in obsessive-compulsive disorder

Major depressive disorder
Posttraumatic stress disorder
Substance use
Impulse-control disorders

TABLE 7–7. Factors influencing suicide attempts in populations with posttraumatic stress disorder

Veterans
Comorbidity with other psychiatric disorders
    Schizophrenia
    Substance abuse
    Depression
Higher IQ
    More severe depression
    Current suicidal ideation
    High levels of combat-related guilt
    Alexithymia
    High rates of dissociation (questionable)
    History of previous suicide attempt
    White race
    Less consistent love from father
    Intense feelings of survivor guilt
    Low sense of purpose in life
    Crying as means of self-expression
    Low levels of spiritual well-being
    High levels of reexperiencing trauma
Civilians
Impulsivity
Poor social support
Depression
Hostility
Comorbid Cluster B personality disorder
Childhood history of abuse
Childhood history of abuse and recent new abuse
Greater life impairment
Poor occupational and social functioning
Loss of employment
Threat to life

Source. Kotler et al. 2001; Oquendo et al. 2005; Panagioti et al. 2011.

cide, exposure to violence, negative coping styles, and alcohol and drug abuse (Ganz and Sher 2010).

Although it is generally known that PTSD is more common after an interpersonal trauma in which one person intentionally injures another, natural disasters can also cause significant distress, resulting in increased rates of PTSD and suicidal ideation. After Hurricane Mitch hit Nicaragua, it was found that 1 in 10 primary health care patients had developed PTSD. Suicidal ideation was considerably more common in the patients who had PTSD (37.9% vs. 9.0% without PTSD, $P=0.000$) (Caldera et al. 2001). Patients who have had accidents or have been assaulted by criminals also have higher rates of PTSD and suicidal thoughts and behaviors, as reviewed by Panagioti et al. (2011). All of these trauma survivors, and still other populations that have survived different kinds of trauma, share common factors that are associated with PTSD and concurrent suicide attempts (Table 7–7).

Comorbidity is a very important part of understanding the connection of suicide with PTSD. Lifetime PTSD in the presence of drug addiction is highly associated with both lifetime suicidal ideation and lifetime suicide attempts. In a population of 729 methadone users, 36.5% with PTSD versus 16.3% without PTSD ($P<0.001$) had suicidal thoughts. Similarly, 26.9% of PTSD patients versus 9.9% of those without PTSD had a lifetime history of suicide attempt

($P<0.001$) (Villagomez et al. 1995). The connection between depression and PTSD is so great that Sher (2009) has proposed a separate condition termed "posttraumatic mood disorder" (PTMD). Sher contends that PTMD is a distinct diagnosis because patients with this comorbidity have more severe symptoms, higher rates of suicidality, and greater difficulty in social and work settings than do patients who have any of these conditions in isolation. Further, there are differences between PTMD and either of the two conditions alone in terms of cerebrospinal fluid, neuroimaging, sleep, and neuroendocrine challenge findings (Sher 2009). Table 7–8 addresses the relationship between PTMD and the development of suicidal behaviors in veterans. Strategies for suicide prevention in veterans with PTMD are outlined in Table 7–9. Both of the following case examples, one depicting PTSD in a civilian and the other in a veteran, demonstrate the importance of comorbidity in exacerbating suicidal impulses in these populations.

Case Example 5

Carla is a 21-year-old white woman who ran away from home at age 17 because her father, who, when drunk, used to molest her eldest sister, had turned to her when that sister married and moved out. Her father had terrified her by telling her that if she told anyone he would slit her throat, and to reinforce his point he gutted the family cat in front of her.

Since her sister had moved out, she had felt acutely isolated. She had no close friends in school because she felt that her problems at home were more than her friends could handle, and she found that she felt more isolated around them than on her own. She ran away to be with Brandon, with whom she had chatted recently over the Internet. He told her that he was 19 and that she could stay with him for a while. Upon meeting him face-to-face, she quickly learned that he was in his 30s and that she could not stay there rent free—he raped her within the first half hour of her arrival and tattooed her bottom with his name. She stayed with him for the next 18 months, enduring his physical, sexual, and emotional abuse.

Brandon did not drink as her father had, but he did use methamphetamine, and she began to use it with him. She found that she could bear his company only when she was high. She felt dissociated when he forced sex on her, and began to cut herself behind her knees just to make

TABLE 7–8.	Posttraumatic mood disorder and suicidal behavior in veterans

Genetic factors

In utero exposures

Biological/psychosocial influences before exposure to combat

Combat stress: physical injury and psychological injury

Stressors encountered upon return, including specific triggers to suicide

Source. Adapted from Sher 2009.

sure she could still feel. At times she would take more meth than she thought she should in hopes that it might kill her, but she never did actually overdose. When he began to beat her to the point where she thought she might die, she called her sister and was invited to stay with her and her sister's husband.

Once safe, Carla immediately had trouble sleeping at night. She would lie in bed thinking about the humiliation she had experienced with Brandon and became afraid he might try to find her and kidnap her or kill her. She would startle whenever the phone rang, and she found that she could not look at people with tattoos on the street without flashing back to the pain and humiliation of the circumstances of her own tattoo. She would wake with horrible nightmares, thinking Brandon was on top of her. As time passed, Carla had trouble getting out of bed, feeling herself a burden on her married sister and feeling too experienced to go back to school but too inexperienced to get any kind of job that would support her. She felt hopeless and worthless and began to think her birth was a mistake. To keep calm, she turned to the alcohol that her sister kept in the liquor cabinet. She would replace the quantities she had drunk with tap water. When none of the bottles could provide her with relief because they were now too dilute, she went into the bathroom, swallowed a full bottle of aspirin, filled the bathtub with very hot water, got in, and slit her wrists. Her sister found her and called 911, and after Carla was stabilized, she was admitted to the psychiatric ward of the community hospital.

On the ward, Carla was treated with an SSRI for her depression and anxiety and with naltrexone for her nightmares and self-abuse. She had

TABLE 7–9.	Suicide prevention in veterans with posttraumatic mood disorder (PTMD)

Recognition of PTMD

Treatment of PTMD

Relapse prevention

Treatment of suicidal ideation

Treatment of comorbid substance abuse (alcohol and drugs) and substance use disorders

Treatment of medical/neurological disorders (i.e., traumatic brain injury)

Social support

Source. Adapted from Sher 2009.

little trouble stopping her drinking once the SSRI kicked in. She joined a trauma group that used dialectical behavior therapy (DBT) techniques and did CBT both for her suicidality and for her PTSD, including exposure and cognitive reprocessing with her individual therapist. When she left the hospital, she was significantly more hopeful and followed up weekly with her outpatient therapist. Her sister let her stay in her apartment while she got a job in a nearby mall, and at night she went to school to get her GED.

Carla's case demonstrates many of the predictive factors for developing PTSD as well as the course of the disease. Carla came from a childhood of chronic abuse, both witnessed and experienced. She was then subject to another trauma that was reminiscent of the first. In the first and second cases, she felt helpless and afraid for her life. In the first, she felt a horror that some believe acts as a kind of "kindling" process that can lead to added vulnerability for PTSD. Carla was lucky to find a supportive environment when she left her abusive boyfriend/captor, but she also had significant comorbidity by then, including drug abuse, major depression, and some emergent Axis II Cluster B pathology. Carla was treated with CBT for her PTSD and DBT for her comorbid Axis II pathology.

Case Example 6

Jim, a 24-year-old white man, decided to join the army to make his dream of becoming a college graduate come true. He thought he would get money for college, see the world, serve his country, and get away from his oppressive and often physically abusive father, with whom he worked at the family auto shop. He was ambivalent about being deployed to Iraq—he was excited to see an exotic land but concerned by stories of suicide bombers. He could not understand how a person would be willing to blow himself up. Within 2 months, he was familiar with his routine and had made some good friends. He was in a unit that was assigned to clear the mines from the roads to let other vehicles safely pass. It was dangerous work, but he had not encountered any major problems. At times he felt as if he were in a video game and enjoyed the work.

One day, he and a friend flipped a coin to see who would go in the dangerous lead vehicle. He took up the rear. The first vehicle hit a road mine and exploded with such force that he only recalled a deafening clap and a burst of heat that felt like a wall slamming into his head. When he regained consciousness, his head throbbed and blood trickled down his temples. His helmet was gone. He and the soldiers from his overturned vehicle crawled out, and he realized he could not hear anything at all. Outside, he saw the body parts of his fellow soldiers and his friend from the first truck scattered along the road ahead. Jim caught sight of his friend's severed head and collapsed. Moments later, when he regained consciousness, he found he had been pulled behind the overturned truck by one of his buddies and that there was firing going on around him. Enemy snipers had been alerted by the explosion and had come to finish their work. Jim tried to discharge his weapon, but his head ached, he was dizzy, and he was terrified. His buddy motioned for him to stay down and smiled just as he received a sniper shot to his head and fell down next to him. Jim passed out again and woke several days later.

Jim was plagued with migraines and remembered nothing that happened after his friend dropped. He was overcome with guilt. Twice that day he had escaped death, and images of his buddy from the first truck haunted him. He wondered if his second buddy would have died if he had been up fighting next to him. Jim could not stop crying and shaking. His hearing gradually returned, but he had some permanent gaps in his memory. He could not remember how to assemble and disassemble his weapon and had lost fine motor control of his hands, which made it impossible to shoot a weapon with accuracy.

As Jim recovered, he realized that he would not be going to college; there was too much damage to his memory from the trauma from the explosion. He realized he might not be so good at the auto shop either. Over the next few months, the psychiatrist at the army base helped him realize that he probably could not have fired his weapon even if he had gotten up, but Jim felt horribly guilty for surviving the encounter that killed his friends. He cried at the slightest provocation, and the medications to cut back on the nightmares and "take the edge off" were useless to him.

Jim went to a rehabilitation facility for traumatic brain injury, and he began to improve dramatically, relearning many of the processes he had lost. He thought he might have a chance at working at his father's shop again but dreaded the loss of his hopes and the thought of returning home, where he would be dependent on his at times brutal father. He began to wonder if God had not made some terrible mistake by forgetting to kill him, too, that day. Although he knew he was having symptoms of PTSD, he could not find the words to express what he was feeling to anyone. He just knew that he was angrier than he had ever been. He took a bat and smashed up his bedroom after he moved back home.

At night especially, but also at random times, he relived the morning caravan ride. He was not doing well at his father's shop. His hands simply would not follow his directions, and he often stared at auto parts, not remembering what to do with them. Because the noises in the shop were continually jerking him back to the image of his friend's head on the ground, he could not work. He stopped going to his therapy sessions and instead began to drink heavily with his father. Drinking helped, but it was something he had sworn that he would never do. When drunk, he would get into terrible physical fights with his father, which he lost. When his father threatened to throw him out on the street because he was "useless," "a crybaby," and "a drunk," he went to his room, found some pleasure in remembering how to reassemble his weapon, and shot himself in the head.

Jim's development of PTSD with suicidality has some similarities to Carla's. There was an early exposure to violence and abuse that increased his susceptibility to develop PTSD. Additionally, he had an erratic pattern of receiving love from his father, a tendency to express himself by crying, and an accompanying alexithymia. It is unclear if the prodrome is derived primarily from genetic or epigenetic phenomena. Jim had a high IQ, which is also a risk factor for suicidality in PTSD. In combat and shortly thereafter, he had significant stressors, including a traumatic brain injury with severe loss of function that sent him into an existential crisis, in which he lost his sense of purpose in life. Additionally, he was plagued by intense feelings of guilt over not having helped in his mission and at having survived his friends who had helped him. The comorbidity, along with depression, that made his PTMD lethal was likely his alcoholism, which increased his impulsivity in the context of a diminished will to live (Table 7–9). A factor that should have been addressed by his health care provider was that there was a firearm in the house of an individual at increased risk for suicide.

Conclusion

Anxiety disorders are among the most commonly diagnosed psychiatric disorders. Data published since the last edition of this volume suggest that anxiety with suicidality is much more prevalent than previously thought, both in isolation and with comorbidities. The presence of an anxiety disorder is significantly associated with suicide attempt, even after adjustment for social and demographic factors and Axis I and Axis II disorders. PTSD, substance abuse, and impulsive disorders are major risk factors for suicide that significantly increase morbidity and mortality when combined with anxiety disorders. Factors discussed in the chapter that distinguish the different anxiety disorders are important for assessment and management of suicidality. Many studies attempt to distinguish suicidal ideation and suicide attempt when evaluating suicidality. Although there is still disagreement about which anxiety disorders cause suicidal ideation and which cause suicide attempt, it is known that suicidal ideation is a risk factor for suicide attempt, and so the clinician must be vigilant in either instance.

Age at onset, gender, severity of symptoms, knowledge of dangerous comorbidities, and presentation in the health care environment are all factors that help clinicians strategize to identify and treat at-risk patients. The tables in this chapter are resources for analyzing risk factors with specific anxiety disorders. It is generally felt that the sooner a diagnosis is made, the less likely a disease is to progress to a suicidal end. It is also assumed that because

anxiety disorders and their comorbidities are factors in suicidality, treatment of them will diminish suicidal thoughts and behaviors; in the majority of cases, however, these are only assumptions that still remain to be proven (Sareen et al. 2005).

It must be remembered that suicidality in anxiety disorders peaks at different ages. A disorder such as OCD, which occurs early in life, has a low risk for suicidality in childhood and adolescence but a higher risk during later stages in life, whereas GAD presents itself most strongly in middle life and contains risk beginning in adolescence and progressing through adulthood (Goldston et al. 2009). This finding suggests that the clinician must be vigilant with patients who have been diagnosed with anxiety disorders and screen for these conditions repeatedly at appropriate times in the life cycle. Perhaps as neuroimaging, neuroendocrinology, and neurogenetics progress, we will gain a greater understanding of which diseases affect what portions of the brain and what modalities palliate and reduce suicide risk.

Key Clinical Concepts

Panic Disorder

- Panic disorder likely confers an increased risk for suicidal ideation and suicide attempt.
- Patients with panic disorder must be screened for comorbidities as well as the severity of panic and comorbidity.
- Suicide assessments belong in the treatment of patients with panic disorder both at the start and during treatment.

Generalized Anxiety Disorder

- The high incidence of patients with generalized anxiety disorder (GAD) presenting to their primary care doctor represents an opportunity for suicide evaluation and referral for treatment.

- GAD becomes more prevalent as patients, especially women, reach middle age, so repeated evaluation may be necessary.
- The frequent presence of comorbidity, especially depression and substance use, significantly increases risk for suicidality.
- Pharmacotherapy that addresses both depression and anxiety together should be considered, such as a selective serotonin reuptake inhibitor (SSRI) or a serotonin-norepinephrine reuptake inhibitor.
- Multiple psychotherapeutic approaches may be necessary to deal with the GAD and comorbid depression or substance use, such as cognitive-behavioral therapy (CBT) and substance abuse counseling.
- Deteriorated function is a warning sign for suicidality.

Social Anxiety Disorder

- Social anxiety disorder (SAD) may carry an independent risk for suicidal ideation and suicide attempt, and this requires a careful suicide screen in patients diagnosed with this disorder.
- The risk for suicidal ideation and suicide attempt caused by SAD appears to be greater in women.
- SAD occurs early in individuals, before the evolution of other comorbidities, and early detection and treatment may help to diminish suicide risk in later years.
- Social phobia should be assessed in patients with bipolar disorder because of their heightened risk for suicide with this comorbidity.
- Caution must be given if treating social phobia in patients with bipolar disorder, because SSRIs must be used with caution in bipolar disorder; however, CBT is an evidence-based approach with fewer side effects.
- Generalized SAD, which predicts worse function, and depression are major risk factors for suicide in patients with SAD.

Obsessive-Compulsive Disorder

- Patients with obsessive-compulsive disorder (OCD) should be assessed for suicide risk and depression. Rating scales such as the Columbia Suicide Assessment Scale, the Scale for Suicide Ideation (worst ever [lifetime] and current), the Hamilton Rating Scale for Depression, the Beck Hopelessness Scale, and the Beck Depression Inventory may be useful tools for assessing suicidality in OCD patients.
- OCD has a high risk for suicidal behavior; hopelessness and severity of symptoms are the correlates for suicidality. The Yale-Brown Obsessive Compulsive Scale is an important tool in assessing severity of OCD symptoms.
- Comorbidities for suicidal behaviors with OCD include lifetime history of major depressive disorder, posttraumatic stress disorder (PTSD), substance use, and impulse-control disorders.

- Religious and sexual obsessions, repeating and reassurance-seeking compulsions, and symmetry/ordering obsessions are independently associated with suicidal behaviors.

- Primary care physicians must be alert to patients with OCD because these patients often present first to them, and early diagnosis and treatment of OCD can substantially improve outcome.

- Clinicians should be alert to the role of withdrawal symptoms in suicidal behaviors.

Posttraumatic Stress Disorder

- Comorbidities in PTSD substantially increase the danger of suicidal ideation and behavior; it is important to do a thorough screen for depression, substance use, and impulsivity, among others.

- Cluster B personality disorders are already associated with high suicidality and even more so in the presence of PTSD.

- CBT can be used to treat both the PTSD and the suicidality caused by it.

- Medication management of the anxiety and the symptoms of PTSD can bring enormous relief and can be used to make a highly traumatized patient more ready for therapy.

- Severity of PTSD symptoms and greater childhood and lifetime trauma are associated with increased suicidality.

- Because improvement of social support is protective for suicidality in patients with PTSD, it is important to help place the individual in a stable, supportive environment.

- Loss of employment is a risk factor for suicidality in patients with PTSD, and special attention must be paid to anticipate impulsive responses to this already stressful life event.

- Relapse prevention must be a strategy for continued management of patients with PTSD.

References

Alonso P, Segalàs C, Real E, et al: Suicide in patients treated for obsessive-compulsive disorder: a prospective follow-up study. J Affect Disord 124:300–308, 2010

Apter N, Horesh D, Gothelf G, et al: Depression and suicidal behavior in adolescent inpatients with obsessive compulsive disorder. J Affect Disord 75:181–189, 2003

Balci V, Sevincok L: Suicidal ideation in patients with obsessive-compulsive disorder. Psychiatry Res 175:104–108, 2010

Bolton JM, Cox BJ, Afifi TO, et al: Anxiety disorders and risk for suicide attempts: findings from the Baltimore Epidemiologic Catchment Area follow-up study. Depress Anxiety 25:477–481, 2008

Butterfield MI, Stechuchak KM, Connor KM, et al: Neuroactive steroids and suicidality in posttraumatic stress disorder. Am J Psychiatry 162:380–382, 2005

Caldera T, Palma L, Penayo U, et al: Psychological impact of the hurricane Mitch in Nicaragua in a one-year perspective. Soc Psychiatry Psychiatr Epidemiol 36:108–114, 2001

Cougle JR, Keough ME, Riccardi CJ, et al: Anxiety disorders and suicidality in the National Comorbidity Survey-Replication. J Psychiatr Res 43:825–829, 2009

Cox BJ, Direnfeld DM, Swinson RP, et al: Suicidal ideation and suicide attempts in panic disorder and social phobia. Am J Psychiatry 151:882–887, 1994

De Bellis MD, Baum AS, Birmaher B, et al: A. E. Bennett Research Award. Developmental traumatology, Part I: biological stress systems. Biol Psychiatry 45:1259–1270, 1999

Fava M, Alpert JE, Carmin CN, et al: Clinical correlates and symptom patterns of anxious depression among patients with major depressive disorder in STAR*D. Psychol Med 34:1299–1308, 2004

Fink M, Akimova E, Spindelegger C, et al: Social anxiety disorder: epidemiology, biology and treatment. Psychiatr Danub 21:533–542, 2009

Friedman S, Smith L, Fogel A: Suicidality in panic disorder: a comparison with schizophrenic, depressed, and other anxiety disorder patients. J Anxiety Disord 13:447–461, 1999

Ganz D, Sher L: Suicidal behavior in adolescents with post-traumatic stress disorder. Minerva Pediatr 62:363–370, 2010

Goldston DB, Daniel SS, Erkanli A, et al: Psychiatric diagnoses as contemporaneous risk factors for suicide attempts among adolescents and young adults: developmental changes. J Consult Clin Psychol 77:281–290, 2009

Hollander E, Kwon JH, Stein DJ, et al: Obsessive-compulsive and spectrum disorders: overview and quality of life issues. J Clin Psychiatry 57 (suppl 8):3–6, 1996

Hollander E, Greenwald S, Neville D, et al: Uncomplicated and comorbid obsessive-compulsive disorder in an epidemiologic sample. Depress Anxiety 4:111–119, 1996–1997

Huang MF, Yen CF, Lung FW: Moderators and mediators among panic, agoraphobia symptoms, and suicidal ideation in patients with panic disorder. Compr Psychiatry 51:243–249, 2010

Kamath P, Reddy YC, Kandavel T: Suicidal behavior in obsessive-compulsive disorder. J Clin Psychiatry 68:1741–1750, 2007

Katzman MA: Current considerations in the treatment of generalized anxiety disorder. CNS Drugs 23:103–120, 2009

Kessler RC, Berglund P, Demler O, et al: Lifetime prevalence and age-of-onset distributions of DSM-IV disorders in the National Comorbidity Survey Replication. Arch Gen Psychiatry 62:593–602, 2005a

Kessler RC, Chiu WT, Demler O, et al: Prevalence, severity, and comorbidity of twelve-month DSM-IV disorders in the National Comorbidity Survey Replication (NCS-R). Arch Gen Psychiatry 62:617–627, 2005b

Kotler M, Iancu I, Efroni R, et al: Anger, impulsivity, social support, and suicide risk in patients with posttraumatic stress disorder. J Nerv Ment Dis 189:162–167, 2001

Krysinska K, Lester D: Posttraumatic stress disorder and suicide risk: a systematic review. Arch Suicide Res 14:1–23, 2010

Ma X, Xiang YT, Cai ZJ, et al: Generalized anxiety disorder in China: prevalence, sociodemographic correlates, comorbidity, and suicide attempts. Perspect Psychiatr Care 45:119–127, 2009

Mazza JJ: The relationship between posttraumatic stress symptomatology and suicidal behavior in school-based adolescents. Suicide Life Threat Behav 30:91–103, 2000

Nepon J, Belik SL, Bolton J, et al: The relationship between anxiety disorders and suicide attempts: findings from the National Epidemiologic Survey on Alcohol and Related Conditions. Depress Anxiety 27:791–798, 2010

Nock MK, Hwang I, Sampson N, et al: Cross-national analysis of the associations among mental disorders and suicidal behavior: findings from the WHO World Mental Health Surveys. PLoS Med 6:e1000123, 2009

Nock MK, Hwang I, Sampson NA, et al: Mental disorders, comorbidity and suicidal behavior: results from the National Comorbidity Survey Replication. Mol Psychiatry 15:868–876, 2010

Norton PJ, Temple SR, Pettit JW: Suicidal ideation and anxiety disorders: elevated risk or artifact of comorbid depression? J Behav Ther Exp Psychiatry 39:515–525, 2008

Noyes R Jr: Comorbidity in generalized anxiety disorder. Psychiatr Clin North Am 24:41–55, 2001

Oquendo M, Brent DA, Birmaher B, et al: Posttraumatic stress disorder comorbid with major depression: factors mediating the association with suicidal behavior. Am J Psychiatry 162:560–566, 2005

Panagioti M, Gooding PA, Dunn G, et al: Pathways to suicidal behavior in posttraumatic stress disorder. J Trauma Stress 24:137–145, 2011

Perroud N, Baud P, Preisig M, et al: Social phobia is associated with suicide attempt history in bipolar inpatients. Bipolar Disord 9:713–721, 2007

Pfeiffer PN, Ganoczy D, Ilgen M, et al: Comorbid anxiety as a suicide risk factor among depressed veterans. Depress Anxiety 26:752–757, 2009

Rasmussen SA, Tsuang MT: Clinical characteristics and family history in DSM-III obsessive-compulsive disorder. Am J Psychiatry 143:317–322, 1986

Sareen J, Cox BJ, Afifi TO, et al: Anxiety disorders and risk for suicidal ideation and suicide attempts: a population-based longitudinal study of adults. Arch Gen Psychiatry 62:1249–1257, 2005

Sareen J, Cox BJ, Stein MB, et al: Physical and mental comorbidity, disability, and suicidal behavior associated with posttraumatic stress disorder in a large community sample. Psychosom Med 69:242–248, 2007

Schmidt NB, Woolaway-Bickel K, Bates M: Evaluating panic-specific factors in the relationship between suicide and panic disorder. Behav Res Ther 39:635–649, 2001

Schneier FR, Johnson J, Hornig CD, et al: Social phobia: comorbidity and morbidity in an epidemiologic sample. Arch Gen Psychiatry 49:282–288, 1992

Sharhabani-Arzy R, Amir M, Kotler M, et al: The toll of domestic violence: PTSD among battered women in an Israeli sample. J Interpers Violence 18:1335–1346, 2003

Sher L: A model of suicidal behavior in war veterans with posttraumatic mood disorder. Med Hypotheses 73:215–219, 2009

Stein MB: Public health perspectives on generalized anxiety disorder. J Clin Psychiatry 65 (suppl 13):3–7, 2004

Stein MB: An epidemiologic perspective on social anxiety disorder. J Clin Psychiatry 67 (suppl 12):3–8, 2006

Strauss J, Birmaher B, Bridge J, et al: Anxiety disorders in suicidal youth. Can J Psychiatry 45:739–745, 2000

Tarrier N, Gregg L: Suicide risk in civilian PTSD patients: predictors of suicidal ideation, planning, and attempts. Soc Psychiatry Psychiatr Epidemiol 39:655–661, 2004

Tidemalm D, Långström N, Lichtenstein P, et al: Risk of suicide after suicide attempt according to coexisting psychiatric disorder: Swedish cohort study with long term follow-up (abstract). BMJ 337:2205, 2008

Torres AR, de Abreu Ramos-Cerqueira AT, Torresan RC, et al: Prevalence and associated factors for suicidal ideation and behaviors in obsessive-compulsive disorder. CNS Spectr 12:771–778, 2007

Torres AR, Ramos-Cerqueira AT, Ferrão YA, et al: Suicidality in obsessive-compulsive disorder: prevalence and relation to symptom dimensions and comorbid conditions. J Clin Psychiatry 72:17–26, 2011

Villagomez RE, Meyer TJ, Lin MM, et al: Posttraumatic stress disorder among inner city methadone maintenance patients. J Subst Abuse Treat 12:253–257, 1995

Warshaw MG, Dolan RT, Keller MB: Suicidal behavior in patients with current or past panic disorder: five years of prospective data from the Harvard/Brown Anxiety Research Program. Am J Psychiatry 157:1876–1878, 2000

Weissman MM, Klerman GL, Markowitz JS, et al: Suicidal ideation and suicide attempts in panic disorder and attacks. N Engl J Med 321:1209–1214, 1989

Wittchen HU, Hoyer J: Generalized anxiety disorder: nature and course. J Clin Psychiatry 62 (suppl 11):15–21, 2001

C H A P T E R   8

Substance-Related Disorders

Martin H. Leamon, M.D.

J. Michael Bostwick, M.D.

During 2009, approximately 42% of the world's population 15 years and older (an estimated 70% in the United States) consumed alcohol, and approximately 4.8% (an estimated 16% in the United States) used illicit substances (Substance Abuse and Mental Health Services Administration 2010; United Nations Office on Drugs and Crime 2011; World Health Organization 2011a). Roughly 19% of the world's population 15 years and older (an estimated 27% in the United States) are current smokers (Substance Abuse and Mental Health Services Administration 2010; World Health Organization 2011b).

Substance use is not rare; it interacts with suicide in many ways. Worldwide, 15%–61% of individuals who died by suicide had alcohol use disorders, and other substance use disorders have been associated with suicide as well (Schneider 2009; Vijayakumar et al. 2011). Substance use disorders also predict suicide attempts, and suicidal ideation can be a component of substance intoxication, substance withdrawal, or substance-induced mood disorders (Nock et al. 2010).

Evidence Base Issues and Terminology

The evidence base on the interactions among suicide, related events, and substance use is substantial, but attempts to compare studies or to extrapolate clinical relevance from individual studies are hampered by confusing and contradictory data. It is worth examining this issue briefly, because readers of this chapter will continue to see future studies or reviews of this topic. Although these issues may be relevant to reading medical literature in general, they hold particular relevance for reading about the relationships between suicide-related events and substance use.

The problems of classification of suicide-related events are dealt with in detail elsewhere in this book (see Chapter 1, "Suicide Risk Assessment: Gateway to Treatment and Management"), but there is only partial overlap between individuals with thoughts of suicide, those who attempt suicide, and those who die by suicide (Nock et al. 2010). For example, study findings on people who die by suicide may not be generalizable to people with suicidal thoughts. In addition, different studies may apply different classifications of suicide-related events depending on instruments used and populations studied.

The degree of clinical relevance can be affected by the time periods for events chosen for a study. Substance use disorders are typically described as 1) lifetime diagnoses (i.e., ever having been present), 2) diagnoses present or absent over the past year, or 3) current, which usually means during the preceding 30 days. Suicide attempts and suicidal ideation may be similarly measured as lifetime, past year, or current. For example, a finding of a relationship between a lifetime diagnosis of a substance use disorder and current suicidal thoughts may have more direct relevance to the assessment of a patient than a finding that patients with substance abuse at sometime in their lives (i.e., lifetime) are more apt to have suicidal thoughts at some point during their lives (also lifetime).

Applicability of studies can also be complicated because of the different populations studied. Studies of substance use disorders in the general population include many participants with less severe substance use disorders, whereas studies recruiting patients from substance use disorder treatment settings tend to have participants with both more severe substance use disorders and more clinically important co-occurring psychiatric disorders. Similarly, one investigation into the relationships among suicide, substance use, and co-occurring psychiatric disorders may look at specific diagnosed co-occurring disorders, whereas another may look at co-occurring symptom clusters that may not reach diagnostic thresholds.

The classification of substance use is somewhat less complicated but affects clinical applicability. The American Psychiatric Association's *Diagnostic and Statistical Manual of Mental Disorders,* 4th Edition, Text Revision (DSM-IV-TR; American Psychiatric Association 2000), separates substance-related disorders into substance-induced disorders and substance use disorders (see Tables 8–1 and 8–2.) The *International Classification of Diseases,* 10th Revision (World Health Organization 1992), uses similar but not identical divisions. DSM-III used slightly different definitions (American Psychiatric Association 1980), and DSM-5 may use different diagnostic criteria as well (American Psychiatric Association 2010). Essentially, none of the substance-related disorder diagnostic criteria except for intoxication mandate acute substance use at the time of diagnosis. Consequently, a study of current alcohol *use* and current suicidal thoughts could have very different clinical implications than a study looking at current diagnoses of alcohol *dependence* and current suicidal thoughts.

In this chapter, we use the DSM-IV-TR classification system for substance use disorders, but (to allow some flexibility of word choice) we may also use the term *addiction* to mean substance dependence and *addict* to mean individuals with substance dependence. We use an encompassing term, *suicide-related events,* to include suicide, suicide attempts, and suicidal thoughts.

Models of Suicide

The constructs of *proximal* and *distal* risk factors for suicide are useful when thinking about the clinical impact of substance use and substance-related disorders on suicide and when thinking about how to intervene therapeutically. Substance dependence is a distal risk factor, and substance intoxication a proximal one. Depending on the

TABLE 8–1.	DSM-IV-TR classification of substance-related disorders

Substance use disorders

    Dependence

    Abuse

Substance-induced disorders

    Intoxication

    Withdrawal

Others (see Table 8–2)

Source. Reprinted from *Diagnostic and Statistical Manual of Mental Disorders*, 4th Edition, Text Revision. Washington, DC, American Psychiatric Association, 2000. Used with permission. Copyright © 2000 American Psychiatric Association.

chronicity and frequency of substance use, substance-induced mood disorders may be either proximal or distal factors. Clinically, one looks at proximal risk factors or stressors as more immediate targets for therapeutic intervention and distal ones as longer-term targets.

The stress-diathesis model of suicidal behaviors is somewhat less immediately clinically applicable. In its original conception, *diathesis* refers to innate constitutional factors more along the lines of temperament than of personality (Mann 2003). In this model, substance dependence would be regarded as a distal stress factor rather than a diathesis component, and intoxication or withdrawal would be considered a proximal stressor. Impulsivity as a predisposing factor for both suicidal behaviors and substance use disorders would be a component of the diathesis, as would, for example, certain genetic haplotypes associated with serotonergic neurotransmission in the brain.

Case Examples

Maria is a 25-year-old woman who has been staying out late and using crack cocaine multiple times a day, and her nonusing fiancé is fed

up with her. Her drug supply runs out, and she is unable to obtain more. Within hours, she is tired, slowed down, and hungry and just wants to sleep. She is also feeling progressively more dysphoric. She tries to return home, but her fiancé will not let her in, yelling through the door that she has had her last chance and that the relationship is over. She goes next door to the market and buys a bottle of cold pills and a soft drink. She walks back outside, sits down on the curb, and swallows the whole bottle of pills. The market owner sees her do this through the window and calls emergency services.

Marcus is a 32-year-old veteran who has been a self-described "functioning alcoholic" since he joined the U.S. Army at age 18. After several tours of duty in combat areas, he was honorably discharged. He has realistic nightmares of combat events, but his heavy daily drinking helps suppress these symptoms and allows him to avoid experiencing them. He successfully completes an outpatient treatment program for alcohol dependence that also addresses his posttraumatic stress symptoms. He remains sober for several years and gets a job teaching college students. The young students, however, increasingly remind him of fellow soldiers he saw killed and was unable to save. The nightmares and other symptoms return, and he resumes dependent drinking. His depression mounts. One night, he drinks a bottle of whiskey and feels overwhelmed with guilt. He puts his pistol to his head and pulls the trigger.

Maria's overdosing on pills occurs during a particular phase of her substance use—during acute cocaine withdrawal, a proximal risk factor. It is likely that when she is intoxicated with cocaine, her mood is quite different. Over a much longer phase, her cocaine dependence, a distal risk factor, has led to relationship problems (another distal risk) that comes to a head during her withdrawal.

Marcus's suicide occurs at a different phase of substance use—while he is actively intoxicated. His resumed drinking precipitates an alcohol-induced mood disorder with depressive features, which augments the worsening symptoms of his co-occurring posttraumatic stress disorder (PTSD). The alcohol that he formerly used to suppress symptoms now fatally reduces his inhibitions.

Neurobiology

The neurobiology of substance dependence and suicide may overlap in terms of neurotransmitter systems and brain regions involved in each (Ross and Peselow 2009; Underwood and Arango 2011; van Heeringen et al. 2011). Impaired executive control from the prefrontal cortex through alterations in excitatory and inhibitory neurocircuitry is a feature of both.

Related to this impaired executive control is impulsivity, which has long been recognized as contributing to both substance use disorders and suicide-related events (Dougherty et al. 2004; Gvion and Apter 2011). Although there is much face validity to and general agreement about the contribution of impulsivity, this factor has been difficult to study. Integrating findings across studies has been difficult, in part due to problems in specifying the exact nature of impulsivity and how best to measure it (Gvion and Apter 2011). Accordingly, the specifics of the underlying neurobiology have yet to be elucidated in a manner that translates meaningfully into clinical care.

Substance-Specific Concerns

General

Overall, individuals with substance use disorders have the same risk factors for suicide-related events as those without substance use. Because of the social and occupational impairments inherently associated with sub-

stance use disorders, however, such individuals are apt to have more proximal risk factors and ones of greater severity (Darke et al. 2007; Wenzel et al. 2008). Additionally, many substances can induce a mood disorder with depressive features, and the withdrawal syndromes of many substances include dysphoria or depressed mood as a component.

Nicotine

In both adult and adolescent populations, there is a highly replicated association between current tobacco smoking (which overwhelmingly means cigarettes) and suicide-related events, with some suggestion of a dose-dependent, positive relationship. A number of different theories and mechanisms of interaction have been proposed (see Hughes 2008 for an excellent review). Given the relationship, a reasonable follow-on hypothesis might be that smoking cessation could reduce the risk of suicide and related behaviors. Although some evidence suggests that this might be the case, more detailed analyses have shown that the association is mediated by the presence of other psychiatric disorders (Berlin et al. 2011; Hughes 2008). Nicotine dependence is probably now best regarded as a general marker for suicidality along with other substance use and other psychiatric disorders. Although former smokers are at lower risk for suicide-related events than current smokers, the difference is likely due to reduction in other risk factors than to the smoking cessation itself.

Dysphoria or depressed mood is one of the DSM-IV-TR criteria for nicotine withdrawal, and patients preparing to quit smoking should at least be educated about withdrawal symptoms and when to ask for additional help with mood symptoms. Nicotine replacement therapy can help alleviate

TABLE 8–2. Diagnoses associated with class of substances

	Dependence	Abuse	Intoxication	Withdrawal	Intoxication delirium	Withdrawal delirium	Dementia	Amnestic disorder	Psychotic disorders	Mood disorders	Anxiety disorders	Sexual dysfunctions	Sleep disorders
Alcohol	X	X	X	X	I	W	P	P	I/W	I/W	I/W	I	I/W
Amphetamines	X	X	X	X	I				I	I/W	I	I	I/W
Caffeine	X		X								I		I
Cannabis	X	X	X		I				I		I		
Cocaine	X	X	X	X	I				I	I/W	I/W	I	I/W
Hallucinogens	X	X	X		I				I*	I	I		
Inhalants	X	X	X		I		P		I	I	I		
Nicotine	X			X									
Opioids	X	X	X	X	I				I	I		I	I/W
Phencyclidine	X	X	X		I				I	I	I		
Sedatives, hypnotics, or anxiolytics	X	X	X	X	I	W	P	P	I/W	I/W	W	I	I/W
Polysubstance	X												
Other	X	X	X	X	I	W	P	P	I/W	I/W	I/W	I	I/W

Note: X, I, W, I/W, or P indicates that the category is recognized in DSM-IV. In addition, I indicates that the specifier With Onset During Intoxication may be noted for the category (except for Intoxication Delirium); W indicates that the specifier With Onset During Withdrawal may be noted for the category (except for Withdrawal Delirium); and I/W indicates that either With Onset During Intoxication or With Onset During Withdrawal may be noted for the category. P indicates that the disorder is Persisting.

*Also Hallucinogen Persisting Perception Disorder (Flashbacks).

mood symptoms of withdrawal and has been shown not to increase rates of suicide-related events. Neither have two of the other medications used, bupropion or nortriptyline, when used for smoking cessation—their warnings against increased risk mandated by the U.S. Food and Drug Administration is a class warning required for all antidepressants. In postmarketing surveillance, there have been concerns that varenicline has an increased risk of a variety of neuropsychiatric side effects, although it is not clear that these include a specific increased risk of suicide-related events either in the general population or in patients with existing psychiatric disorders (Garza et al. 2011; Purvis et al. 2010). Nevertheless, particularly if other risk factors are present, it would be prudent to monitor patients taking varenicline more closely than those undergoing nicotine replacement.

In general, all patients who are smokers should be encouraged and supported in smoking cessation attempts, because all smokers are more likely to die from smoking-related general medical conditions than from suicide, even in the presence of other risk factors for suicide. For example, smokers with alcohol dependence are more likely to die from smoking-related causes than from either alcohol- or suicide-related causes.

Alcohol

The relationship between suicide-related events and alcohol-related disorders has been studied much more than the relationship of such events with other substance-related disorders. Individuals with alcohol use disorders have an approximate overall 7% lifetime risk of dying by suicide, with women being at greater risk than men; the risks are higher if only individuals with al-

cohol dependence are considered (Schneider 2009). Viewed from another perspective, between 15% and 60% of people who die by suicide have been found upon psychological autopsy to have had lifetime alcohol use disorders.

Acute alcohol ingestion is found on autopsy in approximately 35% of people who die by suicide, and the percentage is similar for people who attempt suicide, although in the latter the percentages range from about 10% to 70%, depending on the study.

Cannabis

There is little available information on the interactions between cannabis use or cannabis-related disorders and risk of suicide-related events, and studies yielded discrepant findings (Arendt et al. 2011; Calabria et al. 2010). It would be plausible for cannabis dependence to convey some level of increased risk for suicide, because impulsivity and impaired frontal control are assumed to be components of all substance dependence disorders. One of the criteria proposed for the newly characterized disorder of cannabis withdrawal is depressed mood that potentially may last for weeks (American Psychiatric Association 2010). As with nicotine, it makes good clinical sense to educate individuals undergoing cannabis withdrawal about the syndrome and to monitor them for mood changes that may indicate increased risk.

Cocaine and Amphetamines

Cocaine use disorders increase the risk of suicide-related events, but the magnitude of the increased risk has varied across studies, most of which have been in populations with the additional risk factors of low income and social disadvantage (Degenhardt et al. 2011). Cocaine dependence is a risk factor that seems to cluster with other non–substance-related ones (Roy 2009). Dysphoric mood is a required symptom for the DSM-IV-TR diagnosis of cocaine withdrawal and can confer a proximal risk, as illustrated in the case example of Maria earlier in the chapter. Appropriate assessment, monitoring, and intervention should be performed for any patient with a cocaine-related disorder and especially during withdrawal.

Amphetamine use disorders, primarily involving methamphetamine, probably also increase the risk of suicide, suicide attempts, and suicidal thoughts, but the findings have not always been consistent, perhaps as a result of differences in study design (Marshall and Werb 2010). In one large-scale prospective study (Marshall et al. 2011), injection methamphetamine use was associated with increased risk of earlier suicide attempt, with the increase perhaps greater than that for heroin or cocaine injection use. Symptoms of depression are common in recently abstinent methamphetamine addicts.

Opioids

Similar to cocaine dependence, heroin dependence is associated with increased risk for suicide-related events compared with risk in the general population, but there do not seem to be any risk factors specific to opioid use per se (Darke et al. 2007). As with other substances, polysubstance use, physical and sexual trauma, depressive symptoms, and co-occurring psychiatric disorders all serve to augment risk. Nevertheless, even though the risk factors for attempted suicide do not differ between people addicted to heroin and the general population, the risk in the former is amplified by up to 14 times. As mentioned elsewhere in this chapter, although opioid overdose in opioid addicts is associated with increased risk of sui-

cide attempts, most of these overdoses are not in themselves suicide attempts. People addicted to heroin tend to use means other than opioid overdose during attempts.

Dysphoric mood is one of a number of nonmandatory criteria for the DSM-IV-TR diagnosis of opioid withdrawal. Unassisted opioid withdrawal can be extremely uncomfortable, and patients may develop suicidal thoughts during that kind of withdrawal. Medically managing the withdrawal with symptom amelioration or a substitute-and-taper approach usually relieves the dysphoria.

Pharmacotherapy for opioid dependence includes treatment with the full μ agonist methadone, the partial μ agonist buprenorphine, or the full μ antagonist naltrexone. Buprenorphine is almost always administered compounded with naloxone, and naltrexone is most usually being offered as a monthly depot injection (an implant is available in a few countries). Patients with opioid dependence treated with buprenorphine-naloxone maintenance or methadone maintenance have a much lower rate of suicide than those without medication-assisted treatment. Of patients receiving maintenance therapy, those treated with buprenorphine-naloxone may have a lower risk of suicide compared with those treated with methadone (Soyka et al. 2011). Although there were initial concerns that a long-acting naltrexone preparation might increase the risk of suicide-related events, no such effect has been found (Tait et al. 2008).

Sedative-Hypnotics

Sedative-hypnotics, including the newer nonbenzodiazepine receptor agonists such as zolpidem, are associated with increased risk of suicide-related events, even when controlling for insomnia, which is itself a risk factor (Brower et al. 2011). Benzodiazepines are also frequently used with other substances in suicide by polydrug overdose.

Other Substances

Inhalants

People who use, abuse, or are dependent on inhalants are all at higher risk for lifetime suicide-related events in large general population-based surveys, although the particulars of the relationships have differed between studies (Howard et al. 2010).

MDMA

Lifetime 3,4-methylenedioxymethamphetamine (MDMA/ecstasy) use in adolescents is strongly associated with a past-year suicide attempt, even after other drug use, anxiety disorder, and other factors were controlled for (Kim et al. 2011). MDMA may pose a greater increased risk than other substances.

Patient Assessment

Depending on the setting and urgency, patients may need immediate assessment and intervention to ensure adequate general medical stability and physical safety. Patients with substance-induced toxicity or severe withdrawal symptoms may need poison control management or urgent treatment of withdrawal symptoms before any other assessment. Admission for general medical or psychiatric hospitalization may be required. Once the patient is acutely stabilized, further psychiatric assessment can proceed. Assessment highlights are listed in Table 8–3.

All patients presenting with a suicide attempt, with suicidal thoughts, or with other significant risk factors for suicide should be thoroughly assessed for substance use, regardless of the clinical setting. It is best

TABLE 8–3.	Important suicide assessment items when substance use or use disorders are present

History of suicide attempts

History of overdose

Physical assault before 18 years old

Sexual assault before 18 years old

Living situation (alone, with others, etc.)

Poly substance use

Current substance use

Substance use disorders and their severity

Co-occurring Axis I and Axis II disorders[a]

Depressive symptoms

Sense of belonging

Feelings of self-efficacy or mastery versus feeling overwhelmed

[a]According to the DSM-IV-TR multiaxial conventions.

to ask routinely about all substances in addition to those that the patient mentions and those endemic to the practice location. It is also important to ask about the patient's acute substance use (i.e., over the past week), because substance-induced disorders are proximal risk factors. Many patients, even those without substance use disorders, are uncomfortable discussing their substance use, so a value-neutral, supportive, and empathic approach is essential. A formerly abstinent patient who has resumed substance use even briefly can experience shame and guilt about that use and may require more support during assessment (Larimer et al. 1999). For example, a normalizing, permissive interviewing technique (e.g., "Many patients who are feeling depressed find that their substance use increases. What has your experience been?") may facilitate more open discussion about substance use than more general open-ended inquiries. Once substance use has been discussed, a diagnostic assessment for substance use disorders can be performed, as indicated. Urine toxicology screening can be used, but the practitioner should know exactly which substances the particular assay is capable of detecting. For example, many routine urine drug screens will test only for opioids with morphine metabolites and will not detect methadone or oxycodone.

All patients with substance use disorders, and especially those with substance dependence, should be thoroughly assessed for suicide risk on presentation, at routine intervals during treatment, and as additionally indicated (Center for Substance Abuse Treatment 2009; Wenzel et al. 2008). Although it is important to assess for more distal factors, one must also assess for both proximal risks and potential future risks. Many of the elements of suicide assessment in patients with substance-related disorders are the same as for assessment in other settings and are described elsewhere in this book (see chapters in Part I, "Suicide Risk Assessment," of this book). There are some specific issues that deserve comment, however.

A history of overdose on dependent substances does confer a slightly higher risk for suicide-related events, but most users who overdose on their primary substance do so unintentionally and not with suicidal intent (Bohnert et al. 2010). Most people with substance dependence who attempt or die by suicide use other means, so if thoughts of suicide are present, it is important to ask thoroughly about plans and access to means of suicide.

Addicted patients can be quite interpersonally skilled at deflecting questions about their substance use, even when they are motivated and engaged in substance use disorder treatment, and can become raconteurs with an almost pressured speech when being assessed. At such times, a gently persistent structuring with a directive interview approach may be useful. Similarly, patients with long-standing addictions beginning in their teens or young adulthood may seem almost alexithymic in their inability to describe or label internal states and emotions. Feelings such as depression, worry, mild anger, and disappointment may all be vaguely described as poorly characterized anxiety or tension. Such patients may need to be asked more about their thoughts and actions than about their moods or feelings in order to reduce frustration during the assessment and maintain the therapeutic relationship.

Because patients in early recovery from substance dependence often have difficulty recognizing and labeling internal states as emotions or feelings, their experiencing of strong unfamiliar internal sensations can be disconcerting and overwhelming. Addicted patients usually rely on substances to manage and change their internal states, and so they can be overwhelmed not just by the new sensations themselves but also by the recognition that they do not know how to handle the new feelings and moods and maintain abstinence. The distress can be so severe that patients may develop thoughts of suicide, not out of depression but out of an overwhelming sense of anxiety in the context of having limited other coping skills (Hendin et al. 2010). It can be very helpful for the treating clinician to anticipate such experiences and proactively assess how the patient is handling this aspect of recovery.

Case Example

Jose, a 53-year-old sales manager, comes to your outpatient office at the urging of his wife. A self-described functional alcoholic for 32 years, he stopped drinking a month ago with no symptoms of withdrawal. Several days ago, he scared his wife when he resumed drinking heavily. He began talking about being a failure, how the world would be better off without him, and how he was going to drive his car into a bridge abutment so it would all be over. His wife took away his car keys. Jose told her how he had felt too anxious to lead his daily sales meeting that morning and had had a drink beforehand. He felt horribly guilty for having had one drink but could not take going to any more Alcoholics Anonymous meetings because he felt too uncomfortable and judged by the other members. In his despair, Jose abandoned his attempt at recovery.

During your assessment, a history of social phobia since Jose's college days emerged. He had learned almost inadvertently that a drink or two before a group activity would allow him to come across as more outgoing and relaxed. His drinking gradually became less tied to the anticipation of being in group settings and became more autonomous.

Over the next few months, with the help of a selective serotonin reuptake inhibitor and cognitive-behavioral psychotherapy, Jose was able to maintain sobriety and to feel less anxious in groups. He also learned new ways to interact in social situations without having to be the life of the party, as he had felt before. His wife also learned new ways of being in social situations with her husband. She had formerly focused on monitoring Jose's level of intoxication and on heading off potentially embarrassing situations resulting from his actions while intoxicated.

As the example shows, when substance use is decreased, a co-occurring disorder can be exacerbated, return, or newly arise. It is not uncommon for a patient with PTSD to have a return or worsening of nightmares, feelings of detachment and isolation, hypervigilance, or other symptoms, or for a patient with schizophrenia to have an initial increased level of distress in response to auditory hallucinations. A thorough evaluation of current and past symptoms of other co-occurring psychiatric disorders is essential. The greater the number of additional co-occurring disorders, the greater the additional risk for suicide-related events.

Measures of patient perceptions of social connectedness and "belongingness" have shown predictive value for lifetime (i.e., past) suicide attempts and thoughts. Although it remains to be seen if these attributes are useful as predictors of future behavior, it would seem to be useful to assess these factors (Conner et al. 2007). For example, questions such as "Do you feel close to other people?" or "Do you feel that other people care about you?" could be asked. A related question is whether the patient lives alone, which is easily queried.

Treatment

At least one variation of cognitive-behavioral psychotherapy has been specifically adapted to address issues of substance use disorders and suicidality (Wenzel et al. 2008; see Chapter 13, "Cognitive Therapy for Suicide Prevention"). This therapy focuses on enhancing the patient's self-efficacy and motivation to make positive changes through addressing addiction-related beliefs and suicide-related beliefs together. Dialectical behavior psychotherapy has been shown to be a helpful modality for patients with issues related to suicidal thoughts or behaviors who have borderline personality disorder co-occurring with substance use disorders.

Conceptually, it would seem that motivational enhancement therapy, one of the other manualized psychotherapies for treating substance use disorders, could be adapted to include reduction of suicide-related events as a goal. As with cognitive-behavioral psychotherapy described previously, motivational enhancement therapy targets enhancing motivation to make positive change, in part through enhancing the patient's sense of self-efficacy to do so.

The Center for Substance Abuse Treatment has published a best practices guide and training materials on how to address suicidal thoughts and behaviors during treatment for substance use disorders (Center for Substance Abuse Treatment 2009, 2010a, 2010b). These materials emphasize awareness of proximal risk factors, routine repeated screening for suicide-related events, and utilization of cognitive techniques to increase hope. Although the intended audience is substance abuse counselors, program administrators, and clinical supervisors, the materials, including the sample therapist–patient dialogue, may be helpful for clinicians at all levels of experience.

It is unclear whether addictions treatment reduces subsequent suicide-related events relative to no treatment (Darke et al. 2007; Ilgen et al. 2007). It may be that the risk can be lessened through residential (versus outpatient) treatment and with a longer duration of treatment. In general, however, other prominent risk factors, such as a past history of suicide attempts, are probably more influential than usual substance use disorder treatment per se in determining risk for future suicide-related events.

Often the issue comes up as to whether substance-induced mood disorders with depressed features or withdrawal-related depressive symptoms require the same level of attention as depressive symptoms that are viewed as arising from independent mood disorders or adjustment disorders. Depressive disorders and symptoms are clearly distal and proximal risk factors for suicide-related events. Although the evidence base is of a lower grade, it is probably worth treating symptoms of a major depressive episode, regardless of etiology. Substance-induced and independent depressive episodes have the same prognostic value for future depressive episodes, and ei-

ther type of episode may respond to antidepressant medication (Flensborg-Madsen 2011; Nunes et al. 2006).

Co-occurring psychiatric disorders should always be addressed along with substance-related disorders, using an integrated approach. The combination of bipolar disorder and substance use disorders may place a patient at relatively greater risk. The complexity and uncertainty of making co-occurring disorder diagnoses in patients with substance use disorders can be challenging, and the reader is referred elsewhere for lengthier discussions of this matter (see, e.g., http://www.samhsa.gov/co-occurring/).

Psychopharmacological treatment should adhere to general psychiatric standards, keeping in mind the substance-specific considerations discussed earlier in this chapter. The prescribing clinician should anticipate that the addicted patient will on some level expect that medications will have the same utility as abused substances in quickly modulating mood and arousal. A patient may feel that it is appropriate to adjust dosages up or down on a frequent basis, taking less medication when the mood is better and more when it is worse. Similarly, a patient may prematurely abandon a medication when it is not perceived as producing immediate changes.

Other Patient Populations and Characteristics

Adolescents

Alcohol and other drug use disorders in adolescents are associated with 6–8.5 times greater risk of suicide, and both suicide-related events and substance use disorders are seen as having similar risk factors, precipitating factors, and perpetuating factors that contribute to repeated use/behaviors (Esposito-Smythers and Goldston 2008; Fisher et al. 2011). As with other mental health issues in adolescents, the impact of family relationships, parental mental health (including substance use), peer groups, social relationships, and co-occurring disorders can function as risk or protective factors. The presence and earlier onset (i.e., preteen) of multiple risk factors increase the risks. Treatment should address both issues together and should include family participation. An adaptation of cognitive-behavioral therapy that incorporates these and other elements has been developed and has been shown to be effective in reducing suicide-related events, substance use indicators, and utilization of other healthcare services (Esposito-Smythers et al. 2011).

High Utilizers of Acute and Inpatient Psychiatric Services

A patient familiar to any clinician who has worked in a psychiatric emergency service or inpatient psychiatric unit is the nonpsychotic patient who presents repeatedly with thoughts or plans of suicide and is either intoxicated or in withdrawal. Classically, the concerns of acute high suicidal risk resolve over a day or two, at which point the patient expresses little overt motivation for active substance use disorder or other psychiatric treatment and either wants to or is asked to return to the community. The patient may arouse frustration and anger in the treating clinicians that if acted out can lead to polarized treatment discussions or to therapeutic nihilism.

This group of patients has not been extensively studied, so clinical recommendations backed by a strong evidence base are few (Ries et al. 2009). In one study of male patients, almost all had mood or anxiety disorders, many had borderline personality disorder, and many had at least two Axis I

disorders, according to DSM-IV-TR classification (Spence et al. 2008). Many also had moderate to high levels of alexithymia and so were poorly able to describe their emotional states or to reflect on them. The patients expected the visit to be a negative experience yet felt they had no other options. Acutely, de-escalating patients' affect, validating their distress, and setting reasonable immediate goals that emphasize more adaptive coping skills may be helpful. A longer-term approach, with coordinated treatment planning across disciplines (e.g., general psychiatry/mental health, social work, general medicine, addiction psychiatry, and nonmedical addiction treatment) may help place the recurrent urgent presentations in a framework of more sustained need and distress that can lead to more empathic and effective interventions. Although this level of coordination requires time and effort, it may help reduce symptom intensity and utilization of high-intensity resources, moving the locus of treatment to outpatient or other less intensive settings.

Geriatric Patients

Alcohol use and alcohol-related disorders have been associated with increased risk for suicide in geriatric patients whether in primary care, home health care, or posthospitalization (Blow et al. 2004; Karvonen et al. 2009). Both sedative and hypnotic use has also been associated with increased risk of suicide, even after controlling for psychiatric disorders.

Gender

The literature on gender, substance-related disorders, and suicide-related events is quite heterogeneous. Although suicide-related event differences related to substance use have been found between men and women, studies often are not able to control for baseline gender differences in other known gender-related influences on suicide-related events such as basal suicide rates, income distribution, severity of substance use, co-occurring psychiatric disorders, and others (Wilcox et al. 2004). In women, the combination of substance use disorders, PTSD, and depression may be particularly risky (Cougle et al. 2009; Ilgen et al. 2010). Clinically, all patients with substance use disorders and with suicide-related events should be thoroughly assessed for other co-occurring conditions, as mentioned in the previous section on patient assessment. Other chapters in this book discuss the impact of gender differences on suicide risk assessment and management, and the reader is referred to more specialized texts for impact on the treatment of substance use disorders.

Culture

In 2000 the World Health Organization began conducting the World Mental Health Surveys in 21 developing and developed countries (Harvard Medical School 2005). A study that looked at risk factors for suicide-related events across the culturally diverse sites found that substance use remains one of the prominent ones, although its statistical role in a clinically useful predictive model remains to be determined (Borges and Loera 2010; Borges et al. 2010; Nock et al. 2010). The effect of culture may be particularly important when looking at the relationships between suicide-related events and substance use in adolescents (Fisher et al. 2011).

Conclusion

Substance use, substance use disorders, and suicide-related events are closely associated. Assessment and management of all three conditions are best done together. After physical safety and adequate general medical health is assured, in-depth psychiatric assessment can proceed, attending to the substances involved, the level of acuity, the severity of suicide-related events, and other patient-specific symptoms and features. Treatment is guided by patient history, clinical characteristics, presenting symptoms, and disorder diagnoses.

Key Clinical Concepts

- Substance use and substance-induced disorders can increase the distal and proximal risks for suicide-related events, and suicide-related events often occur with substance use.
- There is insufficient evidence to determine whether use of any particular substance inherently carries greater risk for suicide-related events than use of any other substance.
- It is important to routinely and repeatedly assess for substance use in patients with suicide-related events.
- It is important to routinely and repeatedly assess for suicide-related events in patients with substance use disorders.
- The impact of risk factors is cumulative: the greater the number of risk factors, the greater the risk.

- Clinicians may be able to anticipate typical challenges for patients during recovery from substance use disorders that may pose increased risk of suicide-related events.

- Treatment of patients with substance use disorders and a history of suicide-related events should address both components in an integrated manner. Cognitive-behavioral approaches have been shown to be effective.

References

American Psychiatric Association: Diagnostic and Statistical Manual of Mental Disorders, 3rd Edition. Washington, DC, American Psychiatric Association, 1980

American Psychiatric Association: Diagnostic and Statistical Manual of Mental Disorders, 4th Edition, Text Revision. Washington, DC, American Psychiatric Association, 2000

American Psychiatric Association: Substance use and addictive disorders in DSM-5. 2012. Available at: http://www.dsm5.org/ProposedRevision/Pages/SubstanceUseandAddictiveDisorders.aspx. Accessed January 13, 2012.

Arendt M, Munk-Jørgensen P, Sher L, et al: Mortality among individuals with cannabis, cocaine, amphetamine, MDMA, and opioid use disorders: a nationwide follow-up study of Danish substance users in treatment. Drug Alcohol Depend 114:134–139, 2011

Berlin I, Covey LS, Donohue MC, et al: Duration of smoking abstinence and suicide-related outcomes. Nicotine Tob Res 13:887–893, 2011

Blow FC, Brockmann LM, Barry KL: Role of alcohol in late-life suicide. Alcohol Clin Exp Res 28:48S–56S, 2004

Bohnert ASB, Roeder K, Ilgen MA: Unintentional overdose and suicide among substance users: a review of overlap and risk factors. Drug Alcohol Depend 110:183–192, 2010

Borges G, Loera CR: Alcohol and drug use in suicidal behaviour. Curr Opin Psychiatry 23:195–204, 2010

Borges G, Nock MK, Abad JMH, et al: Twelve-month prevalence of and risk factors for suicide attempts in the World Health Organization World Mental Health Surveys. J Clin Psychiatry 71:1617–1628, 2010

Brower KJ, McCammon RJ, Wojnar M, et al: Prescription sleeping pills, insomnia, and suicidality in the National Comorbidity Survey replication. J Clin Psychiatry 72:515–521, 2011

Calabria B, Degenhardt L, Hall W, et al: Does cannabis use increase the risk of death? Systematic review of epidemiological evidence on adverse effects of cannabis use. Drug Alcohol Rev 29:318–330, 2010

Center for Substance Abuse Treatment: Addressing suicidal thoughts and behaviors in substance abuse treatment. Treatment Improvement Protocol (TIP) Series 50. (HHS Publ No SMA-09-4381). Rockville, MD, Substance Abuse and Mental Health Services Administration, 2009

Center for Substance Abuse Treatment: Addressing suicidal thoughts and behaviors in substance abuse treatment—training video. Treatment Improvement Protocol (TIP) Series 50. (HHS Publ No VA10-TIP50). Rockville, MD, Substance Abuse and Mental Health Services Administration, 2010a

Center for Substance Abuse Treatment: Addressing suicidal thoughts and behaviors in substance abuse treatment: a review of the literature. Update: January 2009 through December 2010. 2010b. Available at: http://kap.samhsa.gov/products/manuals/tips/pdf/TIP50_LitReviewUpdate_July2011.pdf. Accessed January 14, 2012.

Conner KR, Britton PC, Sworts LM, et al: Suicide attempts among individuals with opiate dependence: the critical role of belonging. Addict Behav 32:1395–1404, 2007

Cougle JR, Resnick H, Kilpatrick DG: PTSD, depression, and their comorbidity in relation to suicidality: cross-sectional and prospective analyses of a national probability sample of women. Depress Anxiety 26:1151–1157, 2009

Darke S, Ross J, Williamson A, et al: Patterns and correlates of attempted suicide by heroin users over a 3-year period: findings from the Australian Treatment Outcome Study. Drug Alcohol Depend 87:146–152, 2007

Degenhardt L, Singleton J, Calabria B, et al: Mortality among cocaine users: a systematic review of cohort studies. Drug Alcohol Depend 113:88–95, 2011

Dougherty DM, Mathias CW, Marsh DM, et al: Suicidal behaviors and drug abuse: impulsivity and its assessment. Drug Alcohol Depend 76(suppl):S93–S105, 2004

Esposito-Smythers C, Goldston DB: Challenges and opportunities in the treatment of adolescents with substance use disorder and suicidal behavior. Subst Abus 29:5–17, 2008

Esposito-Smythers C, Spirito A, Kahler CW, et al: Treatment of co-occurring substance abuse and suicidality among adolescents: a randomized trial. J Consult Clin Psychol 79:728–739, 2011

Fisher J, de Mello MC, Izutsu T, et al: Suicidal behaviour in adolescents. Int J Soc Psychiatry 57:40–56, 2011

Flensborg-Madsen T: Alcohol use disorders and depression—the chicken or the egg? Addiction 106:916–918, 2011

Garza D, Murphy M, Tseng L-J, et al: A double-blind randomized placebo-controlled pilot study of neuropsychiatric adverse events in abstinent smokers treated with varenicline or placebo. Biol Psychiatry 69:1075–1082, 2011

Gvion Y, Apter A: Aggression, impulsivity, and suicide behavior: a review of the literature. Arch Suicide Res 15:93–112, 2011

Harvard Medical School: The World Mental Health Survey Initiative. 2005. Available at: http://www.hcp.med.harvard.edu/wmh/. Accessed January 14, 2012.

Hendin H, Al Jurdi RK, Houck PR, et al: Role of intense affects in predicting short-term risk for suicidal behavior: a prospective study. J Nerv Ment Dis 198:220–225, 2010

Howard MO, Perron BE, Sacco P, et al: Suicide ideation and attempts among inhalant users: results from the National Epidemiologic Survey on Alcohol and Related Conditions. Suicide Life Threat Behav 40:276–286, 2010

Hughes JR: Smoking and suicide: a brief overview. Drug Alcohol Depend 98:169–178, 2008

Ilgen MA, Harris AH, Moos RH, et al: Predictors of a suicide attempt one year after entry into substance use disorder treatment. Alcohol Clin Exp Res 31:635–642, 2007

Ilgen MA, Bohnert AS, Ignacio RV, et al: Psychiatric diagnoses and risk of suicide in veterans. Arch Gen Psychiatry 67:1152–1158, 2010

Karvonen K, Hakko H, Koponen H, et al: Suicides among older persons in Finland and time since hospitalization discharge. Psychiatr Serv 60:390–393, 2009

Kim J, Fan B, Liu XH, et al: Ecstasy use and suicidal behavior among adolescents: findings from a national survey. Suicide Life Threat Behav 41:435–444, 2011

Larimer ME, Palmer RS, Marlatt GA: Relapse prevention. An overview of Marlatt's cognitive-behavioral model. Alcohol Res Health 23:151–160, 1999

Mann JJ: Neurobiology of suicidal behaviour. Nat Rev Neurosci 4:819–828, 2003

Marshall BD, Werb D: Health outcomes associated with methamphetamine use among young people: a systematic review. Addiction 105:991–1002, 2010

Marshall BD, Galea S, Wood E, et al: Injection methamphetamine use is associated with an increased risk of attempted suicide: a prospective cohort study. Drug Alcohol Depend 119:134–137, 2011

Nock MK, Hwang I, Sampson NA, et al: Mental disorders, comorbidity and suicidal behavior: results from the National Comorbidity Survey Replication. Mol Psychiatry 15:868–876, 2010

Nunes EV, Liu XH, Samet S, et al: Independent versus substance-induced major depressive disorder in substance-dependent patients: observational study of course during follow-up. J Clin Psychiatry 67:1561–1567, 2006

Purvis TL, Nelson LA, Mambourg SE: Varenicline use in patients with mental illness: an update of the evidence. Expert Opin Drug Saf 9:471–482, 2010

Ries RK, Yuodelis-Flores C, Roy-Byrne PP, et al: Addiction and suicidal behavior in acute psychiatric inpatients. Compr Psychiatry 50:93–99, 2009

Ross S, Peselow E: The neurobiology of addictive disorders. Clin Neuropharmacol 32:269–276, 2009

Roy A: Characteristics of cocaine dependent patients who attempt suicide. Arch Suicide Res 13:46–51, 2009

Schneider B: Substance use disorders and risk for completed suicide. Arch Suicide Res 13:303–316, 2009

Soyka M, Trader A, Klotsche J, et al: Six-year mortality rates of patients in methadone and buprenorphine maintenance therapy: results from a nationally representative cohort study. J Clin Psychopharmacol 31:678–680, 2011

Spence JM, Bergmans Y, Strike C, et al: Experiences of substance-using suicidal males who present frequently to the emergency department. CJEM 10:339–346, 2008

Substance Abuse and Mental Health Services Administration: Results from the 2009 National Survey on Drug Use and Health: detailed tables. 2010. Available at: http://www.drugabusestatistics.samhsa.gov/NSDUH/2k9NSDUH/tabs/TOC.htm. Accessed January 14, 2012

Tait RJ, Ngo HTT, Hulse GK: Mortality in heroin users 3 years after naltrexone implant or methadone maintenance treatment. J Subst Abuse Treat 35:116–124, 2008

Underwood MD, Arango V: Evidence for neurodegeneration and neuroplasticity as part of the neurobiology of suicide. Biol Psychiatry 70:306–307, 2011

United Nations Office on Drugs and Crime: World Drug Report. New York, United Nations, 2011

van Heeringen C, Bijttebier S, Godfrin K: Suicidal brains: a review of functional and structural brain studies in association with suicidal behaviour. Neurosci Biobehav Rev 35:688–698, 2011

Vijayakumar L, Kumar MS, Vijayakumar V: Substance use and suicide. Curr Opin Psychiatry 24:197–202, 2011

Wenzel A, Brown GK, Beck AT: Cognitive therapy for suicidal patients with substance dependence disorders, in Cognitive Therapy for Suicidal Patients: Scientific and Clinical Applications. Washington, DC, American Psychological Association, 2008, pp 283–310

Wilcox HC, Conner KR, Caine ED: Association of alcohol and drug use disorders and completed suicide: an empirical review of cohort studies. Drug Alcohol Depend 76:S11–S19, 2004

World Health Organization: International Statistical Classification of Diseases and Related Health Problems, 10th Revision. Geneva, World Health Organization, 1992

World Health Organization: Global Status Report on Alcohol and Health. Geneva, World Health Organization, 2011a

World Health Organization: WHO Report on the Global Tobacco Epidemic, 2011: Warning About the Dangers of Tobacco. Geneva, World Health Organization, 2011b

C H A P T E R   9

Bipolar Disorder

Ross J. Baldessarini, M.D.

Maurizio Pompili, M.D., Ph.D.

Leonardo Tondo, M.D., M.Sc.

Bipolar (manic-depressive) disorders are prevalent, often severe, disabling, and potentially fatal psychiatric illnesses that are found worldwide (Goodwin and Jamison 2007; Tondo et al. 2003). Lifetime prevalence of type I bipolar disorder (with mania and often psychotic features) is at least 1%, and the total prevalence of bipolar disorder syndromes recognized in DSM-IV-TR (American Psychiatric Association 2000) may be as high as 5% if bipolar II disorder (recurrent major depression with hypomania) and cyclothymia (subsyndromal mood shifts) are included (Kessler et al. 2005b). The prevalence of bipolar disorder among persons seeking psychiatric help for depression has been estimated at 17.4% (Angst et al. 2011). In addition to the risks of cognitive deficits and disability, bipolar disorders present risks of excess mortality due to adverse outcomes of medical disorders, accidents, and complications of comorbid substance use disorders. By far, however, mortality in excess of that expected in the general population is due to suicide (Angst et al. 2005; Ilgen et al. 2010; Pompili 2010; Tondo et al. 2003).

In this chapter, we summarize current knowledge about risks, predictive factors, and treatments related to suicidal behaviors in patients with bipolar disorder, as a contribution to sound clinical management.

Supported, in part, by a grant from the Bruce J. Anderson Foundation and the McLean Private Donors Psychopharmacology Research Fund (to R.J.B.); a grant from the Italian Ministry of University Research–PRIN Project (to M.P.); and an award from the Centro Bini Private Donors Fund (to L.T.). None of the authors has current consulting or research relationships with commercial entities, nor do they or their immediate family members have equity or other financial relationships with pharmaceutical or other commercial entities that might represent potential conflicts of interest.

Suicide Risk in Bipolar Disorder

Comparisons With Other Disorders

The risks of completed and attempted suicide for the general population vary widely among countries and regions, in part owing to differing methods of identification and reporting of such events, and risks are often underestimated. International rates of suicide have averaged 0.014%±0.007% per year (14/100,000 persons per year ± standard deviation [SD]) in the general populations of developed countries (Baldessarini et al. 2007; Tondo et al. 2003). Risks of suicide among persons diagnosed with major affective disorders, on average, are approximately 15–20 times greater than in the general population (Harris and Barraclough 1997). Rates specific to bipolar versus unipolar major depressive or other mood disorders, among bipolar disorder subtypes, or by sex, age, or illness severity, however, are reported inconsistently (Clark and Goebel-Fabbri 1999; Goodwin and Jamison 2007; Ketter 2010; Pompili et al. 2009; "Practice Guideline" 2003; Tondo et al. 2007).

Suicide risks as standardized mortality ratios (SMRs) are reported for psychiatric and medical disorders, and in bipolar disorder (mostly type I), considered separately from other mood disorders. SMR averages 22 times higher than in the general population (Harris and Barraclough 1997; Tondo et al. 2003). SMR for suicide is similar among patients with unipolar major depression sufficiently severe to lead to hospitalization (SMR=20) and patients with polysubstance use disorders (SMR=19), and much greater than in patients with moderately severe depression (SMR=5–9) or other psychiatric or medical disorders (O'Leary et al. 2001; Tondo et al. 2003; Table 9–1). Systematic

comparisons of suicide risk among hospitalized versus less severely ill patients with bipolar disorder are not available.

The weighted mean annual incidence of suicide in patients with bipolar disorder was 0.39%, or 390/100,000 (based on 28 studies reported between the 1970s and early 2000s involving 823 suicides among 21,484 patients with bipolar disorder at risk for an average of 9.93 years) (Tondo et al. 2003). This estimate may be influenced by incompletely controlled effects of various treatments, but it is nearly 28 times higher than the annual suicide rate in the general population (0.39%/0.014%). These findings indicate that suicide risk in patients with bipolar disorder is as high as, if not higher than, risk in patients with any other psychiatric or substance use disorder.

Sex Differences in Suicide Risk

Long-term studies suggest that the proportion of deaths ascribed to suicide among patients with major affective disorder averages 15%–20% (Goodwin and Jamison 2007; Guze and Robins 1970; Tondo et al. 2003), but projections from annual estimates of suicide rates suggest that this proportion may exceed 20% of causes of death among those with bipolar disorder (Table 9–1). In the general population, risk of suicide is several times higher among men than among women, especially among young Caucasian men ("Practice Guideline" 2003). Among patients diagnosed with bipolar disorder, risk of death by suicide appears to be more similar between the sexes than with unipolar major depression. However, the sex-specific proportions for suicide vary widely among studies, ranging from 1.5 to 4 times higher in men, whereas women with bipolar disorders are more likely than men to make suicide attempts (Goodwin and Jamison 2007; Pompili et al. 2009; Tondo et

TABLE 9–1. Risk of suicide in specific disorders

Disorder	Relative risk, SMR	Suicide rate, %/year	Lifetime risk, %
Bipolar disorders	28	0.39	23.4
Severe depression	21	0.29	17.4
Mixed substance abuse	20	0.28	16.8
Severe anxiety disorders	11	0.15	9.0
Moderate depression	9	0.13	7.8
Schizophrenia	9	0.12	7.2
Personality disorders	7	0.10	6.0
Cancer	2	0.03	1.8
General population	1.0	0.014	0.8

Note. SMR=standardized mortality ratio; risk in a specific disorder relative to risk in the general population, adjusted for age and sex. Lifetime risk is based on annual suicide rate multiplied by 60 years of potential risk. Risks in types I and II bipolar disorder are similar, but the rate of completed suicides in men somewhat exceeds that in women diagnosed with bipolar disorder (by 1.85-fold), whereas the male:female risk ratio in the international general population averages 3.24 (according to World Health Organization, 2005). Severe depression involves hospitalization; moderate depression is an estimate for outpatient major depression plus dysthymia. Anxiety disorders include panic disorder with agoraphobia and obsessive-compulsive disorder.
Source. Data from Harris and Barraclough 1997 and Tondo et al. 2003.

al. 2003). A comprehensive review of 60 reports involving 31,814 patients with bipolar disorder found a mean±SD long-term risk of suicide attempts of 26.1%±19.1%, a mean annual rate of 2.13%±2.00%, and a female:male risk ratio of 2.37±1.94 (Pompili et al. 2005). These findings indicate that the great majority of patients with bipolar disorder are likely to make at least one attempt within several decades at risk.

Lethality of Attempts

Another important feature of suicidal behavior among major affective disorder patients is the evidently high *lethality* of suicide attempts (presumably reflecting both intent and means) as reflected in the ratio of estimated rates of suicide attempts to suicides (A:S). This ratio is much *lower* with bipolar disorder than in the general population, in which the A:S ratio varies with age,

sex, ethnicity, and the accuracy of case identification, especially for suicide attempts of varied severity and potential lethality (Tondo et al. 2003). Given these caveats, rates of suicide attempts in the general population are estimated to be 0.14%–0.28% per year, compared with an average suicide rate of 0.014% per year, for a ratio of at least 10:1 and as high as 30:1 (Kessler et al. 2005a; Tondo et al. 2003). This ratio is far lower among patients diagnosed with a major mood disorder, particularly bipolar II disorder, indicating a stronger intent to die in this group than in the general population.

We analyzed suicide risk among 2,826 patients in a Sardinian mood disorder research center to compare lethality in patients with bipolar I, bipolar II, or unipolar depressive disorders (Tondo et al. 2007; Table 9–2). The rate of suicide attempts among all patients with bipolar disorder averaged 1.26% per year, or slightly below the average cited earlier (2.13%). The annualized rate of suicides ranked as follows: bipolar II (0.16%), bipolar I (0.14%), and unipolar (0.05%). The A:S ratio, overall, was 2.68 times lower than in the local general population (9.33 vs. 25.0; Table 9–2).

Other Suicide Risk Factors

Age and Duration of Illness

Suicide risk appears to be particularly high early in the course of bipolar disorder (Dilsaver et al. 1997; Goodwin and Jamison 2007; Ösby et al. 2001; Tondo et al. 1998). In some samples, nearly one-quarter of life-threatening suicidal acts occurred within the first year of illness, and half took place within the first 5 years. Ominously, the average latency from onset of bipolar disorder illness to establishment of the diagnosis and sustained treatment is 5–10 years, in part owing to misdiagnosis as unipolar major depressive disorder. This delay indicates a need to redouble efforts to diagnose and treat the condition earlier, including in juveniles, in whom bipolar disorder may often be unrecognized or misdiagnosed (Faedda et al. 1995; Tondo et al. 1998, 2003).

Diagnostic and Clinical Subtypes

Probably reflecting the wide range of illness severity among persons diagnosed with DSM-IV-TR major depressive disorders, studies differ in their findings on the relative risk of suicide in bipolar disorder versus nonbipolar major depression (Goodwin and Jamison 2007; Tondo et al. 2003). In general, suicide risk is very high in both types of major affective disorders and probably increases with greater illness severity, as reflected in recurrence rates and disability.

In the 1970s Dunner and Fieve (1974) introduced the concept of type II bipolar disorder, with more prominent depressive

than hypomanic phases, and noted a high risk of suicide associated with it. More recently, Rihmer and Pestality (1999) found a high lifetime rate of suicide attempts among patients with bipolar II disorder (61/253, or a 24.1% lifetime risk) that was somewhat greater than that with bipolar I disorder (103/606, or a 17.0% lifetime risk) and far higher than in unipolar depression (143/1,214, or an 11.8% lifetime risk). Similarly high risks in bipolar I and II disorders also were reported by Novick et al. (2010). In our study of 2,826 patients, rates of suicides (%/year) ranked as follows: bipolar II (0.16), bipolar I (0.14), and unipolar major depression (0.05); and that of attempts ranked as follows: bipolar I (1.52), bipolar II (0.82), and unipolar (0.48). Also, the A:S ratio (5.12) was lowest in bipolar II cases, indicating high lethality (Tondo et al. 2007; Table 9–2).

Depressive and dysphoric-irritable states in all types of bipolar disorder appear to be particularly associated with suicide. In a large sample of outpatients with type I or II bipolar disorder who made a serious suicide attempt or who died by suicide, 73% of the suicidal acts were judged to be associated with depression, 16% with dysphoric-mixed manic-depressive states, 11% with mania, and none with hypomania, indicating that 89% of suicidal acts were associated with ongoing depressive or mixed dysphoric mood states (Tondo et al. 1998). Other studies of patients with bipolar disorder also found that 79%–90% of suicides were associated with depressive or mixed dysphoric mood states (Arató et al. 1988; Dilsaver et al. 1997; Isometsä et al. 1994). In addition, previous severe depression was highly predictive of later suicidal behavior (Dilsaver et al. 1997; Tondo et al. 1998), and bipolar mixed states carry a particularly high risk of suicide (Baldessarini et al. 2012; Marneros et al. 2004; Valtonen et al. 2005).

TABLE 9–2. Suicide risk by DSM-IV-TR diagnosis

Measures	Bipolar I	Bipolar II	Unipolar
Cases (n)	529	314	1,983
At-risk (years)	13.2	16.3	9.30
Risk rates (%/year)			
Suicides (S)	0.14	0.16	0.05
Attempts (A)	1.52	0.82	0.48
All suicidal acts (A+S)	1.66	0.98	0.53
Lethality (A:S)	10.9	5.12	9.60
Suicide SMR	12.8	14.7	4.59

Note. Overall risk is based on analysis of clinical records of 2,826 major affective disorder patients in Sardinia (Tondo et al. 2007). SMR=standardized mortality ratio; risk in a specific disorder relative to risk in the general population of Sardinia, whose suicide rate was 0.109%/year, with approximately 25 times more attempts/year. Rates do not differ significantly among ever-hospitalized patients but are markedly lower among more moderately ill, never-hospitalized, unipolar major depressive patients than others.

Demographics

In general and in bipolar disorder specifically, previous suicide attempt is a leading predictor of future suicidal behavior. Caucasian ethnicity and unmarried status also increase risk, along with several clinical factors that are particularly important in bipolar disorder. As noted, these include current depression or dysphoric mixed states, previous severe depression, and hopelessness. Additional risk factors include comorbid anxiety or substance use disorders as well as an irritable temperament and social introversion (Dilsaver et al. 1997; Goodwin and Jamison 2007; Isometsä et al. 1994; Leverich et al. 2003; "Practice Guideline" 2003; Tondo et al. 1998). Impulsivity, a common trait among persons with bipolar disorder, also contributes to risk but probably primarily with attempts of limited lethality rather than completed suicide (Baca-Garcia et al. 2001; Tondo et al. 2003). It is not clear how rates of illness recurrence or presence of rapid cycling (four or more recurrences within a year) contribute quantitatively to suicide risk in mood disorders, but the presence of multiple depressive and mixed episodes is a strong risk factor (Tondo et al. 1998). There may also be a genetic predisposition to suicide, but it has not been proved that this risk is independent of risk for bipolar disorder or depressive illness (Baldessarini and Hennen 2004).

Predisposing factors for suicide probably interact with other stressors that may precipitate suicide even in the absence of a psychiatric disorder. Relevant stressful events identified as suicide risk factors include spousal death and divorce, interpersonal or occupational difficulties, separations and personal or economic losses, retirement, imprisonment or social isolation, and limited access to support or clinical services (Tondo et al. 2006; "Practice Guideline" 2003). In addition, specific affective temperament types may be associated with suicidal behavior in patients with major affective disorder, but more conclusive studies are needed (Akiskal 1996; Akiskal and Pinto 1999; Kochman et al. 2005; Pompili et al. 2011, 2012).

Assessment of Suicide Risk

Effective clinical assessment of suicidal potential requires inquiry into suicidal thinking, the nature of the intent associated with such thoughts, and access to lethal means ("Practice Guideline" 2003). Many physicians and even mental health professionals avoid discussing suicide directly and frankly with patients for fear of "provoking" suicidal behavior or, more likely, because of personal discomfort. Suicidal thoughts rarely are new to suicidal persons; many potential victims are willing to discuss their suicidal thoughts, and the topic needs to be investigated, especially when agitation, severe anxiety, anguish, or psychosis is present. As with any patient at risk for suicide, it is important to evaluate those with bipolar disorder longitudinally, and particularly during depressive or mixed phases of illness, for indications of suicidal intent such as making a specific plan or preparing notes, making a will, giving away possessions or pets, or putting business matters pertaining to survivors in order ("Practice Guideline" 2003).

Key elements in evaluating suicide risk include the following (Brendel et al. 2010; "Practice Guideline" 2003):

1. Assessing the intensity of suicidal ideation
2. Inquiring about details of suicide plans, access to lethal means, and the possibility of rescue
3. Identifying current or recent precipitants for suicidal thinking
4. Screening for the presence of major psychiatric illness, particularly depression
5. Reviewing past suicide attempts and plans
6. Screening for risk and protective factors
7. Evaluating interpersonal and other social supports
8. Administering an adequate mental status examination

A determination of acute high suicide risk calls for family involvement and often requires immediate hospitalization, sometimes by legal commitment, especially if the potentially suicidal patient is not already in treatment or is unwilling to accept help.

Access to Mental Health Care

About 40% of persons with a range of psychiatric diagnoses who eventually died by suicide had contacted a mental health professional within several months of death (Pirkis and Burgess 1998). Among those who died by suicide, 75%–80% had consulted a physician at least once within the year before death, 66% in the month before death, and 20% in the week before (Andersen et al. 2001; Miller and Druss 2001). Only 46% had seen a psychiatrist within the previous month and 36% in the week before death (Pirkis and Burgess 1998).

Little is known about utilization of clinical services by suicidal bipolar disorder patients specifically. However, in one study, 74% of (mainly type II) bipolar disorder patients who died by suicide had been receiving some treatment at the time of death (Arató et al. 1988). Although few studies have specifically addressed the point, these preceding observations and clinical experiences strongly suggest that access to care—and, very likely, the quality of care and of close follow-up—may play a crucial role in suicide prevention (Tondo et al. 2006).

Limitations of Risk Factor Analyses

Interpretation of analyses of risk factors associated with suicide based on case finding only *after* suicide is confounded by lack of knowledge of the proportion of potential suicides that may have been prevented by timely assessment and effective interventions and therefore is not reflected in the data considered. Reliance on routine screening of patients at risk for suicide for risk factors considered earlier can be helpful but is unlikely to predict specific risk and its timing in individual cases ("Practice Guideline" 2003). Such unpredictability may be particularly challenging in the assessment of patients with bipolar disorder, owing to the effects of sometimes rapid shifts in mood (lability), reactivity to losses or other stressors, impulsivity, variable behavioral control, the disinhibiting effects of commonly abused central depressants including alcohol and sedatives, and sometimes erratic adherence to increasingly complex treatment regimens (Centorrino et al. 2010; Goodwin and Jamison 2007).

Treatments Aimed at Limiting Suicide Risk in Patients With Bipolar Disorder

Evidence that specific medical treatments, including use of psychotropic medicines, reduce suicide risk associated with any psychiatric disorder, particularly over the long term, is very limited and largely inconclusive (Baldessarini 2012; Tondo et al. 2003). Moreover, even if some interventions are helpful in limiting suicide risk, use of specific psychiatric treatments in postmortem samples of suicides has been remarkably infrequent, often below 30% and sometimes

as low as 3% of cases, notwithstanding the higher rates of recent clinical consultations noted earlier (Andersen et al. 2001; Miller and Druss 2001; Tondo et al. 2003). The following overview considers pharmacological, physical, and psychosocial interventions aimed at limiting suicidal risk among patients with bipolar disorder.

Psychopharmacological Treatment

Antidepressants

Suicidal behavior is particularly strongly associated with acute depressive illness, and antidepressants have been proven to be moderately effective, at least in the short-term treatment of acute, nonpsychotic major depression of moderate severity (Baldessarini 2012). Antidepressant treatment would seem to be a plausible intervention to prevent suicide in depression associated with major depressive disorder and perhaps also in bipolar disorder (Rihmer and Gonda 2011; Tondo et al. 2008). However, there is considerable uncertainty about the relative efficacy of antidepressant drugs in bipolar depression, especially for long-term prevention of depressive recurrences (Baldessarini 2012; Ghaemi et al. 2004, 2008; Sidor and Macqueen 2011; Yatham 2005). Moreover, risk of dying by an overdose of antidepressants has been reduced greatly since the introduction of serotonin reuptake inhibitors and other modern antidepressants to replace the tricyclic and monoamine oxidase inhibitor antidepressants (Baldessarini 2012). Nevertheless, other lethal means are readily available, and the effects of antidepressant treatment on suicidal behavior remain remarkably uncertain.

International consumption of modern antidepressants has increased strikingly since the 1980s, and their sales have shown suggestive but inconsistent temporal associations with trends toward minor decreases in general population suicide rates in some geographic regions (Baldessarini et al. 2007; Isacsson et al. 2010). Interpretation of such "ecological" correlations is fundamentally limited by the lack of association of relevant variables at the level of individual persons.

Despite widespread clinical use of effective antidepressants for nearly 50 years and broad acceptance of better-tolerated and less toxic modern antidepressants, direct evidence obtained in individually treated patients that antidepressant treatment is associated with a lowering of suicide risk remains inconclusive for major depression and strikingly deficient for bipolar depression (Baldessarini 2012; Baldessarini et al. 2007; Reeves and Ladner 2010). There is even evidence, based on retrospective analyses of age-stratified data from controlled trials submitted for regulatory review, as well as several large clinical cohort or case-control studies involving serotonin reuptake inhibitors, that antidepressant treatment may be associated with suicidal ideation and some behaviors. This association appears to be limited to juveniles and young adults up to age 25, with reduced apparent risk among older adults (Barbui et al. 2009; Hammad et al. 2006). This proposed association led to the U.S. Food and Drug Administration (FDA) requirement of a severe ("black box") warning in the labeling of all drug products used to treat major depression (Laughren 2006; U.S. Food and Drug Administration 2005, 2007).

To some extent the lack of demonstrated effectiveness of antidepressant treatment in reducing suicide risk may reflect continuing low rates of closely supervised adherence to antidepressant treatment, particularly among young men, as well as inadequate dosing and duration of sustained treatment for many depressed patients (Baldessarini 2012). Alternatively, suicidal behavior surely requires more than depressed mood, and other relevant factors, such as anger, aggression, and impulsivity, may be little benefited by antidepressant treatment (Baldessarini 2012; Baldessarini et al. 2007).

Moreover, in some vulnerable patients, including juveniles, mixed dysphoric-agitated states of bipolar disorder can be induced or worsened by antidepressant treatment. Such potentially dangerous reactions may not be recognized and accurately differentiated from worsening depression. Other adverse behavioral responses to antidepressant treatment (such as insomnia, restlessness, irritability, agitation) also may increase risk of aggressive-impulsive acts, perhaps including suicidal behavior, and may be particularly likely among patients with bipolar disorder in depressive or mixed states (Baldessarini 2012; Baldessarini et al. 2007). However, suicidal behavior during treatment with antidepressants seems to be largely confined to early treatment and to a small minority of patients; eventually, suicidal thoughts and acts tend to decrease with continued treatment (Jick et al. 2004; Tondo et al. 2008; Zisook et al. 2011). An association of agitation and aggression with the use of serotonergic antidepressants, particularly serotonin reuptake inhibitors, is counterintuitive in view of substantial evidence associating a deficiency of central serotonergic functioning with violent acts including suicide (Mann et al. 2001).

More generally, as noted, the value of antidepressant treatment in the overall care of patients with bipolar disorder remains controversial, with highly inconsistent evidence of short-term efficacy and very little evidence of long-term prophylactic effectiveness (Baldessarini 2012; Ghaemi et al. 2008; Sidor and Macqueen 2011). Moreover, the effectiveness of mood-stabilizing medicines in preventing agitation, mixed states, or mania during antidepressant treatment is widely assumed but unproved (Tondo et al. 2010). Risks of increased agitation and aggression during antidepressant treatment can be limited by close clinical supervision, especially early in treatment, and removal of the antidepressant or by addition of a mood-stabilizing, antipsychotic, or sedative agent (Pompili et al. 2005).

Lithium Salts

Based on current knowledge about pharmacological interventions and risks of suicide and suicide attempts, prophylactic treatment with lithium carbonate is supported by the strongest available evidence of reduced risk of suicides and attempts of any treatment intervention for bipolar disorder (Baldessarini 2012; Baldessarini and Tondo 2008; Baldessarini et al. 2006; Müller-Oerlinghausen and Lewitzka 2010).

Studies reporting on the association of lithium treatment and suicide in bipolar disorder and other major affective disorders have consistently found lower rates of suicides and attempts during lithium maintenance treatment than without it (Baldessarini and Tondo 2008; Baldessarini et al. 2006). In a study involving 360 Sardinian patients with type I or type II bipolar disorder evaluated before, during, and after discontinuation of maintenance lithium monotherapy, rates of suicide and of life-threatening attempts were reduced by 6.4-fold, or 83% (Tondo et al. 1998). Moreover, in that study, the risk of suicidal acts transiently increased by 20-fold within several months after discontinuation of lithium maintenance treatment, and later fell back to the level encountered before initiation of lithium treatment. This early risk was 2-fold

higher after abrupt or rapid discontinuation of treatment (Tondo et al. 1998).

A more recent, comprehensive meta-analysis of studies of lithium adds additional support to the impression that lithium has major beneficial effects against both suicides and attempts and that these effects are found consistently across almost all trials reported over the past three decades, including trials involving randomization and double-blind assessments, with only rare exceptions (Baldessarini and Tondo 2008; Marangell et al. 2008; Oquendo et al. 2011). Baldessarini and Tondo (2008) reviewed 45 reports involving 53,472 patients with bipolar disorder or more broadly defined manic-depressive disorder (including unipolar recurrent major depressive and schizoaffective disorder) who were treated and evaluated for an average exposure of nearly 348,000 person-years with or without lithium. Risks for both completed suicide and suicide attempts were reduced by nearly fivefold, or 80%, with lithium treatment (see Table 9–3).

Most of the studies analyzed are open to the hypothetical criticism that there may be selection bias if patients who accept a stable, long-term treatment regimen *also* have lower suicide risk than those who find the treatment intolerable or otherwise discontinue early. However, some studies of lithium and suicide risk are based on comparisons of the *same* patients without versus during treatment, or involve random assignment to different treatments (Baldessarini and Tondo 2008; Baldessarini et al. 2006). Even though the same persons are involved under two conditions of treatment or are assigned to treatments at random, those who accept, tolerate, and continue the treatment might differ from other randomly selected patients in subtle ways not readily identified by considering their clinical histories alone. On the other hand,

TABLE 9–3. Lithium treatment versus suicidal risks

Measures	Studies	Risk ratio (95% CI)	P value
All studies	34	4.91 (3.86–6.23)	<0.001
Suicides	25	4.89 (3.46–6.91)	<0.0001
Attempts	20	4.86 (3.58–6.59)	<0.001
Bipolar disorder	15	5.53 (3.75–8.20)	<0.001
Various mood disorders	19	4.58 (3.38–6.21)	<0.001
Randomized trials	8	4.29 (1.46–12.6)	0.008
Open trials	26	5.00 (3.83–6.53)	<0.001

Note. Data are relative risks with versus without lithium treatment with 95% confidence intervals, for suicides or attempted suicides, and for bipolar disorder patients or those with various recurrent major affective disorders (bipolar, unipolar, schizoaffective), all based on random-effects meta-analysis with stratification.
Source. Adapted from Baldessarini et al. 2006; similar findings were obtained in an expanded meta-analysis Baldessarini and Tondo 2008.

it simply is not feasible to evaluate any long-term treatment without substantial acceptance, tolerance of, and adherence to the treatment being investigated. Therefore, we suggest that the available findings on lithium treatment, at a minimum, reflect substantial and consistent reductions in suicide risk among those patients who accept, tolerate, and adhere to long-term prophylactic treatment with lithium salts compared with alternative treatments or a placebo.

The effectiveness of lithium treatment in preventing suicide in broadly defined manic-depressive syndromes may operate through reduction of risk or of severity of recurrences in depression or mixed dysphoric-agitated states. However, some experts have suggested that lithium may have specific effects against suicide independent of its mood-stabilizing actions (Ahrens and Müller-Oerlinghausen 2001; Müller-Oerlinghausen et al. 2002). Specific contributions of lithium treatment may include reduction of impulsive or aggressive behavior, possibly mediated through lithium's reported ability to enhance function-

ing of the central serotonin system (Baldessarini 2012; Mann et al. 2001).

Anticonvulsants

Several anticonvulsants have demonstrated or proposed antimanic efficacy and are used empirically for possible long-term mood-stabilizing effects in patients with bipolar disorder. The potential antisuicidal effects of carbamazepine, lamotrigine, and valproic acid are not established. However, there is evidence that some anticonvulsants (particularly valproic acid and carbamazepine) may be less effective than lithium as mood stabilizers (Dardennes et al. 1995; Denicoff et al. 1997) and possibly less effective against suicide (Baldessarini and Tondo 2009). The evident superiority of lithium over anticonvulsants is unexplained.

Potential beneficial effects of anticonvulsants against suicide risk in conditions other than bipolar disorder have not been investigated, and proposals that some anticonvulsants may increase suicide risk, at least in patients with epilepsy, remain unsubstantiated (Pompili and Baldessarini 2010).

Antipsychotics

A historically important development was regulatory approval of clozapine to reduce suicidal risk in schizophrenia patients (Hennen and Baldessarini 2005; Meltzer et al. 2003). Interestingly, like lithium prophylaxis but in contrast to standard clinical practice in the use of antidepressants, clozapine is employed with unusually close medical supervision and regular blood testing to minimize the risk of potentially lethal side effects. Such interventions might contribute to their antisuicidal effects, although levels of patient-clinician interactions were closely matched in the pivotal randomized trial indicating superior antisuicidal effects of clozapine over olanzapine (Meltzer et al. 2003). Clozapine remains officially in "off-label" (not approved by the FDA) status for all phases of bipolar disorder, but is sometimes used empirically when other treatments prove to be unsatisfactory (Baldessarini 2012). Most antipsychotic agents have short-term antimanic effects, and some modern agents also may have long-term prophylactic effects in bipolar disorders, especially against recurrences of mania (Baldessarini 2012). Their potential for limiting risks of suicidal behavior in mood disorder patients, however, is unknown.

Physical Treatments

Electroconvulsive therapy (ECT) has been considered a treatment of choice in emergencies involving high suicide risk, and it is effective in the short-term treatment of bipolar depression and mania (Read and Bentall 2010). Nevertheless, the effectiveness of ECT for sustained suicide prevention has not been proved and requires further study, including in patients with bipolar disorder ("Practice Guideline" 2003). Other, newer physical treatments, including repeated transcranial magnetic stimulation, vagal nerve stimulation, and deep-brain electrical stimulation, have not been adequately evaluated in the treatment of bipolar disorder, and their potential effects on suicidal behavior are not known (Table 9–4).

Psychosocial Interventions

Specific and comprehensive suicide prevention strategies are required for patients at increased risk and in bipolar disorder in particular. Psychosocial methods may be useful and are widely used clinically, although they have rarely been studied experimentally (Brown et al. 2005; Gray and Otto 2001; Huxley et al. 2000; Krishnan 2005; Rucci et al. 2002). A widely employed clinical tactic involves "contracts for safety" between clinicians and patients, in which the patient agrees to report impending loss of control of suicidal impulses. This approach may seem plausible but frequently fails and has not been adequately tested. It can contribute to decreased vigilance, and it probably offers inadequate protection against legal liability (Garvey et al. 2009). Moreover, its effects with bipolar disorder patients specifically remain unknown. Additional psychosocial interventions include intensive community services and rapid hospitalization, neither of which has been proved to reduce suicidal risk other than in immediate, emergency applications (Huxley et al. 2000). Treatments currently employed for bipolar disorder relevant to suicide prevention are summarized in Table 9–4.

Conclusion

Bipolar disorders with or without mania (types I and II) are prevalent, often severe and disabling, illnesses with greatly increased mortality due to accidents and complications of comorbid substance use and medical illnesses, but particularly to suicide

TABLE 9–4. Effects of treatments for bipolar disorder on suicide risk

Treatments	Comments
Lithium salts	Strong and largely consistent evidence of reducing risk of suicides and attempts in bipolar disorder, and perhaps other recurrent major mood disorders
Anticonvulsants	
Carbamazepine	U.S. Food and Drug Administration (FDA)–approved for acute mania/mixed states; less effective than lithium long-term and probably less protective against suicide
Divalproex	FDA-approved for acute mania; widely used off-label long-term; probably less protective against suicide than lithium
Lamotrigine	Ineffective and impractical for acute mania, FDA-approved for long-term prophylaxis (mainly for bipolar depression); no evidence regarding suicide risk
Others	None (including gabapentin, oxcarbazepine, topiramate) is FDA-approved for any use in bipolar disorder; no evidence regarding suicide risk
Antipsychotics	Chlorpromazine and all modern antipsychotics are FDA-approved for acute mania; aripiprazole (alone or combined with a mood stabilizer), olanzapine (long-term and with fluoxetine short-term), long-acting injected risperidone (alone), and quetiapine and ziprasidone (with lithium or valproate) are approved for long-term treatment; evidence for protection against suicide only for clozapine (probably more effective than olanzapine) in schizophrenia only
Antidepressants	Widely used empirically; evidence for short-term antidepressant efficacy in bipolar depression is conflicted and weak long-term; suicide risk may increase with agitated-dysphoric or mixed states associated with antidepressants (especially in bipolar I patients); evidence that mood stabilizers avoid such risk is limited
Physical treatments	
ECT	Probably effective against suicide in the short term; evidence of long-term benefit is lacking
Repeated TMS	Effects on suicide remain untested
VNS	Experimental; effects on suicide unknown
DBES	Experimental; effects on suicide unknown
Psychosocial interventions	May contribute to improved treatment adherence and overall clinical outcomes, but effects on suicide remain little tested

Note. DBES=deep-brain electrical stimulation; ECT=electroconvulsive therapy; TMS=transcranial magnetic stimulation; VNS=vagal nerve stimulation.
Source. Based on evidence summarized by Baldessarini and Tondo 2008; and Baldessarini 2012.

in younger persons. Suicide rates in bipolar disorder patients average 0.4% per year, at least 25 times higher than rates in the general population (approximately 0.014% per year). Suicidal acts often occur early in bi-polar illness, particularly in association with bipolar depression and dysphoric-agitated mixed phases, and following repeated, severe depressions, particularly with comorbid substance abuse. High lethality of suicide attempts is suggested by the much lower ratio (A:S) of attempts to completed suicides among bipolar disorder patients (approximately 5:1) than in the general population (about 20:1). Consideration of associated or risk factors helps to identify patients at increased risk for suicide but has very limited power to predict the timing and circumstances of suicide attempts in individuals. Ongoing, adequate clinical assessment is essential to limit suicidal outcomes, particularly in newly ill patients or those who are not well evaluated or well known to the responsible clinicians.

Widely employed short-term interventions to manage acute suicidal risks in bipolar disorder patients range from close clinical supervision and rapid hospitalization to ECT. Remarkably, however, evidence of long-term effectiveness of any treatment against mortality associated with bipolar and other psychiatric disorders is sparse. A notable exception is lithium prophylaxis, which is associated with compelling and quite consistent evidence of sustained reduction of risk of suicides and attempts, and a decreased ratio of attempts to suicides. Such effects are less likely, or remain untested, for emerging pharmacological treatments for bipolar and other mood disorders, including anticonvulsants, second-generation antipsychotics, and modern antidepressants, as well as magnetic and vagal stimulation, or psychosocial and administrative interventions. For now, treatment aimed at reducing suicide risk in patients with bipolar or other major affective disorders can be enhanced by applying current knowledge systematically, with close and sustained clinical supervision of patients who are well evaluated and well known to responsible clinicians.

Key Clinical Concepts

- Bipolar disorder is highly prevalent internationally, often severe, sometimes disabling, and potentially fatal.

- Bipolar disorder is associated with very high risks of suicide and relatively lethal attempts, especially early in the illness when sustained clinical interventions, and even the diagnosis, may not have been established.

- Suicide risk in bipolar disorder continues over many years, with suicide accounting for at least 15% of eventual deaths.

- The epidemiology of suicide risk has been confounded by inconsistent separation of bipolar disorder from unipolar major depression or of type I from type II bipolar disorder.

- Depressive and dysphoric-agitated, mixed phases of bipolar disorder are especially life-threatening as well as challenging to diagnose and to treat effectively and safely.

- Bipolar disorder is associated with high rates of substance use, anxiety disorders, impulsivity, lack of insight, and poor treatment adherence— all adding to suicide risk and complicating treatment.

- Short-term interventions that are widely accepted empirically for managing acute suicidality include close clinical supervision, rapid hospitalization, and use of ECT.

- These and other treatments, including most specific mood-altering medicines and widely accepted psychosocial therapies, have little evidence of sustained effectiveness in reducing *long-term* suicide risk in patients with bipolar disorder.

- Lithium maintenance treatment is a unique exception, with abundant research support for consistent, substantial, and sustained reduction of risk of suicide and both rates and lethality of attempts in bipolar disorder and possibly in other mood disorders.

- Anticonvulsants, modern antipsychotics, and less toxic modern antidepressants are widely employed in the treatment of bipolar disorder, but their potential ability to limit suicide risk either is unsupported by preliminary evidence or requires further study.

- Long-term prophylactic effectiveness of available treatments for bipolar disorder, especially against depression, mixed states, sustained dysthymia, rapid cycling, comorbidity, demoralization, and dysfunction, in addition to mania and psychosis, as well as for suicide prevention, largely remains to be demonstrated and compared critically over realistically prolonged observation times.

- Efforts to reduce suicide risk among patients with bipolar disorder can usefully include improved and earlier diagnosis and optimized and sustained clinical management. This process requires greater dissemination and more systematic application of knowledge, as well as improved access to care by clinicians skilled in clinical management of patients with major, complex, life-threatening psychiatric illnesses.

References

Ahrens B, Müller-Oerlinghausen B: Does lithium exert an independent antisuicidal effect? Pharmacopsychiatry 34:132–136, 2001

Akiskal HS: Temperamental foundations of mood disorders, in Interpersonal Factors in the Origin and Course of Affective Disorders. Edited by Mundt CH. London, Gaskell, 1996, pp 3–30

Akiskal HS, Pinto O: The evolving bipolar spectrum. Psychiatr Clin North Am 22:517–534, 1999

American Psychiatric Association: Diagnostic and Statistical Manual of Mental Disorders, 4th Edition, Text Revision. Washington, DC, American Psychiatric Association, 2000

Andersen UA, Andersen M, Rosholm JU, et al: Psychopharmacological treatment and psychiatric morbidity in 390 cases of suicide with special focus on affective disorders. Acta Psychiatr Scand 104:458–465, 2001

Angst J, Angst F, Gerber-Werder R, et al: Suicide in 406 mood-disorder patients with and without long-term medication: a 40 to 44 years' follow-up. Arch Suicide Res 9:279–300, 2005

Angst J, Azorin JM, Bowden CL, et al: Prevalence and characteristics of undiagnosed bipolar disorders in patients with a major depressive episode. Arch Gen Psychiatry 68:791–800, 2011

Arató M, Demeter E, Rihmer Z, et al: Retrospective psychiatric assessment of 200 suicides in Budapest. Acta Psychiatr Scand 77:454–456, 1988

Baca-Garcia E, Diaz-Sastre C, Basurte E, et al: Prospective study of the paradoxical relationship between impulsivity and lethality of suicide attempts. J Clin Psychiatry 62:560–564, 2001

Baldessarini RJ: Chemotherapy in Psychiatry, 3rd Edition. New York, Springer, 2012

Baldessarini RJ, Hennen J: Genetics of suicide: an overview. Harv Rev Psychiatry 12:1–13, 2004

Baldessarini RJ, Tondo L: Lithium and suicidal risk. Bipolar Disord 10:114–115, 2008

Baldessarini RJ, Tondo L: Meta-analytic comparison of antisuicidal effects of lithium vs. anticonvulsants. Pharmacopsychiatry 42:72–75, 2009

Baldessarini RJ, Tondo L, Davis P, et al: Decreased risk of suicides and attempts during long-term lithium treatment: a meta-analytic review. Bipolar Disord 8:625–639, 2006

Baldessarini RJ, Tondo L, Strombom I, et al: Analysis of ecological studies of relationships between antidepressant utilization and suicidal risk. Harv Rev Psychiatry 15:133–145, 2007

Baldessarini RJ, Undurraga J, Vázquez GH, et al: Predominant recurrence polarity among 928 adult international bipolar I disorder patients. Acta Psychiatr Scand 125:293–302, 2012

Barbui C, Esposito E, Cipriani A: Selective serotonin reuptake inhibitors and risk of suicide: a systematic review of observational studies. CMAJ 180:291–297, 2009

Brendel RW, Wei M, Lagomasino IT, et al: Care of the suicidal patient, in Massachusetts General Handbook of General Hospital Psychiatry, 6th Edition. Edited by Stern TA, Fricchione GL, Cassem NH, et al. Philadelphia, PA, Saunders-Elsevier, 2010, pp 541–554

Brown GK, Ten Have T, Henrigues GR, et al: Cognitive therapy for the prevention of suicide attempts: a randomized controlled trial. JAMA 294:563–570, 2005

Centorrino F, Ventriglio A, Vincenti A, et al: Changes in medication practices for hospitalized psychiatric patients: 2009 versus 2004. Hum Psychopharmacol 25:179–186, 2010

Clark DC, Goebel-Fabbri AE: Lifetime risk of suicide in major affective disorders, in The Harvard Medical School Guide to Suicide Assessment and Intervention. Edited by Jacobs DG. San Francisco, CA, Jossey-Bass, 1999, pp 270–286

Dardennes R, Even C, Bange F, et al: Comparison of carbamazepine and lithium in the prophylaxis of bipolar disorder. A meta-analysis. Br J Psychiatry 166:378–381, 1995

Denicoff KD, Smith-Jackson EE, Disney ER, et al: Comparative prophylactic efficacy of lithium, carbamazepine, and the combination in bipolar disorder. J Clin Psychiatry 58:470–478, 1997

Dilsaver SC, Chen Y-W, Swann AC, et al: Suicidality, panic disorder and psychosis in bipolar depression, depressive-mania and pure mania. Psychiatry Res 73:47–56, 1997

Dunner DL, Fieve RR: Clinical factors in lithium carbonate prophylaxis failure. Arch Gen Psychiatry 30:229–233, 1974

Faedda GL, Baldessarini RJ, Suppes T, et al: Pediatric-onset bipolar disorder: a neglected clinical and public health problem. Harv Rev Psychiatry 3:171–195, 1995

Garvey KA, Penn JV, Campbell AL, et al: Contracting for safety with patients: clinical practice and forensic implications. J Am Acad Psychiatry Law 37:363–370, 2009

Ghaemi SN, Rosenquist KJ, Ko JY, et al: Antidepressant treatment in bipolar vs. unipolar depression. Am J Psychiatry 161:163–165, 2004

Ghaemi SN, Wingo AP, Filkowski MA, et al: Long-term antidepressant treatment in bipolar disorder: meta-analysis of benefits and risks. Acta Psychiatr Scand 118:347–356, 2008

Goodwin FK, Jamison KR: Manic-Depressive Illness, 2nd Edition. New York, Oxford University, 2007

Gray SM, Otto MW: Psychosocial approaches to suicide prevention: applications to patients with bipolar disorder. J Clin Psychiatry 62(suppl):56–64, 2001

Guze SB, Robins E: Suicide and primary affective disorders. Br J Psychiatry 117:437–438, 1970

Hammad TA, Laughren TP, Racoosin JA: Suicidality in pediatric patients treated with antidepressant drugs. Arch Gen Psychiatry 63:332–339, 2006

Harris EC, Barraclough B: Suicide as an outcome for mental disorders: meta-analysis. Br J Psychiatry 170:205–208, 1997

Hennen J, Baldessarini RK: Suicidal risk during treatment with clozapine: a meta-analysis. Schizophr Res 73:139–145, 2005

Huxley NA, Parikh SV, Baldessarini RJ: Effectiveness of psychosocial treatments in bipolar disorder: state of the evidence. Harv Rev Psychiatry 8:126–140, 2000

Ilgen MA, Bohnert AS, Ignacio RV, et al: Psychiatric diagnoses and the risk of suicide in veterans. Arch Gen Psychiatry 67:1152–1158, 2010

Isacsson G, Rich CL, Jureidini J, et al: Increased use of antidepressants has contributed to the worldwide reduction in suicide rates. Br J Psychiatry 196:429–433, 2010

Isometsä ET, Henriksson MM, Aro HM, et al: Suicide in bipolar disorder in Finland. Am J Psychiatry 151:1020–1024, 1994

Jick H, Kaye JA, Jick SS: Antidepressants and the risk of suicidal behaviors. JAMA 292:338–343, 2004

Kessler RC, Berglund P, Borges G, et al: Trends in suicide ideation, plans, gestures, and attempts in the United States, 1990–1992 to 2001–2003. JAMA 293:2487–2495, 2005a

Kessler RC, Chiu WT, Demler O, et al: Prevalence, severity, and comorbidity of 12-month DSM-IV disorders in the National Comorbidity Survey Replication. Arch Gen Psychiatry 62:617–627, 2005b

Ketter TA: Diagnostic features, prevalence, and impact of bipolar disorder. J Clin Psychiatry 71:e14, 2010

Kochman FJ, Hantouche EG, Ferrari P, et al: Cyclothymic temperament as a prospective predictor of bipolarity and suicidality in children and adolescents with major depressive disorder. J Affect Disord 85:181–189, 2005

Krishnan KR: Psychiatric and medical comorbidities of bipolar disorder. Psychosom Med 67:1–8, 2005

Laughren TP: Overview of a meeting of the Psychopharmacology Drug Advisory Committee (PDAC) [concerning suicidal risk in trials of antidepressant drugs in juvenile and adult patients]. November 16, 2006. Available at: http://www.fda.gov/ohrms/dockets/ac/06/briefing/2006-4272b1-index.htm.

Leverich GS, Altshuler LL, Frye MA, et al: Factors associated with suicide attempts in 648 patients with bipolar disorder. J Clin Psychiatry 64: 506–515, 2003

Mann JJ, Brent DA, Arango V: The neurobiology and genetics of suicide and attempted suicide: a focus on the serotonergic system. Neuropsychopharmacology 24:467–477, 2001

Marangell LB, Dennehy EB, Wisniewski SR, et al: Case-control analyses of the impact of pharmacotherapy on prospectively observed suicide attempts and completed suicides in bipolar disorder. J Clin Psychiatry 69:916–922, 2008

Marneros A, Rottig S, Wenzel A, et al: Affective and schizoaffective mixed states. Eur Arch Psychiatry Clin Neurosci 254:76–81, 2004

Meltzer HY, Alphs L, Green AI, et al: Clozapine treatment for suicidality in schizophrenia: International Suicide Prevention Trial (InterSePT). Arch Gen Psychiatry 60:82–91, 2003

Miller CL, Druss B: Suicide and access to care. Psychiatr Serv 52:1566–1567, 2001

Müller-Oerlinghausen B, Lewitzka U: Lithium reduces pathological aggression and suicidality: a mini-review. Neuropsychobiology 62:43–49, 2010

Müller-Oerlinghausen B, Berghöfer A, Bauer M: Bipolar disorder. Lancet 359:241–247, 2002

Novick DM, Swartz HA, Frank E: Suicide attempts in bipolar I and bipolar II disorder: a review and meta-analysis of the evidence. Bipolar Disord 12:1–9, 2010

O'Leary D, Paykel E, Todd C, et al: Suicide in primary affective disorders revisited: a systematic review by treatment era. J Clin Psychiatry 62:804–811, 2001

Oquendo MA, Galfalvy HC, Currier D, et al: Treatment of suicide attempters with bipolar disorder: a randomized clinical trial comparing lithium and valproate in the prevention of suicidal behavior. Am J Psychiatry 168:1050–1056, 2011

Ösby U, Brandt L, Correia N, et al: Excess mortality in bipolar and unipolar disorder in Sweden. Arch Gen Psychiatry 58:844–850, 2001

Pirkis J, Burgess P: Suicide and recency of health care contacts: a systematic review. Br J Psychiatry 173:462–474, 1998

Pompili M: Exploring the phenomenology of suicide. Suicide Life Threat Behav 40:234–244, 2010

Pompili M, Baldessarini RJ: Suicidal risk associated with antiepileptic drug treatment. Nature Rev Neurology 6:651–653, 2010

Pompili M, Tondo L, Baldessarini RJ: Suicidal risk emerging during antidepressant treatment: recognition and intervention. Clin Neuropsychiatry 2:66–72, 2005

Pompili M, Rihmer Z, Innamorati M, et al: Assessment and treatment of suicide risk in bipolar disorders. Exp Rev Neurother 29:109–1036, 2009

Pompili M, Rihmer Z, Akiskal H, et al: Temperaments mediate suicide risk and psychopathology among patients with bipolar disorders. Compr Psychiatry June 2, 2011 [Epub ahead of print]

Pompili M, Innamorati M, Rihmer Z, et al: Cyclothymic-depressive-anxious temperament pattern is related to suicide risk in 346 patients with major mood disorders. J Affect Disord 136:405–411, 2012

Practice guideline for the assessment and treatment of patients with suicidal behaviors. Am J Psychiatry 160 (suppl 11):1–60, 2003

Read J, Bentall R: The effectiveness of electroconvulsive therapy: a literature review. Epidemiol Psichiatr Soc 19:333–347, 2010

Reeves RR, Ladner ME: Antidepressant-induced suicidality: an update. CNS Neurosci Ther 16:227–234, 2010

Rihmer Z, Gonda X: Antidepressant-resistant depression and antidepressant-associated suicidal behaviour: the role of underlying bipolarity. Depress Res Treat April 3, 2011 [Epub ahead of print]

Rihmer Z, Pestality P: Bipolar II disorder and suicidal behavior. Psychiatr Clin North Am 22:667–673, 1999

Rucci P, Frank E, Kostelnik B, et al: Suicide attempts in patients with bipolar I disorder during acute and maintenance phases of intensive treatment with pharmacotherapy and adjunctive psychotherapy. Am J Psychiatry 159:1160–1164, 2002

Sidor MM, Macqueen GM: Antidepressants for the acute treatment of bipolar depression: a systematic review and meta-analysis. J Clin Psychiatry 72:156–167, 2011

Tondo L, Baldessarini RJ, Hennen J, et al: Lithium treatment and risk of suicidal behavior in bipolar disorder patients. J Clin Psychiatry 59:405–414, 1998

Tondo L, Isacsson G, Baldessarini RJ: Suicidal behaviour in bipolar disorder: risk and prevention. CNS Drugs 17:491–511, 2003

Tondo L, Albert M, Baldessarini RJ: Suicide rates In relation to health care access in the United States: an ecological study. J Clin Psychiatry 67:517–523, 2006

Tondo L, Lepri B, Baldessarini RJ: Suicidal risks among 2826 Sardinian major affective disorder patients. Acta Psychiatr Scand 116:419–428, 2007

Tondo L, Lepri B, Baldessarini RJ: Suicidal status during antidepressant treatment in 789 Sardinian patients with major affective disorder. Acta Psychiatr Scand 118:106–115, 2008

Tondo L, Vázquez G, Baldessarini RJ: Mania associated with antidepressant treatment: comprehensive meta-analytic review. Acta Psychiatr Scand 121:404–414, 2010

U.S. Food and Drug Administration: Public health advisory: suicidality in adults being treated with antidepressant medications. June 30, 2005. Available at: http://www.fda.gov/Drugs/DrugSafety/Postmarket DrugSafetyInformationforPatientsand Providers/DrugSafetyInformationfor HeathcareProfessionals/PublicHealth-Advisories/ucm053169.htm.

U.S. Food and Drug Administration: Antidepressant use in children, adolescents, and adults. May 2, 2007. Available at: http://www.fda.gov/Drugs/DrugSafety/Informationby DrugClass/ucm096273.htm. Accessed February 3, 2012.

Valtonen H, Suominen K, Mantere O, et al: Suicidal ideation and attempts in bipolar I and II disorders. J Clin Psychiatry 66:1456–1462, 2005

Yatham LN: Diagnosis and management of patients with bipolar II disorder. J Clin Psychiatry 66(suppl):13–17, 2005

Zisook S, Lesser IM, Lebowitz B, et al: Effect of antidepressant medication treatment on suicidal ideation and behavior in a randomized trial: an exploratory report from the Combining Medications to Enhance Depression Outcomes Study. J Clin Psychiatry 72:1322–1332, 2011

CHAPTER 10

Schizophrenia

Jong H. Yoon, M.D.
Cameron S. Carter, M.D.

The management of suicidality in patients with schizophrenia represents a common but highly challenging problem for clinicians. The lifetime prevalence of completed suicide and suicide attempts in this patient group is much higher than in the general population, with a generally accepted range of 5%–10% for completed suicides and 25%–50% for suicide attempts (Palmer et al. 2005). The basics of proper assessment and management of suicidal patients with schizophrenia share many features with treatment of suicidality in other patient populations. For example, factors such as previous attempts, comorbid depression or substance abuse, and male gender confer higher suicide risk in individuals with schizophrenia (Hawton et al. 2005; Limosin et al. 2007), mirroring important risk factors in the general population. However, the unique constellation of symptoms in schizophrenia and their sequelae present special challenges in the implementation of assessment and treatment

strategies. Some clinical features of schizophrenia also offer specific factors that may be especially helpful in assessing risk and guiding treatment in this patient population.

Our goal in this chapter is to highlight these disease-specific assessment and treatment strategies through the use of two representative case studies, which are augmented by a limited review of empirical studies focusing on schizophrenia and suicide. It must be emphasized that despite progress in identifying predictive factors of suicide in schizophrenia, we are still far from identifying any risk factor that has a high degree of sensitivity or specificity. Thus, the proper detection and management of suicidality in this patient population require the same common sense approach required by other specialties that deal with rare but lethal conditions—namely, a high index of suspicion and an aggressive approach to instituting the appropriate evaluation and treatment modalities.

Case Example 1: Elevated Suicide Risk in a Newly Diagnosed Patient With Schizophrenia

C.M. came from a solidly middle- to upper-middle-class family without any history of major mental illness. His birth, childhood development, and adolescence were unremarkable, with no evidence of cognitive, behavioral, or emotional abnormalities. C.M. was a talented, bright young male with a record of academic as well as extracurricular achievements in high school that gained him entry into an exclusive undergraduate school. During his freshman year, he was social, was well liked by peers and teachers, and enjoyed a large circle of friends. In short, C.M. appeared to be a typical high-achieving young adult with a very bright future and with no warning signs of impending severe mental illness.

During his sophomore year in college, C.M. began to exhibit what his friends considered to be manifestations of mild depression, characterized by social withdrawal, blunting of affect, sluggishness, and poor personal hygiene. He also became overly concerned about his popularity and how others viewed him. He began to experience nonspecific cognitive problems such as the inability to concentrate and a tendency for vagueness in his speech. Consequently, he began to receive uncharacteristically poor grades and he was barely able to complete his courses that semester. While at home during winter break, at the urging of his parents, he began seeing a psychiatrist, who diagnosed him with major depression and treated him with antidepressants.

On his return to college for the spring semester, his friends did not notice any significant improvement in his condition. As the semester wore on, C.M. became more reclusive and erratic. He limited his social contacts to a few select peers. In public, he often appeared upset, anxious, and fearful. To his closest confidants, he started to express concerns that people were making fun of him or talking about him behind his back. Soon, his friends could not convince C.M. that he was being overly sensitive to perceived insults or just imagining that people were doing this. His grades were failing, and he feared being placed on academic probation. Scholastic failure was an entirely new situation for him and caused him

significant anxiety. His increasing preoccupation with being singled out for ridicule by his peers and his worsening academic situation caused him to stay up late at night worrying. His dormitory mates noted that he could be heard talking to himself in his room. C.M.'s concerns about others' treatment of him started to affect his behavior in public. On a few occasions, he abruptly interrupted a conversation between strangers to accuse them of talking about him. In one of these confrontations, he threatened to kill one of the students. It was at this point that C.M. was taken by the university's security officers for an evaluation by a counselor at the university. C.M. was deemed to present an imminent risk of harm to others, and he was placed on a 72-hour psychiatric hold and admitted to the local psychiatric hospital for further evaluation.

During the evaluation in the hospital, C.M. reports to the inpatient psychiatric attending his firm conviction that other students have been singling him out for persecution in a variety of ways, including plotting to get him expelled from school. He also relates that he is hearing male voices that frequently make derogatory comments about him. He is reluctant to tell anyone about the voices because he has all along realized that these voices are not real and that their presence may signal that he has a major mental illness. After a couple of days in the hospital, C.M. begins to express some doubts about the veracity of his prior claims. C.M. initially refuses all psychiatric medications except anxiolytics. However, after meeting with his parents, the patient reluctantly agrees to a trial of haloperidol. Within 1 week of hospitalization, C.M. notes decreased auditory hallucinations and less concern about being persecuted by classmates. C.M. is discharged to his parents, and he takes a leave of absence from school.

C.M. remains compliant with medications for a brief period after discharge. However, as his symptoms improve, C.M. believes that he no longer requires medications, and he stops all of his psychiatric medications despite his parents' admonishments. He attempts to take on various jobs in his neighborhood, but for one reason or another he is not able to keep them for any length of time. C.M. communicates with his college friends by phone or mail, but otherwise he does not socialize much, and he spends most of his time in his room. When asked about any of his symptoms, he categorically denies them, but his parents have the distinct feeling that he is not being truthful. C.M.'s condition remains in this quasi-stable state for the remainder of his time with his parents. C.M. is feeling well enough to return to college the following fall semester. However, it becomes very apparent soon after start of classes that C.M. cannot manage. He begins exhibiting overt signs of paranoia and internal preoccupation. He takes another leave of absence and returns home to his parents. This time, C.M.'s parents are able to convince him of the need to continue to take psychiatric medications, and he begins regular visits to his psychiatrist. He reluctantly continues to take neuroleptics but complains about many side effects, including sedation, weight gain, and restlessness. His parents notice that he has become even more reclusive and less talkative. He also appears to be sleeping more than usual. Then, one morning, when C.M. does not respond to repeated requests for him to come to breakfast, his parents go into C.M.'s room, where they find him lying dead in his bed. They find an empty bottle of tricyclic antidepressants in his room.

The case of C.M. highlights several important issues in the assessment and management of the suicidal patient with schizophrenia. First, patients with the diagnosis of schizophrenia represent a high-risk group with a substantially higher rate of suicide compared with the general population. The lifetime prevalence of suicide has generally been taken to be 5%–10% (Palmer et al. 2005).

Second, the timing of his suicide in relation to the onset of his illness is very pertinent. Within the context of overall higher lifetime prevalence of suicide, studies have clearly documented that the period after initial diagnosis of schizophrenia represents an especially vulnerable period. Palmer et al. (2005) showed in a meta-analysis that the risk of suicide among cohorts of first-episode schizophrenia patients is nearly three times the rate of a chronic cohort. Other studies have also documented

the greatest risk within the first few years of illness (Black and Winokur 1988; Kua et al. 2003).

This increased suicide rate early in the course of illness likely represents the despair experienced by these individuals in anticipating future years filled with disability and downward drift in socioeconomic status associated with this condition. In the case of C.M., he came from a privileged background with a history of academic and social achievement and high expectations for his future. It is noteworthy that the suicide occurred after he acknowledged having a major mental illness, inferred by his willingness voluntarily to accept treatment. For individuals like C.M., the transition in their expectations for themselves in terms of level of functioning before and after the onset of schizophrenia most likely prove too difficult to manage. This is consistent with the results of a recent large, multicenter study that demonstrated a relationship between a patient's insight into his or her illness and higher risk of committing suicide (Bourgeois et al. 2004). Interestingly, the authors of this and another related study (Kim et al. 2003) further suggested that the positive correlation between increased insight and suicide may be mediated by depression and a sense of hopelessness.

These results highlight the important role the clinician can play in allaying some of the fears that may be fueling a patient's sense of hopelessness about the future. In the course of educating the patient and the family about the likelihood that this illness will result in significant disability, the clinician may find that the fears may be based on commonly held misconceptions about schizophrenia. The patient with new-onset schizophrenia and family members may not be aware that this illness can have a highly variable course (Davidson and Mc-Glashan 1997) and that there are now many medications that can significantly ameliorate many of the symptoms. Additionally, they may not be aware that early treatment of psychosis may have a significant impact on short- and long-term level of functioning (Bottlender et al. 2000, 2003).

Second, the importance of comorbid depression in individuals with chronic schizophrenia, or what has often been described as "postpsychotic" depression, as a risk factor for suicide cannot be overemphasized, particularly around the initial episodes of illness. As with other medical conditions, the presence of comorbid depression increases substantially the risk of suicide. A 10-year prospective study (Limosin et al. 2007) and one of the most comprehensive meta-analyses to date (Hawton et al. 2005) of suicide and schizophrenia have both identified comorbid depression as one of the major predictors of suicide in individuals with schizophrenia. Consequently, the appearance of depressive symptoms should be seen as a red flag to prompt the clinician to directly assess this risk.

The assessment of depression in schizophrenia does, however, present some unique challenges. Core features of the illness can render the usual signs and symptoms of depression difficult to detect. Affective blunting and other negative symptoms of schizophrenia can mimic, and therefore mask, the symptoms of depression. People with schizophrenia can appear affectively blunted and unreactive, uninterested in activity, or may avoid social situations. Masking of symptoms of depression can be further exacerbated by the side effects of neuroleptics, especially the typical neuroleptics with their ability to induce parkinsonian symptoms. For these reasons, clinicians should rely on additional strategies to assess depression in schizophrenia.

Studies conducted by Kring and colleagues (Earnst and Kring 1999; Kring et al. 1993) on the capacity for experiencing pleasure among individuals suffering from schizophrenia suggest an efficient strategy for the assessment of depression in these patients. Contrary to the commonly held view that people with schizophrenia do not experience pleasure, Kring's studies have shown that they are in fact capable of experiencing the same degree of enjoyment as healthy people while engaged in pleasurable activity (Kring and Moran 2008). These studies do, however, document a deficit in the anticipation of enjoyment in the future, which may be in part due to impairments in prefrontal cortex functioning that is normally required to implement the mental processes necessary for the anticipation of enjoying future events (Ursu et al. 2011).

For the above-cited reasons, the proper assessment of depression in schizophrenia, in general, should de-emphasize the usual manifestations of depression observable in a mental status exam, such as affective blunting, because the illness itself or antipsychotics could be causing or worsening these symptoms. Instead, the assessment should emphasize the reporting of internal hedonic states. Furthermore, the questions that the clinician uses to screen for the presence of the anhedonic symptoms of depression should be modified to de-emphasize the anticipatory aspects and focus on the here and now. Consequently, instead of asking "Do you look forward to going to the movies?" the clinician should rephrase this question to focus on an in-the-moment experience of pleasure, as in "Yesterday, when you went to see the movie, did you enjoy it?" Consistent with the idea that the outward observable signs of emotion may not be a good indicator of the patient's internal state was a finding from a study conducted by Cohen et al. (1990), in which a patient's subjective sense of emotional distress, and not the clinician's observation of distress, was significantly predictive of suicide risk.

Another effective strategy to assess the presence of depression may be to gather collateral observational information from the patient's family or case manager, or others who are in a position to directly observe the patient's ability to engage in and enjoy activities. Another option is to rely on symptom rating scales such as the Calgary Depression Scale, which was specifically developed to assess the presence of depression in individuals with schizophrenia (Addington et al. 1993).

Once depression is suspected, the psychiatrist should aggressively treat it. If the patient appears to be depressed as a consequence of having insight into his or her illness, supportive psychotherapy and psychoeducation, for both the patient and his or her family support system, are indicated.

As for pharmacological treatment, emerging evidence on the neurobiology of the brain's reward system provides guidance in effectively treating psychosis while addressing the presence of depressive symptoms in schizophrenia. The neural circuitry of reward, the ventral tegmental area–nucleus accumbens circuit, is dependent on dopamine and signaling through the dopamine D_2 receptor subtype to convey pleasurable experiences (Di Chiara et al. 2004). Consequently, typical neuroleptics with high D_2 antagonism, such as haloperidol, at high doses may block the function of the reward circuitry in patients. This blockade could explain why negative symptoms may develop or worsen after initiation of the older, typical antipsychotics (King 1998). One study also found that the degree of D_2 antagonism by typical neuroleptics is highly positively correlated with the presence of depressive symptoms in patients with schizophrenia (Bressan et al. 2002). Additionally, there may be a therapeutic window of optimal D_2 receptor occupancy by the neuroleptic that balances the antipsychotic efficacy and the dysphoric side effects of D_2 antagonism (de Haan et al. 2000).

The newer, atypical antipsychotics are often cited for their lower affinity for the D_2 receptor. Consequently, one of the advantages in using atypical antipsychotics as compared with a typical agent to treat individuals with schizophrenia may be the preservation of the function of the reward circuitry. Additionally, several lines of evidence suggest that these agents are in fact effective in the treatment of depression. There is now a fairly large body of evidence demonstrating the efficacy of atypical antipsychotics in cases of treatment-refractory depression in major depressive disorder. A recent meta-analysis demonstrated significant efficacy for olanzapine, risperidone, quetiapine, and aripiprazole when each agent was used to augment first-line antidepressants (Nelson and Papakostas 2009). Additionally, several studies have demonstrated that atypical antipsychotics have differential benefits in comparison with typical antipsychotics in treating depression in schizophrenia (Csernansky et al. 2002; Levinson et al. 1999; Marder et al. 1997; Tollefson et al. 1998). The American Psychiatric Association practice guideline recommended the use of atypical antipsychotics for the treatment of depression in schizophrenia (Lehman et al. 2004).

Among the atypical antipsychotics, two deserve special mention regarding the treatment or prevention of suicide in schizophrenia. The first is clozapine, which is often cited in the scientific literature as being associated with reduction in the suicide rate among people with schizophrenia. Prospective studies have demonstrated that clozapine reduces impulsive aggression and suicidality compared with haloperidol treatment (Spivak et al. 2003). One multicenter, prospective, randomized treatment trial also demonstrated superior efficacy of clozapine compared with olanzapine in reducing suicidal behavior (Meltzer et al. 2003). The second atypical agent, aripiprazole, deserves special mention because of its unique pharmacodynamic property. Aripiprazole is a partial D_2 receptor agonist in that it is a D_2 antagonist under hyperdopaminergic conditions and a D_2 agonist under hypodopaminergic conditions (Burris et al. 2002). The antidepressant property of aripiprazole may also be attributable to the partial-agonist activity at serotonin type 1A (5-HT_{1A}) and antagonist activity at 5-HT_{2A} receptors (Jordan et al. 2004). It is currently the only antipsychotic approved by the U.S. Food and Drug Administration for augmentation in treatment of treatment-refractory depression. A recent meta-analysis (Janicak et al. 2009) of the efficacy of aripiprazole in schizophrenia found that aripiprazole was significantly more effective for depressive symptoms compared with haloperidol and placebo.

More basic and clinical research are required to specify the mechanism of action of clozapine in minimizing suicidality in this high-risk group. Nonetheless, these studies offer yet another reason for the consideration of atypical neuroleptics as first-line agents in the treatment of schizophrenia.

Case Example 2: Elevated Suicide Risk in a Patient With Chronic Schizophrenia and Comorbid Substance Abuse

L.C. is a 35-year-old single male with schizophrenia since the age of 21. His psychiatric treatment has been sporadic and characterized by brief periods of treatment with neuroleptics inside and outside of the hospital. L.C. has had difficulty maintaining a treatment alliance with virtually every psychiatrist he has encountered. Consequently, L.C. has been chronically without a consistent primary psychiatrist or mental health treatment. His illness is also exacerbated by his inability to control his dependence on cocaine. L.C.'s parents, one of whom is a surgeon, became worn out by his inability to maintain abstinence and to consistently follow through with his psychiatric treatment. The parents now refuse to provide housing for him in their home, and they maintain only distant involvement in L.C.'s life and psychiatric care. Without a stable support network, L.C. is often homeless and abusing drugs.

For this particular episode, L.C. brings himself to the emergency room reporting suicidal urges brought on by derogatory auditory hallucinations that constantly tell him to kill himself and depressed mood that began after the end of a cocaine binge. On examination, L.C. appears very disheveled and malodorous, gaunt, internally preoccupied, and guarded. He is also withdrawn, with psychomotor slowing and diminished spontaneity in speech and movements. Urine toxicology is positive for cocaine. L.C. is placed on an involuntary 72-hour hold and admitted to the dual-diagnosis psychiatric unit.

The staff at the emergency room and the hospital's dual-diagnosis unit know L.C. very well, because this is one of many contacts with him involving psychostimulant abuse, psychosis, and suicidal ideation. What is especially noteworthy about his hospitalizations is the high degree of ambivalence L.C. displays toward psychiatric treatment. Typically, at the time of admission, L.C. voluntarily seeks out care and is compliant with recommendations for the initiation of neuroleptics to control his psychosis. However, after 2 days of treatment, he typically becomes increasingly resistant, negative, oppositional, and frankly paranoid toward clinicians, challenging his diagnosis of schizophrenia and the need for long-term psychotropic treatment. He equates psychiatric medications with mind control and accuses clinicians of merely complying with his father's orders. At the end of the 72-hour period of involuntary detainment, L.C. petitions for his release from the psychiatric hospital. In most instances, L.C. is granted his petition over the objections of his treating psychiatrists. Once discharged, L.C. does not follow up with outpatient treatment appointments and loses contact with mental health services until his next inpatient admission.

At baseline, L.C. frequently experiences auditory hallucinations and many forms of persecutory delusions. However, he does not display prominent thought disorder. He can hold long conversations that are goal directed, and he can appear rational when he is discussing topics unrelated to his paranoia. His mental status is also notable for a high degree of hostility toward others, especially authority figures. However, he does not have any history of severe physical violence toward others.

Each time L.C. is admitted to the dual-diagnosis unit, he engenders strong antipathy from the staff. The attending psychiatrist is often given subtle and not-so-subtle suggestions by staff members to discharge the patient quickly. Some staff members openly deride L.C.'s suicidality and accuse him of manipulating the system. A strong sense of futility surrounds his admissions, with staff members expressing their belief that any effort by them to help L.C. would not have any appreciable benefit on L.C.'s short- or long-term course. Despite this skepticism and animosity, the emergency department staff treats L.C.'s suicidal threats very seriously because of the increased risk of suicide posed by his documented history of past suicide attempts of high potential lethality, ongoing substance abuse, and depression.

In the case of C.M., we discussed some of the unique suicide risk factors and treatment issues related to new-onset schizophrenia, such as the increased risk associated with postpsychotic depression and the difficulties of detecting depression in patients with schizophrenia. The case of L.C. illustrates some of the pertinent factors in assessing and treating suicidality in the patient with established-diagnosis schizophrenia and comorbid substance abuse.

Patients with schizophrenia are much like others in that the expression of suicidality has many layers of meaning. In this case, suicidality may in fact be a way for L.C. to temporarily obtain food and shelter. On a more psychodynamic level, threats of suicide may also represent L.C.'s primitive means of expressing anger toward self and others and ambivalence about his life. Despite these potential layers of meaning, it is clear that L.C. is at very high risk for suicide for a variety of reasons. Before discussing these risk factors, a critical aspect of providing care for a patient such as this is to be mindful of not minimizing his or her risks due to negative countertransference or giving into the strong sense of futility engendered by his or her many intractable problems.

One strategy to combat the bias that negative countertransference may have on clinical decision making is to rely on clinical rating scales in assessing suicide risk. There are now a number of validated clinical rating scales that are available to assist the clinician in gauging suicide risk in patients with schizophrenia. The Columbia Suicide Severity Rating Scale offers a comprehensive set of scales suitable for research and clinicians (Mundt et al. 2010). (Information on obtaining training in use of the scales and copies of the scales is available at www.cssrs.columbia.edu.) The InterSePT Scale for Suicidal Thinking (Lindenmayer et al. 2003) is an interview-based instrument that has been specifically developed for the assessment of suicide risk in schizophrenia.

One of the most important factors to consider in assessing suicide risk in this case is comorbid substance abuse. A number of studies have documented that comorbid substance abuse is a risk factor for suicide in this condition (Hawton et al. 2005; Limosin et al. 2007; Palmer et al. 2005; Potkin et al. 2003). The rate of substance abuse among individuals with schizophrenia remains very high, with a lifetime prevalence in the United States estimated to approach 50% (Regier et al. 1990). As in other patient populations, individuals with schizophrenia are at high risk of committing suicide in the acute intoxicated state because of impaired judgment and impulse control. People with schizophrenia are especially vulnerable to the disinhibiting properties of drugs, because a core feature of the illness itself may be dysfunction of the prefrontal cortex (Yoon et al. 2008), a region of the brain thought to subserve impulse control and judgment.

Substance abuse with psychostimulants such as cocaine or amphetamine increases suicide risk not only during the acute intoxication phase but also in the withdrawal phase. It is common for psychostimulant abusers to experience a depressive syndrome after a period of sustained drug intake (Kosten 2002). This withdrawal-related depression can be severe, with prominent vegetative symptoms such as psychomotor slowing, increased sleep, and diminished appetite, as well as increased suicidal ideation (Sofuoglu et al. 2003). However, the withdrawal syndrome is usually time limited. Given the high prevalence of comorbid substance abuse in this patient population and the important role of substance abuse in suicide risk, the treatment of suicidality in patients with schizophrenia and comorbid substance abuse must involve the coordinated treatment of both conditions.

Paradoxically, intact higher-order cognitive capacity may be a relative risk factor for suicide in individuals with schizophrenia. Cognitive deficits in schizophrenia are characterized by abnormalities in executive functions such as planning. Consequently, individuals with severe cognitive deficits may lack the ability to effectively plan and execute suicidal acts. Conversely, individuals such as L.C., with relatively intact cognitive abilities as evidenced by lack of disorganization or formal thought disorder, would have the ability to plan successfully and carry out a suicidal act.

Finally, this case should be taken as a cautionary tale highlighting the importance of early intervention and treatment of psychosis and schizophrenia. The cause of L.C.'s hostility toward mental health clinicians and authority figures is most likely complex and multifactorial. Regardless of the etiology, his maladaptive pattern of relating to health care providers has become ingrained, and it would be very difficult for any one clinician or single point of contact to undo this. This emphasizes the importance of establishing a more productive pattern of relating to and engaging with mental health providers and services early in the course of the illness so that the necessary treatment and services can be mobilized to minimize the negative outcomes that can result from this illness.

There is accumulating evidence that the duration of untreated psychosis early in the course of illness can have tremendous impact on various levels and indices of functioning (Bottlender et al. 2000, 2003). In the case of L.C., early and aggressive treatment of his persecutory delusions would have maximized his chances of establishing a more productive relationship with clinicians, who could then have been in a better position to assist L.C.. One meta-analysis identified poor therapeutic alliance and inadequate discharge planning as major factors associated with poor treatment compliance (Lacro et al. 2002). It appears that a multidisciplinary approach that addresses behavioral, psychological, psychoeducational, and social needs of the patient with schizophrenia early in the illness can have significant benefits in terms of improved adherence to treatment (Dolder et al. 2003).

Key Clinical Concepts

- Have a high index of suspicion and a low threshold for assessment and treatment of patients with schizophrenia, who represent a high-risk group.

- Remember that a window of especially high risk exists in the first few years after diagnosis.

- In addition to the presence of depression, substance abuse, and hopelessness, more disease-specific risk factors for suicide may include higher cognitive ability, awareness of loss of function imposed by illness, and difficulty accepting decline in socioeconomic status.

- In meeting the special challenges in detecting depression in schizophrenia, use suicidality rating scales and strategies that gauge patients' in-the-moment experience of pleasure to assess anhedonia and depression.

- In early intervention, minimize the duration of psychosis, and promote a more healthy pattern of engagement with the mental health system and its professionals.

- Use lowest effective dosages of neuroleptics to minimize dopamine D_2 receptor blockade.

- Consider that clozapine may have a special role in management of suicide risk in patients with schizophrenia.

References

Addington D, Addington J, Maticka-Tyndale E: Assessing depression in schizophrenia: the Calgary Depression Scale. Br J Psychiatry Suppl 22:39–44, 1993

Black DW, Winokur G: Age, mortality and chronic schizophrenia. Schizophr Res 1:267–272, 1988

Bottlender R, Strauss A, Moller HJ: Impact of duration of symptoms prior to first hospitalization on acute outcome in 998 schizophrenic patients. Schizophr Res 44:145–150, 2000

Bottlender R, Sato T, Jäger M, et al: The impact of the duration of untreated psychosis prior to first psychiatric admission on the 15-year outcome in schizophrenia. Schizophr Res 62:37–44, 2003

Bourgeois M, Swendsen J, Young F, et al; InterSePT Study Group: Awareness of disorder and suicide risk in the treatment of schizophrenia: results of the International Suicide Prevention Trial. Am J Psychiatry 161:1494–1496, 2004

Bressan RA, Costa DC, Jones HM, et al: Typical antipsychotic drugs: D2 receptor occupancy and depressive symptoms in schizophrenia. Schizophr Res 56:31–36, 2002

Burris KD, Molski TF, Xu C, et al: Aripiprazole, a novel antipsychotic, is a high-affinity partial agonist at human dopamine D2 receptors. J Pharmacol Exp Ther 302:381–389, 2002

Cohen LJ, Test MA, Brown RL: Suicide and schizophrenia: data from a prospective community treatment study. Am J Psychiatry 147:602–607, 1990

Csernansky JG, Mahmoud R, Brenner R, et al: A comparison of risperidone and haloperidol for the prevention of relapse in patients with schizophrenia. N Engl J Med 346:16–22, 2002

Davidson L, McGlashan TH: The varied outcomes of schizophrenia. Can J Psychiatry 42:34–43, 1997 de Haan L, Lavalaye J, Linszen D, et al: Subjective experience and striatal dopamine D2 receptor occupancy in patients with schizophrenia stabilized by olanzapine or risperidone. Am J Psychiatry 157:1019–1020, 2000

Di Chiara G, Bassareo V, Fenu S, et al: Dopamine and drug addiction: the nucleus accumbens shell connection. Neuropharmacology 47 (suppl 1):227–241, 2004

Dolder CR, Lacro JP, Leckband S, et al: Interventions to improve antipsychotic medication adherence: review of recent literature. J Clin Psychopharmacol 23:389–399, 2003

Earnst KS, Kring AM: Emotional responding in deficit and non-deficit schizophrenia. Psychiatry Res 88:191–207, 1999

Hawton K, Sutton L, Haw C, et al: Schizophrenia and suicide: systematic review of risk factors. Br J Psychiatry 187:9–20, 2005

Janicak PG, Glick ID, Marder SR, et al: The acute efficacy of aripiprazole across the symptom spectrum of schizophrenia: a pooled post hoc analysis from 5 short-term studies. J Clin Psychiatry 70:25–35, 2009

Jordan S, Koprivica V, Dunn R, et al: In vivo effects of aripiprazole on cortical and striatal dopaminergic and serotonergic function. Eur J Pharmacol 483:45–53, 2004

Kim CH, Jayathilake K, Meltzer HY: Hopelessness, neurocognitive function, and insight in schizophrenia: relationship to suicidal behavior. Schizophr Res 60:71–80, 2003

King DJ: Drug treatment of the negative symptoms of schizophrenia. Eur Neuropsychopharmacol 8:33–42, 1998

Kosten TR: Pathophysiology and treatment of cocaine dependence, in Neuropsychopharmacology: The Fifth Generation of Progress. Edited by Davis K, Charney D, Coyle JT, et al. Baltimore, MD, Lippincott Williams & Wilkins, 2002, pp 1461–1473

Kring AM, Moran EK: Emotional response deficits in schizophrenia: insights from affective science. Schizophr Bull 34:819–834, 2008

Kring AM, Kerr SL, Smith DA, et al: Flat affect in schizophrenia does not reflect diminished subjective experience of emotion. J Abnorm Psychol 102:507–517, 1993

Kua J, Wong DI, Kua EH, et al: A 20-year follow-up study on schizophrenia in Singapore. Acta Psychiatr Scand 108:118–125, 2003

Lacro JP, Dunn LB, Dolder CR, et al: Prevalence of and risk factors for medication nonadherence in patients with schizophrenia: a comprehensive review of recent literature. J Clin Psychiatry 63:892–909, 2002

Lehman AF, Lieberman JA, Dixon LB, et al: Practice guideline for the treatment of patients with schizophrenia, second edition. Am J Psychiatry 161:1–56, 2004

Levinson DF, Umapathy C, Musthaq M: Treatment of schizoaffective disorder and schizophrenia with mood symptoms. Am J Psychiatry 156:1138–1148, 1999

Limosin F, Loze J, Philippe A, et al: Ten-year prospective follow-up study of the mortality by suicide in schizophrenic patients. Schizophr Res 94:23–28, 2007

Lindenmayer JP, Czobor P, Alphs L, et al: The InterSePT Scale for Suicidal Thinking reliability and validity. Schizophr Res 63:161–170, 2003

Marder SR, Davis JM, Chouinard G: The effects of risperidone on the five dimensions of schizophrenia derived by factor analysis: combined results of the North American trials. J Clin Psychiatry 58:538–546, 1997

Meltzer HY, Alphs L, Green AI, et al; International Suicide Prevention Trial Study Group: Clozapine treatment for suicidality in schizophrenia: International Suicide Prevention Trial (InterSePT). Arch Gen Psychiatry 60:82–91, 2003

Mundt JC, Greist JH, Gelenberg AJ, et al: Feasibility and validation of a computer-automated Columbia-Suicide Severity Rating Scale using interactive voice response technology. J Psychiatr Res 44:1224–1228, 2010

Nelson JC, Papakostas GI: Atypical antipsychotic augmentation in major depressive disorder: a meta-analysis of placebo-controlled randomized trials. Am J Psychiatry 166:980–991, 2009

Palmer BA, Pankratz VS, Bostwick JM: The lifetime risk of suicide in schizophrenia: a reexamination. Arch Gen Psychiatry 62:247–253, 2005

Potkin SG, Alphs L, Hsu C, et al; InterSePT Study Group: Predicting suicidal risk in schizophrenic and schizoaffective patients in a prospective two-year trial. Biol Psychiatry 54:444–452, 2003

Regier DA, Farmer ME, Rae DS, et al: Comorbidity of mental disorders with alcohol and other drug abuse: results from the Epidemiologic Catchment Area (ECA) study. JAMA 264:2511–2518, 1990

Sofuoglu M, Dudish-Poulsen S, Brown SB, et al: Association of cocaine withdrawal symptoms with more severe dependence and enhanced subjective response to cocaine. Drug Alcohol Depend 69:273–282, 2003

Spivak B, Shabash E, Sheitman B, et al: The effects of clozapine versus haloperidol on measures of impulsive aggression and suicidality in chronic schizophrenia patients: an open, nonrandomized, 6-month study. J Clin Psychiatry 64:755–760, 2003

Tollefson GD, Sanger TM, Lu Y, et al: Depressive signs and symptoms in schizophrenia: a prospective blinded trial of olanzapine and haloperidol. Arch Gen Psychiatry 55:250–258, 1998

Ursu S, Kring AM, Gard MG, et al: Prefrontal cortical deficits and impaired cognition-emotion interactions in schizophrenia. Am J Psychiatry 168:276–285, 2011

Yoon JH, Minzenberg MJ, Ursu S, et al: Association of dorsolateral prefrontal cortex dysfunction with disrupted coordinated brain activity in schizophrenia: relationship with impaired cognition, behavioral disorganization, and global function. Am J Psychiatry 165:1006–1014, 2008

C H A P T E R   1 1

Personality Disorders

Juan J. Carballo, M.D., Ph.D.

Barbara Stanley, Ph.D.

Beth S. Brodsky, Ph.D.

Maria A. Oquendo, M.D.

The prevalence of personality disorders in the general population of the United States has been the subject of recent investigations, which have estimated the point prevalence of any personality disorder to be in the range of 9%–15.7% (Crawford et al. 2005; Lenzenweger et al. 1997, 2007; Samuels et al. 2002). Similar rates have been reported in two different European community samples (Coid et al. 2006; Torgersen et al. 2001). Studies of the prevalence of personality disorders have also been conducted in clinical populations. Using structured interviews, Zimmerman et al. (2005) reported a rate of 45.5% for any personality disorder in an outpatient setting. Among hospitalized patients, the rates may be even higher—as high as 91% (Linehan et al. 1991).

Suicide is currently understood as a multidimensional disorder that results from a complex interaction of biological, genetic, psychological, sociological, and environmental factors. According to the World Health Organization (WHO), suicide is a crucial public health problem and is among the three leading causes of death among those ages 15–44 years in some countries, and is the second leading cause of death among persons ages 10–24 years. Risk factors for suicide include mental disorders such as personality disorders. In fact, personality disorders are associated with estimated lifetime rates of suicide ranging from 3% to 9% (American Psychiatric Association 2003). Compared with the general population, the estimated risk for suicide is about 7 times greater in persons with personality disorder (Harris and Barraclough 1997) and about 13-fold for formerly hospitalized patients with personality disorders (Black and Winokur 1986; Zilber et al. 1989).

Psychological autopsy studies have helped demonstrate the importance of personality disorder as a risk factor for completed suicide. One meta-analysis has shown that as many as 57% of those who die by suicide had at least one personality disorder (Isometsä 2001). Among adolescent and young adult suicide completers, nearly half had a personality disorder (Apter et al. 1993; Brent et al. 1994; Lesage et al. 1994; Linehan et al. 2005). Similarly, among psychiatric outpatients, half of patients who died by suicide had a personality disorder (Baxter and Appleby 1999; Brown et al. 2000). Nevertheless, actual rates might be even higher. Some authors cite a bias toward giving an Axis I principal diagnosis instead of an Axis II diagnosis when a suicide has occurred (Linehan et al. 2005), which may lead to underreporting of personality disorder diagnoses among suicide completers.

The occurrence of suicide attempts and self-injurious behavior is an equally staggering clinical problem. Personality disorders are the second group of disorders among suicide attempters in the WHO/ EURO Multicentre Study of Suicidal Behavior. Moreover, it is estimated that among those with personality disorders, suicide attempts may occur in up to 84% (Black et al. 2004). This estimation varies depending on the type of personality disorder (Cluster A, B, or C or individual disorders) or the presence of comorbidities, especially mood and substance use disorders. Of note, self-injurious behavior is an important risk factor for suicidal behavior, because 55%–85% of patients with self-injurious behavior have made at least one suicide attempt (Stanley and Brodsky 2005).

Suicidal Behavior in Personality Disorders

The ability of clinicians to evaluate correctly suicidality has been challenged by a lack of well-defined terminology and understanding as to what constitutes suicidal behavior (Posner et al. 2007a). In this vein, the use of a standardized method of classifying the spectrum of suicidal ideation and behavior has been recommended (De Leo et al. 2006). Adherence to a standardized system promotes the use of reliable terminology that may help 1) follow variation in a patient's suicidal behavior over time, 2) avoid the use of erroneous synonyms for suicidal behavior, and 3) foster communication between clinicians (Posner et al. 2007a).

We recently (Posner et al. 2007b) developed a classification system that provides definitions for a spectrum of suicidal behaviors and thoughts, the Columbia Classification Algorithm for Suicide Assessment. *Suicide* is a death resulting from an individual's own actions, in which the individual intended to end his or her life (Posner et al. 2007a). A *suicide attempt* is a potentially self-destructive act performed with at least some intent to die. Although this definition is apparently straightforward, *intent* may be difficult to determine through direct inquiry, because retrospective reports can be influenced by reinterpretation of motivation and outcome and may no longer represent accurate descriptions of the individual's state of mind at the time of the self-injury. In some cases, suicidal intent may be concealed or denied. Clinically, suicidal intent is often deduced from external behaviors or factors, such as how medically lethal the self-injury was, or the circumstances surrounding the act, such as the likelihood of discovery during and immediately following the act. Any amount of intent to die, however, is sufficient to label an act as suicidal. This strategy for determining suicidal intent can lead to erroneous assumptions, particularly among individuals with borderline personality disorder (BPD) who have a history of self-injury without intent to die and in whom intent to die may be ambiguous. Perception of intent can also be distorted by a history of previous nonlethal attempts (Stanley et al. 2001).

Self-injurious behavior is defined as intentional self-destructive behavior performed with no intent to die (i.e., if the individual committing the act is doing it purely for reasons other than to end his or her life). Suicidal behavior and nonsuicidal self-injury are therefore distinguished by the presence or absence of suicidal intent. Self-injurious behavior with no suicidal intent can be understood as an effort to regulate emotions. Although these behaviors are often interpreted by clinicians and family members as representing suicidal intent, individuals who engage in such behaviors are often quite clear that the behaviors "help" them feel better.

The distinction between suicidal and nonsuicidal behavior has led to proposals for new diagnostic categories for the upcoming DSM-5 classification system: nonsuicidal self-injury and suicidal behavior. The rationale for this proposal is, in part, that the disorder has "clinical value, improving accurate identification and/or treatment; and [is] prevalent, impairing, and distinctive" (American Psychiatric Association, DSM-5 Development; available at: http://www.dsm5.org/ProposedRevision/Pages/proposedrevision.aspx?rid=443#).

Two other terms warrant mention: self-mutilation and parasuicide. Although *self-mutilation* is used to describe nonsuicidal self-harm, some forms of self-injury such as head banging and hitting oneself do not involve mutilation. Thus, this definition is not inclusive enough. The term *parasuicide* was originally defined as any self-injurious behavior with or without suicidal intent that does not result in death. However, the term is often mistakenly used to include only behaviors without suicidal intent. We do not use these two terms in this chapter, as rec-

ommended by the Centers for Disease Control and Prevention.

We have proposed two different types of models to understand suicidal acts and self-injurious behavior, respectively. For understanding suicidal acts in the context of Axis I and II psychiatric disorders, we have proposed a stress-diathesis model (Corbitt et al. 1996; Mann and Arango 1992; Mann et al. 1999; Oquendo et al. 1997, 2004) that explains how different risk factors interact, resulting in suicide or suicide attempts (see Figure 11–1 for example of this model in the context of BPD).

According to this model, the diathesis refers to the propensity for manifesting suicidal behavior, is considered trait related, and appears to be independent of the main psychiatric diagnosis (Mann 2003). In contrast, triggers are precipitants or stressors that determine the timing and probability of suicidal acts. Thus, triggers may be considered state related.

In this vein, risk factors for suicidal behavior in patients with personality disorder may be categorized according to whether they affect the diathesis or the trigger (Oquendo et al. 1997). Some personality traits, such as aggression and impulsivity, are important components of the diathesis for suicidal behavior regardless of the presence of personality disorder (Mann et al. 1999). Familial, genetic, and biological factors; substance and alcohol abuse; early traumatic experiences; early parental loss; social isolation; low self-esteem; sex; religion; and other factors also influence the diathesis for suicidal behavior. In contrast, major depressive episode; acute substance intoxication; social, financial, or family crises; and contagion may act as triggers (see Oquendo et al. 1997) in individuals with personality disorder.

Stanley and Brodsky (2005) proposed a parallel model for understanding the intra-

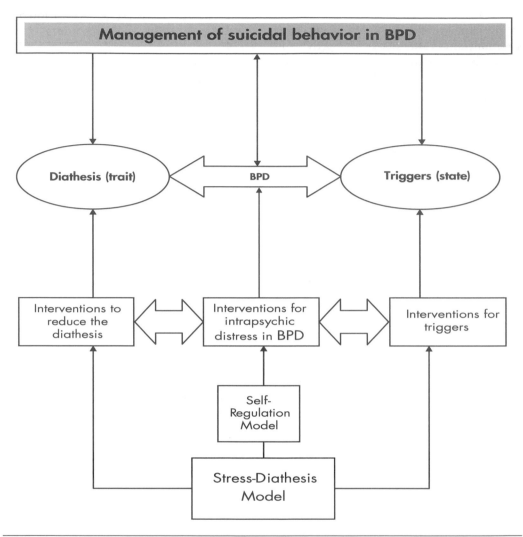

FIGURE 11–1. Management of suicidal behavior in patients with borderline personality disorder (BPD).

psychic phenomena that lead to suicidal behavior and self-injury in BPD. The Self-Regulation Model posits that self-injury and suicidal behavior serve a dual function in BPD. They both inflict physical harm and regulate the self, particularly emotions, to restore a sense of equilibrium and well-being. In this model, unbearable emotions, particularly anxiety, and thoughts are experienced as out of control and as never-ending, even though they may last only a few hours. Self-condemnation for feeling out of control frequently ensues. In response to this state, individuals feel they must act to alter how they feel. Suicide attempt or self-injury is perceived as a reasonable solution. After the episode, individuals usually feel calmer and often regain a sense of emotional equilibrium. Thus, the suicide attempt or self-injury episode is "successful." This may explain why individuals with BPD feel better after self-injury episodes and suicide attempts and frequently repeat the be-havior. It also explains why, in some cases, hospitalization after a self-destructive epi-sode may not be clinically indicated.

Cluster A Personality Disorders

In a psychological autopsy study (Apter et al. 1993), the most common Axis II person-ality disorder in completed suicide was schizoid personality disorder (37.2%), al-though this finding was not replicated in other samples of suicide completers (Cheng et al. 1997; Schneider et al. 2006). Conversely, Schneider et al. (2006) found a higher risk of suicide completion in subjects with para-noid or schizotypal personality disorder, but not in subjects with schizoid personality disorder, compared with population-based control persons. Cluster A personality dis-orders (paranoid, schizoid, schizotypal; Table 11–) are also reported to be associated with suicide attempt (Markar et al. 1991), even after adjustment for the presence or se-verity of depression (Chioqueta and Stiles 2004). Another study (Bornstein et al. 1988) showed that 60% of subjects with schizo-typal personality disorder report at least one suicide attempt in their lifetime, whereas Lentz et al. (2010), using data from the Na-tional Epidemiologic Survey on Alcohol and Related Conditions ($N=34,653$), showed that individuals with schizotypal personal-ity disorder are more likely to attempt sui-cide than the general population. Thus, a re-lationship between Cluster A personality disorders and both suicide completion and attempts exists.

Cluster C Personality Disorders

Few studies have investigated the associa-tion between Cluster C personality disor-ders (obsessive-compulsive, avoidant, and dependent) and suicidal behavior. A psycho-

TABLE 11–1. DSM-IV-TR classification of personality disorders

Cluster A	Cluster B	Cluster C
Paranoid	Antisocial	Avoidant
Schizoid	Borderline	Dependent
Schizotypal	Histrionic Narcissistic	Obsessive-compulsive

logical autopsy study of adolescents (Brent et al. 1994) showed a higher prevalence of probable or definite Cluster C personality disorders among persons who completed suicide compared with community control subjects. Similarly, in an adult psychological autopsy study (Isometsä et al. 1996), 10% of all individuals who died by suicide in Fin-land in a 1-year period met the criteria for a Cluster C personality disorder. In terms of suicide attempts, a longitudinal study of a community sample (Johnson et al. 1999) found that patients with Cluster C personal-ity disorders were at increased risk for sui-cide attempts and suicidal thoughts, even after affective disorders were controlled for. However, in a clinical sample, Chioqueta and Stiles (2004) showed that dependent personality disorder, but not avoidant or ob-sessive-compulsive personality disorder, was significantly associated with suicide at-tempts, although this association did not re-main significant after controlling for lifetime depressive disorder and severity of depres-sion. Dervic et al. (2007) compared de-pressed inpatients with and without "pure" Cluster C personality disorders (CCPD) and found that those with comorbid CCPD had higher levels of suicidal ideation but not more previous suicide attempts compared with patients without CCPD, whereas Dia-conu and Turecki (2009) reported greater suicidal ideation and frequency of attempts in subjects with obsessive-compulsive personality disorder compared with normal control subjects. Thus, there appears to be greater risk for suicidal ideation, suicide attempts, and suicide completions in individuals with Cluster C personality disorders than in the general population.

Cluster B Personality Disorders

Cluster B personality disorders (antisocial, narcissistic, histrionic, and borderline) are associated with suicide completion (Corbitt et al. 1996; Engstrom et al. 1997; Isometsä et al. 1996; Lecrubier 2001; Zanarini et al. 2004). Moreover, patients with these disorders are generally prone to affective disorders (Engstrom et al. 1997; Zanarini et al. 2004), which may also increase their risk for suicidal acts. Studying the co-occurrence of suicidal behavior and Cluster B personality disorders poses problems, especially given that BPD has suicidal behavior as one of its diagnostic criteria. We review suicidal behavior in all the Cluster B personality disorders except histrionic personality disorder, for which we could find no data separate from those for Cluster B personality disorder, using a computerized literature search.

Antisocial Personality Disorder

Only a few studies have documented the lifetime risk of suicide of individuals with antisocial personality disorder. Maddocks (1970) estimated a 5% lifetime risk of suicide during a 5-year follow-up study, and in a psychological autopsy study conducted in Finland, antisocial behavior was reported among 43% of the adolescent victims (Marttunen et al. 1994). However, among causes of death of 1,000 delinquent and nondelinquent males ages 14–65 years, suicide occurred in equal proportions in each group (Laub and Vaillant 2000), contradicting findings from the previously mentioned studies. The relationship between antisocial personality disorder and suicide attempts

appears to be more consistent. Beautrais et al. (1996) found that subjects with antisocial personality disorder were 3.7 times more likely to attempt suicide than the general population. Interestingly, when analyses were restricted to subjects under 30 years of age, the likelihood of attempting suicide among subjects with antisocial personality disorder was 9 times higher. Although as many as 72% of patients with antisocial personality disorder attempt suicide (for review, see Pompili et al. 2004), it is possible that it is the presence of comorbid antisocial personality disorder and BPD that actually increases the risk of suicidal acts (Stone et al. 1987). Additional risk factors among subjects with antisocial personality disorder include separation from parent, parental alcohol abuse, parental violence, alcohol abuse or dependence, and comorbid mental disorder, especially cocaine and hallucinogen use disorder (Links et al. 2003).

Narcissistic Personality Disorder

Narcissistic personality disorder patients are significantly more likely to die by suicide than are those without a narcissistic personality disorder diagnosis or narcissistic traits (Stone 1989). At present, there are no reliable estimates of suicidal behavior for this population, and some authors postulate that suicidal behavior is an underestimated cause of mortality in narcissistic personality disorder (Blasco-Fontecilla et al. 2009a). Of note, a study of adolescents (Links et al. 2003) found that patients with antisocial personality disorder and BPD are at risk for suicidal behavior when depressed, whereas patients with narcissistic personality disorder are also at suicide risk when not depressed. A recent study by Blasco-Fontecilla et al. (2009a) reported that subjects with narcissistic personality disorder show specific features of suicidal behavior compared with the rest of Cluster B personality disorders. In their study, suicide attempters diagnosed with narcissistic personality disorder were less impulsive and made suicide attempts characterized by higher lethality, which is in agreement with the reported association between narcissism and aggression, violence, depression, and suicidality (Svindseth et al. 2008).

Borderline Personality Disorder

BPD is the only personality disorder in which suicidal behavior and self-injurious behavior are part of the DSM-IV-TR (American Psychiatric Association 2000) diagnostic criteria ("recurrent suicidal behavior, gestures, or threats, or self-mutilating behavior"; p. 710). Patients with BPD represent 9%–33% of all completed suicides (Black et al. 2004), suggesting that BPD is one of the most important psychiatric disorders related to suicide (Ahrens and Haug 1996). Furthermore, as many as 84% of subjects with BPD report at least one previous suicide attempt (Black et al. 2004), and many individuals with BPD experience frequent nonsuicidal self-injury, along with chronic suicidal ideation, suicide threats, and intermittent nonlethal suicide attempts. It is not surprising, then, that most research on suicidality in personality disorders has focused on this group.

Psychiatric comorbidity is one of the most important risk factors for suicide attempt in BPD (see Black et al. 2004 for a review). Depressed borderline patients attempt suicide more frequently than depressed patients, both with or without other Axis II disorders (Corbitt et al. 1996). Comorbid antisocial personality disorder or substance abuse is reported to be a risk factor for suicide attempts in BPD (Black et al. 2004). Moreover, comorbid major depression and substance abuse have been shown to increase both the number and seriousness of suicide attempts (Black et al. 2004).

In addition, several clinical characteristics have been identified as risk factors for suicidal behavior in BPD and include impulsivity (Brodsky et al. 1997), the number of previous suicide attempts (Black et al. 2004), childhood physical or sexual abuse (Brodsky et al. 1997; Soloff et al. 2002), early childhood parental loss, parental separation, and higher level of education. School and/or legal problems, longer hospitalizations, lack of treatment, and violating the treatment contract have been associated with suicide completion in BPD (Black et al. 2004).

Moreover, the intrapsychic experience in BPD also contributes to the risk of deliberate self-harm. Compared with individuals with other personality disorders, those with BPD spend a higher percentage of time feeling overwhelmed, worthless, angry, empty, abandoned, betrayed, or enraged (Zanarini et al. 1998). It has been estimated that individuals with BPD spend about 44% of the time experiencing cognitions of being misunderstood, thinking that no one cares, thinking about killing themselves, or thinking that they are "bad" or damaged. Thus, self-worth is tenuous, and they rely on external proof of worthiness. This reliance on others for self-worth results in magnification of the pain experienced in the context of interpersonal difficulties. Frantic distress in response to interpersonal conflict and dysregulated anger at both the cause of upset and the self are common responses. These feelings of "badness," anger at self, and self-criticism for being so vulnerable often lead to suicidality and self-injury. Thus, clinical, environmental, and intrapsychic factors in BPD contribute to the risk for self-injurious behavior and suicide attempts.

A 27-year follow-up study (Paris and Zweig-Frank 2001) indicated that roughly 10% of patients with BPD die by suicide, with suicides being more commonly observed during the first years of follow-up and at younger ages. This is an intriguing finding because most BPD patients showed significant improvement over time, which may signal the importance of early recognition and adequate treatment or that those with more severe pathology die by suicide, leaving the healthier part of the cohort available for follow-up. In a case-control study, McGirr et al. (2007) suggested that BPD individuals who die by suicide may be a distinct group of BPD patients and hypothesized an interaction between impulsivity and features associated with Cluster B comorbidity.

Comorbidity

It is worth noting that studies of suicidal acts and personality disorders generally have not excluded other, comorbid personality disorders, such as Cluster B personality disorders. This is critical because comorbidity of two or more personality disorders could affect the association of a given personality disorder with suicidal behavior. Indeed, this methodological problem is underscored by findings from a community sample (Johnson et al. 1999), in which 32% of those meeting criteria for any personality disorder had diagnoses in two or more personality disorder clusters.

Blasco-Fontecilla et al. (2009b) took another perspective when analyzing the relationship between personality disorders and suicidal behavior. In that study, the authors postulated that severity of personality disorders may be of greater utility in estimating suicide risk than the diagnosis of specific personality disorders. The authors classified personality disorder according to Tyrer and Johnson's (1996) classification of severity (no personality disorder, simple personality disorder, diffuse personality disorder) and found that young females with severe

(diffuse) personality disorder were more likely to make repeated suicide attempts. However, the severity of personality disorder was not related to the severity/lethality of suicide attempts (Blasco-Fontecilla et al. 2009b).

Case Examples

Case Example 1

Ms. A is a 22-year-old woman with BPD who has made more than eight suicide attempts since adolescence. The bulk of these attempts required emergency department or hospital admission. Many of the suicide attempts occurred in the absence of depressive symptoms. Ms. A views suicide attempts and suicidal ideation as a way to manage overwhelming feelings and to avoid confrontation and responsibility.

Regarding her latest attempt, Ms. A reports that after a telephone conversation with her mother, she became enraged at her mother but did not want to confront her. She could not stop thinking about how thoughtless and inconsiderate her mother had been, and instead of feeling better with the passage of time, Ms. A felt increasingly angry. The anger soon became overwhelming, and Ms. A became anxious and fearful that she was going to "lose it." She felt she could not tolerate feeling this way and decided to "get it over with." She decided to take an overdose of her medications and began ingesting pills one after the other. After taking about 35 pills, Ms. A "realized I blew it" and called her therapist. She did not tell the therapist directly what had happened but hinted that she was in trouble. She reports she cannot remember what happened after that. The therapist, unable to reach Ms. A when she called later in the day to check on her, contacted emergency services. The medics arrived and took Ms. A for medical care at the local emergency department.

Paradoxically, as was often the case, Ms. A felt less anxious and almost "bright" after the suicide attempt. Ms. A stated that she was motivated for change and was willing to set goals for the future. Of note, Ms. A reported regret that she had hurt and worried her loved ones. Ms. A's mother seemed more interested in her daughter's feelings and appeared to be trying hard to understand her. Thus, as a consequence of the attempt, Ms. A felt closer to her mother and less lonely and overwhelmed.

Case Example 2

Ms. B is a 31-year-old woman with BPD who uses self-injurious behavior to manage overwhelming feelings of anger, anxiety, and guilt. She states that when she is angry, she feels immediately guilty and that she does not have the right to be so mad. These feelings of guilt make her feel worthless and loathsome. As these feelings intensify, Ms. B becomes convinced that she cannot tolerate the self-hate. It is in this context that she scratches her skin to elicit physical pain. Sometimes the intense scratching draws blood. The sight of the blood gives her relief, and she reports that it feels that she now has "something to show" for how badly she feels. Ms. B feels "back in control" after the scratching. She is quite clear that this behavior has nothing to do with wanting to die; rather, she is just seeking relief.

Ms. B also describes a suicide attempt that she distinguishes from the self-injurious behavior. On the anniversary of her father's death, she became angry that her boyfriend appeared to have "no clue" that this was a very difficult day for her. Ms. B felt that not only was her boyfriend unable to understand her that day but also that he would never "get it." She felt hopeless, convinced that she would always feel the aching loss of her father. She could not imagine that anyone could help her recover from that loss. It seemed insurmountable. Overcome with grief, feelings of loss, emptiness, and anger, she decided to take an overdose to kill herself. However, after taking a handful of pills, she felt relieved. The suicide attempt was an action that helped her feel like she did have some control and that she could "do something." Feeling more in control, Ms. B found that her wish to die had subsided. She fell asleep until the next morning, when she felt much better.

Discussion

Following the Self-Regulation Model, several aspects of the self-destructive behavior should be evaluated. Rather than assuming that the intent of nonsuicidal self-injury is purely manipulative and attention-seeking,

evaluation to detect other functions of the self-injury, such as emotion regulation, self-punishment, and self-validation, may be useful. Awareness of the multiple functions of self-harm behavior, as was illustrated in the case of Ms. B in her wish to die and to escape unbearable feelings, can target treatment approaches focused on the development of skills to address these functions.

Moreover, patients may have distorted beliefs that lead to self-injury. For example, as mentioned by both Ms. A and Ms. B in the vignettes, patients may believe they cannot tolerate emotional pain or that the only way to handle their emotional state is through self-injury. Such beliefs can be modified through cognitive restructuring. The therapeutic dyad can work together to understand how intense emotional arousal leads to distorted cognitions or interpretations of external events. Therapeutic interventions can increase awareness of how past traumatic events can distort perceptions of current reality.

On the other hand, identifying reinforcing consequences of the behavior, as was observed in Ms. A's case, in which her mother became more interested in Ms. A's feelings after the self-harm, provides information about ways to modify these reinforcement patterns so as to promote more skillful behaviors. Distinguishing between intended and unintended consequences can help both patient and clinician to clarify original intent compared with learned intent. Patients can gain insight into how their behaviors affect people in their lives, providing an opportunity for improved interpersonal effectiveness.

Risk Assessment and the Decision to Hospitalize

In deciding whether to hospitalize a patient, the twin goals of decreasing suicide risk and increasing the patient's capacity to safely tolerate chronic suicidal ideation on his or her own are paramount. Decisions regarding hospitalization can be complicated in cases in which there is chronic suicidal ideation and/or nonsuicidal self-injurious behavior. On the one hand, if the family or the clinician experiences the self-harm as attention-seeking, regardless of the patient's intention, reduced sensitivity to risk may ensue. Similarly, becoming inured to the day-to-day emotional pain experienced by individuals with BPD can lead to under-recognition of suicide risk. On the other hand, chronic suicidal ideation and nonsuicidal self-injury can lead to multiple hospitalizations that severely disrupt the individual's ability to function, in addition to not being always helpful in decreasing suicide risk (Stanley and Brodsky 2005). Thus, assessment of the subjective experience of deliberate self-harm can aid in the decision to hospitalize.

As illustrated in the two cases, suicidal ideation and self-injurious behavior in BPD do not necessarily indicate a strong intent to die. Instead, they may be the patient's attempt to relieve an intolerable emotional state. An outpatient treatment that addresses the need for relief and provides support for the individual to manage these states safely can reduce the need for frequent hospital admissions. However, if hospitalization or emergency department admission is to be used, as was the situation with Ms. A, brief stays during times of extreme distress that would normally lead to a suicide attempt are optimal. Thus, hospitalization would block self-harm and help the individual to tolerate the emotions until they subside.

Empirically Tested Treatments for Self-Harm in Borderline Personality Disorder

Psychosocial Interventions

The effectiveness of psychosocial interventions for personality disorder patients has received more attention in recent years, and an increasing number of well-controlled studies have been conducted (McMain 2007). Evidence from a meta-analysis and a systematic review has indicated that two treatment models have been shown to lower rates of attempted suicide among BPD patients: psychodynamically oriented day treatment involving a mentalization-based model, and dialectical behavior therapy (Binks et al. 2006; Brazier et al. 2006). Nevertheless, caution is suggested by the authors of these studies, given the limited number of trials and the small sample sizes of the studies included, which limits drawing firm conclusions about the effectiveness of such psychosocial interventions. Both treatments have some elements in common: weekly meetings with an individual therapist, one or more weekly group sessions, and meetings of therapists for consultation and/or supervision (American Psychiatric Association 2001).

Psychodynamic Therapy

The effectiveness of a psychodynamically oriented day treatment program for personality disorders has been evaluated in only a few studies. A randomized controlled trial compared the effectiveness of psychoanalytically oriented partial hospitalization with standard care for patients with BPD (Bateman and Fonagy 1999). Patients who were partially hospitalized showed improvement in depressive symptoms, a decrease in suicidal and self-injurious acts, and reduced inpatient days compared with the other group. Improvement in social and interpersonal function began at 6 months and continued until the end of treatment at 18 months. Patients who completed the partial hospitalization program not only maintained substantial gains at an 18-month follow-up evaluation but also showed continued improvement on most measures, in contrast with patients treated with standard psychiatric care (Bateman and Fonagy 2001). In addition, fewer patients who completed the partial hospitalization program attempted suicide or carried out self-injuring acts.

The effectiveness of a twice-weekly psychodynamic therapy for outpatients with BPD (Stevenson and Meares 1992) has been evaluated by comparing 1 year of the patient's life before treatment with 1 year after. The most frequently observed changes were reductions in impulsivity, affective instability, anger, and suicidal behavior, when comparing the same outpatients with an outpatient waiting-list control group (Meares et al. 1999). Patients who received the psychodynamic intervention had a better outcome than control subjects. However, it is unclear whether better outcome was due to the type of therapy or the greater amount of treatment received (American Psychiatric Association 2001).

Chiesa et al. (2004) used a step-down treatment approach to evaluate the effectiveness of a specialized psychodynamic program combined with a postdischarge analytic psychotherapy group in patients with primarily Cluster B personality disorders. After 2 years, a significant reduction in suicidal behaviors was observed in this group compared with individuals who received 1 year of a specialized psychodynamic inpatient program and compared with those who received standard care in the community.

Dialectical Behavior Therapy

Most published reports of cognitive-behavioral treatment for patients with BPD are uncontrolled clinical or single case studies (American Psychiatric Association 2001). However, in recent decades several controlled studies have been done, particularly of a form of cognitive-behavioral therapy called *dialectical behavior therapy* (DBT).

DBT was developed as a treatment for women who are chronically suicidal and/or self-injuring (Linehan 1987). The most fundamental dialectic addressed by the treatment is that of acceptance and change. Treatment attempts to help these patients, who ordinarily have trouble accepting themselves and others, to develop acceptance-oriented skills and change-oriented skills. The results of several randomized controlled trials conducted over the past 15 years support the efficacy of this approach in treating BPD patients with self-injurious behaviors. Some of these trials evaluated standard outpatient DBT (Linehan et al. 1991; Stanley et al. 2001; Verheul et al. 2003). These studies indicate that DBT is helpful in reducing self-injury and suicidal behavior and related traits in BPD, whereas two follow-up studies have shown sustained efficacy (Linehan et al. 1993; van den Bosch et al. 2005). However, it is possible that the superior effects of DBT are related to weakness in the treatment-as-usual condition (Robins and Chapman 2004). To overcome such limitations, Linehan et al. (2006) conducted a study assigning 101 patients to either DBT or "community treatment by experts" and found that patients receiving DBT were one-half as likely to make a suicide attempt and had lower medical risk associated with self-injurious behaviors and suicide attempts. Two other controlled studies, however, did not replicate these findings (Clarkyn et al. 2007; McMain et al. 2009).

Cognitive Therapy

Another psychotherapy that has been adapted to treat BPD is *cognitive therapy*. Cognitive therapy has been empirically tested to treat a variety of Axis I disorders, such as depression, and has been reported to be useful in the treatment of patients with personality disorders (see Brown et al. 2004 for a review). In an open clinical trial, Brown et al. (2004) reported that BPD patients who received weekly cognitive therapy over a 1-year period showed significant decreases on measures of suicidal ideation, hopelessness, depression, number of borderline symptoms, and dysfunctional beliefs at termination and at 18-month assessment interviews. Similarly, in a randomized controlled trial by Davidson et al. (2006), patients who received cognitive-behavioral therapy were less likely to attempt suicide and showed greater improvement in dysfunctional beliefs, state anxiety, and distress.

Other Psychosocial Interventions

Brief skills-based interventions for patients with BPD have shown promising evidence for addressing self-injurious behavior in BPD (Black et al. 2004; van Wel et al. 2006; Weinberg et al. 2006). However, a manual-based group treatment program for outpatients with BPD that combines cognitive-behavioral elements and skills training with a systems component was not superior to standard care for suicide attempts, self-harm acts, or hospitalizations (Blum et al. 2008). On the other hand, a 3-year randomized trial of schema-focused therapy (SFT) versus transference-focused therapy showed greater improvement in suicidal and/or self-injuring behaviors in patients receiving SFT (Giesen-Bloo et al. 2006), a finding that appears to offer preliminary support for the effectiveness of SFT. Interestingly, this study was the first of its kind to compare a cognitive-oriented approach with psychodynamic

therapy. Like Giesen-Bloo et al. (2006), Bateman and Fonagy (2009) conducted a randomized controlled trial of two active treatments, testing outpatient mentalization-based treatment (MBT) versus structured clinical management for BPD, and found a difference between them but over a shorter period and unrelated to amount of therapist contact. Subjects assigned to MBT had fewer suicide attempts and hospitalizations—results that extend previous findings of the superiority of MBT to standard care and of positive long-lasting effects (Bateman and Fonagy 2008).

Early Intervention

Although diagnosing adolescent personality pathology remains controversial, preliminary findings from a randomized controlled trial and a quasi-experimental follow-up study (Chanen et al. 2008, 2009) suggest that active interventions such as cognitive analytic therapy could be effective in reducing suicidal behavior in adolescents diagnosed with BPD. As noted by the study authors, there is a need for longer-term follow-up of these samples, to show whether the gains made through early intervention are sustained throughout adulthood.

Pharmacotherapy

Because there are no pharmacological treatment studies on BPD and suicide, in the following discussion we summarize medication trials that have found effects on suicidal behavior or on behaviors related to the likelihood of suicidal acts such as aggression or impulsivity.

Selective Serotonin Reuptake Inhibitors

Studies of selective serotonin reuptake inhibitors (SSRIs) suggest that aggression, irritability (Coccaro and Kavoussi 1997), depressed mood, and self-injury respond to SSRIs. Of note, improvement in impulsive behaviors may appear as early as the first week of treatment, independent of effects on depression and anxiety (Coccaro and Kavoussi 1997), and if discontinuation or nonadherence occurs, improvement disappears (American Psychiatric Association 2001). There have been several randomized controlled trials of SSRIs in treating BPD. Results of these trials suggest that SSRIs may lessen symptoms of affective instability, anger, and impulsivity in subjects with BPD, although a recent meta-analysis found little evidence of effectiveness for antidepressant treatment in BPD (Lieb et al. 2010).

Mood Stabilizers

Divalproex is one of the most-studied pharmacological therapies to date used in BPD. Reductions in aggression and depression have been reported among patients treated with divalproex sodium, although the exclusion of subjects with suicidal ideation and the lack of suicidality as an outcome measure limit the generalization to suicidal patients (Frankenburg and Zanarini 2002; Hollander et al. 2001). Lamotrigine has been useful in reducing suicidal behavior in a open-label trial (Pinto and Akiskal 1998), whereas a randomized controlled trial found a reduction in anger and aggression among BPD subjects (Tritt et al. 2005) that, according to a later follow-up study of this group, was maintained over time (Leiberich et al. 2008). Three randomized controlled trials have studied the effectiveness of topiramate in the treatment of BPD subjects, with promising results in treating symptoms of anger, including impulsive aggression (see Lieb et al. 2010 for a review). On the other hand, there is evidence that carbamazepine is not beneficial in treating patients with BPD.

Antipsychotics

A continuation study of recurrently suicidal and/or self-injuring patients with BPD and histrionic personality disorder treated with flupenthixol 20 mg once a month reported a significant decrease in suicidal behaviors compared with the placebo group (Montgomery et al. 1979). Notably, this was the first study to report a positive effect of pharmacotherapy (or any other therapy) in reducing suicidal behavior. However, findings from this important study await replication.

There is support for the use of low-dose antipsychotics for the acute management of global symptom severity (American Psychiatric Association 2001), schizotypal symptoms, psychoticism, anger, and hostility. In BPD, randomized controlled trials have suggested that olanzapine may reduce obsessive-compulsive symptoms, interpersonal sensitivity, depression, anger-hostility, anxiety, paranoia, psychoticism, and overall psychopathology (see Lieb et al. 2010 for a review), but suicidal behavior per se was not used as an outcome variable in such studies. Similar reports exist from open studies of risperidone and quetiapine use, although controlled trials are not available to verify these effects (Lieb et al. 2010). A double-blind placebo-controlled study evaluated the role of aripiprazole in the treatment of BPD (Nickel et al. 2006) and found aripiprazole to have significant effects in the reduction of the core pathological symptoms of BPD such as anger and impulsivity and in the prevalence of self-injury in the medication group. On the other hand, a controlled study did not show any benefit from ziprasidone in the treatment of BPD (Pascual et al. 2008).

Other Medications

Opiate antagonists have been used in an attempt to diminish self-injury-induced analgesia and euphoria associated with self-injurious behavior. However, there is no clear evidence that they are effective in reducing self-injurious behavior among BPD patients (Cardish 2007). Two double-blind placebo-controlled studies showed positive effects of supplementation of omega-3 fatty acids in the treatment of BPD, including reducing self-harm and depression (Hallahan et al. 2007; Zanarini and Frankenburg 2003).

Summary

Only a few controlled studies of medication report benefits against suicidal behavior. Clinicians are therefore in the position of having to base treatment on expert consensus practice guidelines. In January 2009, the National Institute for Health and Clinical Excellence's (2009) clinical guideline for BPD noted that "drug treatment should not be used specifically for borderline personality disorder or for the individual symptoms or behaviour associated with the disorder (e.g., repeated self-harm, marked emotional insta-

bility, risk-taking behaviour and transient psychotic symptoms)" (p. 21). Similarly, the American Psychiatric Association's (2001) practice guideline for treatment of patients with BPD states that the primary treatment for BPD is psychotherapy, complemented by symptom-targeted pharmacotherapy.

In addition, management includes establishing and maintaining a therapeutic framework and alliance as well as providing crisis intervention and monitoring patient safety. Providing education about BPD and its treatment, coordinating treatment provided by multiple clinicians (with attention to potential problems involving splitting and boundaries), monitoring progress, and reassessing the effectiveness of the treatment plan are also key (American Psychiatric Association 2001). Suicidal and self-destructive behaviors should be addressed as the highest priorities, along with conducting ongoing risk assessment and helping the patient find ways to maintain safety (American Psychiatric Association 2001).

Key Clinical Concepts

- Cluster B personality disorders have an increased suicide risk. Up to 84% of subjects with borderline personality disorder (BPD) report at least one previous suicide attempt.

- Deliberate self-harm includes two forms of self-destructive behavior: one with an intent to die and one in which the self-inflicted damage does not have this intent. A *suicide attempt* is defined as a potentially self-injurious act performed with at least partial intent to die. *Nonsuicidal self-injury*, sometimes called *self-mutilation*, is defined as intentional self-destructive behavior performed with no intent to die.

- In the treatment of BPD, self-harm behaviors must be addressed as the highest priorities, with an effort from the therapist to both evaluate risk for these behaviors and help the patient find ways to maintain safety.

- Recognizing the various functions of deliberate self-harm, and not simply assuming the intent to be solely manipulative, while maintaining awareness of the day-to-day emotional pain experienced by individuals with BPD, can reduce the underrecognition of suicide risk.

References

Ahrens B, Haug HJ: Suicidality in hospitalized patients with a primary diagnosis of personality disorder. Crisis 17:59–63, 1996

American Psychiatric Association: Diagnostic and Statistical Manual of Mental Disorders, 4th Edition, Text Revision. Washington, DC, American Psychiatric Association, 2000

American Psychiatric Association: Practice guideline for the treatment of patients with borderline personality disorder. Am J Psychiatry 158(suppl):1–52, 2001

American Psychiatric Association: Practice guideline for the assessment and treatment of patients with suicidal behaviors. Am J Psychiatry 160(suppl):1–60, 2003

Apter A, Bleich A, King RA, et al: Death without warning? A clinical postmortem study of suicide in 43 Israeli adolescent males. Arch Gen Psychiatry 50:138–142, 1993

Bateman A, Fonagy P: Effectiveness of partial hospitalization in the treatment of borderline personality disorder: a randomized controlled trial. Am J Psychiatry 156:1563–1569, 1999

Bateman A, Fonagy P: Treatment of borderline personality disorder with psychoanalytically oriented partial hospitalization: an 18-month follow-up. Am J Psychiatry 158:36–42, 2001

Bateman A, Fonagy P: 8-year follow-up of patients treated for borderline personality disorder: mentalization-based treatment versus treatment as usual. Am J Psychiatry 165:631–638, 2008

Bateman A, Fonagy P: Randomized controlled trial of outpatient mentalization-based treatment versus structured clinical management for borderline personality disorder. Am J Psychiatry 166:1355–1364, 2009

Baxter D, Appleby L: Case register study of suicide risk in mental disorders. Br J Psychiatry 175:322–326, 1999

Beautrais AL, Joyce PR, Mulder RT, et al: Prevalence and comorbidity of mental disorders in persons making serious suicide attempts: a case-control study. Am J Psychiatry 153:1009–1014, 1996

Binks CA, Fenton M, McCarthy L, et al: Psychological therapies for people with borderline personality disorder. Cochrane Database of Systematic Reviews 2006, Issue 1. CD005652. DOI: 10.1002/14651858.CD005652.

Black DW, Winokur G: Prospective studies of suicide and mortality in psychiatric patients. Ann N Y Acad Sci 487:106–113, 1986

Black DW, Blum N, Pfohl B, et al: Suicidal behavior in borderline personality disorder: prevalence, risk factors, prediction, and prevention. J Pers Disord 18:226–239, 2004

Blasco-Fontecilla H, Baca-Garcia E, Dervic K, et al: Severity of personality disorders and suicide attempt. Acta Psychiatr Scand 119:149–155, 2009a

Blasco-Fontecilla H, Baca-Garcia E, Dervic K, et al: Specific features of suicidal behavior in patients with narcissistic personality disorder. J Clin Psychiatry 7:1583–1587, 2009b

Blum N, St John D, Pfohl B, et al: Systems Training for Emotional Predictability and Problem Solving (STEPPS) for outpatients with borderline personality disorder: a randomized controlled trial and 1-year follow-up. Am J Psychiatry 165:468–478, 2008

Bornstein RF, Klein DN, Mallon JC, et al: Schizotypal personality disorder in an outpatient population: incidence and clinical characteristics. J Clin Psychol 44:322–325, 1988

Brazier J, Tumur I, Holmes M, et al: Psychological therapies including dialectical behaviour therapy for borderline personality disorder: a systematic review and preliminary economic evaluation. Health Technol Assess 10:iii, ix–xii, 1–117, 2006

Brent DA, Johnson BA, Perper J, et al: Personality disorder, personality traits, impulsive violence, and completed suicide in adolescents. J Am Acad Child Adolesc Psychiatry 33:1080–1086, 1994

Brodsky BS, Malone KM, Ellis SP, et al: Characteristics of borderline personality disorder associated with suicidal behavior. Am J Psychiatry 154:1715–1719, 1997

Brown GK, Beck AT, Steer RA, et al: Risk factors for suicide in psychiatric outpatients: a 20-year prospective study. J Consult Clin Psychol 68:371–377, 2000

Brown GK, Newman CF, Charlesworth SE, et al: An open clinical trial of cognitive therapy for borderline personality disorder. J Pers Disord 18:257–271, 2004

Cardish RJ: Psychopharmacologic management of suicidality in personality disorders. Can J Psychiatry 52:115–127, 2007

Chanen AM, Jackson HJ, McCutcheon LK, et al: Early intervention for adolescents with borderline personality disorder using cognitive analytic therapy: randomised controlled trial. Br J Psychiatry 193:477–484, 2008

Chanen AM, Jackson HJ, McCutcheon LK, et al: Early intervention for adolescents with borderline personality disorder: quasi-experimental comparison with treatment as usual. Aust N Z J Psychiatry 43:397–408, 2009

Cheng AT, Mann AH, Chan KA: Personality disorder and suicide: a case-control study. Br J Psychiatry 170:441–446, 1997

Chiesa M, Fonagy P, Holmes J, et al: Residential versus community treatment of personality disorders: a comparative study of three treatment programs. Am J Psychiatry 161:1463–1470, 2004

Chioqueta AP, Stiles TC: Assessing suicide risk in cluster C personality disorders. Crisis 25:128–133, 2004

Clarkin JF, Levy KN, Lenzenweger MF, et al: Evaluating three treatments for borderline personality disorder: a multiwave study. Am J Psychiatry 164:922–928, 2007

Coccaro EF, Kavoussi RJ: Fluoxetine and impulsive aggressive behavior in personality-disordered subjects. Arch Gen Psychiatry 54:1081–1088, 1997

Coid J, Yang M, Tyrer P, et al: Prevalence and correlates of personality disorder in Great Britain. Br J Psychiatry 188:423–431, 2006

Corbitt EM, Malone KM, Haas GL, et al: Suicidal behavior in patients with major depression and comorbid personality disorders. J Affect Disord 39:61–72, 1996

Crawford TN, Cohen P, Johnson JG, et al: Self-reported personality disorder in the children in the community sample: convergent and prospective validity in late adolescence and adulthood. J Pers Disord 19:30–52, 2005

Davidson K, Norrie J, Tyrer P, et al: The effectiveness of cognitive behavior therapy for borderline personality disorder: results from the Borderline Personality Disorder Study of Cognitive Therapy (BOSCOT) trial. J Pers Disord 20:450–465, 2006

De Leo D, Burgis S, Bertolote JM, et al: Definitions of suicidal behavior: lessons learned from the WHO/EURO multicentre Study. Crisis 27:4–15, 2006

Dervic K, Grunebaum MF, Burke AK, et al: Cluster C personality disorders in major depressive episodes: the relationship between hostility and suicidal behavior. Arch Suicide Res 11:83–90, 2007

Diaconu G, Turecki G: Obsessive-compulsive personality disorder and suicidal behavior: evidence for a positive association in a sample of depressed patients. J Clin Psychiatry 70:1551–1556, 2009

Engstrom G, Alling C, Gustavsson P, et al: Clinical characteristics and biological parameters in temperamental clusters of suicide attempters. J Affect Disord 44:45–55, 1997

Frankenburg FR, Zanarini MC: Divalproex sodium treatment of women with borderline personality disorder and bipolar II disorder: a double-blind placebo-controlled pilot study. J Clin Psychiatry 63:442–446, 2002

Giesen-Bloo J, van Dyck R, Spinhoven P, et al: Outpatient psychotherapy for borderline personality disorder: randomized trial of schema-focused therapy vs transference-focused psychotherapy. Arch Gen Psychiatry 63:649–658, 2006

Hallahan B, Hibbeln JR, Davis JM: Omega-3 fatty acid supplementation in patients with recurrent self-harm: single-centre double-blind randomised controlled trial. Br J Psychiatry 190:118–122, 2007

Harris EC, Barraclough B: Suicide as an outcome for mental disorders: a meta-analysis. Br J Psychiatry 170:205–228, 1997

Hollander E, Allen A, Lopez RP, et al: A preliminary double-blind, placebo-controlled trial of divalproex sodium in borderline personality disorder. J Clin Psychiatry 62:199–203, 2001

Isometsä ET: Psychological autopsy studies—a review. Eur Psychiatry 16:379–385, 2001

Isometsä ET, Henriksson MM, Heikkinen ME, et al: Suicide among subjects with personality disorders. Am J Psychiatry 153:667–673, 1996

Johnson JG, Cohen P, Skodol AE, et al: Personality disorders in adolescence and risk of major mental disorders and suicidality during adulthood. Arch Gen Psychiatry 56:805–811, 1999

Laub JH, Vaillant GE: Delinquency and mortality: a 50-year follow-up study of 1,000 delinquent and nondelinquent boys. Am J Psychiatry 157:96–102, 2000

Lecrubier Y: The influence of comorbidity on the prevalence of suicidal behaviour. Eur Psychiatry 16:395–399, 2001

Leiberich P, Nickel MK, Tritt K, et al: Lamotrigine treatment of aggression in female borderline patients, Part II: an 18-month follow-up. J Psychopharmacol 22:805–808, 2008

Lentz V, Robinson J, Bolton JM: Childhood adversity, mental disorder comorbidity, and suicidal behavior in schizotypal personality disorder. J Nerv Ment Dis 198:795–801, 2010

Lenzenweger MF, Loranger AW, Korfine L, et al: Detecting personality disorders in a nonclinical population: application of a 2-stage procedure for case identification. Arch Gen Psychiatry 54:345–351, 1997

Lenzenweger MF, Lane MC, Loranger AW, et al: DSM-IV personality disorders in the National Comorbidity Survey Replication. Biol Psychiatry 62:553–564, 2007

Lesage AD, Boyer R, Grunberg F, et al: Suicide and mental disorders: a case-control study of young men. Am J Psychiatry 151:1063–1068, 1994

Lieb K, Völlm B, Rücker G, et al: Pharmacotherapy for borderline personality disorder: Cochrane systematic review of randomised trials. Br J Psychiatry 196:4–12, 2010

Linehan MM: Dialectical behavior therapy for borderline personality disorder: theory and method. Bull Menninger Clin 51:261–276, 1987

Linehan MM, Armstrong HE, Suarez A, et al: Cognitive-behavioral treatment of chronically parasuicidal borderline patients. Arch Gen Psychiatry 48:1060–1064, 1991

Linehan MM, Heard HL, Armstrong HE: Naturalistic follow-up of a behavioral treatment for chronically parasuicidal borderline patients. Arch Gen Psychiatry 50:971–974, 1993

Linehan MM, Rizvi SL, Welch SS: Psychiatric aspects of suicidal behaviour: personality disorders, in The International Handbook of Suicide and Attempted Suicide. Edited by Hawton K, van Heering K. Chichester, UK, Wiley, 2005, pp 147–178

Linehan MM, Comtois KA, Murray AM, et al: Two-year randomized controlled trial and follow-up of dialectical behavior therapy vs therapy by experts for suicidal behaviors and borderline personality disorder. Arch Gen Psychiatry 63:757–766, 2006

Links PS, Gould B, Ratnayake R: Assessing suicidal youth with antisocial, borderline, or narcissistic personality disorder. Can J Psychiatry 48:301–310, 2003

Maddocks PD: A five year follow-up of untreated psychopaths. Br J Psychiatry 116:511–515, 1970

Mann JJ: Neurobiology of suicidal behaviour. Nat Rev Neurosci 4:819–828, 2003

Mann JJ, Arango V: Integration of neurobiology and psychopathology in a unified model of suicidal behavior. J Clin Psychopharmacol 12:2S–7S, 1992

Mann JJ, Waternaux C, Haas GL, et al: Toward a clinical model of suicidal behavior in psychiatric patients. Am J Psychiatry 156:181–189, 1999

Markar HR, Williams JM, Wells J, et al: Occurrence of schizotypal and borderline symptoms in parasuicide patients: comparison between subjective and objective indices. Psychol Med 21:385–392, 1991

Marttunen MJ, Aro HM, Henriksson MM, et al: Antisocial behaviour in adolescent suicide. Acta Psychiatr Scand 89:167–173, 1994

McGirr A, Paris J, Lesage A, et al: Risk factors for suicide completion in borderline personality disorder: a case-control study of cluster B comorbidity and impulsive aggression. J Clin Psychiatry 68:721–729, 2007

McMain S: Effectiveness of psychosocial treatments on suicidality in personality disorders. Can J Psychiatry 52:103–114, 2007

McMain SF, Links PS, Gnam WH, et al: A randomized trial of dialectical behavior therapy versus general psychiatric management for borderline personality disorder. Am J Psychiatry 166:1365–1374, 2009

Meares R, Stevenson J, Comerford A: Psychotherapy with borderline patients, I: a comparison between treated and untreated cohorts. Aust N Z J Psychiatry 33:467–472, 1999

Montgomery SA, Montgomer DB, Rani SJ, et al: Maintenance therapy in repeat suicidal behaviour: a placebo controlled trial. Proceedings of the Tenth International Congress for Suicide Prevention, Ottawa, Ontario, Canada, 1979, pp 227–229

National Institute for Health and Clinical Excellence: Borderline personality disorder: treatment and management (NICE Clinical Guideline 78). January 2009. Available at: http://www.nice.org.uk/nicemedia/pdf/CG78FullGuideline.pdf. Accessed August 15, 2011.

Nickel MK, Muehlbacher M, Nickel C, et al: Aripiprazole in the treatment of patients with borderline personality disorder: a double-blind, placebo-controlled study. Am J Psychiatry 163:833–838, 2006

Oquendo MA, Malone KM, Mann JJ: Suicide: risk factors and prevention in refractory major depression. Depress Anxiety 5:202–211, 1997

Oquendo MA, Galfalvy H, Russo S, et al: Prospective study of clinical predictors of suicidal acts after a major depressive episode in patients with major depressive disorder or bipolar disorder. Am J Psychiatry 161:1433–1441, 2004

Paris J, Zweig-Frank H: A 27-year follow-up of patients with borderline personality disorder. Compr Psychiatry 42:482–487, 2001

Pascual JC, Soler J, Puigdemont D, et al: Ziprasidone in the treatment of borderline personality disorder: a double-blind, placebo-controlled, randomized study. J Clin Psychiatry 69:603–608, 2008

Pinto OC, Akiskal HS: Lamotrigine as a promising approach to borderline personality: an open case series without concurrent DSM-IV major mood disorder. J Affect Disord 51:333–343, 1998

Pompili M, Ruberto A, Girardi P, et al: Suicidality in DSM-IV Cluster B personality disorders: an overview. Ann Ist Super Sanita 40:475–483, 2004

Posner K, Melvin GA, Stanley B, et al: Factors in the assessment of suicidality in youth. CNS Spectr 12:156–162, 2007a

Posner K, Oquendo MA, Gould M, et al: Columbia Classification Algorithm of Suicide Assessment (C-CASA): classification of suicidal events in the FDA's pediatric suicidal risk analysis of antidepressants. Am J Psychiatry 164:1035–1043, 2007b

Robins CJ, Chapman AL: Dialectical behavior therapy: current status, recent developments, and future directions. J Pers Disord 18:73–89, 2004

Samuels J, Eaton WW, Bienvenu OJ, et al: Prevalence and correlates of personality disorders in a community sample. Br J Psychiatry 180:536–542, 2002

Schneider B, Wetterling T, Sargk D, et al: Axis I disorders and personality disorders as risk factors for suicide. Eur Arch Psychiatry Clin Neurosci 256:17–27, 2006

Soloff PH, Lynch KG, Kelly TM: Childhood abuse as a risk factor for suicidal behavior in borderline personality disorder. J Pers Disord 16:201–214, 2002

Stanley B, Brodsky B: Suicidal and self-injurious behavior in borderline personality disorder: a self-regulation model, in Understanding and Treating Borderline Personality Disorder: A Guide for Professionals and Families. Edited by Gunderson JG, Hoffman PD. Washington, DC, American Psychiatric Publishing, 2005, pp 43–63

Stanley B, Gameroff MJ, Michalsen V, et al: Are suicide attempters who self-mutilate a unique population? Am J Psychiatry 158:427–432, 2001

Stevenson J, Meares R: An outcome study of psychotherapy for patients with borderline personality disorder. Am J Psychiatry 149:358–362, 1992

Stone MH: Long-term follow-up of narcissistic/borderline patients. Psychiatr Clin North Am 12:621–641, 1989

Stone MH, Stone DK, Hurt SW: Natural history of borderline patients treated by intensive hospitalization. Psychiatr Clin North Am 10:185–206, 1987

Svindseth MF, Nøttestad JA, Wallin J, et al: Narcissism in patients admitted to psychiatric acute wards: its relation to violence, suicidality and other psychopathology. BMC Psychiatry 8:13, 2008

Torgersen S, Kringlen E, Cramer V: The prevalence of personality disorders in a community sample. Arch Gen Psychiatry 58:590–596, 2001

Tritt K, Nickel C, Lahmann C, et al: Lamotrigine treatment of aggression in female borderline-patients: a randomized, double-blind, placebo-controlled study. J Psychopharmacol 19:287–291, 2005

Tyrer P, Johnson T: Establishing the severity of personality disorder. Am J Psychiatry 153:1593–1597, 1996

van den Bosch LM, Koeter MW, Stijnen T, et al: Sustained efficacy of dialectical behaviour therapy for borderline personality disorder. Behav Res Ther 43:1231–1241, 2005

van Wel B, Kockmann I, Blum N, et al: STEPPS group treatment for borderline personality disorder in the Netherlands. Ann Clin Psychiatry 18:63–67, 2006

Verheul R, Van Den Bosch LM, Koeter MW, et al: Dialectical behaviour therapy for women with borderline personality disorder: 12-month, randomised clinical trial in the Netherlands. Br J Psychiatry 182:135–140, 2003

Weinberg I, Gunderson JG, Hennen J, et al: Manual assisted cognitive treatment for deliberate self-harm in borderline personality disorder patients. J Pers Disord 2:482–492, 2006

Zanarini MC, Frankenburg FR: Omega-3 fatty acid treatment of women with borderline personality disorder: a double-blind, placebo-controlled pilot study. Am J Psychiatry 160:167–169, 2003

Zanarini MC, Frankenburg FR, Dubo ED, et al: Axis I comorbidity of borderline personality disorder. Am J Psychiatry 155:1733–1739, 1998

Zanarini MC, Frankenburg FR, Hennen J, et al: Axis I comorbidity in patients with borderline personality disorder: 6-year follow-up and prediction of time to remission. Am J Psychiatry 161:2108–2114, 2004

Zilber N, Schufman N, Lerner Y: Mortality among psychiatric patients: the groups at risk. Acta Psychiatr Scand 79:248–256, 1989

Zimmerman M, Rothschild L, Chelminski I: The prevalence of DSM-IV personality disorders in psychiatric outpatients. Am J Psychiatry 162:1911–1918, 2005

PART III

Treatment

Psychopharmacotherapy and Electroconvulsive Therapy

H. Florence Kim, M.D., M.A.

Frank Chen, M.D.

Stuart C. Yudofsky, M.D.

Suicide and suicidal behavior can be devastating emotionally to affected individuals and their families. As detailed in previous chapters of this book, suicide is also an enormous public health problem. Suicide was the eleventh most common cause of death in the United States in 2007 (Centers for Disease Control and Prevention 2011). The annual incidence of completed suicide was 11.3 for every 100,000 persons per year, and for every completed suicide another 11 nonfatal suicide attempts are estimated to occur (Centers for Disease Control and Prevention 2011).

The risk of suicide and suicidal behaviors increases dramatically in psychiatric populations. Among individuals with mood disorders, including unipolar major depression and bipolar disorder, the lifetime suicide risk is 15–20 times greater than the risk in the general U.S. population (Harris and Barraclough 1997). As for primary psychotic disorders, the risk of suicide is estimated to be 8.5 times higher for patients with schizophrenia than for the general U.S. population (Harris and Barraclough 1997). The most significant risk factor for suicide is the presence of a psychiatric disorder; in one study, 93% of those who completed suicide met the criteria for at least one psychiatric diagnosis at postmortem psychological autopsy (Henriksson et al. 1993). Mood disorders specifically, including unipolar major depression and bipolar disorder, are the diagnoses most often found in completed suicide (Henriksson et al. 1993).

Thus, it is of utmost importance that suicidal individuals receive treatment for underlying psychiatric disorders. In fact, two studies have shown that most individuals who complete suicide were not taking antidepressants immediately prior to death. In a Swedish study of 3,400 of 4,000 suicides for which forensic data in 1990–1991 were available, antidepressants were detected via toxicological screen in less than 16% (542 of 3,400 cases) (Isacsson et al. 1994b). A smaller U.S. study showed that only 19 (8%) of 247 individuals who completed suicide between 1981 and 1983 in the San Diego area had been using tricyclic or tetracyclic antidepressants as detected by postmortem toxicology (Isacsson et al. 1994a). Of 97 subjects who met the criteria for major depression, bipolar depression, or atypical depression by postmortem research analysis, in the 90 days preceding suicide only 52 (54%) had seen a physician, 33 (34%) had been diagnosed with depression, and 20 (21%) had been prescribed tricyclic or tetracyclic antidepressants. Finally, 9 of these 97 subjects (9%) had antidepressants present by postmortem toxicology (Isacsson et al. 1994a). Thus, it appears that at least in the case of depression, most individuals were not taking antidepressants immediately prior to their completed suicide, implying possible undertreatment or insufficient treatment for underlying psychiatric disorders (Licinio and Wong 2005).

Management of suicide and suicidal behaviors is complex and multidisciplinary and includes aggressive pharmacotherapy in conjunction with a strong psychotherapeutic alliance with the affected individual. As illustrated in preceding chapters, a thorough clinical assessment, early detection of risk factors and suicidal ideation, aggressive reduction of reversible risk factors and methods of suicide, careful consideration of hospitalization, and establishment of a strong therapeutic alliance with concomitant interpersonal and/or cognitive-behavioral therapy go hand in hand with careful but aggressive pharmacological treatment and/or electroconvulsive therapy (ECT). Medications to treat symptoms such as psychic pain, anxiety and turmoil, panic attacks, agitation, impulsiveness, aggression, and feelings of hopelessness can be extremely helpful in managing the patient with suicidal tendencies.

Long-term psychopharmacological treatment is associated with a decreased suicide rate. A Swiss long-term follow-up study of almost 400 patients hospitalized for affective disorders showed that patients who received long-term treatment (longer than 6 months' duration) with psychotropic medications, including antidepressants, lithium, and neuroleptics, had significantly lower suicide rates than those who did not receive treatment with psychotropic medications over the 22-year follow-up period (Angst et al. 2002). However, in the acute phases of treatment with antidepressants, suicidal thoughts and behaviors may increase. This is of particular concern in children and adolescents, as articulated in warnings from the U.S. Food and Drug Administration (FDA) and the European Committee for Medicinal Products for Human Use in 2005. These risk assessments were based on 24 placebo-controlled clinical trials among children and adolescents treated with antidepressants—trials that, in aggregate, demonstrated a risk of suicidal thinking or behavior in 4% of participants treated with antidepressants compared with 2% of participants given placebo. There were no completed suicides, and all trials were less than 4 months in duration. These warnings apply to all antidepressant medications and were expanded to include young adults between the ages of 18 and 24 in 2007. A study by Jick et al. (2004) does suggest that caution is warranted in the first few weeks of treatment. These investigators evaluated 555 cases of first-time nonfatal suicidal behavior or ideation (ages 10–69) and reported that the relative risk of suicidal behavior was four times greater for patients within 1–9 days of starting an antidepressant compared with patients who had started taking an antidepressant more than 90 days before developing nonfatal suicidal behavior (Jick et al. 2004). However, given the long-term benefit of antidepressants, these warnings are not intended to prevent the use of these medicines but rather underscore the need for close monitoring in the early phases of treatment.

Case Examples

The following two cases illustrate the importance of treatment with pharmacotherapy and ECT as well as the complexity underlying treatment of these psychiatric disorders, of which suicidal ideation and behavior are symptoms. Evidence for clinical efficacy of psychotropic medications and ECT in prevention of suicide and suicidal behaviors is presented after the cases, although clinical trial data are rather disparate and often limited.

Case Example 1

Mr. A is a 64-year-old certified public accountant who lost his job 2 years prior to psychiatric hospitalization. He had worked in the business office of a multinational company for 36 years and was told that his position was eliminated because of "a consolidation in the central office." Mr. A believed that the real reason that he was fired was because of his seniority and the cost savings associated with replacing him with a far younger accountant. For about 1 year he tried in vain to find another position, and ultimately reluctantly decided to retire.

For most of Mr. A's adult life, his passion had been his work, and consequently he had few hobbies or recreational interests. Upon retiring, he spent most of his time around the house and was bored. For the first time in his life, he began to drink scotch during the daytime hours and drank even more heavily at dinner and before bedtime. He rarely left home, became argumentative with his wife, lost his appetite and stopped eating regular meals, and could only fall asleep if he was intoxicated.

Without trying to diet, Mr. A lost 35 pounds in a period of 8 months. He became preoccupied

with his former boss from work. He confided to his wife that his boss "always had it in for me, had me fired, and won't be happy until I'm dead." His wife was alarmed when Mr. A told her that he had found "evidence" that his former boss had placed listening devices around the house "in order to monitor my habits." He became fearful that his food was being poisoned by this man. Although his wife encouraged him to see a psychiatrist, Mr. A staunchly refused: "I am not crazy, so there is no need for me to see some headshrinker." Finally, his wife arranged to have their family physician evaluate her husband at home. This physician diagnosed major depression and prescribed paroxetine, 20 mg/day. Over the next 3 weeks, Mr. A became increasingly more agitated and confused. He began to talk to himself, and it appeared to his wife that he was having conversations with people who were not in the house. She called the family physician, who told her to be patient and to be sure that her husband took the medication, because it "might take two or three more weeks before it becomes effective." Mr. A was now remaining in his room most of the time, staying in his bed, refusing to eat or drink—except the scotch, into which his wife would empty the capsule of paroxetine. Five weeks after the medication was initiated, Mrs. A heard a gunshot in her husband's bedroom and found him lying motionless in bed in a pool of blood. She called 911 and the emergency medical services (EMS) arrived within several minutes.

Mr. A was stabilized by the EMS team and general hospital emergency department physicians and staff and required 7 hours of surgery to repair the damage of the gunshot wound to his chest. Fortunately, the .22-caliber bullet missed his heart and vital blood vessels. Six days later he was transferred from the surgical service of the general hospital to the inpatient psychiatric service.

At the time of his admission to the psychiatry service, Mr. A was not speaking, not interacting with family or staff, and not accepting food or medication. Although he did not demonstrate waxy flexibility, he barely moved and seemed to be in a catatonic state. With the cooperation and approval of Mrs. A, the psychiatric service successfully petitioned the local court for permission to treat their patient with intramuscular haloperidol, but his mental status did not change. Although Mr. A was on intravenous fluids and received nasogastric feedings, his psychiatric condition did not improve over the next 2 weeks. The psychiatric team returned to court to seek permission to administer a course of 7–10 ECT treatments, and this request was granted by the judge. Following his second treatment, Mr. A began to speak with family and staff, to walk about the psychiatry unit, and to feed himself. He acknowledged having felt so frightened, sad, and desperate that he had tried to kill himself at home by shooting himself in the chest. He stated, "At this point, I just don't know what got into me. I felt I was in great danger, I was hearing the voice of my former boss talking to me and threatening me, and I felt hopeless. I guess I really lost it." Following the course of 7 ECT treatments, Mr. A denied feeling hopeless, suicidal, or even sad. He willingly and productively participated in psychotherapy and group treatments. He was discharged with twice-weekly psychiatric follow-up and family counseling once a week with a social worker.

Mr. A exhibited many biopsychosocial risk factors for suicide:

- Being a Caucasian male over 60 years old
- Having recently been fired from a job
- Not accepting or adapting to retirement
- Abusing alcohol
- Having major depression with psychotic features
- Refusing psychiatric treatment

Although the family practitioner correctly diagnosed major depression and prescribed an antidepressant, he failed to recognize the concomitant psychotic symptoms and alcohol abuse or to take into account their significance with regard to treatment. People with depression accompanied by psychosis are at increased risk of suicide, and they do not respond nearly as well to antidepressants as do people with depression without psychosis. Alcohol abuse may have occurred as the result of depression or may have affected his brain in ways that intensified Mr. A's depression. Treatment with antidepressants, without the concomitant alcohol abuse first being diagnosed and treated, was destined to fail. Psychiatric hospitalization was indicated at the time of Mr. A's initial evaluation by the family practitioner, in order to monitor him closely as medications were initiated and to facilitate the safe withdrawal from alcohol. In addition, an antipsychotic medication should have been initiated along with the antidepressant, because this approach is virtually always required in patients with both depression and psychosis.

Monitoring severely depressed patients closely and regularly for suicidal ideation and intent is imperative during the early phases of antidepressant treatment. After his suicide attempt and surgical treatment, Mr. A became catatonic. ECT is highly effective in treating major depression, psychosis, and catatonia and may do so more rapidly and reliably than medication treatment. Given Mr. A's deteriorating mental status and physical state during his hospitalization, ECT was clearly indicated at that point in his care. After his ECT and his resulting euthymia, the psychiatric team considered prescribing a course of antidepressants. The team noted that this was Mr. A's first episode of depression and that he had stopped abusing alcohol and was being compliant in regular psychotherapeutic follow-up. They also noted that psychosocial interventions, including exercise and structured socialization, had been initiated. For these reasons, and given the concern of eliciting further psychotic symptoms and other side effects with medication use, the psychiatric team chose to follow the patient closely without initiating antidepressant medications.

Case Example 2

Ms. E was a 26-year-old employee of a commercial airline company when she entered treatment with a social worker for "anxiety and failures in all my important relationships." Her father, who had mood swings, irritability, and chronic alcoholism, abandoned the family when Ms. E was 5 years old, and her mother remarried 2 years later to a man who had two teenage sons from a previous marriage. Ms. E's stepfather was critical and stern, and her mother, who chronically complained of back pain and fatigue, was often bedridden and unable or unavailable to care for Ms. E throughout her childhood. From the time Ms. E was 8 years old until she left home at age 17, she was recurrently abused sexually by both of her stepbrothers. Ms. E entered treatment with the social worker after the breakup of a 2-year relationship with a coworker. Her therapist initially diagnosed her as having "grief reaction, moderate depression, and intermittent anxiety." The thrust of treatment involved insight-oriented psychotherapy intended to help Ms. E connect her low self-esteem and dysfunctional behavioral patterns with the traumatic events of her childhood.

During the first year of twice-weekly psychotherapy, Ms. E became increasingly dependent on her psychotherapist for support and guidance in her personal life. Approximately once a month Ms. E experienced what she termed "the worst anxiety of my life." During those episodes, she became terrified that she was going to have a heart attack and die, had racing of her heart, experienced tingling about her face and in the fingers of both hands, and felt as though she had "separated from my body." Because she feared having another attack when alone and unable to get help, Ms. E began restricting her activities, eventually limiting them to work and her therapy sessions. When the psychotherapist left for a planned holiday, Ms. E cut her left wrist deeply with a razor blade. Several hours later, she went of her own accord to a general hospital emergency department "to be sewn up." She was referred by the surgeon to the emergency department psychiatrist following the closure of her wound. She told the psychiatrist, "When I cut myself, I fully intended to kill myself, but I changed my mind several hours later. Now I feel fine and have no plans to hurt myself." The psychiatrist also learned that this was not Ms. E's first suicide attempt: she had taken overdoses of over-the-counter sedatives on at least three occasions during adolescence and in her early 20s. All suicide attempts were made at times when Ms. E believed that she was being abandoned by

important people in her life. Ms. E also revealed that on occasion, she would cut the trunk of her body with razor blades and disclosed that "cutting makes me feel real and sometimes reduces my anxiety." Ms. E also told the psychiatrist of her "anxiety episodes" and how she had limited her activities as a consequence thereof. The psychiatrist made the diagnoses of panic disorder with agoraphobia and borderline personality disorder. The psychiatrist made the following recommendations to the patient and her psychotherapist:

1. Begin the antidepressant sertraline, 50 mg/day, to treat panic disorder and agoraphobia.
2. Transfer Ms. E's outpatient care to a senior social worker with special expertise in treating patients with borderline personality disorder.

The patient and her psychotherapist accepted this recommendation. On this regimen, Ms. E did not experience the recurrence of panic attacks or suicidal behavior. In addition, she became progressively less withdrawn, confident in social situations, and engaged in a fulfilling relationship that ultimately led to marriage.

Two important principles are illustrated in this case. The first principle is that *diagnosis comes before effective treatment.* Although Ms. E's first psychotherapist recognized that his patient had anxiety, he failed to make the correct diagnoses of borderline personality disorder and panic disorder with agoraphobia. His treatment was not sufficiently attentive to the establishment of appropriate boundaries with his patient, who believed that the supportive and involved therapist could replace intimacies in her personal life. Ms. E regressed and became dangerously dependent on her therapist to meet all her life's needs. The vacation of the therapist enraged the patient, who believed that she was being "led on to feel that he cared for me more than he really did." Additionally, Ms. E's dependencies on her therapist were intensified by her social withdrawal related to her undiagnosed and untreated panic disorder with agoraphobia. The use of sertraline not only treated Ms. E's panic attacks but also reduced her anxiety in general and the extreme level of her emotional responses to such stressors as perceived rejection.

A second principle of care illustrated by the case of Ms. E is that *experienced and knowledgeable psychotherapists are required for treating people with severe personality disorders.* Working with a psychotherapist experienced in the treatment of people with borderline personality disorder enabled Ms. E to derive the benefit of understanding the implications of her childhood trauma without becoming overly dependent on her therapist, psychologically regressed, and socially withdrawn. Under this therapeutic regimen Ms. E's suicidal or self-mutilating behavior has not recurred. For a detailed presentation of how such psychotherapeutic treatment is conceptualized and implemented in combination with psychiatric medications, the reader may refer to Chapter 6 in the book *Fatal Flaws: Navigating Destructive Relationships With People With Disorders of Personality and Character* (Yudofsky 2005).

Pharmacological Treatment

Antidepressants

Antidepressant medications such as selective serotonin reuptake inhibitors (SSRIs), serotonin-norepinephrine reuptake inhibitors (SNRIs), tricyclic antidepressants (TCAs), and monoamine oxidase inhibitors (MAOIs) are proven first- and second-line treatments for mood and anxiety disorders. It has been assumed that because they treat the affective and anxiety disorders often underlying suicidal behavior, these medications should inferentially treat the suicidal behaviors and thoughts that are symptoms of these disorders.

Clinical data are lacking as to antidepressants' proven efficacy in the reduction of suicide or suicidal behaviors in the short and long term, partly because available data are derived from studies whose primary focus is on the treatment of affective disorders or from meta-analyses, as few studies exist that examine suicidal behaviors as their primary endpoint (Müller-Oerlinghausen and Berghöfer 1999; Tondo et al. 2001).

Long-term prospective studies of the effects of antidepressant medications on suicide and suicidal behaviors do not exist (Baldessarini 2001). What data that do exist are derived from meta-analyses of randomized clinical trials of antidepressant efficacy and retrospective observational studies, neither of which have successfully demonstrated a consistent association between antidepressant treatment and suicidality. Patients at risk for suicide are largely excluded from randomized controlled trials of antidepressant efficacy, and sample size is small in these trials. Retrospective studies require large patient populations and long follow-up times in order to achieve sufficient statistical power, because suicide is such a rare occurrence and is underreported (Tiihonen et al. 2006a). Furthermore, data on suicide risk with antidepressant treatment are largely for patients with major depressive disorder, with little data reported on antidepressant use and suicide risk and behaviors in other psychiatric disorders, such as anxiety disorders and primary psychotic disorders.

Several early case reports suggested that SSRI antidepressants may be associated with *increased* risk of impulsivity, aggression, and suicidal behaviors (Mann and Kapur 1991; Teicher et al. 1990). As a result, several researchers carried out retrospective analyses to determine whether treatment with

SSRIs may in fact be associated with an increase in suicide and suicidal behaviors, but with differing results.

A meta-analysis by Khan et al. (2003) of controlled clinical trials of antidepressant treatment in depression from the FDA database showed no significant differences in rates of suicide for patients treated with SSRIs, non-SSRI antidepressants, and placebo. However, in another meta-analysis, Fergusson et al. (2005) compared randomized controlled trials of an SSRI versus placebo, TCAs, and other active non-SSRI/TCA medication and reported differing results. In this analysis, although no between-group difference in fatal suicide attempts was found, the SSRI treatment group had a statistically significant increase in nonfatal suicide attempts compared with the placebo group. There was no significant difference in suicide attempts in the SSRI treatment group compared with the TCA treatment group or the other active medication control group.

The picture is further clouded by a few meta-analyses of single SSRI agents showing a decrease in suicidal ideation in treated patients. A meta-analysis of controlled trials with fluoxetine demonstrated reduced suicidal ideation, although no significant difference in suicide attempts was found in patients receiving fluoxetine versus patients receiving placebo (Beasley et al. 1991). Meta-analyses of short-term controlled clinical trials with paroxetine showed significant decreases in suicidal ideation and completed suicides with paroxetine treatment compared with placebo or the active control arms (Montgomery et al. 1995). A meta-analysis of fluvoxamine treatment trials found a significant improvement in suicidal ideation in patients receiving fluvoxamine compared with those receiving placebo (Letizia et al. 1996).

Tiihonen et al. (2006a) retrospectively studied suicide attempts in a cohort of nonpsychotic patients who were hospitalized for a suicide attempt over a 6-year period and followed for a mean of 3.4 years. There was no significant difference in completed suicide risk in patients who were treated with SSRIs, SNRIs, or TCAs compared with those patients who did not use antidepressants. However, the relative risk of nonfatal suicide attempt was higher for patients treated with any antidepressant compared with those not treated with antidepressants.

In a long-term, prospective, open-label study of 400 patients with heterogeneous affective disorders treated for at least 6 months with multiple medications, including antidepressants, Angst and colleagues (2002) found a reduction in suicide rates in the group receiving medication compared with patients who were not treated with medications. Unfortunately, the study did not examine antidepressants alone; hence, no definitive conclusions could be made concerning their possible benefits in reducing suicidal behavior.

Some information about the effect on suicidal behaviors is available from clinical trials of SSRI antidepressant use in personality disorders. In a double-blind, placebo-controlled study, personality disorder patients with a history of recurrent suicide attempts and without a history of major depression or bipolar disorder who were treated with paroxetine showed a significant decrease in suicide attempts over a 1-year follow-up period compared with those receiving placebo (Verkes et al. 1998). This study substantiates data from smaller open-label trials of fluoxetine in patients with personality disorder who were at high risk for suicide.

Even though there is inconclusive evidence for improvement in suicide rates and suicidal behaviors with antidepressant treatment, antidepressants are still effective treatments for mood disorders often underlying suicidal behaviors and have established benefit in the acute short and long term for patients with affective disorders. Any potential risk of antidepressants inducing suicidal behaviors cannot outweigh the importance of effectively treating a patient's depression with antidepressants and thereby reducing fatal suicide risk.

Close monitoring by the clinician and patient education are critical to ensuring the safety of the suicidal patient treated with antidepressants. Upon initiation of treatment with antidepressants, the clinician must closely monitor patients for symptoms of increased anxiety, restlessness, agitation, sleep disturbance, and the precipitation of mixed states or psychotic episodes. Furthermore, the patient should be educated about the delay in symptom relief, because the effects of antidepressants may not manifest until weeks after initiation of treatment.

Patients should also be closely monitored for and educated about a possible increase in suicidal impulses in the initial phases of recovery, when they have more energy to act on these impulses. Fortunately, overdose risk is lessened with the SSRIs and newer antidepressants. TCAs and MAOIs can be lethal in overdose and thus should be prescribed in limited quantities for patients at high risk for suicide (Baldessarini 2001). However, because TCAs and MAOIs may be efficacious in depressed individuals whose illness has been resistant to the newer antidepressants, the risks associated with acute overdose should not preclude use of these medications.

Table 12–1 lists adverse effects associated with overdose of antidepressant and other psychotropic medications.

Mood Stabilizers

Lithium

Much better data exist for lithium's effect on suicide and suicidal behaviors. Long-term maintenance trials with lithium have established its significant reduction of suicide and suicide attempts in individuals with affective disorders (Baldessarini et al. 2003; Tondo et al. 2003). Meta-analyses of long-term lithium maintenance treatment in patients with affective disorders showed a highly significant decrease in completed suicides and suicide attempts of up to 14-fold in patients during lithium treatment compared with when they were not taking lithium (Schou 1998; Tondo et al. 2003). In another, larger meta-analysis of 33 studies of patients with bipolar disorder, major depression, or schizoaffective disorder, completed suicide rates decreased by more than 80% and suicide attempts decreased by more than 90% in patients during lithium treatment compared with when they were not being treated with lithium. The risk of all suicidal acts for lithium-treated patients was reduced to 0.21 suicidal acts per 100 person-years from 3.10 suicidal acts per 100 person-years for those patients who did not receive lithium. A similar suicide risk reduction was seen across all psychiatric disorders represented in the meta-analysis (Baldessarini et al. 2003). A similar reduction in suicide deaths and deliberate self-harm events was seen in another large meta-analysis of 32 trials comparing lithium with placebo or other medications used in the treatment of mood disorders (Cipriani et al. 2005).

Controlled, prospective clinical trials of the effects of lithium, compared with other treatments, on suicidal behaviors are few but generally point to lithium's protective effect on suicide risk (Thies-Flechtner et al. 1996; Tondo and Baldessarini 2000). One

TABLE 12–1. Adverse effects associated with overdose, by class of medication

Class	Medication	Effects of overdose
Antidepressants		
Selective serotonin reuptake inhibitors (SSRIs)	Citalopram/escitalopram, fluoxetine, fluvoxamine, paroxetine, sertraline	Serotonin syndrome can occur with any drug with serotonergic action (SSRIs, MAOIs, TCAs, and other nonpsychotropic medications). Symptoms typically include restlessness, hyperreflexia, muscle twitches, tremor, and autonomic dysfunction. More severe intoxication can progress to seizures and coma. Death can occur rarely with overdosage.
Serotonin-norepinephrine reuptake inhibitors (SNRIs)	Venlafaxine/desvenlafaxine, duloxetine	Same as for SSRIs.
Dopamine-norepinephrine reuptake inhibitors	Bupropion	Same as for SSRIs.
Serotonin modulators	Nefazodone, trazodone	Same as for SSRIs.
Norepinephrine-serotonin modulators	Mirtazapine	Same as for SSRIs.
Tricyclic/tetracyclic antidepressants (TCAs)	Imipramine, amitriptyline, doxepin, clomipramine, desipramine, nortriptyline, amoxapine	Severe intoxication occurs at doses of imipramine above 1 g. Deaths have been reported with doses of imipramine of 2 g or more. Acute overdose can result in delirium, hypotension, cardiac arrhythmias, and seizures, followed by rapid development of coma and depressed respiration. Anticholinergic delirium is a medical emergency requiring full supportive care.
Monoamine oxidase inhibitors (MAOIs)	Phenelzine, tranylcypromine, moclobemide	Toxic reactions from overdose of an MAOI may occur in a matter of hours, despite the long delay in onset of a therapeutic response. Effects of overdose include agitation, hallucinations, hyperreflexia, hyperpyrexia, and convulsions. Both hypotension and hypertension also occur. Treatment of such intoxication is problematic, but conservative treatment is often successful. Hypertensive crisis can occur with concomitant ingestion of foods with high tyramine content, resulting in headache, hypertension, and possible intracerebral hemorrhage.

TABLE 12–1. Adverse effects associated with overdose, by class of medication *(continued)*

Class	Medication	Effects of overdose
Mood stabilizers		
	Lithium	Symptoms consist of tremor, ataxia, vomiting, diarrhea, seizures, cardiac arrhythmias, and hypotension and may progress to coma and death. Neurotoxic side effects may be irreversible. Supportive treatment is recommended. Dialysis is recommended for serum lithium concentrations greater than 4.0 mEq/L in acute overdoses and greater than 1.5 mEq/L in chronic overdoses.
Antiepileptics	Valproate	Toxicity results in sedation, confusion, hyperreflexia/hyporeflexia, seizures, respiratory suppression, and supraventricular tachycardia and may progress to coma. Treatment consists of gastric lavage, cardiac monitoring, respiratory support, and treatment of seizures.
	Carbamazepine	Symptoms of toxicity include nausea and vomiting, urinary retention, myoclonus, hyperreflexia, nystagmus, cardiac conduction problems, seizures, and coma. Treatment consists of induction of vomiting, gastric lavage, cardiac monitoring, and supportive care.
	Lamotrigine	Toxicity may result in ataxia, nystagmus, altered mental status, intraventricular conduction delay, seizures, and coma. Overdose can result in death.
	Oxcarbazepine	Isolated cases of overdose up to 24 g have been reported; recovery in all cases with symptomatic treatment.

TABLE 12–1. Adverse effects associated with overdose, by class of medication (continued)

Class	Medication	Effects of overdose
Antipsychotic agents		
First-generation/typicals	Chlorpromazine, thioridazine, pimozide, trifluoperazine, fluphenazine, perphenazine, thiothixene, loxapine, haloperidol	Death is rare in overdose if supportive care is given and there is no concomitant ingestion of other central nervous system (CNS) drugs or alcohol. Fatalities have occurred due to respiratory compromise related to dystonia and neuroleptic malignant syndrome (NMS). NMS is more likely to occur with high-potency neuroleptics and consists of autonomic instability, tremor, catatonia, fluctuating mental status, creatine kinase elevation, and myoglobinemia.
Second-generation/atypicals	Clozapine, aripiprazole, olanzapine, quetiapine, risperidone, ziprasidone, asenapine, iloperidone, lurasidone	Toxicity results in CNS depression, hypotension, tachycardia. Seizures occur most commonly with clozapine overdose. Anticholinergic side effects are most common with clozapine and olanzapine. QT prolongation can occur. Significant extrapyramidal symptoms are less likely than with typical antipsychotics but can occur and are dose related. NMS can occur with atypical antipsychotic overdose. Deaths occur infrequently with overdose, related to cardiovascular complications, although fatalities can occur from pulmonary, endocrine, gastrointestinal, and neurological complications. Treat with supportive measures and cardiac monitoring.
Anxiolytics		
Benzodiazepines		Dangerous in overdose because of synergistic effects with other CNS depressants and alcohol. Treat with respiratory support and benzodiazepine antagonist flumazenil.
Buspirone		Symptoms of overdose include dizziness, vomiting, sedation. No reported deaths with overdose.

Source. Information in this table comes from Baldessarini 2001; Baldessarini and Tarazi 2001; Marangell et al. 2003; and drug manufacturer prescribing information.

large, noncontrolled retrospective study of completed and attempted suicides in patients with bipolar disorder over a mean follow-up period of 2.9 years compared suicidal behaviors among three groups (those treated with lithium, valproate, and carbamazepine, respectively). Lithium-treated patients had a significantly lower rate of suicide attempts and completed suicides compared with those patients taking valproate. Comparisons with carbamazepine were not possible because of the relatively low number of patients being treated with carbamazepine (Goodwin et al. 2003).

Lithium treatment does not completely negate the effects of psychiatric disorder on suicidality. The suicide rate among patients receiving lithium, although lower than the rate among patients receiving no treatment, is still much higher than the rate in the general population (0.0107%; Tondo and Baldessarini 2000). Furthermore, samples in studies of the effects of lithium on suicide risk are largely limited to bipolar disorder patients. However, a few small studies of lithium treatment for major depression have found a significant decrease in suicidal acts (to almost 0%, compared with 1.33% per year in non-lithium-treated patients; Baldessarini et al. 2003).

The pathophysiological mechanism by which lithium decreases suicide risk is unknown. It is possible that lithium reduces the impulsivity, aggression, or anger that may precipitate a suicide attempt. Or lithium may exert general mood-stabilizing qualities that decrease severity of depression or mixed dysphoric states. It is also possible that patients benefit from the close medical and laboratory monitoring associated with lithium treatment (Tondo and Baldessarini 2000).

Lithium in overdose can have significant toxicity; thus, the prudent clinician should consider prescribing conservative quantities of this medication to patients at risk for suicide. This potential toxicity should not prevent lithium treatment of suicidal patients, especially given lithium's association with suicide risk reduction. When weighing the risks and benefits of first-line treatments for a bipolar disorder patient with significant suicide risk factors, the clinician should certainly consider lithium's association with suicide risk reduction.

Antiepileptic Mood Stabilizers

Valproate, carbamazepine, and lamotrigine are also first-line treatments for the prophylaxis and acute episodes of bipolar disorder. However, studies of the effects of mood stabilizers other than lithium are limited, with even fewer controlled prospective studies of these medications' effects on suicidal behavior.

Much interest in these medications and their relation to suicidality has been spurred by a recent FDA warning. In 2008, the FDA reported a significant association between 11 antiepileptics and increased suicidality but stopped short of recommending a black box warning. This report was based on a meta-analysis of 199 placebo-controlled trials of 11 antiepileptic medications; suicidal thoughts or behaviors were reported in 0.43% of patients treated with antiepileptics, compared with 0.22% of patients receiving placebo (U.S. Food and Drug Administration 2008). This warning applied to all 11 antiepileptic medications: carbamazepine, divalproex, felbamate, gabapentin, lamotrigine, levetiracetam, oxcarbazepine, pregabalin, tiagabine, topiramate, and zonisamide. However, treatment with only two of these medications, lamotrigine and topiramate, showed significant association with suicidal behaviors or thoughts, with the nine other medications showing no significant association (Gibbons et al. 2009).

A retrospective database review of patients with bipolar disorder compared data on suicidal behaviors for the year prior to diagnosis with the year after diagnosis. After treatment, there was no statistically significant difference in suicide attempts or suicidal behaviors in patients who received one of 11 antiepileptic medications ($n=$ 13,385) compared with those who were not treated with an antiepileptic medication or lithium ($n=25,432$). Analyzed individually, each antiepileptic medication showed similar results except for topiramate and carbamazepine, which both showed a significant increase in suicidality in the 1 year after diagnosis compared with the 1 year prior (Gibbons et al. 2009).

In a retrospective chart review, Yerevanian et al. (2003) examined completed suicides and suicide attempts while patients were, first, treated with lithium and, then, treated with either valproate or carbamazepine. No significant difference was observed in suicide attempt rate between lithium and either divalproex or carbamazepine (2.94 attempts/100 patient-years for lithium vs. 3.75 attempts/100 patient-years for divalproex/carbamazepine) (Yerevanian et al. 2003). Similar results were reported by Yerevanian et al. (2007) in a larger retrospective study of 405 veterans with bipolar disorder. More importantly, patients who discontinued treatment with lithium or divalproex or carbamazepine were 16 times more likely to have a nonlethal suicidal event after discontinuation than patients who continued treatment (55.89 vs. 3.48 events/100 patient-years).

However, Goodwin et al. (2003) found significantly higher risk of suicide attempts and completed suicides in patients treated with valproate compared with those treated with lithium. Comparisons with carbamazepine were not possible because of the small sample treated with carbamazepine included in this study. Likewise, a retrospective review of 12,662 Medicaid patients with bipolar disorder showed significantly greater suicide attempts for patients treated with divalproex compared with lithium but nonsignificant increases in those treated with gabapentin or carbamazepine (Collins and McFarland 2008). Results of both studies are limited by nonrandomization of treatment groups, and it is unclear whether illness severity may have influenced practitioners' choice of medication (i.e., less acutely suicidal and less severely ill patients may have been put on lithium rather than antiepileptic mood stabilizers).

Although the degree of beneficial effect that antiepileptic mood stabilizers have on suicidality is not yet defined, the use of these medications is still superior to no medications at all in the prevention of suicidal ideation and behavior in bipolar disorder.

Antipsychotics

First-generation antipsychotics, although quite effective for treatment of acute psychosis, agitation, and aggression, are clearly understudied with respect to their effect on suicidal behaviors. The limited data that are available about these medications suggest that they may be beneficial in attenuating suicidal behavior.

Second-generation, or atypical, antipsychotic agents are somewhat better studied and in fact have become very helpful in the treatment of suicidal patients with psychotic disorders, due to their effects in terms of lessening anxiety as well as curbing impulsivity, agitation, and mania. Second-generation antipsychotic medications, which include aripiprazole, clozapine, olanzapine, quetiapine, risperidone, ziprasidone, asenapine, and lurasidone, are first-line treatments for primary psychotic disorders, and most have indications for the treatment of bipolar disorder. They are generally preferred for clinical use over first-generation, or typical, antipsychotic agents because of their favorable side-effect profile, with fewer extrapyramidal symptoms, and improved cognition (Meltzer and McGurk 1999).

Again, the second-generation antipsychotics have not been systematically and prospectively evaluated with respect to their effect on suicidal behaviors. The limited retrospective data that exist about suicidality and antipsychotic use are somewhat mixed. Two meta-analyses of suicide and suicide attempts in clinical trials of atypical antipsychotics showed no difference in rate of completed suicide and suicide attempts between medication-treated and placebo groups (Khan et al. 2001; Storosum et al. 2003). On the other hand, a retrospective cohort study followed 2,230 newly hospitalized adults with schizophrenia or schizoaffective disorder for a mean of 3.6 years to assess mortality associated with treatment with 10 commonly prescribed first-generation and second-generation antipsychotic medications (i.e., olanzapine, clozapine, risperidone, oral perphenazine, thioridazine, perphenazine depot, chlorprothixene, chlorpromazine, haloperidol, and levomepromazine). Although no significant differences were found between groups treated with each antipsychotic medication, mortality was increased 10-fold in patients not taking antipsychotic medications at all compared with those being treated with antipsychotic medication. Only one completed suicide occurred in the group treated with antipsychotics, compared with 26 suicides in the group not taking antipsychotics (Tiihonen et al. 2006b). In a more recent retrospective cohort study conducted in Finland by Tiihonen et al. (2009), mortality data on outpatients with schizophrenia were examined

with respect to any antipsychotic medication use or not, as well as the use of the six most frequently prescribed antipsychotic medications (clozapine, olanzapine, thioridazine, risperidone, haloperidol, quetiapine) compared with perphenazine use. As in the earlier study, overall mortality risk was significantly lower in patients using antipsychotic medications long term (7–11 years) compared with those who never used antipsychotics. Compared with outpatients using perphenazine, those using quetiapine had the highest overall risk of death, and those using clozapine had the lowest risk. In addition, patients taking clozapine had the lowest risk of suicide compared with patients taking any other typical or atypical antipsychotic medication studied.

The most data on risk reduction of suicidal behaviors exist for the atypical antipsychotic clozapine, the only treatment approved by the FDA for suicide risk reduction, although this indication is limited to patients with schizophrenia. The use of clozapine is limited, and it is generally prescribed when primary psychosis does not respond to the other antipsychotic agents available, because of possible hematological complications. Yet strong evidence exists in schizophrenia and schizoaffective disorders for an association between clozapine use and decreased rates of suicidal behaviors (Reid et al. 1998; Walker et al. 1997). Data from the Texas Department of Mental Health and Mental Retardation, as well as from the Clozapine National Registry, show that the annual suicide rate was decreased by 75%–80% for clozapine-treated patients with schizophrenia and schizoaffective disorder (Reid et al. 1998). Additionally, in a long-term study of 88 patients with chronic schizophrenia or schizoaffective disorder receiving clozapine monotherapy, the annual number of suicide attempts decreased 12-fold in the 6-month to 7-year follow-up period compared with the 2 years prior to clozapine treatment (Meltzer and Okayli 1995). Furthermore, patients reported improvement in depression and hopelessness symptoms.

A randomized, controlled open-label study, the International Suicide Prevention Trial (InterSePT), compared the effects of clozapine and another atypical antipsychotic, olanzapine, on suicidal behavior. Schizophrenia and schizoaffective patients considered at high risk for suicide based on previous suicide attempts in the 3 years prior to enrollment or current suicidal ideation were included and treated with either open-label clozapine or olanzapine. Although this study was not specifically powered to study the reduction in suicide deaths as an endpoint, the study nonetheless showed that clozapine-treated patients experienced a significant reduction in the rate of all suicidal events. Clozapine-treated patients had a significantly lower rate of suicide attempts compared with olanzapine-treated patients, although there was no statistical difference in completed suicide rate. In fact, the rate of suicide attempts for the olanzapine-treated patients was half that prior to enrollment. Thus, olanzapine is also associated with a decreased risk of suicidal behaviors, although not perhaps as great as that for clozapine (Meltzer et al. 2003).

Thus, clozapine may have preventive effects on suicidal behavior in schizophrenia and schizoaffective disorder, more so than other antipsychotics, both typical and atypical agents. However, clozapine's effect on suicidal behavior in other psychiatric disorders is not available. Clearly, it is useful for suicidal patients with schizophrenia and schizoaffective disorder (Meltzer et al. 2003). When assessing whether a patient should be treated with clozapine, the clinician must weigh the potential antisuicide effects as well as the other benefits of treatment with clozapine against potential adverse effects, including fatal agranulocytosis, cardiomyopathy, and myocarditis.

Olanzapine also appears to have preventive effects on suicidal behavior, although not as great as those for clozapine. Few other studies exist about olanzapine and the other atypical antipsychotics' effects on suicidal behaviors in primary psychotic disorders and in other psychiatric disorders. One study of note followed 339 patients with schizophrenia, schizoaffective disorder, and schizophreniform disorder treated with short-term olanzapine or risperidone. Secondary analysis of the suicide attempt rates found that patients given olanzapine had significantly lower rates of suicide attempts than those treated with risperidone during the 28-week follow-up period (Tran et al. 1997). Another 5-year retrospective study of 378 case-controlled schizophrenia/schizoaffective pairs showed an overall similar protective effect of risperidone and olanzapine, with fewer suicide attempts among both groups receiving these antipsychotics (Barak et al. 2004). There are no known studies examining the effects on suicidal behavior for the other atypical antipsychotics (i.e., ziprasidone, aripiprazole, asenapine, iloperidone, lurasidone).

Anxiolytics

Psychic anxiety, panic, agitation, and insomnia are commonly associated with suicide risk in depression (Fawcett et al. 1990). Thus, it would be expected that anxiolytic medications such as benzodiazepines, antidepressants, low-dose atypical antipsychotics, and mood stabilizers might have a calming and beneficial effect on suicidal patients. However, the limited clinical trial data do not support this assumption for either short-term or long-term treatment with anxiolytic medications. A meta-analysis of controlled clinical trials of treatments for several different anxiety disorders found little difference in rates of completed suicide and suicide attempts in patients treated with anxiolytic medications compared with those given placebo (Khan et al. 2002). Very few studies exist on the effects of anxiolytics on suicidal behavior.

It would seem clinically prudent to continue to target directly anxiety symptoms such as intrapsychic distress, anxiety, agitation, and insomnia in order to limit suicide risk, especially given earlier reports that benzodiazepine discontinuation may be associated with increased risk of suicidal behavior (Gaertner et al. 2002; Joughin et al. 1991). Thus, short-term benzodiazepine treatment for the acute treatment of anxiety symptoms can be helpful, with longer-acting agents preferable to shorter-acting agents to prevent rebound anxiety. Gradual discontinuation through dose titration, accompanied by vigilant monitoring for increasing suicidality, agitation, anxiety, or depression, is recommended. Patients treated with benzodiazepines should also be monitored for disinhibition, increased aggressive behaviors and impulsivity (Cowdry and Gardner 1988), and interaction with other prescribed drugs, illicit drugs, and alcohol.

Electroconvulsive Therapy

ECT is an established therapeutic modality for severe major depression with or without psychotic features as well as for the treatment of manic or mixed episodes of bipolar disorder and acute episodes of schizoaffective disorder or schizophrenia. It can be extremely useful for acutely sui-

cidal patients because of its rapid antidepressant response and associated rapid reduction in short-term suicidal ideation (Ciapparelli et al. 2001; Kellner et al. 2005; Prudic and Sackeim 1999; Rich et al. 1986).

The few studies that have assessed the short-term effects of ECT on suicidality (suicidal ideation or intent) all show rapid, significant improvement in suicide ratings with ECT (Ciapparelli et al. 2001; Kellner et al. 2005; Prudic and Sackeim 1999; Rich et al. 1986). However, no studies exist of ECT effects on suicide attempts or completed suicides or of the long-term effects of ECT.

Based on the limited data available for the short-term effects of ECT, ECT can be helpful for severe major depressive episodes accompanied by suicidal behavior, especially when a delay in treatment response would be life-threatening, such as for patients who are overtly psychotic, catatonic, or refusing to eat. ECT may also be helpful for pregnant patients who are at risk for suicide and whose illness is resistant to medications or who are unable to tolerate medications. Because of the lack of data regarding the long-term effects of ECT on suicidality, it is recommended that after acute treatment with ECT, maintenance treatment be continued with psychotropic medication or further ECT.

Neuropsychiatric Medical Devices

Transcranial magnetic stimulation (TMS) is a recently approved (2008), noninvasive treatment for adult patients with major depressive disorder who have not experienced improvement from at least one prior treatment with an antidepressant at the standard treatment dose and duration (George et al. 2010). The treatment uses the pulsed electromagnetic induction of electric currents in the brain. Repetitive, or rapid-rate, TMS delivers up to 50 stimuli per second and has been proposed as being effective in the treatment of both major depression and other neuropsychiatric disorders (Dlabac-de Lange et al. 2010). Both procedures require anesthesia and have been proposed as having fewer side effects than ECT.

Vagus nerve stimulation (VNS) was approved in 2005 for the adjunctive treatment of treatment-resistant depression in adult patients who have not had adequate response to at least four antidepressant medication trials. Electrical pulses generated from a permanent pulse stimulator implanted in the superficial chest wall are transmitted via electrode to the left vagus nerve, which in turn transmits these electrical pulses to purported mood centers in the brain. VNS was originally pioneered as a treatment for medication-resistant epilepsy but was investigated for the treatment of depression when mood improvement in epilepsy patients was observed anecdotally to occur independent of seizure control. Based on limited data summed from two pilot studies and one large controlled, multicenter trial of patients with treatment-resistant depression treated with VNS ($N= 345$), rates of suicide attempts in patients with treatment-resistant depression treated with VNS appear to be comparable to those among depressed patients treated with antidepressants (O'Reardon et al. 2006).

Deep brain stimulation (DBS) is not approved for the treatment of any of the mood disorders, although it is FDA approved for the treatment of chronic, severe, treatment-resistant obsessive-compulsive disorder, adjunctive treatment of advanced Parkinson's disease, and chronic, intractable dystonia and essential tremor. DBS is currently being investigated in the treatment of treatment-resistant depression. It involves sur-

gical implantation of a medical device in the brain to deliver electrical pulses to anatomical areas believed to be important to the neural circuitry of depression, including the anterior limb of the internal capsule, the ventral capsule/ventral striatum, the nucleus accumbens, and the subcallosal cingulate gyrus. Very limited data exist for DBS in treatment-resistant depression. In an open-label study of 20 patients with treatment-resistant depression, 2 completed suicides and 2 other suicide attempts occurred in the mean 3.5-year follow-up period after DBS implantation in the subcallosal cingulate gyrus (Kennedy et al. 2011). Although it is unlikely that the high rate of suicide and suicidal behaviors is related to the DBS rather than to the severity of the treatment-resistant depression in these patients, further research is certainly needed to investigate not only the efficacy of DBS as a treatment modality but also its potential effects on suicidal behaviors.

Given the strong association of untreated major depression and suicide, one might infer that any effective treatment of major depression would reduce the risk of suicidal ideation and behavior. However, in absence of specific data regarding the prevention of suicidal behaviors with TMS, VNS, and DBS to confirm this inference, we believe that it is premature to come to this conclusion. Thus, we continue to recommend psychopharmacological interventions and ECT for the somatic treatment of patients with major depression and the risk of suicide.

Conclusion

Treatment of suicide and suicidal behaviors is complex, requiring aggressive pharmacotherapy in conjunction with a strong psychotherapeutic alliance with the affected individual. Although variable data exist as to their short-term and long-term efficacy in decreasing rates of suicide and suicidal behaviors, psychotropic medications and/or ECT to treat symptoms such as psychic pain, anxiety and turmoil, panic attacks, agitation, impulsiveness, aggression, and feelings of hopelessness can be extremely helpful in managing the patient with suicidal tendencies. Aggressive pharmacological treatments and/or ECT used in conjunction with early identification and reduction of risk factors for suicide, thorough clinical assessment and diagnosis, close monitoring by the treatment team, careful consideration of hospitalization, and a strong therapeutic alliance are essential components of successful management of the suicidal patient.

Key Clinical Concepts

- ▪ Treatment of suicide and suicidal behaviors is complex and multidisciplinary and includes aggressive pharmacotherapy in conjunction with a strong psychotherapeutic alliance with the affected individual.

- ▪ Medications to treat symptoms such as psychic pain, anxiety and turmoil, panic attacks, agitation, impulsiveness, aggression, and feelings of hopelessness can be extremely helpful in managing the patient with suicidal tendencies.

- ▪ Good short-term and long-term data are lacking regarding the clinical effectiveness of psychiatric medications and electroconvulsive therapy (ECT) on suicidal behaviors, largely because data on suicidal behaviors are obtained through secondary analyses of treatment efficacy studies and meta-analyses. Despite this, lithium and the atypical antipsychotic agent clozapine appear to exert a positive effect on suicidal behaviors. Data are accruing for effects of the newer atypical antipsychotic agents and antiepileptic mood stabilizers on suicidal behaviors.

- ▪ Even though there is inconclusive evidence for improvement in suicide rates and suicidal behaviors with antidepressant treatment, antidepressants are still effective treatments for the affective disorders often underlying suicidal behaviors and have established benefit in the acute short and long term for patients with affective disorders.

- ▪ Close monitoring by the clinician and patient education, especially during initiation of therapy with an antidepressant medication, are critical to ensuring the safety of the suicidal patient treated with antidepressants.

- ▪ Although data are limited as to the effects of ECT on suicide rates, ECT can be helpful for severe major depressive episodes accompanied by suicidal behavior, especially when a delay in treatment response would be life-threatening, such as for patients who are overtly psychotic, catatonic, or refusing to eat.

References

Angst F, Stassen HH, Clayton PJ, et al: Mortality of patients with mood disorders: follow-up over 34–38 years. J Affect Disord 68:167–181, 2002

Baldessarini RJ: Drugs and the treatment of psychiatric disorders: antidepressant and antianxiety agents, in Goodman & Gilman's The Pharmacological Basis of Therapeutics, 10th Edition. Edited by Goodman LS, Hardman JG, Limbird LE, et al. New York, McGraw-Hill, 2001, pp 447–484

Baldessarini RJ, Tarazi FI: Drugs and the treatment of psychiatric disorders: psychoses and mania, in Goodman & Gilman's The Pharmacological Basis of Therapeutics, 10th Edition. Edited by Goodman LS, Hardman JG, Limbird LE, et al. New York, McGraw-Hill, 2001, pp 485–520

Baldessarini RJ, Tondo L, Hennen J: Lithium treatment and suicide risk in major affective disorders: update and new findings. J Clin Psychiatry 64(suppl):44–52, 2003

Barak Y, Mirecki I, Knobler HY, et al: Suicidality and second generation antipsychotics in schizophrenia patients: a case-controlled retrospective study during 5-year period. Psychopharmacology (Berl) 175:215–219, 2004

Beasley CM, Dornseif BE, Bosomworth JC, et al: Fluoxetine and suicide: a meta-analysis of controlled trials of treatment for depression. BMJ 303:685–692, 1991

Centers for Disease Control and Prevention, National Center for Injury Prevention and Control: Web-based Injury Statistics Query and Reporting System (WISQARS). Available at: http://www.cdc.gov/injury/wisqars/index.html. Accessed August 9, 2011.

Ciapparelli A, Dell'Osso L, Tundo A, et al: Electroconvulsive therapy in medication-nonresponsive patients with mixed mania and bipolar depression. J Clin Psychiatry 62:552–555, 2001

Cipriani A, Pretty H, Hawton K, et al: Lithium in the prevention of suicidal behavior and all-cause mortality in patients with mood disorders: a systematic review of randomized trials. Am J Psychiatry 162:1805–1819, 2005

Collins JC, McFarland BH: Divalproex, lithium and suicide among Medicaid patients with bipolar disorder. J Affect Disord 107:23–28, 2008

Cowdry RW, Gardner DL: Pharmacotherapy of borderline personality disorder: alprazolam, carbamazepine, trifluoperazine, and tranylcypromine. Arch Gen Psychiatry 45:111–119, 1988

Dlabac-de Lange JJ, Knegtering R, Aleman A: Repetitive transcranial magnetic stimulation for negative symptoms of schizophrenia. J Clin Psychiatry 71:411–418, 2010

Fawcett J, Scheftner WA, Fogg L, et al: Time-related predictors of suicide in major affective disorder. Am J Psychiatry 147:1189–1194, 1990

Fergusson D, Doucette S, Glass KC, et al: Association between suicide attempts and selective serotonin reuptake inhibitors: systematic review of randomised controlled trials. BMJ 330:396, 2005

Gaertner I, Gilot C, Heidrich P, et al: A case control study on psychopharmacotherapy before suicide committed by 61 psychiatric inpatients. Pharmacopsychiatry 35:37–43, 2002

George MS, Lisanby SH, Avery D, et al: Daily left prefrontal transcranial magnetic stimulation therapy for major depressive disorder: a sham-controlled randomized trial. Arch Gen Psychiatry 67:507–515, 2010

Gibbons RD, Hur K, Brown CH, et al: Relationship between antiepileptic drugs and suicide attempts in patients with bipolar disorder. Arch Gen Psychiatry 66:1354–1360, 2009

Goodwin F, Fireman B, Simon G, et al: Suicide risk in bipolar disorder during treatment with lithium, divalproex, and carbamazepine. JAMA 290:1467–1473, 2003

Harris EC, Barraclough B: Suicide as an outcome for mental disorders: a meta-analysis. Br J Psychiatry 170:205–228, 1997

Henriksson MM, Aro HM, Marttunen MJ, et al: Mental disorders and comorbidity in suicide. Am J Psychiatry 150:935–940, 1993

Isacsson G, Bergman U, Rich CL: Antidepressants, depression, and suicide: an analysis of the San Diego study. J Affect Disord 32:277–286, 1994a

Isacsson G, Holmgren P, Wasserman D, et al: Use of antidepressants among people committing suicide in Sweden. BMJ 308:506–509, 1994b

Jick JH, Kaye JA, Jick SS: Antidepressants and the risk of suicidal behaviors. JAMA 292:338–343, 2004

Joughin N, Tata P, Collins M, et al: Inpatient withdrawal from long-term benzodiazepine use. Br J Addict 86:449–455, 1991

Kellner CH, Fink M, Knapp R, et al: Relief of expressed suicidal intent by ECT: a Consortium for Research in ECT study. Am J Psychiatry 162:977–982, 2005

Kennedy SH, Giacobbe P, Rizvi SJ, et al: Deep brain stimulation for treatment-resistant depression: follow-up after 3–6 years. Am J Psychiatry 168:502–510, 2011

Khan A, Khan SR, Leventhal RM, et al: Symptom reduction and suicide risk among patients treated with placebo in antipsychotic clinical trials: an analysis of the Food and Drug Administration database. Am J Psychiatry 158:1449–1454, 2001

Khan A, Leventhal RM, Khan S, et al: Suicide risk in patients with anxiety disorders: a meta-analysis of the FDA database. J Affect Disord 68:183–190, 2002

Khan A, Khan S, Kolts R: Suicide rates in clinical trials of SSRIs, other antidepressants, and placebo: analysis of FDA reports. Am J Psychiatry 160:790–792, 2003

Letizia C, Kapik B, Flanders WD: Suicidal risk during controlled clinical investigations of fluvoxamine. J Clin Psychiatry 57:415–421, 1996

Licinio J, Wong ML: Depression, antidepressants and suicidality: a critical appraisal. Nat Rev Drug Discov 4:165–172, 2005

Mann JJ, Kapur S: The emergence of suicidal ideation and behavior during antidepressant pharmacotherapy. Arch Gen Psychiatry 48:1027–1033, 1991

Marangell LB, Silver JM, Goff DC, et al: Psychopharmacology and electroconvulsive therapy, in The American Psychiatric Publishing Textbook of Clinical Psychiatry, 4th Edition. Edited by Hales RE, Yudofsky SC. Washington, DC, American Psychiatric Publishing, 2003, pp 1047–1149

Meltzer HY, McGurk SR: The effects of clozapine, risperidone, and olanzapine on cognitive function in schizophrenia. Schizophr Bull 25:233–255, 1999

Meltzer HY, Okayli G: Reduction of suicidality during clozapine treatment of neuroleptic-resistant schizophrenia: impact on risk-benefit assessment. Am J Psychiatry 152:183–190, 1995

Meltzer H, Alphs L, Green A, et al: Clozapine treatment for suicidality in schizophrenia: International Suicide Prevention Trial (InterSePT). Arch Gen Psychiatry 60:82–91, 2003

Montgomery SA, Dunner DL, Dunbar GC: Reduction of suicidal thoughts with paroxetine in comparison with reference antidepressants and placebo. Eur Neuropsychopharmacol 5:5–13, 1995

Müller-Oerlinghausen B, Berghöfer A: Antidepressants and suicidal risk. J Clin Psychiatry 60 (suppl 2):94–99, 1999

O'Reardon JP, Cristancho P, Peshek AD: Vagal nerve stimulation (VNS) and treatment of depression: to the brainstem and beyond. Psychiatry (Edgmont) 3:54–63, 2006

Prudic J, Sackeim HA: Electroconvulsive therapy and suicide risk. J Clin Psychiatry 60(suppl):104–110, 1999

Reid WH, Mason M, Hogan T: Suicide prevention effects associated with clozapine therapy in schizophrenia and schizoaffective disorder. Psychiatr Serv 49:1029–1033, 1998

Rich CL, Spiker DG, Jewell SW, et al: Response of energy and suicidal ideation to ECT. J Clin Psychiatry 47:31–32, 1986

Schou M: The effect of prophylactic lithium treatment on mortality and suicidal behavior: a review for clinicians. J Affect Disord 50:253–259, 1998

Storosum JG, van Zwieten BJ, Wohlfarth T, et al: Suicide risk in placebo vs active treatment in placeb-controlled trials for schizophrenia. Arch Gen Psychiatry 60:365–368, 2003

Teicher MH, Glod C, Cole JO: Emergence of intense suicidal preoccupation during fluoxetine treatment. Am J Psychiatry 147:207–210, 1990

Thies-Flechtner K, Müller-Oerlinghausen B, Seibert W, et al: Effect of prophylactic treatment on suicide risk in patients with major affective disorder. Pharmacopsychiatry 29:103–107, 1996

Tiihonen J, Lönnqvist J, Wahlbeck K, et al: Antidepressants and the risk of suicide, attempted suicide, and overall mortality in a nationwide cohort. Arch Gen Psychiatry 63:1358–1367, 2006a

Tiihonen J, Wahlbeck K, Lönnqvist J, et al: Effectiveness of antipsychotic treatments in a nationwide cohort of patients in community care after first hospitalisation due to schizophrenia and schizoaffective disorder: observational follow-up study. BMJ 333:224, 2006b

Tiihonen J, Lönnqvist J, Wahlbeck K, et al: 11-year follow-up of mortality in patients with schizophrenia: a population-based cohort study (FIN11 study). Lancet 374:620–627, 2009

Tondo L, Baldessarini RJ: Reduced suicide risk during lithium maintenance treatment. J Clin Psychiatry 61(suppl):97–104, 2000

Tondo L, Ghiani C, Albert M: Pharmacologic interventions in suicide prevention. J Clin Psychiatry 62(suppl):51–55, 2001

Tondo L, Isacsson G, Baldessarini RJ: Suicidal behavior in bipolar disorder: risk and prevention. CNS Drugs 17:491–511, 2003

Tran PV, Hamilton SH, Kuntz AJ, et al: Double-blind comparison of olanzapine versus risperidone in the treatment of schizophrenia and other psychotic disorders. J Clin Psychiatry 17:407–418, 1997

U.S. Food and Drug Administration: Statistical review and evaluation: antiepileptic drugs and suicidality. 2008. Available at: http://www.fda.gov/ohrms/dockets/ac/08/briefing/2008-4372b1-01-FDA.pdf. Accessed August 10, 2011.

Verkes RJ, van der Mast RC, Hengeveld MW, et al: Reduction by paroxetine of suicidal behavior in patients with repeated suicide attempts but not major depression. Am J Psychiatry 155:543–547, 1998

Walker AM, Lanza LL, Arellano F, et al: Mortality in current and former users of clozapine. Epidemiology 8:671–677, 1997

Yerevanian BI, Koek RJ, Mintz J: Lithium, anticonvulsants and suicidal behavior in bipolar disorder. J Affect Disord 73:223–228, 2003

Yerevanian BI, Koek RJ, Mintz J: Bipolar pharmacotherapy and suicidal behavior. Part I: lithum, divalproex and carbamazepine. J Affect Disord 103:5–11, 2007

Yudofsky SC: Fatal Flaws: Navigating Destructive Relationships With People With Disorders of Personality and Character. Washington, DC, American Psychiatric Publishing, 2005

C H A P T E R   1 3

Cognitive Therapy for Suicide Prevention

Gregory K. Brown, Ph.D.

Jesse H. Wright, M.D., Ph.D.

Michael E. Thase, M.D.

Aaron T. Beck, M.D.

Cognitive Therapy for Suicide Prevention (CT-SP) is a type of psychotherapy that is based primarily on the assumption that individuals who are suicidal or who attempt suicide lack specific cognitive or behavioral skills for coping effectively with suicidal crises (Wenzel et al. 2009). CT-SP targets suicidal ideation and behavior directly rather than focusing on the treatment of other psychiatric disorders that include suicide behavior as a symptom. Although there are many motivations and distal risk factors for suicide, the principal aim of this treatment is first to identify the specific triggers and proximal risk factors that occur during a suicidal crisis and then to identify specific coping and problem-solving skills that could be used to help individuals survive future crises. CT-SP is similar to Cognitive Therapy (CT) that was developed specifically for the treatment

of depression (A.T. Beck et al. 1979). Like CT for depression, CT-SP is based on the cognitive model, which posits that individuals who experience negative mood states also experience negative automatic thoughts and engage in unhelpful behaviors. Given that individuals who die by suicide were likely to report a higher level of hopelessness and suicidal thinking than those who die for other reasons (A.T. Beck et al. 1990; Brown et al. 2000), CT-SP focuses on helping patients to learn specific skills for mitigating hopelessness and suicide risk.

CT-SP is recognized as one of the few evidence-based psychotherapy interventions specifically for suicide prevention (Mann et al. 2005). Another evidence-based psychotherapy for suicide prevention, dialectical behavior therapy (DBT), has also been shown to prevent suicide attempts

(Linehan et al. 2006). DBT is similar to CT-SP in that both treatments focus on preventing suicidal behavior by teaching high-risk patients specific skills. CT-SP has been found to be efficacious for preventing suicide attempts as well as for decreasing other risk factors for suicide, such as depression and hopelessness. In a study by Brown and colleagues (2005), patients who made a recent suicide attempt and who were evaluated at a medical or psychiatric emergency department (ED) were recruited for participation. In addition to making a suicide attempt within 48 hours of being evaluated at the ED, participants must have met the following inclusion criteria: 1) 16 years of age or older, 2) English speaking, 3) able to complete a baseline assessment, 4) able to provide at least two verifiable contacts to improve tracking for subsequent assessments, and 5) able to understand and provide informed consent. Potential participants were excluded if they had a medical disorder that would prevent participation in an outpatient clinical trial.

After a baseline research assessment was completed, participants were randomly assigned to receive CT-SP or not to receive this treatment (control group). Patients who were assigned to the CT-SP condition were scheduled to receive approximately 10 outpatient, individual therapy sessions. Patients who were assigned to either study condition were allowed to receive usual care as provided in the community as well as treatment referral and engagement services that were provided by a study case manager. The sample consisted of 120 participants whose ages ranged from 18 to 66 years and 61% of whom were female. At baseline, 92% were diagnosed with major depressive disorder, 68% were diagnosed with a substance use disorder, and 85% had more than one psychiatric disorder. The

majority of patients (58%) had attempted suicide by overdosing with prescription, over-the-counter, or illicit substances. Other methods of varying lethality that were used included cutting oneself (17%); jumping (7%); and hanging, shooting, or drowning (4%).

This study found that 24% of the individuals who received CT-SP, compared with 42% of the individuals who received only usual care, made another suicide attempt during an 18-month follow-up period. Thus, patients who received CT-SP were approximately 50% less likely to make a repeat suicide attempt during the follow-up period than those who did not receive CT-SP. Additionally, patients who received CT-SP also were significantly less depressed and hopeless than patients who received only usual care over the course of the follow-up period. Post hoc analyses indicated that patients who received CT-SP had lower scores on the Beck Depression Inventory at the 6-, 12-, and 18-month follow-up periods and significantly lower scores on the Beck Hopelessness Scale at the 6-month follow-up period than patients who received only usual care (Brown et al. 2005). This study supported the conclusion that cognitive therapy was efficacious for preventing suicide attempts and that the effect was above and beyond that of the case management services that were provided.

In this chapter, we provide an overview of the most important aspects of the intervention used during the clinical trial. We describe each of the major phases of cognitive therapy specifically adapted for preventing suicide: 1) early phase of treatment, 2) cognitive case conceptualization and treatment planning, 3) middle phase of treatment, and 4) later phase of treatment. A full description of CT-SP is available elsewhere (Wenzel et al. 2009).

Early Phase of Treatment

The early phase of treatment is the most crucial component of CT-SP, given that patients who are evaluated in acute care settings and who recently attempted suicide or experienced acute suicidal ideation are the most vulnerable to dropping out of outpatient treatment as well as making another suicide attempt. The principal aims of the early phase of CT-SP are 1) to explain CT-SP and obtain consent, 2) to develop a commitment to treatment, 3) to conduct a comprehensive suicide risk assessment, 4) to develop a safety plan, and 5) to develop hopefulness and reasons for living.

Explaining CT-SP and Obtaining Consent

Providing patients with specific information about the structure and process of CT-SP, the limits of privacy and confidentiality, and the potential risks and benefits of treatment is especially important with suicidal patients (Rudd et al. 2009). Educating patients about these issues and then giving them the opportunity to ask questions is critical, given suicidal patients' propensity to feel hopeless about treatment or to drop out of treatment altogether (see, e.g., Berk et al. 2004; Kreitman 1979; Morgan et al. 1975; O'Brien et al. 1987).

In describing the details of the format and structure of CT-SP, the therapist may outline the CT session structure, including conducting a mood check, assessing clinical symptoms (including suicidal ideation and behavior), providing a summary of the previous session, setting a prioritized agenda, providing a summary of the current session, collaborating on a self-help assignment, and obtaining feedback regarding the helpfulness of the session. After explaining the basic elements of CT-SP, the therapist then asks for the patient's consent to be treated with this form of therapy. A crucial task of the consent process is to obtain an explicit commitment to treatment, including the patient's agreement to consistently attend and participate in the sessions, to work toward achieving the treatment goals, to complete homework assignments, and to actively participate in other aspects of treatment in order to better manage his or her suicidal crises. In our experience, using these methods to increase patients' motivation for treatment also will help to decrease the likelihood that they will drop out treatment.

Developing a Commitment to Treatment

Suicidal patients often have a poor treatment history or feel hopeless that (any) treatment will be helpful to them. One set of strategies for addressing these concerns involves listening closely to patients' descriptions of their previous experiences in treatment and assessing the degree to which any negative treatment experience contributes to a negative attitude toward the current treatment. Giving patients the opportunity to describe the helpful and unhelpful aspects of prior treatments allows clinicians to tailor the CT-SP intervention by emphasizing specific aspects of the intervention that are likely to increase treatment effectiveness. For example, perhaps a patient did not find previous therapy helpful because specific reasons for living or practical skills for managing crises were never discussed. Such issues would then be emphasized in the current treatment.

An additional strategy for enhancing motivation for treatment is to emphasize that CT-SP specifically focuses on preventing suicide. In this regard, the therapist may ask patients to refrain from acting on their suicidal urges and to fully engage in the treatment process for a given number of sessions. The idea is to have patients fully commit to treatment for a limited period of time while they are learning specific coping skills and to make an explicit agreement to refrain from attempting suicide while they are learning these skills. Patients are informed that after they complete the agreed-on number of sessions, the therapist and patients will evaluate whether treatment was helpful for them. Patients are also told that if therapy is to be successful, it is important that they commit to the treatment process fully by attending a reasonable number of sessions and engaging in any self-help assignments before concluding that CT-SP will not be helpful to them.

It is essential that when working with suicidal patients, clinicians also reach out and contact patients, especially with regard to attending treatment sessions. Specifically, we have found that maintaining frequent contact with patients by making reminder telephone calls, as well as by sending reminder and nondemanding letters, helps minimize dropping out of treatment. Assisting patients by helping them to problem solve any practical or psychological barriers to treatment will also help to increase attendance. In this regard, therapists who work with high-risk patients are encouraged to be more flexible in how treatment is provided. For example, telephone sessions could be arranged, especially when patients are in crisis or when they are unable to attend treatment sessions.

One of the problems that is often encountered by clinicians who work with high-risk patients involves feeling overwhelmed or even hopeless about successfully treating the patient. This problem may arise when the therapist is working with patients who have chronic or reoccurring episodes of suicidal ideation or who make repeated suicide attempts or intentionally injure themselves. Therapists who hold such negative beliefs about treatment or who feel hopeless about helping their patients need to be keenly aware of these thoughts and seek consultation from a trusted colleague or supervisor when they occur. If we, as therapists, have no hope for helping our patients, then how can we expect that patients will have hope about being helped?

In our clinical trial, we used a "team approach" for providing treatment. In this context, treatment teams typically consisted of therapists, supervisors, and case managers. In our experience, therapists found the treatment team approach useful for solving difficulties encountered during treatment and for maintaining hopefulness about their patients. Therapists also found the study case managers to be especially helpful, since they assisted the therapists in maintaining contact with patients, reminding patients about their appointments, providing referrals for mental health and social services, and serving as a second supportive contact person (Brown et al. 2005). Most importantly, case managers assisted clinicians when they experienced problematic feelings by offering support or by interacting with patients to build a sense of hope about the treatment. All of these activities, such as calling and sending reminders, allowing for flexible scheduling, and utilizing case management services, help to convey to patients that there are clinicians who genuinely care about their well-being and who are concerned about building a sense of commitment to the treatment process. In a clinical setting that does not have a treatment team with case managers, we recommend that the therapist make the contact with patients as described above by himself or herself or work with office staff (if available) to maintain close contact with high-risk patients and promote session attendance.

Conducting a Comprehensive Suicide Risk Assessment

During the early phase of treatment, a comprehensive psychological assessment should be conducted that includes 1) gathering information to formulate current psychiatric diagnoses, 2) obtaining detailed histories of previous psychiatric and addiction treatment, 3) obtaining a medical and psychosocial history, and 4) conducting a mental status examination (Wenzel et al. 2009). Because suicidal individuals constitute a high-risk population, it is essential that clinicians conduct a comprehensive suicide risk assessment at the beginning of treatment as well as briefer assessments of suicide risk at each subsequent session. A comprehensive suicide risk assessment includes direct questioning about patients' current mental status, administration of self-report measures, review of medical records, and clinical observation of patients' behavior (American Psychiatric Association 2003; see Chapter 1, "Suicide Risk Assessment: Gateway to Treatment and Management," in this volume). Often the comprehensive risk assessment is conducted because it assists the clinician in determining the most appropriate level of care so that patients remain safe. However, this assessment is also important in outpatient treatment because it provides for the opportunity to identify possible risk factors, such as hopelessness, that have the potential to be modifiable with treatment.

In addition to identifying specific risk and protective factors during the risk assess-ment, clinicians should elicit further information about the specific characteristics of the most recent suicidal crisis to help identify helpful strategies to mitigate suicide risk (see Chapter 2, "The Interpersonal Art of Suicide Assessment: Interviewing Techniques for Uncovering Suicidal Intent, Ideation, and Actions" and Chapter 3, "The Clinical Risk Assessment Interview," in this volume). To assess these characteristics, clinicians should ask patients to "tell their story" of their most recent suicidal crisis. Obtaining this narrative information serves several aims that are relevant to this treatment. First, the narrative informs the suicide risk assessment by focusing on the risk and protective factors that were most proximal to the recent suicidal crisis. Second, having patients describe the sequence of events that led to the crisis helps them to feel understood by the clinician, which is vital for developing a strong therapeutic alliance. Third, the narrative information can be very useful for developing a case conceptualization of the proximal risk factors that are associated with the occurrence of a suicidal crisis, as well as for identifying those factors that may be modifiable using CT-SP.

When patients tell their story, there are several specific points during the narrative that should be a focus of the interview. Initially, most patients describe their crisis as beginning following a stressful event or situation. For example, patients may report that they began to feel suicidal following an intense argument with their partner. Patients may describe the events that occurred in detail but typically do not describe their reactions to those events. These reactions may include specific thoughts, feelings, or behaviors that occurred during the crisis. The role of the CT-SP therapist is to identify and understand the activating events as well as the patients' reactions to these events. For patients who attempted suicide, a critical point occurred at the moment that the patients had intent to end their lives. When focusing on this moment, clinicians should help patients to identify the automatic thoughts that occurred prior to this decision. Automatic thoughts are usually quick, evaluative thoughts that patients often do not recognize when they occur during an intense mood shift (A.T. Beck et al. 1979). According to the cognitive model, automatic thoughts mediate emotional and behavioral distress and are targets of the CT-SP intervention. Teaching patients to ask themselves the question "What was going through my mind?" during the point at which they were most distressed facilitates patients' awareness of these suicide-related cognitions. For example, many patients have reported thoughts of helplessness or hopelessness, such as "I can't take it anymore," during these moments. At this point, therapists should also assist patients in identifying the corresponding emotion(s), such as despair, sadness, or fear. It is important that patients learn to differentiate their thoughts from their feelings, because this skill is required for cognitive restructuring strategies. More importantly, a clear understanding of the thoughts, feelings, and behaviors that were present during the suicidal crisis is essential for developing an accurate conceptualization of the suicidal crisis that can be used to guide selection of the most helpful cognitive and behavioral strategies to prevent future crises.

In addition to identifying the thoughts, feelings, and behaviors that precede the crisis, therapists should identify patients' reactions to the attempt as well as the reactions of others to the attempt. The reaction of regret that the suicide attempt did not result in death has been found to increase the risk for suicide (Henriques et al. 2005),

and such regret should be taken into account when evaluating suicide risk.

While patients are telling their stories, it is recommended that therapists not challenge the accuracy or reasonableness of the story, attempt to engage in problem solving to mitigate the crisis, or give advice on how to better cope with the crisis. Rather, therapists should carefully listen to patients as they describe their "stories" and provide empathic statements. This therapeutic approach will assist patients to feel understood and will facilitate a more detailed account of the suicidal crisis. Offering suggestions for dealing with the crisis may lead some patients to be reluctant to describe the crisis fully, or even to drop out of treatment, because they do not feel understood. Another common reason that patients may be reluctant to fully describe a crisis involves the fear of reexperiencing negative emotions or thoughts. In such cases, therapists should solicit feedback throughout the interview. Therapists may need to directly address unpleasant feelings that are likely to occur during the session and discuss potential solutions for handling these feelings, such as letting the therapist know about the feelings or taking a break from talking about the crisis. Such a therapeutic approach communicates to patients that the therapist understands their difficulties when discussing sensitive topics.

Developing a Safety Plan

Following the suicide risk assessment, the clinician works with the patient early in treatment to develop a safety plan to assist in reducing suicide risk. It is crucial that the therapist conduct an intervention to specifically prevent suicide during the first session of treatment because patients who recently attempted suicide are most vulnerable to subsequent attempts shortly after an attempt. The safety plan is a written list of prioritized coping strategies that patients agree to implement and resources that patients agree to use during a suicidal crisis (Stanley and Brown 2012). Given that it is often difficult for patients to use problem-solving skills during a time of crisis, the purpose of the safety plan is to develop a set of coping strategies while they are not in crisis so that these strategies will be readily available to prevent suicide. The basic components of the Safety Plan are as follows:

1. Recognizing warning signs that precede the suicidal crisis.
2. Identifying coping strategies that can serve as a distraction and that can be used without contacting another person.
3. Identifying people or social settings that serve as a distraction from the crisis.
4. Contacting friends or family members for help with the crisis.
5. Contacting mental health professionals or agencies.
6. Removing access to lethal means.

One of the most important features of the safety plan is to identify clear and specific warning signs of an impending crisis that can serve as cues for patients to retrieve and follow their written safety plan. Patients are coached to follow each step on their safety plan until the crisis is resolved. If the first strategy does not alleviate the crisis or reduce the level of ideation, patients should proceed to the next step(s) on the plan until the crisis is resolved.

Many of the steps in the safety plan may be derived from the crisis that the patient previously described. For example, the warning signs that were identified in the narrative could be written down in the safety plan. Therapists then work with patients in a collaborative manner to identify those activities that are going to be the most distracting to them during a crisis. Such coping strategies should have the potential to be used without involving another person. Here, it is important to convey to patients that they may use a skill to survive (and potentially resolve) a crisis on their own. Patients should be asked about specific distracting activities that they have used in the past that do not place them at increased risk. Working together as a team, the therapist and patient can ascertain whether such strategies are realistic or useful and whether the patient would be likely to employ them during a crisis, and can address any barriers to implementing them.

Another key feature of the safety plan is an explicit discussion about making the environment safe. Sometimes patients are reluctant to limit their access to lethal means such as firearms because they perceive that having a lethal method readily available is one way of coping with extreme distress. However, patients may be more cooperative in limiting their access to such methods when they are provided with other specific techniques for dealing with such distress. Given that death by firearm is a common method of suicide, it is preferable that all guns and ammunition be removed and stored in a place that is not accessible to patients (Simon 2007). However, asking patients to remove the firearm themselves and turn it over to a family member is problematic because patients' risk for suicide will increase further when they have direct contact with the firearm. Instead, an optimal plan would be to have the firearm removed from the patient's possession by a designated responsible person—usually a family member or trusted friend (Simon 2007). We have found that the best safety plans use the patients' own words and are located where they are readily available, such as in a wallet, purse, cell phone, desk drawer, or glove compartment. During CT-SP, the safety plan is revised throughout treatment as new skills are learned or as the social or health care network is expanded.

The safety plan intervention has also been used as a stand-alone intervention, independent of CT-SP. It has been widely used in acute care settings, such as psychiatric inpatient units, crisis lines, and ED settings, and has become a standard of care for veterans who are identified as being at high risk for suicide (Stanley and Brown 2008). The safety plan intervention has been included in the Best Practices Registry by the Suicide Prevention Resource Center and the American Foundation for Suicide Prevention.

Developing Hopefulness and Reasons for Living

Although building hope is an important characteristic of all approaches to treatment, it is essential that suicide prevention strategies specifically target hopelessness, because it is a significant predictor of suicide (Brown et al. 2000). One method that assists patients in developing hope is to discuss their reasons for living and their reasons for dying (Jobes 2006). This process is initiated in the early phase of treatment, and a list of reasons to live is often an important part of the safety plan developed at the beginning of CT-SP. As therapy progresses, the list of reasons for living can be expanded and strengthened.

Together, the patient and clinician identify and review the patient's reasons for dying, which should be written down so that the patient can reflect on them. After these reasons have been discussed and the patient feels understood, the therapist would then ask about the patient's reasons

for living. Often, when beginning this exercise, patients are unable to generate many reasons for living, given their recent suicidal crisis. However, in most cases patients can identify at least a few possible reasons (e.g., "I don't want to hurt my children," "I'd like to see grandchildren someday," "I'd like to finish school"). If any reasons are identified, the therapist can ask Socratic questions to draw out and amplify the reasons to live.

Typically, patients who are depressed and who are in a suicidal crisis have intensely negative and dysfunctional cognitions about their reasons to live. They may minimize their value to others (e.g., "My children would be better off with another mother... They would forget me and move on") or ignore evidence that life could be better for them in the future (e.g., "I'll never be happy...I'll never be able to live with the shame of what happened...I'll never get another job"). These types of dysfunctional cognitions can provide excellent opportunities for change as therapists work with patients to develop a rational and fully realized list of reasons to live. By questioning such dysfunctional conclusions, using methods such as examining the evidence and exploring alternative viewpoints, therapists can help patients move toward a life-sustaining conceptualization of truly meaningful reasons to live now and into the future.

In cases where a patient cannot identify reasons to live or has a very limited response to this question, the therapist may need to give prompts or hints that may uncover some important reasons to live that have been obscured by depression or substance abuse. For example, the therapist could ask about important people in the patient's life and how the patient's death might affect these people. Inquiries could be made about activities that the patient used to enjoy or that brought him or her a sense of mastery or accomplishment. Another strategy is to ask patients about reasons they might have had to live before they became depressed or how they might see things differently if the depression or current life problem was resolved.

The reasons for living are written down, and the clinician asks the patient to reflect upon both the reasons for living and the reasons for dying. Homework assignments to expand or develop more detail in the list of reasons for living are commonly suggested for patients in CT-SP. The clinician and patient may also agree to include the most important reasons for living on their safety plan to remind the patient of these reasons during a suicidal crisis.

Cognitive Case Conceptualization and Treatment Planning

As previously discussed, an important component of CT that begins in the early phase of treatment is the cognitive case conceptualization (J.S. Beck 1995), which involves identification of specific events, automatic thoughts, and beliefs that were activated during the suicidal crisis (for a more detailed description of this approach, see Wenzel et al. 2009). The cognitive case conceptualization will be modified throughout the course of treatment as more information emerges; however, the information that is revealed when patients describe their crisis provides the foundation of the case conceptualization as early as the first session. Not only does the conceptualization characterize the automatic thoughts and beliefs that are directly relevant to suicidal behavior, it also incorporates early experiences, compensatory behavioral strategies, and key life events that triggered the crisis. Based on the case conceptualization, the

clinician and patient identify the relevant strategies that are most likely to help prevent an attempt.

Using the case conceptualization, the clinician and patient then identify specific treatment goals that will help to minimize suicide risk. Although the primary goal of CT-SP is to prevent a suicide attempt and/or to decrease the severity and frequency of suicidal ideation, there may be other treatment goals that can help reduce the risk for suicide. These additional goals are usually formulated in behavioral terms so that it is clear whether patients have achieved the goals. For example, patients may initially disclose that they do not feel connected to others and that this belief makes them vulnerable to feeling suicidal. Instead of just noting that the goal of treatment would be to improve the patient's perceived connectedness to others, the therapist would ask the patient, "How would you or others be able to recognize that you were more connected? What would you be doing differently?" This line of questioning would then lead the patient to formulate this particular goal in more behavioral terms, such as spending a specific number of hours per week doing a social activity with another specific person. It is acknowledged from the beginning of treatment that CT-SP is short-term and time-limited, which contrasts with the complex, usually chronic difficulties experienced by the patient. Thus, clinician and patient collaboratively prioritize the problems and develop a framework for addressing them.

Middle Phase of Treatment

The middle phase of treatment consists of developing specific skills to manage suicidal thoughts and behaviors, which are guided by the patient's individualized cognitive case conceptualization. During the middle phase, the clinician follows the same general session structure as previously described. This includes a brief assessment of the patient's suicidal ideation and behavior during each session. Any change in suicide risk status would prompt a more detailed risk assessment. Methods used in the middle phase of treatment include the application of cognitive and behavioral strategies. In addition, treatment focuses on increasing compliance with adjunctive medical, substance abuse, psychiatric, and social interventions. Although CT-SP includes many strategies that we will not be able to describe here because of space limitations (see Wenzel et al. 2009), some of the more commonly used cognitive and behavioral strategies are discussed in the following subsections.

Cognitive Strategies

Clinicians assist patients in developing skills to identify negative thoughts and core beliefs and in helping patients understand the manner in which these cognitions affect their feelings and behavior. Through the use of cognitive restructuring, patients begin to understand the core beliefs that were active at the time of the suicidal crisis by examining recurrent themes in their automatic thoughts and by exploring early memories and experiences related to their viewpoints of themselves or others (Wenzel et al. 2009). For example, patients may have the recurring thought that they "cannot take it anymore" when they experience distress and observe that this thought is followed by thoughts of suicide. The therapist would assist the patient in recognizing the core beliefs that underlie such thoughts by asking, "What does that mean, that you 'cannot take it anymore'?" The patient might

then respond, for example, that he or she was defective in some way and, upon further discussion with the therapist, recognize that this core belief about being defective began in childhood when the patient was verbally abused by the father.

Once patients are able to identify the key automatic thoughts and associated beliefs that are most associated with suicidal crises, there are several strategies that they can use to develop more adaptive ways of thinking, especially during a suicidal crisis. Success with these tasks often strengthens the therapeutic relationship, as patients develop confidence that their distress can be mitigated and that the clinician has helpful tools to offer them.

Putting Together a Hope Kit

The Hope Kit is a concrete memory aid to be used in times of crisis that utilizes patients' resourcefulness and creativity. The Hope Kit is a collection of items that reminds patients of reasons to live during suicidal crises. Patients should review the reasons for living that were listed during the initial phase prior to constructing a Hope Kit. Patients may then locate something as simple as a shoebox, envelope, or scrapbook where they can store mementos such as pictures, postcards, letters, and inspirational or religious sayings or poems (Wenzel et al. 2009). The Hope Kit can be adapted for teenagers by including pictures, stories, texts, or music that remind them of reasons for living on a Web page or on a cellular phone. We have found that this exercise is quite enjoyable for patients and is one of the most meaningful strategies learned in therapy to address their suicidal thoughts and behaviors. Moreover, during the course of constructing a Hope Kit, patients often find that they are able to identify reasons for living that they had previously overlooked.

Using Coping Cards

Another simple cognitive strategy that embodies these principles is to develop coping cards (Wenzel et al. 2009). Coping cards contain adaptive coping statements that patients can review during a time of distress. We have found that coping cards are most likely to be located and used when they are developed during the session and then laminated.

There are several types of coping cards that can be used in this intervention. For example, patients could list a suicide-relevant thought or belief on one side of the card, such as "I can't take it anymore." The other side of the coping card would contain a more balanced or adaptive statement, such as "I know that I experience some periods of time that I find very difficult, but I know that these feelings do not last for a long time and that I have been able to recover from them in the past on my own." Other types of coping cards might contain statements that motivate patients to take specific steps toward reaching specific goals that prompt them to practice adaptive coping skills and that list their reasons for living or positive self-affirmations.

Some patients find that completing thought records may also be a very helpful cognitive restructuring activity (J.S. Beck 1995). In CT, thought records are a commonly used intervention that involves patients noting the situation, emotion, and automatic thought and examining the evidence in order to generate an adaptive response and noting the outcome of using the adaptive response. Although thought records are very effective for helping patients modify their negative thinking, they are more difficult to complete during a time of crisis because of the level of concentration and effort that is required for this task. An advantage of developing laminated coping cards is that they may be more likely to be used during a crisis period.

Developing Problem-Solving Skills

Helping patients improve their problem-solving skills for managing suicidal crises is a hallmark of CT (A.T. Beck et al. 1979). Using a collaborative approach, the clinician and patient identify problems that may increase the patient's vulnerability to suicide, prioritize the problems, and then establish a behavioral goal for each problem (Wenzel et al. 2009).

When addressing specific problems, the clinician helps the patient brainstorm as many potential solutions as possible without weighing the costs or benefits of each solution. After patient and therapist list as many potential solutions as possible, the therapist may encourage the patient to examine the advantages and disadvantages or the pros and cons for each of the proposed solutions. Patients should be asked to consider both the short- and long-term consequences of the potential solutions and the manner in which their proposed decisions would affect the lives of others and themselves. After weighing the pros and cons, the patient chooses the best solution. Next, therapist and patient identify specific tasks that can be reasonably accomplished for the chosen solution. A useful homework assignment may be to anticipate and plan for difficulties in carrying out the tasks by identifying any barriers or challenges to accomplishing the tasks as well as any solutions to potential problems (Wenzel et al. 2009).

Behavioral Strategies

Increasing Social Support

Suicidal patients often have the belief that they are alone or that they have no emotional support (Fridell et al. 1996). Thus, helping patients to have increased contact with others in their natural social network is a key component of this intervention. For some patients, this simply means turning their attention toward the people who are most caring in their lives and who would be glad to help if only the patient would be more forthcoming and responsive. For other patients, it may be necessary to build a support system. Clinicians may help patients to do this by first identifying others who are already in the patients' support network or people that the patients may see on a regular basis. Patients can be urged to contact old friends, neighbors, or members of their church and to access other community resources.

A useful homework assignment involves asking patients to make a list of individuals who already are or could be part of their support system. Patients can then be encouraged to use a calendar or activity schedule to schedule as many positive social activities as possible with individuals on their list. When patients are scheduling such activities, it is important that they understand the rationale for increasing social activities and identify whether they think it would be helpful for them. Additionally, it is useful to obtain patients' feedback about whether the activity is reasonable for them and the degree to which they think they could engage in the activity. Any barriers or challenges to completing such activities would also be reviewed, and a firm commitment to complete the activity should be obtained if possible.

We have noted that patients who attempt suicide typically underutilize their family re-sources. For example, patients who have attempted suicide often report that "no one cares" and that "I am all alone." Upon questioning, however, many patients have family members who, in fact, do care and are willing to make efforts to be more involved in the patients' lives. These family members may have given up on trying to help the patient because they are overwhelmed by their own sense of helplessness or because repeated efforts are not reciprocated or acknowledged. Thus, one method that we have found helpful to mobilize patients' family resources is to devote one or two sessions to a family session with the patient. The family meeting helps the clinician to determine whether a patient's belief that he or she is alone is accurate or largely a distortion (Wenzel et al. 2009). The session can also be helpful to educate family members about what to do if the patient becomes suicidal by reviewing the patient's safety plan with them. Family sessions should be scheduled only with the patient's permission and only if the patient and therapist believe that such meetings would be helpful.

Increasing Adherence to Adjunctive Treatments

Patients who are at high risk for suicide often face a number of psychiatric, substance abuse, and physical health problems as well as social and economic problems. Although such problems may or may not be the reason for the recent suicidal crisis, it is likely that patients may benefit from a range of psychiatric, substance abuse, medical or social services.

Suicidal patients may also seek services from EDs and then are referred for outpatient care after they are discharged from the hospital. However, rates of adherence to pharmacotherapy for depression and other psychiatric problems and use of medical and social services among discharged patients who have attempted suicide are often quite low (Kreitman 1979; Morgan et al. 1975; O'Brien et al. 1987).

In many cases, the need for medical and social services is urgent. For example, patients with a serious chronic health problem may require referral for specialist treatment, patients who abuse substances may require referral to addiction counseling, and unemployed or homeless patients may require referral to a social worker for housing or vocational services. In each of these cases, the problems (unemployment, homelessness, and substance use) are often proximal risk factors for suicide. Increasing patients' utilization of appropriate medical and social services should be an integral part of any suicide prevention treatment.

The clinician and patient should collaboratively establish goals regarding adherence to adjunctive medical, psychiatric, substance abuse treatments and social services. Given that suicidal patients may have a history of past and current adherence problems, it is recommended that clinicians play a greater role in monitoring their adherence with other treatments than with nonsuicidal patients. For example, an early intervention can be either providing information about the problem and its treatment or problem solving with the patient how he or she can obtain more information about the problem and its treatment.

Methods for enhancing medication adherence can include eliciting and modifying dysfunctional automatic thoughts and beliefs about medication use and a range of helpful behavioral strategies for making medication regimens a routine part of daily activities (Wright et al. 2010). Clinicians also may use graded-task assignments to help patients achieve ultimate goals, such as finding employment or housing. In these cases, the clinician would use a step-by-step ap-proach and develop specific goals that could then be easily completed by the patient within a short period of time (Wenzel et al. 2009).

Later Phase of Treatment

When the clinician believes that the patient has made significant gains in therapy and has significantly reduced suicide risk, a formal assessment of the cognitive and behavioral skills that the patient has learned during treatment is indicated. To do this, a relapse prevention task is introduced in which patients have an opportunity to actively demonstrate that they are able to implement the skills developed throughout the course of treatment. Other key elements of the later phase of treatment are efforts to consolidate skills and maintain treatment gains (Wenzel et al. 2009).

Consolidation of Skills

A couple of weeks before termination, clinicians should ask patients to read through and organize any notes that they have taken so they can easily refer to them in the future. If patients have not taken notes throughout the sessions, they might focus on making a therapy notebook or Hope Kit during the last few sessions. The clinician and patient can review and summarize the important points of therapy. Sometimes patients will resist writing or may not be able to write. In this case, the clinician can provide a written summary of the skills the patient has learned, because it is helpful for the patient to have a written record of the salient points from therapy that can be used in the future.

Relapse Prevention Task

Following the consolidation of specific skills, the therapist uses this information to work on preventing relapse (or a suicide attempt). The relapse prevention task consists of several guided-imagery exercises in which the patient imagines past suicide crises as well as crises that may occur in the future. The primary aim of this intervention is to have the patient describe in detail how he or she would cope with similar crises. This provides the patient with an opportunity to practice his or her suicide-management skills in a safe environment before applying them in a state of distress. It also facilitates "overlearning" of a specific skill so that the patient remembers to use it during a crisis. This task also serves as an assessment of treatment progress and of whether termination is appropriate (Wenzel et al. 2009). If the patient has difficulty successfully completing the relapse prevention task, the clinician understands that more work needs to be done in therapy and termination is delayed.

Prior to conducting the relapse prevention task, the clinician must prepare patients to experience memories and aversive emotions. First, the clinician obtains consent from patients to conduct the task. Patients are advised that this task has the potential to elicit negative feelings but that the clinician will guide them through the activity and assist them in resolving such emotions by the end of the session. In addition, it is important to provide a sound rationale for this task in order to motivate patients to actively engage in this potentially aversive procedure. Patients are informed that by imagining the suicidal crisis and reliving the emotional turmoil that they experienced, they will assess whether they can implement the coping strategies discussed in therapy. After a discussion of the risks and benefits of completing this task, some patients may prefer not to do it. In this case, the patients' preference is respected, but the clinician may review with patients the coping skills the patients have learned as previously described and the manner in which they might apply them in the future.

During the relapse prevention task, the clinician uses guided imagery to help patients imagine in detail the events leading up to the suicidal crisis. Patients are encouraged to close their eyes and describe the sequences of events out loud to the clinician and attempt to reexperience the emotions and thoughts that occurred at the time of the crisis. At the completion of this exercise, the clinician again leads patients through a similar task but this time encourages them to describe how they will use the CT skills to cope with the event in order to mitigate suicide risk. Next, patients are instructed to imagine in detail a future suicidal crisis and outline the manner in which they would apply the skills learned in treatment to cope with any suicidal ideation that is activated. After completing these guided imagery exercises, the clinician debriefs the patient, commending him or her for successfully engaging in such a difficult activity, and obtains feedback on whether that task was helpful. If suicidal ideation emerged during the task, the clinician assesses for suicide risk and uses the strategies presented in this chapter to address it (e.g., reviewing the safety plan). The clinician also poses additional crisis scenarios to ensure that patients have adequate flexibility in applying the skills learned in treatment to specific situations. In addition, we have found that new information about the suicidal crisis is often revealed during this task. It is possible that the patient feels more secure in revealing such information near the end of treatment, after a strong therapeutic alliance has been established.

Maintenance of Treatment Gains

Patients who attempt suicide are very vulnerable to relapse of their suicidal ideation and behavior as well as their psychiatric disorder(s) because they often face multiple chronic stressors, such as financial problems, housing problems, drug and alcohol problems, unstable relationships, and lack of social support. Although the high rate of chronic stressors may increase the likelihood of a relapse of a psychiatric disorder, the primary aim of CT-SP is to reduce the likelihood of another suicide attempt in spite of such a setback. When the clinician and patient have determined that the patient will be able to utilize his or her new skills to prevent or cope effectively with future suicidal crises, then they may prepare for termination. After treatment goals have been attained, therapy is gradually tapered, on a trial basis, to once every 2 weeks and then to once per month. In addition, "booster" sessions may be scheduled for several months after termination to allow for evaluation of the patient's suicide risk and review of coping skills, including the safety plan.

The clinician needs to assess the patient's expectations for what is considered to be satisfactory maintenance of his or her progress and prepare the patient for mood fluc-

tuations and setbacks. The clinician must caution the patient against "catastrophic" and "all-or-none" thinking if the patient experiences a setback or relapse of his or her symptoms. The therapist may alert the patient to avoid making conclusions about the degree of success of the treatment (e.g., "therapy didn't work") when the patient experiences setbacks.

When the therapist is discussing tapering or terminating treatment with a patient, it is crucial to obtain the patient's feedback, especially given that suicidal patients may have a limited social network and have become accustomed to relying on the therapists for emotional support. There are several strategies for helping patients to cope effectively with termination, including 1) weighing the advantages and disadvantages of ending treatment, 2) scheduling booster sessions, 3) coaching patients to be their own therapist using the skills that they have learned, and 4) expanding their social network. Finally, therapists should help patients to recognize specific symptoms, behaviors, or other warning signs that would serve as a cue for scheduling subsequent mental health evaluations.

Key Clinical Concepts

- Cognitive Therapy for Suicide Prevention (CT-SP) is a type of psychotherapy that has been adapted for patients at high suicide risk.

- CT-SP comprises a specific set of cognitive and behavioral interventions for suicidal behavior, derived from general principles of cognitive theory and therapy for emotional disorders. CT-SP can be applied to a wide variety of clinical problems that are associated with suicide attempts.

- CT-SP is based primarily on the assumption that individuals who are suicidal or who attempt suicide lack specific cognitive or behavioral skills for coping effectively with suicidal crises. CT-SP targets suicidal ideation and behavior directly rather than focusing on the treatment of other psychiatric disorders that include suicide behavior as a symptom.

■ Innovative aspects of the intervention include the individualized cognitive case conceptualization, the safety plan, the Hope Kit, and the relapse prevention task, which directly targets suicide behavior rather than focusing on the treatment of a specific psychiatric disorder.

■ An important goal of the National Strategy for Suicide Prevention (U.S. Public Health Service 2001) is to translate evidence-based treatments into community-based settings. The strong evidence for effectiveness of the CT-SP approach, as well as the practical nature of its methods and its roots in the widely practiced and empirically supported methods of cognitive therapy, suggests that CT-SP could be used extensively in outpatient treatment to reduce the risk of suicide.

References

American Psychiatric Association: Practice Guideline for the Assessment and Treatment of Patients With Suicidal Behaviors. Arlington, VA, American Psychiatric Association, 2003

Beck AT, Rush AJ, Shaw BF, et al: Cognitive Therapy of Depression. New York, Guilford, 1979

Beck AT, Brown G, Berchick RJ, et al: Relationship between hopelessness and ultimate suicide: a replication with psychiatric outpatients. Am J Psychiatry 147:190–195, 1990

Beck JS: Cognitive Therapy: Basics and Beyond. New York, Guilford, 1995

Berk MS, Henriques GR, Warman DM, et al: A cognitive therapy intervention for suicide attempters: an overview of the treatment and case examples. Cog Behav Pract 11:265–277, 2004

Brown GK, Beck AT, Steer RA, et al: Risk factors for suicide in psychiatric outpatients: a 20-year prospective study. J Consult Clin Psychol 68:371–377, 2000

Brown GK, Tenhave T, Henriques GR, et al: Cognitive therapy for the prevention of suicide attempts: a randomized controlled trial. JAMA 294:563–570, 2005

Fridell EJ, Ojehagen A, Träskman-Bendz L: A 5-year follow-up study of suicide attempts. Acta Psychiatr Scand 93:151–157, 1996

Henriques G, Wenzel A, Brown GK, et al: Suicide attempters' reaction to survival as a risk factor for eventual suicide. Am J Psychiatry 162:2180–2182, 2005

Jobes D: Managing Suicidal Risk. New York, Guilford, 2006

Kreitman N: Reflections on the management of parasuicide. Br J Psychiatry 135:275–277, 1979

Linehan MM, Comtois KA, Murray AM, et al: Two-year randomized controlled trial and follow-up of dialectical behavior therapy vs therapy by experts for suicidal behaviors and borderline personality disorder. Arch Gen Psychiatry 63:757–766, 2006

Mann JJ, Apter A, Bertolote J, et al: Suicide prevention strategies: a systematic review. JAMA 294:2064–2074, 2005

Morgan HG, Burns-Cox CJ, Pocock H, et al: Deliberate self-harm: clinical and socioeconomic characteristics of 368 patients. Br J Psychiatry 127:564–574, 1975

O'Brien G, Holton AR, Hurren K, et al: Deliberate self-harm and predictors of out-patient attendance. Br J Psychiatry 150:246–247, 1987

Rudd MD, Joiner TE, Brown GK, et al: Informed consent with suicidal patients: rethinking risks in (and out of) treatment. Psychotherapy: Theory, Research, Practice, Traiing 46:459–468, 2009

Simon RI: Gun safety management with patients at risk for suicide. Suicide Life Threat Behav 37:518–526, 2007

Stanley B, Brown GK (with Karlin B, Kemp J, von Bergen H): Safety Plan Treatment Manual to Reduce Suicide Risk: Veteran Version. Washington, DC, U.S. Department of Veterans Affairs, 2008

Stanley B, Brown GK: Safety planning intervention: a brief intervention to mitigate suicide risk. Cognitive and Behavioral Practice 19:256–264, 2012

U.S. Public Health Service: National Strategy for Suicide Prevention: Goals and Objectives for Action. Rockville, MD, U.S. Department of Health and Human Services, 2001

Wenzel A, Brown GK, Beck AT: Cognitive Therapy for Suicidal Patients: Scientific and Clinical Applications. Washington, DC, American Psychological Association, 2009

Wright JH, Sudak D, Turkington D, et al: High-Yield Cognitive-Behavior Therapy Methods for Brief Sessions: An Illustrated Guide. Washington, DC, American Psychiatric Publishing, 2010

CHAPTER 14

Psychodynamic Treatment

Glen O. Gabbard, M.D.

Andreea L. Seritan, M.D.

Sara E. Allison, M.D.

Treatment of the suicidal patient may be likened to negotiating the perils of a mine-field—with each step, one is terrifyingly aware of the potential lethality underfoot. Because most, if not all, psychiatrists will eventually find themselves attempting to guide a patient through this terrain fraught with risk and uncertainty, a psychodynamically informed road map may be helpful to both strengthen the clinician's footing and identify hazards on the path to recovery.

Psychodynamic treatment of the suicidal patient refers not only to psychotherapy but to a broader approach to treatment in general. This conceptual model is used by the clinician to determine the most appropriate interventions designed to alter the patient's fundamental wish to die. The patient-specific psychodynamic treatment strategy is largely derived from the clinician's exploration of the patient's internal world, including unconscious conflicts, deficits and distortions of intrapsychic structures, and internal object relations (Gabbard 2005). This understanding must, of

course, be integrated with contemporary findings from the neurosciences and psychopharmacology.

Psychodynamic psychiatry, as a whole, is shaped by a number of theoretical models, including ego psychology, with its central notion of unconscious conflict; object relations theory; self psychology; and attachment theory. From the outset of each therapeutic relationship, the psychiatrist undertakes a dynamic assessment of the patient's needs and uses the findings to construct a coherent conceptual framework from which all future interventions are prescribed. The dynamic psychiatrist employs a wide range of treatment modalities, including pharmacotherapy, risk factor assessment and modification, mobilization of social support, and psychotherapy. Regardless of whether the patient's plan of care includes dynamic psychotherapy, the treatment is, by definition, *dynamically informed*.

A set of time-honored principles guides the dynamic psychiatrist's approach to the treatment of the suicidal patient. These ideological cornerstones include the beliefs that suicidality may have unconscious meanings, that the past repeats itself in the present, that unconscious motivations may lead to patient resistance, that transference to the clinician may have a major impact on the treatment, and that countertransference responses of the treater to the patient must be taken into account to avoid potential errors.

Research on Psychodynamic Therapy With Patients at Risk for Suicide

Efficacy

Although there is a good deal of research on the efficacy of dynamic psychotherapy in the treatment of complex psychiatric disorders (Leichsenring and Rabung 2008; Leichsenring et al. 2004), there is little elucidation of the direct effect this form of therapy may have on *suicidality* in major depression. Psychodynamic therapy is used in the treatment of suicidal patients in both inpatient and outpatient settings. According to a recent study, adolescents discharged from psychiatric hospitals after a suicide attempt or severe suicidal ideation attended on average eight therapy sessions, with 18% terminating treatment against therapist advice within the first 3 months (Spirito et al. 2011). The therapists surveyed in this study utilized psychodynamic, cognitive-behavioral, and family systems techniques about equally. Guthrie et al. (2001, 2003) randomly assigned 119 patients who presented to the emergency department following deliberate self-poisoning to receive either brief psychodynamic interpersonal therapy or treatment as usual (outpatient follow-up with a general practitioner). Those patients who received the therapy demonstrated a significantly greater reduction in

suicidal ideation and were less likely to report repeat self-harm attempts at 6-month follow-up compared with control subjects.

In contrast to the relative lack of empirical evidence demonstrating the efficacy of dynamic psychotherapy in the treatment of suicidality in major depression, data have shown this modality's promise in the care of those with borderline personality disorder (BPD). Research involving the treatment of BPD using a randomized controlled trial of psychodynamically based partial hospitalization (in which dynamic individual therapy and group therapy were the foundation of the program) demonstrated dramatic reductions in suicidality (Bateman and Fonagy 2001, 2003). Although 95% of the sample of 38 patients with BPD had attempted suicide in the 6 months prior to the beginning of the study, only 5.3% had made attempts in the 6 months after treatment at the investigators' 18-month follow-up. In a randomized clinical trial of 104 women with BPD treated for 1 year either with transference-focused therapy or by an experienced community psychotherapist, significantly fewer patients in the transference-focused therapy group attempted suicide, although self-harm behavior was not reduced in either group (Doering et al. 2010).

Expanding the framework to include other personality disorders, Petersen et al. (2008) examined the outcomes of 38 patients enrolled in a 5-month-long day treatment program combining psychodynamic and cognitive-behavioral therapy in group and individual settings. The intervention group showed a significant reduction in acute and prolonged hospitalizations and suicide attempts and improved social functioning as compared with 28 wait-listed patients. Chiesa et al. (2009) explored the effectiveness of a community-based psychodynamic therapy program by prospectively following for 2 years a group of 68 patients with severe personality disorders. The community-based sample improved to a significantly greater degree with regard to three clinical outcome measures (hospital admissions, self-mutilation, and suicide attempts) and had significantly lower early dropout rates as compared with 38 inpatients from a long-term residential treatment program at the same institution.

Psychodynamic Themes

Further studies have sought to delineate the psychodynamic themes relevant to suicidal patients. Kaslow et al. (1998) compared 52 inpatients following a suicide attempt with 47 inpatients with no history of suicidal behavior. Their results highlighted the importance of recent losses in the context of a history of childhood loss, a pattern found to be significantly more common in the population of suicide attempters. More impaired object relations were also demonstrated within the suicidal group as compared with the control group.

Preexisting psychological variables may increase the likelihood of acting on suicidal thoughts. Projective tests allow expression of intrapsychic conflicts and object relations schemas, even though individuals may not consciously acknowledge them. Through the use of projective psychological testing, researchers (Smith 1983; Smith and Eyman 1988) have identified four patterns of ego functioning and internal object relations paradigms that differentiate individuals who made serious attempts from those who merely made gestures to control significant others (see Table 14–1). A similar hypothesis has been formulated regarding suicidality in elderly men, highlighting the core conflict between fusion and separation wishes (Lindner 2010). Although this pattern applies more to men than to women

TABLE 14–1. Psychodynamic themes in serious suicide attempters

Conflict between fusion and separation wishes
Sober but ambivalent view toward death
Excessively high self-expectations
Overcontrol of affect, particularly aggression

Source. Adapted from Lindner 2010; Smith 1983; Smith and Eyman 1988.

(Smith and Eyman 1988), an inhibitory attitude toward aggression distinguishes serious female attempters from those who make mild gestures. Other clinicians have utilized the Rorschach and Thematic Apperception Test, in conjunction with follow-up soon after the hospitalization and 1 year later, to monitor the psychological functioning of teenagers who attempted or threatened suicide (de Kernier et al. 2010). These findings imply that the preexisting psychological structures that favor suicide are more consistent across individual patients than are the various motivations behind a particular suicidal act.

Recently, a great deal of attention has been directed toward the field of implicit cognition, which can reveal unconsciously held beliefs through the Implicit Association Test (IAT). The IAT is a brief computer-administered test that uses subjects' reaction times when classifying semantic stimuli to measure automatic mental associations on various topics (Nosek et al. 2011). In a study of 157 patients seeking treatment at a psychiatric emergency department, the implicit association of death/suicide with self was significantly stronger in individuals who presented after suicide attempts than in those seen for other reasons. Furthermore, patients who held implicit associations of death/suicide with self had a sixfold increased risk of making a suicide attempt in the next 6 months (Nock et al. 2010).

Empirical studies have consistently linked high levels of perfectionism with suicidal ideation (Beevers and Miller 2004; Blatt et al. 1995; Hamilton and Schweitzer 2000). In fact, one study (Beevers and Miller 2004) demonstrated the impact of perfectionism to be both independent of and equal in significance to hopelessness, a factor commonly regarded as the best cognitive predictor of suicidal ideation (Weishaar 1996). Moreover, high levels of perfectionism were discovered to have a negative impact on all four brief treatment strategies for depression (cognitive-behavioral therapy, interpersonal therapy, imipramine, and placebo) investigated in the National Institute of Mental Health Collaborative Study (Blatt et al. 1995).

Psychodynamic clinicians have developed a substantial literature that provides useful exploration of the varying meanings of the wish to die as well as the formidable obstacles that may be encountered as one attempts to treat the suicidal patient. Operating under the assumption that the ego could kill itself only by treating itself as an object, Freud (1917/1963) postulated that suicide results from displaced murderous impulses—destructive wishes toward an internalized object that are instead directed against the self. However, more recent studies have not supported this theory (Kaslow et al. 1998); specifically, a sample of 99 suicide attempters did not acknowledge more self-directed or externally targeted anger as compared with control subjects. After the development of the structural model (Freud 1923/1961), Freud redefined suicide as the victimization of the ego by a sadistic superego. Karl Menninger's (1933) conceptualization was a bit more complex, with a view of the suicidal act as consisting of at least three wishes—the wish to kill, the wish to be killed, and the wish to die. Object relations theorists have noted the recurrent theme of a struggle between a sadistic, persecuting internal object, dubbed the "hidden executioner" (Asch 1980), and a tormented victim who may grow to believe that the only method of escape is through the act of suicide. In other cases, aggression plays less of a role and the patient's motivation is instead fulfillment of a reunion wish (Fenichel 1945)—that is, a fantasy involving the joyous and magical rejoining with a lost loved one or a narcissistic union with a loving superego figure. When an individual's self-esteem and self-integrity depend on attachment to a lost object, suicide may seem to be the only way to restore self-cohesion. The pursuit of perfectionism or an idealized view of the self, held to rigidly despite repeated disappointments, may also lead to the belief that suicide is the only way out (Gabbard 2005).

Countertransference Pitfalls

Psychodynamic clinicians (Gabbard and Wilkinson 1994; Maltsberger and Buie 1974) have also stressed the countertransference pitfalls associated with treatment of suicidal patients, particularly those with significant Axis II pathology. Hate, rescue fantasies, and narcissistic vulnerability are among the most prominent responses. There is little doubt that intensive psychotherapy of suicidal patients stirs sadistic and murderous wishes in the therapist, a reaction noted to be the flip side of the fervent wish to rescue the patient (Chessick 1977). When the therapist assumes the role of savior or omnipotent rescuer who will go to all forms of self-sacrifice to save the patient, countertransference hate and resentment are often the unfortunate by-products. This may take the form of aversion, leading the therapist to abandon the patient in subtle ways (forgetting appointments, withdrawing emotionally), or malice, filling the therapist with impulses to respond to the patient in overtly hostile or sarcastic ways. Therapists may fear that a patient's suicide will make them look bad to their colleagues, and this recognition of the patient's power over them may breed resentment. In addition, borderline patients often realize that the therapist's narcissism is on the line when a patient is contemplating suicide. They may exploit this vulnerability by enjoying the sadistic power they wield over the therapist. The most useful principle of managing these countertransference pitfalls is prevention. By refusing to take the role of the patient's rescuer, the therapist can avoid the resentment and hatred often accompanying that role. Monitoring one's responses and the defensive postures assumed to deal with such hateful feelings is also essential in managing countertransference.

Treatment Steps

Navigation of the perilous landscape of psychodynamic treatment of the suicidal patient is best conducted in a series of deliberate, carefully placed steps (see Table 14–2).

First and foremost, a solid therapeutic alliance between the patient and clinician must be established to ensure honest communication of any suicidal threat. Second, differentiating between the *fantasy of suicide* as a means of escape and the intent to carry out the *act of suicide* is of the utmost importance and may be useful in determining whether the psychodynamic treatment will be conducted on an outpatient basis or within the safe confines of the inpatient psychiatric unit. Third, the clinician and patient must have a frank discussion about the limits of treatment. It should be made clear to patients that the therapist cannot stop the patient from committing suicide. Moreover, there must be a clear differentiation between

TABLE 14–2. Steps in the psychodynamic treatment of the suicidal patient

Establish a therapeutic alliance.

Differentiate between the fantasy and the act of suicide.

Discuss the limits of treatment.

Investigate precipitating events.

Explore fantasies of the interpersonal impact of suicide.

Establish level of suicidality present at baseline.

Monitor transference and countertransference.

the therapist's responsibilities and the patient's responsibilities within the context of the therapeutic alliance. Fourth, the therapist must investigate precipitating events that may have triggered the patient's suicidality. These stressors may provide hints about the relevant dynamic themes that inform the meaning of suicide. Exploring the patient's fantasy about the specific interpersonal impact of suicide may also be productive. In the chronically suicidal patient, a baseline level must be established so that a descent into an acute risk state can be detected. Finally, as treatment progresses, the therapist must carefully monitor both transference and countertransference. Hendin et al. (2006) interviewed therapists for 36 patients who died by suicide while receiving open-ended therapy and medication. Based on this, six potential problem areas were identified: 1) poor communication with another provider involved in the case, 2) permitting patients or relatives to control the therapy, 3) avoidance of issues related to sexuality, 4) ineffective or coercive actions resulting from the therapist's anxieties about a patient's potential suicide, 5) not recognizing the meaning of the patient's communications, and 6) untreated or undertreated symptoms. Paying close attention to these critical areas may help optimize the treatment of suicidal patients, although one cannot entirely prevent tragic outcomes.

Case Example 1: Acute Suicidality

Ms. A, a 34-year-old single female with no previous history of suicide attempts, was in psychotherapy twice a week for long-standing difficulties in romantic relationships. She came to a session one day in considerable distress. She said that the man she was dating had told her on their second date that he was not ready to commit to a relationship so soon after his recent divorce. She said he had been very considerate to her and had behaved "like a gentleman." She found herself deeply wounded by his wish to end their budding relationship. She even said that she no longer wanted to date. She said she felt hopeless about ever finding the right man. She looked at Dr. B, her therapist, and asked poignantly, "Do you think any man is ever going to want me?"

Her therapist sputtered a bit, knowing that he was on potentially perilous ground, and tried his best to respond in a helpful way: "Well, it's a hard question for me to answer with any certainty, but I definitely don't think it's hopeless like you do. You've had some very positive relationships."

Ms. A replied, "Yeah, but they never go anywhere."

Dr. B then said, attempting to reassure Ms. A, "But most relationships don't result in marriage. It doesn't mean that there aren't positive things about them."

A pause ensued, and Ms. A then told her therapist, with some hesitation: "When I was lying awake last night, I kept thinking about committing suicide. I couldn't get it out of my mind."

Dr. B was taken aback by this revelation. Unable to suppress his surprise, he expressed his frank amazement (somewhat unempathetically): "I don't understand. You've known this man for a few weeks and been on two dates with him. Is he worth committing suicide over?"

Ms. A responded: "I know it makes no sense. I can't understand why I'm reacting this intensely."

Her therapist asked what it was about him that made the loss so unbearable. Ms. A thought for a moment and said, "He just seemed like a great catch. He was caring, thoughtful, and financially well off. He's worldly, too. He's been everywhere, has a kind of class about him, and he's older and wiser than most of the men I've dated."

The therapist knew that Ms. A had lost her father when she was 10, which led the therapist to formulate in his mind the possibility that the current loss reawakened the pain and longing from the childhood loss. He posed a tentative interpretive understanding in the form of a simple observation: "Old enough to be your father."

Ms. A hesitated: "Yeah, but he's different than my father—at least the way I remember him."

"Yes, of course he's not exactly like your dad. But sometimes one loss reawakens feelings about an earlier loss," Dr. B responded.

Ms. A responded with reflectiveness this time. She noted, "There must be something like that going on. It just doesn't make sense that I'd feel this much pain over the end of our relationship. I didn't even know him that well."

The therapy then continued to explore the meaning of the precipitating event: the linkage—previously unconscious, now more conscious—between the much older romantic partner and Ms. A's father. Recognizing that the patient's hopelessness and suicidality were serious, Dr. B engaged the patient in further discussion in order to establish her potential threat to self. Although Ms. A admitted to fantasizing about suicide, she denied any specific plan or intent to carry out the act. Dr. B felt that outpatient care with frequent follow-up was most appropriate and, after discussion with the patient, recommended Ms. A begin an antidepressant medication.

This case of acute suicidality in a woman who had never considered suicide before supports the findings of Kaslow et al. (1998) that one may be at high risk if a recent loss is superimposed on a history of childhood loss. The therapist explored the meaning of the triggering event and helped the patient to understand how a previous loss was amplifying the impact of the current loss.

Case Example 2: Chronic Suicidality in Borderline Personality Disorder

Ms. G was a 23-year-old patient with BPD who was admitted to a psychiatric inpatient unit after the latest in an extensive history of suicide attempts, this time by overdose. She was then referred to Dr. H for psychotherapy. She met with Dr. H while still hospitalized. Dr. H asked Ms. G if she wanted to work on the reasons for her chronic suicidality. Ms. G said that she really did not want to work on it. She just wanted to die. Dr. H asked her why she was intent on dying. Ms. G told her that it was impossible for her to live up to her parents' expectations. She went on to say that her parents, both academics, had raised her to follow in their footsteps. Throughout her childhood, they had gone over homework assignments with her, corrected her grammar on her English papers, and helped her memorize material for her exams. She said she knew they loved her, but she could not measure up to what they thought she should be. She contrasted herself to her brother, who was a Ph.D. candidate at a prestigious university. She had graduated from college with a reasonably good grade point average but had been denied admission to the highly competitive program to which she had then applied. Hence she had started graduate school in comparative literature at what she regarded as a "mediocre university." She explained that her chronic level of suicidality had become worse when she had received a B on her first essay in a graduate course in an area of great interest to her.

Dr. H made a simple observation: "A B is a pretty decent grade."

Ms. G replied, "No it isn't. In grad school you really have to get As or you'll never get a job."

Dr. H argued a bit with her and noted, "But it's only your first paper. Most professors grade a little lower at first and expect improvement in the course of the semester."

"My professor hates me. There is no way she will ever give me an A. My parents would be so upset if they knew I was getting Bs," Ms. G insisted.

Dr. H began to note the combination of intense perfectionism and the borderline tendency to see "bad objects" everywhere. She asked, "Do you think your parents hate you, too?"

Ms. G thought for a moment and said, "Well, I know they think I'm a failure and a brat for giving up and trying to kill myself. I hate them for what they've done to me."

Dr. H observed quietly, "Well, suicide is one way to get back at them." She then went on, "They must be terribly worried about you right now."

Ms. G's face became twisted with scorn: "They couldn't care less. I think they'd be glad if I died because I'm such a pain in the ass for them."

Dr. H asked, "Is it possible that they might think differently than you imagine they do?"

Ms. G was puzzled: "What do you mean?"

Dr. H replied, "Well, you said earlier that you knew they loved you when they tried to help you with your homework as a child. I'm sure that no matter how much of a pain in the ass you have been recently, they still have feelings of love for you."

Ms. G said, "How do *you* know that?"

"I don't know for sure, but in my experience, parents rarely stop loving their kids. Has it occurred to you that they might be devastated if you killed yourself and might never get over it?"

Dr. H continued to stress this approach of helping the patient see that her parents' reaction to her suicide might be quite different than what she might have imagined. Ultimately, with the help of meetings with her parents and the social worker on the inpatient unit, she realized that she had misread her parents' attitude toward her. She told Dr. H, "I realize now that if I killed myself, I wouldn't be eliminating my pain. I'd simply be passing it on to them." Dr. H also helped her realize that she had internalized her parents' expectations so that now her perfectionism reflected her own internal expectations of what she should do. Her parents made it clear to her that they would love her "even if she was a ditchdigger."

After helping her own her perfectionism and her need to berate herself for never achieving her excessively high self-expectations, the therapist then focused on the need to mourn this tormenting and idealized view of herself and settle for more reasonable goals. Ms. G gradually began to accept that she could be a worthwhile person despite having flaws. At the same time she could see that she could achieve excellence in her writing while still being less than perfect.

The case of Ms. G illustrates a number of key principles in the psychodynamic treatment of suicidal patients. First, one must differentiate acute suicidality from the chronic baseline of suicide risk in patients with BPD. Second, as with many borderline patients, Ms. G's ability to mentalize was impaired (Bateman and Fonagy 2004a, 2004b). *Mentalization* refers to the capacity to understand that one's own and others' thinking is representational in nature and that one's own and others' behavior is motivated by internal states, such as thoughts and feelings (Fonagy 1998). Ms. G demonstrated impairment in this function because she found it difficult to imagine how the mind of her parents might be different from her own mind. Dr. H worked in therapy to help her appreciate that the impact of her suicide on her parents would be much more devastating than she thought. Similarly, the therapist helped her see that one meaning of her wish to die was that it was a way of seeking revenge against her parents. She could make them suffer and get back at them for driving her to perform at a level that met their expectations. Dr. H also helped Ms. G see that her parents' perfectionistic expectations were now internalized as her own. She had to take responsibility for them and recognize that they were so unreasonable that they led to feelings of hopelessness and a wish to die. She had to mourn her fantasized achievements to ultimately lead a more realistic existence.

Although the first two cases are examples of how psychodynamic therapy can be useful in treating suicidal patients, the following case illustrates the value of applying psychodynamic thinking when treatment becomes seriously misguided.

Case Example 3: Countertransference and Boundary Violations

Ms. X was a chronically suicidal female who came to treatment at the age of 32 with Dr. Y, an experienced female psychotherapist. Ms. X had seen three previous therapists but had "fired" all three of them for what she perceived as their failings—specifically, their inability to help her with her feelings of hopelessness and helplessness. She had struggled with romantic relationships and work for her entire adult life and had frequently felt like giving up and taking her own life. She had never actually attempted suicide, but she thought about it every day.

In her first meeting with Dr. Y, Ms. X told her that she had been a victim of multiple episodes of childhood incest perpetrated by her father and had felt like a "whore" and a "slut" ever since. She thought of herself as "damaged goods" and worried that no man would want her. She also had intense anger at her mother for not protecting her from her father. Her parents were divorced, and she had not seen her father for years. She and her mother had an intensely conflictual relationship, so she often felt that she had no familial support. Her previous psychiatrist had diagnosed her as having dysthymia with major depressive episodes periodically superimposed, or "double depression."

Dr. Y suggested that they have twice-weekly therapy sessions and also started Ms. X on paroxetine. About 4 weeks into the treatment, Ms. X told her that she was not taking the medication. Dr. Y asked her why she had stopped it. Ms. X replied, "I've had every drug in the book for depression and not a single one has helped." Dr. Y suggested that she try it anyway, because she didn't think therapy alone would be enough. Ms. X looked at Dr. Y with contempt and said, "You're not listening to me. You're treating me from a textbook instead of listening to what I need. Please hear what I'm saying. These drugs don't work with me." Dr. Y then backed off and agreed not to press the issue of medication.

The therapy continued twice a week, but Ms. X continued to feel suicidal and hopeless. At the end of the sessions, when Dr. Y said, "We have to stop now," Ms. X would seem terribly wounded, and she would often say that she was right in the middle of a story. Sometimes she would ask if she could finish. Dr. Y would reluctantly extend the hour even though she was then late for her next patient. As therapy continued, Dr. Y began to feel that her observations were not helping Ms. X, and she told her so. Ms. X gave her a piercing look and said, "Words don't help me. I need to be loved. I wasn't loved as a child, and I need someone to love me now to heal." Dr. Y replied that therapy was all about understanding and she had to convey that understanding with words. Ms. X became intensely angry and told her therapist, "You're not listening again. Words don't help me. You're just like my mother. You're more interested in yourself than you are in me. What I really need is a hug." Dr. Y felt pangs of guilt. She had wanted to provide a different parenting experience for Ms. X and didn't want to be considered a "bad mother" in the same way that the real mother was regarded by Ms. X. She reluctantly agreed to hug Ms. X. Her patient thanked her and seemed to feel better.

The patient still felt terrible, however, and she regularly asked Dr. Y for a hug. Pretty soon the hug was a regular occurrence in each session. Dr. Y felt guilty about it since she knew that hugs were not ordinarily part of psychotherapy. She also felt that she should not be extending the length of the sessions, but she feared that Ms. X would be deeply wounded if she tried to stop what she had started. She even worried that her patient would become more suicidal if she denied her the hugs; thus, she continued them.

The hugs became more prolonged and more intense. On one occasion, Dr. Y actually feared that Ms. X wouldn't let go so that the session could end. The patient frequently talked about horrific sexual episodes with her father where she felt trapped and unable to escape from him. She told her therapist that during the incestuous sexual relations with her father, she would often imagine how suicide was her only way out. She knew her mother would not rescue her, so suicide was her only option. Dr. Y felt a good deal of empathy for her dilemma, and she vowed to be a different kind of mother in her therapeutic role.

Ms. X told Dr. Y that she wanted to call her "Mom." With some hesitation, Dr. Y consented to this request, fearing that to turn her down would be devastating. She began to get calls from her patient nearly every night, usually around 10 or 11 P.M. Dr. Y felt she had to talk with her or she might kill herself. Dr. Y was feeling tormented at this point. She felt that her life was completely controlled by the patient and that she had no recourse but to continue the course she had begun.

At one point Dr. Y contacted a consultant. She confided that she felt she was in the patient's grip and that the patient would never let her go. To make matters worse, she had dramatically reduced the fee because the patient had been fired from a job, and Dr. Y felt that she was being paid a pittance to treat an extraordi-narily difficult patient. The consultant told her that she must be furious about it. Dr. Y recognized that she had been burying her rage at the patient because she was intent on being a good mother to her, and she really felt she loved her patient at some level. The consultant pointed out that it is common to hate someone you love. Dr. Y felt freed up by the consultation and realized how much she had allowed herself to be utterly controlled by the patient. She told the patient that she was no longer able to continue under the circumstances and offered a referral to a trainee in a local clinic where, after an appropriate transitional period to end her work with Dr. Y, she could continue to receive low-fee care. Ms. X was furious and told her that she felt deeply betrayed. She stomped out of the office without saying good-bye. Dr. Y later heard from the trainee at the clinic who took over the case that the patient was still coming to therapy and still had not attempted suicide.

Several lessons can be learned from this terribly misguided treatment. First, many patients who have experienced severe child abuse and neglect will approach psychotherapy with the expectation that they deserve to be compensated for their tragic past by extraordinarily special treatment on the part of the therapist (Davies and Frawley 1992). The ordinary professional boundaries of therapists' work are felt as depriving and even sadistic. Therapists may feel coerced into desperate efforts to demonstrate that they are completely different from the abusive object from the past, an approach that has been termed "disidentification with the aggressor" (Gabbard 2003). One reason this strategy fails is that the patient is searching for a "bad-enough object" (Gabbard 2000; Rosen 1993). In other words, such patients desperately need the therapist to take on characteristics of the abusive internal object that they carry within themselves, because abusive object relations are both predictable and familiar to these patients. If therapists do not allow themselves to be transformed into the bad object role, the patient will need to continue to escalate the demands until he or she finally provokes the therapist into exasperation. Dr. Y, much like her patient, began to lose the capacity to mentalize. Her own sense of reflective analytic space got lost in the flurry of concern about what action should be taken to prevent the suicide. This collapse of reflective space paralleled the patient's failure to distinguish between impulsive actions and fantasy (Gabbard and Wilkinson 1994; Lewin and Schulz 1992). Suicidality and the act of suicide are not the same thing. It is noteworthy, in this regard, that Ms. X never attempted suicide despite thinking about it every day. The anxiety about keeping the patient alive may lead to a frantic effort to take away the suicidality, which may be a valuable source of escape for the patient. For this patient, it was the only way out of horrific incest. As Nietzsche (1886/1966) once noted, "The thought of suicide is a great source of comfort: with it a calm passage is to be made across many a bad night."

The case of Ms. X also illustrates the dangers of encouraging the patient to think of the therapist as a real parent who is always available. This implied promise fills the patient with false hopes that will ultimately be dashed and lead to further contemplation of suicide. The patient will also assign the responsibility for keeping himself or herself alive to the therapist, one of the most lethal features of suicidal patients (Hendin 1982).

When therapists place themselves in bondage to the patient, they soon find their omnipotent wishes to heal are thwarted. Furthermore, under this intense confinement, therapists may find themselves in the grips of countertransference hate and the powerful urge to enact these feelings. Whether in the more subtle form of aversion (forgetting appointments, withdrawing emotionally) or outright acts of malice (sarcastic or hostile responses), these behaviors communicate the therapist's unconscious wish to abandon or even kill the patient, often serving only to heighten or acutely worsen the patient's suicidality. The case also illustrates the problem with surrendering good judgment on such issues as the need for medication, the prohibition of hugging, and the charging of reasonable fees for care.

Finally, Dr. Y wisely sought consultation before the pattern of boundary violations dragged her down the slippery slope to a point of more severe ethical transgressions. Consultation with a colleague on a regular basis should be a routine part of the treatment of chronically suicidal borderline patients. In addition, Dr. Y returned to her own psychotherapy in order to more fully explore her vulnerabilities. Personal therapy or analysis for clinicians who do intensive dynamic therapy with suicidal patients serves as a further protective measure, providing the therapist useful insight and perspective on the limits of the art.

Key Clinical Concepts

- *Suicidality* has meanings that vary from patient to patient. These meanings may be multiple and complicated; thus, they require careful exploration in the context of a strong therapeutic alliance.

- Suicidal patients create intense countertransference feelings, ranging from anxiety to despair to hatred and beyond, in those who treat them. These feelings can lead to boundary violations as well as life-threatening errors if they are disavowed.

- Thoughtful reflection on the transference/countertransference developments in psychotherapy often reveals the major interpersonal themes relevant to the patient's suicidality.

- Patients who are suicidal must be cautioned that no one can save them from suicide. They are ultimately responsible for their own safety while they are working in psychotherapy to find ways to live with pain.

References

Asch SS: Suicide and the hidden executioner. Int Rev Psychoanal 7:51–60, 1980

Bateman AW, Fonagy P: Treatment of borderline personality disorder with psychoanalytically oriented partial hospitalization: an 18-month follow-up. Am J Psychiatry 158:36–42, 2001

Bateman AW, Fonagy P: Health service utilization costs for borderline personality disorder patients treated with psychoanalytically oriented partial hospitalization versus general psychiatric care. Am J Psychiatry 160:169–171, 2003

Bateman AW, Fonagy P: Mentalization-based treatment of BPD. J Pers Disord 18:36–51, 2004a

Bateman AW, Fonagy P: Psychotherapy for Borderline Personality Disorder: Mentalization-Based Treatment. Oxford, UK, Oxford University Press, 2004b

Beevers CG, Miller IW: Perfectionism, cognitive bias, and hopelessness as prospective predictors of suicidal ideation. Suicide Life Threat Behav 34:126–137, 2004

Blatt SJ, Quinlan DM, Pilkonis PA, et al: Impact of perfectionism and need for approval on the brief treatment of depression: the National Institute of Mental Health Treatment of Depression Collaborative Research Program revisited. J Consult Clin Psychol 63:125–132, 1995

Chessick RD: Intensive Psychotherapy of the Borderline Patient. New York, Jason Aronson, 1977

Chiesa M, Fonagy P, Gordon J: Community-based psychodynamic treatment program for severe personality disorders: clinical description and naturalistic evaluation. J Psychiatr Pract 15:12–24, 2009

Davies JM, Frawley MG: Dissociative processes and transference-countertransference paradigms in the psychoanalytically oriented treatment of adult survivors of childhood sexual abuse. Psychoanalytic Dialogues 2:5–36, 1992

de Kernier N, Canouï P, Golse B: Taking care of teenagers hospitalized after a suicidal gesture or a suicidal threat [in French]. Arch Pediatr 17:435–441, 2010

Doering S, Hörz S, Rentrop M, et al: Transference-focused psychotherapy v. treatment by community psychotherapists for borderline personality disorder: randomised controlled trial. Br J Psychiatry 196:389–395, 2010

Fenichel O: The Psychoanalytic Theory of Neurosis. New York, WW Norton, 1945

Fonagy P: An attachment theory approach to treatment of the difficult patient. Bull Menninger Clin 62:147–169, 1998

Freud S: Mourning and melancholia (1917), in The Standard Edition of the Complete Psychological Works of Sigmund Freud, Vol 14. Translated and edited by Strachey J. London, Hogarth, 1963, pp 237–260

Freud S: The ego and the id (1923), in The Standard Edition of the Complete Psychological Works of Sigmund Freud, Vol 19. Translated and edited by Strachey J. London, Hogarth Press, 1961, pp 1–66

Gabbard GO: On gratitude and gratification. J Am Psychoanal Assoc 48:697–716, 2000

Gabbard GO: Miscarriages of psychoanalytic treatment with suicidal patients. Int J Psychoanal 84:249–261, 2003

Gabbard GO: Psychodynamic Psychotherapy in Clinical Practice, 4th Edition. Washington, DC, American Psychiatric Publishing, 2005

Gabbard GO, Wilkinson SM: On victims, rescuers, and abusers, in Management of Countertransference With Borderline Patients. Washington, DC, American Psychiatric Press, 1994, pp 47–70

Guthrie E, Kapur N, Mackway-Jones K, et al: Randomised controlled trial of brief psychological intervention after deliberate poisoning. BMJ 323:135–138, 2001

Guthrie E, Kapur N, Mackway-Jones K, et al: Predictors of outcome following brief psychodynamic-interpersonal therapy for deliberate self-poisoning. Aust N Z J Psychiatry 37:532–536, 2003

Hamilton TK, Schweitzer RD: The cost of being perfect: perfectionism and suicide ideation in university students. Aust N Z J Psychiatry 34:829–835, 2000

Hendin H: Psychotherapy and suicide, in Suicide in America. New York, WW Norton, 1982, pp 160–174

Hendin H, Pollinger Hass A, Maltsberger J, et al: Problems in psychotherapy with suicidal patients. Am J Psychiatry 163:67–72, 2006

Kaslow NJ, Reviere SL, Chance SE, et al: An empirical study of the psychodynamics of suicide. J Am Psychoanal Assoc 46:777–796, 1998

Leichsenring F, Rabung S: Effectiveness of long-term psychodynamic therapy: a meta-analysis. JAMA 300:1551–1565, 2008

Leichsenring F, Rabung S, Leibing E: The efficacy of short-term psychodynamic psychotherapy in specific psychiatric disorders: a meta-analysis. Arch Gen Psychiatry 61:1208–1216, 2004

Lewin RA, Schulz CG: Losing and Fusing: Borderline Transitional Object and Self Relations. Northvale, NJ, Jason Aronson, 1992

Lindner R: Psychodynamic hypothesis about suicidality in older men. Psychother Psychosom Med Psychol 60:290–297, 2010

Maltsberger JT, Buie DH: Countertransference hate in the treatment of suicidal patients. Arch Gen Psychiatry 30:625–633, 1974

Menninger KA: Psychoanalytic aspects of suicide. Int J Psychoanal 14:376–390, 1933

Nietzsche F: Beyond Good and Evil: Prelude to a Philosophy of the Future (1886). Translated by Kaufman W. New York, Random House, 1966

Nock MK, Park JM, Finn CT, et al: Measuring the suicidal mind: implicit cognition predicts suicidal behavior. Psychol Sci 21:511–517, 2010

Nosek BA, Banaji MR, Greenwald AG: Project Implicit. 2011. Available at: https://implicit.harvard.edu/implicit. Accessed June 22, 2011.

Petersen B, Toft J, Christensen NB, et al: Outcome of a psychotherapeutic programme for patients with severe personality disorders. Nord J Psychiatry 62:450–456, 2008

Rosen IR: Relational masochism: the search for a bad-enough object. Presented to the Topeka Psychoanalytic Society, Topeka, KS, January 1993

Smith K: Using a battery of tests to predict suicide in a long term hospital: a clinical analysis. Omega 13:261–275, 1983

Smith K, Eyman J: Ego structure and object differentiation in suicidal patients, in Primitive Mental States of the Rorschach. Edited by Lerner HD, Lerner PM. Madison, CT, International Universities Press, 1988, pp 175–202

Spirito A, Simon V, Cancilliere MK, et al: Outpatient psychotherapy practice with adolescents following psychiatric hospitalization for suicide ideation or a suicide attempt. Clin Child Psychol Psychiatry 16:53–64, 2011

Weishaar ME: Cognitive risk factors in suicide, in Frontiers of Cognitive Therapy. Edited by Salkovskis PM. New York, Guilford, 1996, pp 226–249

CHAPTER 15

Split Treatment

Coming of Age

Donald J. Meyer, M.D.

Traditionally, *split treatment* has referred to mental health treatment by two clinicians in which one has provides pharmacotherapy and the other provides psychotherapy (Balon and Riba 2001; Meyer 2002). In contrast to the collaborative treatment between physician specialists that is typically driven by the patient's medical diagnoses, split treatment historically has been driven primarily by socioeconomic and professional forces unrelated to the patient's illness. In most jurisdictions, the right to prescribe is limited to medically trained professionals, thereby requiring nonmedical psychotherapists to collaborate with their medically trained colleagues when their patients require somatic therapies.

Although the clinical borders of medical specialties roughly mirror the human body's own pathophysiologic borders, mental illness cannot be similarly parsed between mental health disciplines. Split treatment's lack of a fundamental patient-centered, biological, or medical raison d'être highlights the origin of many of the interprofes-

sional conflicts and risks frequently encountered. The necessity of addressing these risks and conflicts is heightened with suicidal patients, who present clinical high-risk uncertainty for assessment, treatment, and management.

Third-party payers have been a prominent force in promoting split treatment, in which the psychotherapy is provided by a nonmedical therapist who is reimbursed at a lower rate than a psychiatrist. In a recent *New York Times Magazine* article (Harris 2011), a hapless adult psychiatrist who formerly provided both psychotherapy and pharmacotherapy explained that the repricing of psychotherapy had increasingly driven him to the more delimited role of psychopharmacologist. In the National Ambulatory Medical Care Survey (Mojtabai and Olfson 2008), researchers found that psychiatrists in 2005 provided verbal therapy to 10.8% of their patients. Although the *Times* article neglected to point out that 60% of psychiatrists continue to do psychotherapy (Pies 2011), third-party payers' low reimbursement of psychotherapy has promoted split treatment for patients needing somatic and nonsomatic therapies.

In spite of the decades-long reimbursement policy by third-party payers, medical research has not clearly supported that split treatment is either more cost-effective or more clinically effective than the administration of those same treatments by a single psychiatrist (Dewan 1999; Goldman et al. 1998). It is possible that a split-treatment prescriber's more delimited clinical contacts translate to less timely recognition of clinical changes and side effects, resulting in a longer, less clinically responsive, and more expensive term of treatment and, more importantly, a longer period of illness for the patient. There is insufficient research about whether split treatment or another treatment paradigm is the most clinically effective and cost-effective for patients requiring a combination of somatic and verbal therapies.

Patients at Risk for Suicide

In the United States, 90% of patients who complete suicide have a diagnosed mental disorder (Goldsmith et al. 2002). Disorders of affect, depression, bipolar illness, anxiety disorders, and disorders of thought such as schizophrenia confer particularly high rates of risk for suicidality and for completed suicide (Goldsmith et al. 2002). Comorbidity with a second Axis I mental disorder compounds risk. One-quarter of those who complete suicide are intoxicated (Centers for Disease Control and Prevention 2009a). Borderline personality disorder, the only personality disorder in which suicidality is a named diagnostic feature, confers risk on par with that of a thought disorder (Goldsmith et al. 2002).

Split-treatment patients by definition require multiple concurrent therapies. As a general rule, patients requiring multiple therapies have more complex, relatively treatment-resistant disease. Patients in split treatment who are also suicidal will, by virtue of these two clinical demographics, be among the most clinically ill and clinically challenging.

Mental health treatments do not rely on the costly technological procedures that third-party payers often seek to regulate to mitigate medical-surgical costs in health care. In the absence of being able to contain mental health treatment costs by the regulation of procedures, managed care third-party payers have focused on authorization of inpatient and outpatient treatment time to regulate costs. High levels of third-party administrative oversight, treatment denials, and low rates of reimbursement have in turn motivated all mental health clinicians to reduce unreimbursed clinical time, a motivation that is a barrier to the interprofessional clinical bridges that must be constructed if split treatment is to be clinically sound.

Many split-treatment therapies have their beginnings with a "cold call" from a hospital social worker or third-party payer care coordinator trying to find two available, willing, in-network clinicians who will agree to assume the care of a psychiatric inpatient who is soon to be discharged, clinicians who may have no preexisting professional relationship. Patients who are admitted to psychiatric inpatient units have a higher level of morbidity and acuity than in the past. When these patients are discharged 5–6 days later, they may have been stabilized, but their conditions cannot have been fully treated. Patients are at especially greater risk for suicide immediately following discharge from a hospital, a risk factor that does not fully diminish for a year.

Outpatients may also turn to their third-party payers to find willing clinicians for split treatment. Some are patients already in psychotherapy with a therapist who is not linked to an established network of medical providers that include psychopharmacologists. Some psychotherapists, rather than appropriately assuming the responsibility of finding a pharmacologist collaborator, will wrongly delegate that important clinical task to the patient, not appropriately appreciating the stake the therapist has in which pharmacologist is chosen.

In the end, many split-treatment pairs of clinicians may know nothing of each other. Unlike a team of medically trained professionals who typically are members of a shared health care agency (e.g., a hospital, an independent practice association), split-treatment "teams" are often independent providers who are ignorant of each other's professional training, experience, and clinical methods. Making that acquaintance takes time and clarification, time that typically is unreimbursed. Nevertheless, there are several key issues in split treatment to address if clinical risk management and effective treatment are to prevail.

Interprofessional Considerations

Licensure

Medical professionals who prescribe medications must be licensed by both the state and the federal government. Being a *psychotherapist*, in a generic sense, does not require licensure in many jurisdictions. In many communities there are individuals who proffer themselves as psychotherapists but who are lawfully unlicensed. Individuals who have an interest in psychotherapy but are without formal training, those with an alternative or holistic health background, and those who have pursued religious studies may all lawfully represent themselves as psychotherapists in many jurisdictions. Because of the shared clinical responsibility and the shared liability exposure, medical professionals are advised to limit their split-treatment partners to those with appropriate training jurisdictional licensure, and liability insurance.

Clinical Training, Experience, and Knowledge

What is the colleague's training and experience? A clinician seeking answers to this question of a professional colleague can mitigate the potential risk of sounding intrusive or condescending by first volunteering that information about him- or herself. It makes for a more egalitarian framework when asking for information from a colleague if the questioner has already been forthcoming with his or her own information.

Is there a specialized knowledge required for the treatment of this particular patient? If the patient has a substance abuse problem, is that a skill set possessed by at least one of the split-treatment team? If the patient has an eating disorder, what range of clinical expertise will be required? Will the split-treatment team also need the involvement of an internist or neurologist for the patient in question? Will this patient also need group treatment or partial hospitalization? What institutional affiliations may be needed to facilitate those services?

What if the colleague does not have the training or experience, licensure, and liability insurance that are, in the clinician's opinion, required for this patient to meet the clinician's individual standard of care? Clinicians are not obliged to work with and share responsibility with just anyone. Rather, they have the responsibility to make a good-faith effort to ascertain that their colleague has the requisite competence. The decision to work together is a choice for each clinician that should be made "eyes open" and a decision that even once made is still open to prospective review, based on their experience together with this patient. Clinicians may terminate a split treatment that has become unworkable so long as they avoid abandonment of the patient by providing a good-faith effort to find alternative sources of psychopharmacology and psychotherapy (Gutheil and Simon 2003).

Urgent Access

How will the clinicians access each other, and how will the patient access them, in the event of an emergency? It is common to provide answering machines with messages that ask patients to leave a message and instruct that for an emergency the patient go to the nearest emergency facility. These are not prudent for the care of suicidal patients. Responsibility for clinical care of patients who may become acutely ill cannot be assigned to an unknowing hospital emergency department.

Clinicians who treat more severely disordered patients need to provide urgent access to patients whose clinical status is foreseeably fluid. Clinicians do not individually have to be available 24/7, although the patients should have easy, transparent guidance on how to access the covering clinician. In this age of telecommunications, clinicians have a panoply of choices for arranging access.

The word *emergency* itself may also impose an unwitting clinical barrier to a patient and can be usefully replaced by the word *urgent*. Depressed, obsessive patients may refrain from seeking care when they should, reasoning that they were not sure it was a "true emergency." Patients who are in crisis typically have diminished, not enhanced, skills at reasoning about their level of clinical acuity and their clinical choices.

Patients can be encouraged to call their clinician over something that *they* perceive as *urgent,* regardless of whether it ultimately proves to be a true medical or psychiatric emergency. Therapists can educate patients who overuse that access. It is easier and safer to intervene with a problem of overuse than with patients who are not calling when they should.

In split treatment, the clinician who sees the patient most may take first call and triage. However, patients may independently decide that their problem is a medical one, regardless of the arrangement between clinicians. Emergencies that are principally medical do occur. Medical clinicians who are directly, prospectively providing ongoing pharmacotherapy are primary treaters, not consultants. Regardless of the arrangement with the psychotherapist, both psychotherapists and medical clinicians or their covering surrogates must be reachable to respond to urgent clinical developments. On no account can clinicians assume that their responsibility for the patient is proportional to the frequency or duration of time spent with the patient.

Coverage for Weekends, Holidays, and Vacations

It follows that coverage for weekends, holidays, and vacations also needs to be addressed. Even though each clinician will typically have an individual coverage arrangement for his or her patients, it is also possible that a psychotherapist may ask the collaborating pharmacotherapist to cover the patient they share rather than simply being accessible to the covering surrogate psychotherapist. Each arrangement is clinically sensible for patient care. The psychotherapist, lacking medical training, cannot return the favor in kind when the pharmacotherapist goes on vacation.

Inequities of time and money are part of the basic fabric of split treatment. They often do not pass the "What's in it for me?" test and can foster resentment over time. If not addressed or simply forgiven, these resentments can unconsciously leak and contaminate the professionals' working relationship and their patient's treatment.

In successful split-treatment teams, the two clinicians both feel that they have each other's support and that they are in it together. Voice mail and e-mail updates can foster both the relational and informational aspects of the patient's treatment without being unduly burdensome. Reviewing the e-mail updates directly with the patient or having the patient listen in to voice mails as they are being left can also convey to the patient that there is an ongoing collaboration between treating clinicians and the nature of the data of that collaboration. Including this activity during the time spent with the patient appropriately frames the activity as part of the therapy and also provides for legitimate reimbursement for the time. Clinicians should be aware that their interprofessional e-mails are a part of the patient's medical record and that the text and content should reflect that fact.

Ideological Conflicts

Although "I don't like the idea of medication" is a comment often heard from patients, it can also be a position held by clinicians, medical and nonmedical alike. Within psychiatry, there was at one time a debate about whether prescribing medication for symptoms was wrongly putting a Band-Aid on a wound that in fact needed exploration and reconstruction. Fortunately, research has repeatedly demonstrated that the combination of pharmacotherapy and psychotherapy is preferable to either alone for myriad psychiatric disorders.

However, the negative valence of psychologically active medications persists with some mental health professionals, who feel their patient's integrity and independence are tarnished by pharmacotherapy. This attitude can understandably lead to interprofessional conflicts and to patient nonadherence with medications.

Alternatively, strongly biologically oriented mental health professionals may wrongly hold the belief that psychoactive drugs, not talk therapy, are the true agents of treatment. These ideological conflicts, if undetected and not addressed, will prevent two clinicians from becoming one team and commonly will lead to an acting out of the conflict by their shared patient.

Acknowledging That Job Descriptions Overlap

Neither mental illness nor its treatment is clearly divisible into its medical and nonmedical parts, nor is it separable by mental health discipline. In split treatment, there are overlapping areas of professional responsibility. Risk assessment of a suicidal patient is not assignable to one therapist or the other. They each must both assess and then resolve differences of opinion and judgment. Diagnosis and treatment formulation are shared responsibilities even when the responsibility for the implementation of some facets of that treatment rests with each clinician individually.

Even psychotherapy itself cannot be parsed with a clinical bright white line by discipline between the two split-treatment clinicians. For example, although clarification and interpretations of the patient's psychodynamics are part of the patient's psychotherapy, it is nevertheless expectable that the patient will have transference reactions both to the medicating clinician and to the medication itself. The practice of all psychopharmacology involves psychotherapy. A patient who eschews all dependency in his or her personal life can also be expected to have psychological reactions to having to see a doctor regularly, if only briefly, and to having to take a medication daily. A patient who fears being controlled should be expected to have those dynamics arise with the medicating therapist and with the medication itself.

The psychotherapist can legitimately expect that most interpretation and clarification will be in the domain of the psychotherapy. However, that same therapist must also recognize that all appropriate treatment of patients with psychiatric disorders will involve psychotherapeutic management of the relationship by the application of psychotherapeutic understanding and techniques.

Alternatively, experienced psychotherapists have treated many patients who have received medications, and may have a reasonable basis for suggesting to a patient that they should call the prescribing clinician for assessment of akathisia, hypomanic symptoms, or panic. Sometimes the therapist may mention a medicine or a class of medicines. Here, too, the team needs to work together without being unduly prideful or territorial.

Informed Consent and Release of Information

The patient needs to be apprised of the expected bidirectional flow of clinical information that is essential in split treatment. Appropriate prospective releases are needed so that sharing of information between therapists is unrestricted. Patients who find this change from a formerly dyadic therapy model troubling have the right to refuse it, but clinicians have a responsibility not to acquiesce to patient requests and conditions that are below the clinicians' standard of care. Mental health practitioners are at times unduly conflicted about being assertive with patients, even when the practitioners know that a patient's care will be compromised.

Access and involvement of patient family members or other important individuals to the patient have been shown to be effective mitigators of suicidal risk. The patient should provide a release to the clinicians to contact important individuals in the event of an urgent clinical development.

Split Treatment by Institutionally Based Clinicians

For simplicity, it was assumed in the preceding text that the split-treatment clinicians were independently licensed and in solo practice. If one or both clinicians are part of an institution—for example, a hospital or independent group clinic—that institution may have policies that preempt what the two therapists might otherwise work out on their own. Departure by an employee from accepted institutional policies and procedures can be the basis for negligence per se in the event of malpractice litigation. Clinic managers and supervisors who have the authority to direct the treating clinician(s) also have liability exposure. By the legal doctrine of *respondeat superior* (let the master respond), supervisors' liability exposure flows from their clinical authority, regardless of whether they directly examined the patient or actually sought to direct the patient's care (*Andrews v. United States* 1984).

Split Treatment by Trainee Clinicians

In the preceding text it was also assumed that the split-treatment clinicians were independently licensed. Trainee clinicians are dependently licensed to practice within their jurisdiction through the training heath care facility that has been designated by the state to provide the requisite supervision. In mental health education, *supervision* is a linguistically ambiguous term of art, sometimes indicating an educational process without managerial authority, and sometimes identifying an individual who has the authority to direct the supervisee's actions.

In the latter case, it is the responsibility of the managing supervisor to be the guarantor of the quality of care the patient receives from the dependently licensed trainee clinician. It is the responsibility of the managing supervisor to assess both the clinical needs of the patient being treated and the clinical capacities of the trainee clinician and to make sure the former do not exceed the latter (*Cohen v. State of New York* 1976). Under the law in most jurisdictions, clinicians are required to meet a standard of care of an average, prudent clinician in similar circumstances. In some jurisdictions, that standard of care is not that of the average trainee clinician but rather that of the average clinician (*St. Germain v. Pfeifer* 1994). Teaching hospitals do not proffer a substandard level of health care to the public by virtue of their having trainees. They therefore can be held to the same standards to which other institutions and practitioners are held.

In addition to these intra-institutional policies, procedures, and legal requirements that may have bearing on split treatment, institutionally driven psychological forces may affect treatment. A psychotherapist in private practice working with a hospital-based psychopharmacologist may rightly or wrongly be viewed as an outsider, with lower status, or as less reliable. The therapist may rightly or wrongly view the institution-

ally based prescriber as aloof, condescending, and unreachable. If institutionally based clinicians are trainees, what appears to be a two-clinician team in fact involves a larger cast of supervisors and also may involve interdepartmental institutional tensions—for example, psychiatry and psychology or psychiatry and social work. Trainees can find themselves trying to negotiate with staff-level clinicians, and the power differential may negatively influence clinical decisions. In these circumstances, as in others in split treatment in which there are conflicting agendas, clinical care and the individual clinician's standard of care are each unimpeachable foundations for an open, if tense, discussion.

Case Example 1

A resident presented the new case of a suicidal patient from her psychopharmacology clinic. The patient had been referred by the patient's primary care physician, who no longer wanted to prescribe both antidepressants and stimulants for the patient.

The patient was a 34-year-old single woman who had reported symptoms of depression and anxiety, beginning 3 years previously when she and her boyfriend broke off their relationship. The patient had commenced treatment with a psychotherapist who specialized in eye movement desensitization and reprocessing (EMDR). However, the EMDR therapist did not feel the patient was ever sufficiently stable to begin that specialty treatment. The therapist thought the patient had been "traumatized" by a borderline mother and had a posttraumatic stress disorder variant. The EMDR therapist asked the patient's primary care physician for a medication evaluation. The patient, who had symptoms of anxiety, depression, impaired attention, and rejection sensitivity, was ultimately prescribed both a selective serotonin reuptake inhibitor (SSRI) and methylphenidate.

Because the psychiatric resident had taken over doing the patient's medication backup, the EMDR therapist had also, without consultation, enlisted an additional psychotherapist from a community mental health clinic who could be more available to the patient than the EMDR therapist was prepared to be.

The resident reported that the patient would page her and report suicidal feelings and at the same time assure the resident that she would never "do anything." The patient explained that she paged the resident because the resident was the most accessible of the three mental health clinicians. The patient was also irregularly attending her psychotherapy.

There is insufficient information to know whether it will be possible for this patient to be contained and treated in split treatment, but the information does justify the resident's worry. The patient's diagnosis is in doubt. The severity of her suicidal risk is unassessed. The appropriateness of the medication regimen is in question. Equally important, the "team" responsible for making these determinations is not in it together. The EMDR therapist is responding as though the patient is more than she can handle. The case involves clinicians from two institutions and a third who is a solo practitioner. The patient is attending treatment erratically and selecting the trainee as the clinician in charge of emergencies.

Ironically, it is the most junior member of the team who is the most clinically concerned, and her concerns are appropriate. These clinicians, either through their own collaboration or through use of a consultant, need to agree on a working diagnosis, perform an adequate risk assessment, and then formulate a treatment plan.

It is possible but not clear whether the patient has character traits (a tendency to split and act out) that will prove a contraindication for split treatment. If the clinicians go forward with split treatment, they need to parse the clinical tasks "in accordance with the qualifications and limitations of each therapist's discipline and abilities" (American Psychiatric Association 1980). The EMDR therapist cannot delegate her

availability to another clinician. She may have to resign from the case. The resident may need additional supervisory support in the event that the appropriate clinical goals are not supported by the more senior clinicians.

Split Treatment Is Not for Every Patient

Certain psychiatric disorders of themselves may be especially challenging in split treatment. Disorders that significantly impair the patient's capacity to form and sustain a relationship with health care providers and/ or cause unheralded severe swings in mental status and conduct may not be appropriate for split treatment.

For example, personality disorders that are characterized by reliance on projective identification, splitting, projection, and denial may be a poor fit for a split-treatment team. Having two mental health clinicians can provide a larger, divided arena in which the patient may act out those pathological defenses.

One therapist may be idealized while the other is devalued. The patient's capacity to be an accurate historian with a consistent story may be challenged by the patient's seeing the two clinicians in very different affective lights. Split-treatment teams may find that a patient of this description has unilaterally, summarily fired one of the clinicians, leaving the other clinician in an untenable situation with which he or she cannot and should not abide. Clinicians are responsible for guarding their own clinical standards of care, independent of the patient's preferences and demands.

Schizoid or paranoid suicidal patients with few relational skills may also be poorly suited to split treatment because they may be hard-pressed to relate to a team of mental health clinicians when relating to one person is challenge enough. Patients who have a history of lying about or withholding important clinical facts will be better served by one clinician than a team in which the patient has the opportunity to tell too many inaccurate stories.

Patients with a history of rapid-cycling bipolar illness are also less well suited to a treatment paradigm, in which essential, rapidly evolving clinical information that needs to be consolidated may be at risk for being divided between two clinicians.

Patients with a history of a psychotic transference to a health care provider present an interesting clinical problem. They may find the management of two clinical relationships doubles the opportunity for transferential misalignment. A legitimate counterargument can be made that with an effective split-treatment team, the two therapists may dilute the intensity of the transference and provide some added relational ballast for the patient. This author does not feel that there is a generally applicable rule for this class of patients, and a realistic dialogue with the patient about the risks and benefits is a better choice.

Clinical Assessment of the Suicidal Patient in Split Treatment

Conceptualizing Suicidal Thinking and Intent and Suicide Risk

As clinicians, when we use the word *suicidal*, it is with the awareness that this psychological state of mind is strongly associated with mental illness (Goldsmith et al. 2002; Merikangas et al. 2011). There is no psychiatric disorder, save for mental retardation, that does not raise the risk of suicide (American Psychiatric Association 2003).

However, the proven association of mental illness and suicidality is not to say that mental illness is the cause per se.

Epidemiological research has documented the importance and potency of nonpsychopathological factors in shaping the patient's inner experience and clinical trajectory in managing or acting on suicidal feelings. A patient's age and ethnic, social, religious, geographic, and financial demographics all play a role in shaping an individual patient's suicidality and risk for completing suicide (Centers for Disease Control and Prevention 2011a, 2011b; Mann et al. 2005). The increased risk of completed suicide conferred by patient access to highly lethal means of suicide has also been demonstrated by research, as has the benefit of removing that easy access (Gunnell and Miller 2010; Hawton and van Heeringen 2009).

Some research has borne out observations that have made intuitive sense to clinicians. Social engagement and a sense of purpose, on balance, mitigate suicidality (Malone et al. 2000). Substantial loss makes suicidality worse. Although money will not buy happiness, financial reversals and poverty are associated with greater mental health problems. Attendance at a house of worship is a mitigator of suicidality, regardless of whether the individual actually believes in a supreme being.

Many minority immigrant ethnic groups have a lower incidence of suicide (Centers for Disease Control and Prevention 2009b) than Caucasian Americans. Native Americans, an ethnic minority, have among the highest rates of suicide until old age (Centers for Disease Control and Prevention 2009c) when, paradoxically, their rates are more similar to those of other minority ethnic groups. The stark contrast between the impulsive phenomenology of teenage suicidality and the premeditated quality of suicide by aging Caucasian men is a reminder of how profoundly the psychology of the individual's developmental stage influences the experience of and response to a suicidal thought.

Clinicians cannot change the age, gender, or ethnicity of their patient. They cannot alter the fact that the patient has attempted suicide in the past, even as they note these factors may increase future risk for suicide. These are static factors that raise or lower the level of clinical concern but as data are immutable.

On the other hand, psychiatric disorders, comorbid medical and substance abuse disorders, social isolation, and some known suicide-activating psychological affects are not immutable. Intervention can lower the likelihood that suicidal intent will segue to suicidal conduct. All require clinician attention. The transition from suicidal intent to action is often precipitated by affective innervation. Regardless of the origin of a patient's suicidality, a patient's experiencing unrelenting anxiety (Sareen et al. 2005), agitation, severe drug-induced akathisia (Rothschild and Locke 1991), escalating paranoia, or acute shame and humiliation may be infused with the energy of activation for suicidal conduct.

Unambivalent suicidal intent is very hard to sustain. Patients who are so resolved intentionally diminish opportunities for clinical intervention and in fact view clinicians as the enemy to their goal (Resnick 2002). It is the patients who have some residual degree of ambivalence about their suicidal intent who offer clinicians the greatest opportunity not only to treat and mitigate illness but also to militate for the patient's positive side of the ambivalence—that is, for those relational and existential anchors that have the power to hold the patient in the world of the living.

In 2006, addressing the American Psychiatric Association, John Kevin Hines, a rare survivor of a suicidal jump from the Golden Gate Bridge, narrated his recollection of the event to attendee psychiatrists. Robert Simon, M.D. (2007), chronicled the story.

> He jumped. On the way down, he changed his mind. He remembered thinking, "I want to live. Why am I doing this?" It was too late. Severely injured, Mr. Hines [reported he] was kept afloat by a sea lion until rescuers arrived. Mr. Hines is now gainfully employed as an activities coordinator at a high school. He is a frequent speaker at high schools and other interested groups about his experience with mental illness and suicide. Mr. Hines is a strong advocate for physical barriers on the Golden Gate Bridge and other bridges. It is his contention that suicides are impulsive, overcoming the ambivalence about dying that is present to the last moment.

Clinicians have learned from research the importance of the individual patient's reasons for living (Malone et al. 2000) to fostering the positive side of the patient's ambivalence and to mitigating impulsivity. Relational ties and obligations, a sense of purpose, and a sense of engagement are not easily thrown off, even at times of enormous psychic distress. They can be sources of solace and altruism that can help a patient successfully contend with grave psychological suffering.

Split-Treatment Assessment of Suicidality

In contrast to the potential interprofessional patient-specific pitfalls of split treatment, a potential benefit conferred by split treatment to the care of suicidal patients is that two heads can sometimes assess better than one. In a best-case scenario, the separate assessments from two clinicians can provide clinical parallax. The two clinicians usually have somewhat differing clinical skills and thereby can offer a more diversified therapeutic intervention for the patient.

Clinicians each need to do their own independent assessment, based on their knowledge and their differing training and orientation. Determining diagnosis is important but of itself is not determinative of the risks, weaknesses, and strengths patients have in their contending with suicidal intent.

The following questions are offered as a way of operationalizing the therapists' inquiry with their patient and assuring that both clinicians know and share the concretized warning signs, interventions, and urgent responses specific to this individual patient:

1. Do both therapists and patient have a shared view of this patient's premonitory signs and symptoms of relapse?
2. Have the clinicians assessed the patient for the patient's current willingness and capacity to prospectively self-monitor for those premonitory symptoms? (As opposed to an attestation of "no harm," this is an attestation of therapeutic engagement by the patient.)
3. Do clinicians and patient have a shared list of those activities, persons, and environments to which the patient typically can turn for comfort, solace, and restraint?
4. Do all three—both the clinicians and the patient—have a shared stepwise plan that addresses clinician access and clinician intervention up to and including the use of an emergency room and access to hospitalization should the premonitory signs and symptoms prove unyielding?

5. Do all three have an appreciation that things can and do change and that assessment of suicidality is an iterative process over time and not an event?

Clinical Deterioration

The therapist and psychopharmacologist need to provide each other timely notice of a patient's worsening clinical status. Together they can formulate a hypothetical explanation of the patient's deterioration.

Clinicians are typically attuned to the psychological ramifications of various changes in the patient's real and psychological environment: changes in relationships, work and living situations, and financial status may all affect the patient's clinical status. Even positive developments such as a promotion or a more substantive or deepening relationship may provoke patient anxiety, acting out, or regression.

Clinicians also need to be mindful that the very psychotherapeutic and pharmacologic tools on which we rely for benefit to a patient also have the capacity to make patients worse. A patient who is given a neuroleptic may then develop a severe akathisia 2 weeks later. A deepening exploration of an earlier trauma could lead to a recurrence of symptoms of posttraumatic stress disorder. The second antidepressant that was supposed to help with symptoms of anxiety or depression may instead provoke a manic switch or a serotonin syndrome. Some of these potential risks are foreseeable. One clinician informing the other of an anticipated change in some facet of the patient's treatment is notice of the possibility of iatrogenic side effects from a well-intentioned therapeutic intervention.

Case Example 2

A 33-year-old lesbian woman in individual and couples treatment was referred for medication consultation for symptoms of depression. She was diagnosed by the medicating psychiatrist with major depressive disorder and treated with an SSRI. The individual therapist and psychiatrist, each in private practice, knew each other professionally from a common institutional affiliation, an affiliation that also attested to the professionals' training, experience, and insurance. The patient was seen in follow-up 2 weeks later by the psychiatrist and appeared to be responding to treatment. The patient was scheduled for a medication backup visit in 2 months.

Two weeks later the individual therapist noted that the patient's mood was continuing to improve and that the patient seemed more able to assert herself in the couples setting. However, after another 2 weeks, the couples therapist informed the individual therapist that the patient seemed to have crossed the line from being assertive to being enraged and intolerant. She was "fed up and not going to be shortchanged." The individual therapist noted the patient was reporting insomnia and presumed it to be secondary to the acrimony in the relationship. The patient called the psychiatrist for additional medication for the sleeplessness. Trazodone was phoned in without patient reassessment.

In the subsequent 3 weeks, the patient's dysphoric manic switch became full-blown but remained undiagnosed. She precipitously had an affair that she then announced to her partner. Her partner threatened to leave. Soon after, the partner came home to find the patient had hung herself.

Several issues are highlighted by this case. The therapists had not been alerted by the prescriber about the risks of mania from treatment of depression. The patient's sudden assertiveness, short temper, and sleeplessness were not diagnostically appreciated to be early symptoms of a manic switch.

The patient's medication appointment in 8 weeks might have been all right as long as the patient remained on a stable trajectory. However, the prescriber did not assess either on the phone or in person the significance of the patient's new-onset insomnia and wrongly assumed it must be simply a reaction to the couple's acrimony or a medication side effect. In fairness, each mistaken conclusion about the cause of the patient's new symptoms would often be correct.

Because her medicating psychiatrist did not take that opportunity for reassessment and was not informed by the patient's therapist of the patient's hypomanic behavior, the patient went undiagnosed. She became more disinhibited, angry, and hypersexual. In a dysphoric state, she felt intense shame and guilt for her infidelity and for the loss of the relationship and died by suicide. The patient's estate sued all three for malpractice.

Nonadherence: Medical and Psychological Factors

Health care providers may assume that a medication prescribed is a medication being taken as directed. A recent Centers for Disease Control and Prevention survey indicated that 75% of patients (U.S. Surgeon General Regina Benjamin 2011) do not take their medications as prescribed. Although some nonadherence is minor—an occasional forgotten dose—many instances are not.

Psychotropic medications may cause a host of side effects that may lead to nonadherence. Almost all classes of antidepressants may cause sexual side effects. Almost all classes of neuroleptics, new and old, can cause akathisia. Almost all psychotropic medications carry the risk of weight gain. Many can negatively alter mental sharpness and the ability to acquire new information. Many cause sexual side effects, disturb sleep, or cause intense, unwanted dreams. Many medications bring future medical risks such as tardive dyskinesia, renal or hepatic damage, and drug-drug interactions when a patient is treated for a new, unrelated medical disorder.

As part of informed consent, patients are informed of both significant and common side effects at the inception of pharmacotherapy. They also need to be queried further down the clinical road for the actual occurrence of problems and asked whether they have been able to take medications as directed. Asking the question makes it clear that the clinician knows that adherence cannot be presumed (Osterberg and Blaschke 2005; Vergouwen et al. 2003).

In addition to unwanted medical effects as a cause of patient nonadherence with psychotropic medications, there are also psychological bases. For most patients, taking any medication long term accurately evokes some feeling of being reliant on something outside of themselves and as such is an affront to their sense of self-sufficiency. Many patients can tolerate the narcissistic injury of being a little more dependent than they would wish. Many cannot.

The problem is not limited to psychiatric patients. Medical patients on chronic drug regimens for hypertension, epilepsy, cardiovascular disease, or diabetes, despite clear cognitive knowledge of the rationale for those regimens and the risks of discontinuation, will nevertheless stop their medications.

However, psychiatric patients, having a higher proportion of maladaptive personality traits, are even more vulnerable to discontinuation of treatments in response to the perceived narcissistic injury. Moreover, medications are often viewed as the symbolic documentation of an illness that is socially and personally stigmatizing. Alternatively, patients may view their improvement in psychological symptoms as synthetic and not genuinely them. As both the heart and the sexual reproductive organs are known as intense objects of narcissistic psychological investment, so too is a patient's mind. Feeling one's mind will not function adequately without medical therapy is a diffi-

cult psychological "pill" for many patients to swallow.

Patients also fear that if they are treated with psychotropic medications, they will appear drugged or feel blunted, or will in some important way no longer be the person they have known themselves to be. Patients who have suffered from long-term major mental illness have typically incorporated that experience into their sense of identity. Although positive effects of treatment may be welcomed, it is very common that patients will have some concern that this is no longer "the real me." Illness often has become a distinguishing feature of who a person is and, in that perspective, a part of what the patient views as making him or her different and special. Patients whose illness goes into partial or complete remission may feel that the clinical improvement unacceptably makes them just like everyone else: being well may involve no longer being different and special.

Patients who are treated with medications and as a result are no longer suffering from anxiety or depression may struggle with whether they have become less empathic to people and events as opposed to less symptomatic to them. Patients who were socially avoidant as a result of untreated symptoms of depression and anxiety may feel that the more socially confident, capable person they have become is not really them. Patients who have been used to struggling with feeling profoundly needy and panicked may have psychological resistance to integrating their newfound resilience.

These psychodynamic issues stemming from patient improvement from pharmacotherapy are counterintuitive for patients. If not addressed by the split-treatment team, they may undermine adherence with the medication regimen and account for unforeseen clinical deterioration.

Split Treatment in the New Millennium

Split treatment's initial paradigm was a psychiatrist and psychotherapist working in tandem (American Psychiatric Association 1980; Sederer et al. 1998). Although that original paradigm still remains, there are more recent permutations on the theme as a result of new developments in health care. First among these is the increasing number of potential prescribers.

Primary care physicians can and do prescribe psychotropic medications to their patients (Katon et al. 2005), who may or may not be concurrently receiving a form of psychotherapy from a mental health clinician. Primary care physicians are accustomed to backing up and collaborating with a variety of health care professionals in a shared responsibility for a patient in common.

Increasingly, primary care physicians are using "physician extenders" to widen patient access and to provide chronic disease management and lower cost. These auxiliary health care providers follow up with patients on the phone or at home, assessing patient adherence to a variety of clinical measures. As with medical disorders such as diabetes and hypertension, many psychiatric disorders may ultimately find a fit within this model of primary care chronic disease management (Katon et al. 2010), a model that is finding increasing favor in the medical health care community.

The clinical benefit to patients of primary care physicians performing split treatment is the increased patient access to psychotropic medications for common psychiatric disorders that have high community rates of both prevalence and lack of treatment (Bao et al. 2011; Kessler et al. 2003). The risk posed by this evolving model of split treatment is that the psychopharmacologic and psychotherapeutic training and experience of a primary care physician and the physician extenders may be insufficient to address the complexity of the patient's psychiatric condition.

Primary care physicians without extensive psychiatric training may prudently avoid prescribing psychotropics for patients with complex or off-label psychopharmacologic regimens, bipolar disorder, psychotic disorders, comorbid substance abuse, and severe personality disorders. Split treatment by primary care physicians may also suffer from underfunding of the time allocated for the doctor-patient interaction. Primary care physicians may be expected to squeeze in treatment of a psychiatric disorder among other medical disorders rather than being able to allocate additional time for a mental health problem. Time for the doctor-patient relationship is one of the most endangered species in the current health care climate.

Psychiatric nurse specialists and nurse practitioners are another group of medically trained clinicians who provide psychopharmacologic treatment with nonmedical psychotherapists. Although the supervisory requirements may vary by jurisdiction, typically these practitioners are required by their state medical board to have supervision from a psychiatrist.

In addition to the changing professional face of clinicians who provide psychopharmacology, psychotherapy itself has also changed (Comtois and Linehan 2006). Increasingly novel therapies that are symptom (Brown et al. 2005; Fountoulakis et al. 2009) or syndrome specific are being offered to patients. Dialectical behavior therapies for patients who self-mutilate; cognitive-behavioral therapy for depression, anxiety, and eating disorders; interpersonal therapy for depression; and life skills training for undersocialized patients are but a few examples of the treatments available today.

Sometimes these therapies are in addition to a broader general psychotherapy and sometimes they are in lieu of it. Many of these newer therapies have become somewhat standardized through the use of workbooks and intersession homework assignments.

The potential benefit to patients of novel disease- or symptom-specific therapies is clear. The risk is that the practitioners of these novel treatments may, as might be true of any split-treatment clinician, wrongly assume that responsibility for the patient is circumscribed by the practice of their novel therapy or, even worse, that it is assignable to another clinician. No matter the development of new therapies, clinician responsibility for the patient is unassignable.

Conclusion

The past may be prologue to the future of split treatment. The success or failure of split treatment has always centered on relational and informational collaboration, in spite of other economic and interprofessional disincentives. Currently, the most substantial political and economic forces in the nation's history are being applied to the delivery of health care. Accountable care organizations (Berwick 2011) and a virtual medical home are newly proposed models to raise health care quality and diminish cost. Although the effects on the infrastructure of delivery of medical and surgical care are not clear, the plan for the delivery of mental health care in this paradigm is largely unaddressed.

The new health care delivery concepts propose that patient care be centered within a group of collaborating health care professionals responsible for an identified patient population and reimbursed by funds prospectively estimated on that population's anticipated needs rather than retrospectively on units of service actually provided. Because mental illness is responsible for such a major share of the disease burden borne by patients (World Health Organization 2002), mental health practitioners will, of necessity, have to participate in many so-called medical homes in what will be the next iteration of split treatment. Then, as now, success will depend on clinicians finding a way to be in it together, in touch, regularly, for the patient's best treatment interests with an endorsable standard of care.

Key Clinical Concepts

- Split treatment of suicidal patients can offer a multidimensional therapy by combining the skills of clinicians with differing expertise. In some health care systems and some geographic areas, split treatment may be the only practical way to provide patient access to psychopharmacological therapies.

- No single treatment paradigm is right for every patient. Patients' biologically based diagnoses, their character defenses, the complexity of their pharmacological regimens, the histories of impulsivity and suicidality, and their historic patterns of relating to health care providers are all important determinants of suicidal patients' suitability for split treatment.

- Risk assessment/risk management of a suicidal patient in split treatment is an iterative process to be performed repeatedly and collaboratively by a team of mental health clinicians sharing clinical data and clinical decision making.

- Clinicians need to assess themselves and each other for their respective availability and competence and the interpersonal fit required to work collaboratively, even in the face of financial and administrative disincentives for that required collaboration.

- Chronic disease management, accountable care organizations, and the virtual medical home are current conceptual strategies that may alter the paradigm of split treatment of psychiatric patients in the United States.

- Mental health clinicians who are truly a team can provide each other with consultation and emotional ballast during the sometimes grueling process of treating suicidal patients.

References

American Psychiatric Association: Guidelines for psychiatrists in consultative, supervisory, or collaborative relationships with nonmedical therapists. Am J Psychiatry 137:1489–1491, 1980

American Psychiatric Association: Practice guideline for the assessment and treatment of patients with suicidal behaviors. Am J Psychiatry 160(suppl):1–60, 2003

Andrews v United States, 732 F2d 366 (1984)

Balon R, Riba MB: Improving the practice of split treatment. Psychiatr Ann 31:594–596, 2001

Bao Y, Alexopoulos GS, Casalino LP: Collaborative depression care management and disparities in depression treatment and outcomes. Arch Gen Psychiatry 68:627–636, 2011

Berwick D: Launching accountable care organizations—the proposed rule for the Medicare Shared Savings Program. N Engl J Med 364:e32, 2011

Brown GK, Ten Have TR, Henriques GR, et al: Cognitive therapy for the prevention of suicide attempts: a randomized controlled trial. JAMA 294:563–570, 2005

Centers for Disease Control and Prevention: Alcohol and suicide among racial/ethnic populations—17 states, 2005–2006. June 19, 2009a. Available at: http://www.cdc.gov/mmwr/preview/mmwrhtml/mm5823a1.htm. Accessed August 10, 2011.

Centers for Disease Control and Prevention: Suicide rates among persons ages 25–64 years, by race/ethnicity and sex, United States, 2002–2006. September 2009b. Available at: http://www.cdc.gov/violenceprevention/suicide/statistics/rates04.html. Accessed August 10, 2011.

Centers for Disease Control and Prevention: Suicide rates among persons ages 65 years and older, by race/ethnicity and sex, United States, 2002–2006. September 2009c. Available at: http://www.cdc.gov/violenceprevention/suicide/statistics/rates05.html. August 10, 2011.

Centers for Disease Control and Prevention: National suicide statistics at a glance: U.S. map of suicide. 2011a. Available at: http://www.cdc.gov/violenceprevention/suicide/statistics/aag.html#2. Accessed August 10, 2011.

Centers for Disease Control and Prevention: Suicide: risk and protective factors. 2011b. Available at: http://www.cdc.gov/violenceprevention/suicide/riskprotectivefactors.html. Accessed August 10, 2011.

Cohen v State of New York, 382 NYS 2nd 128 (1976)

Comtois KA, Linehan MM: Psychosocial treatments of suicidal behaviors: a practice-friendly review. J Clin Psychol 62:161–170, 2006

Dewan M: Are psychiatrists cost-effective? An analysis of integrated versus split treatment. Am J Psychiatry 156:324–326, 1999

Fountoulakis KN, Gonda X, Siamouli M, et al: Psychotherapeutic intervention and suicide risk reduction in bipolar disorder: a review of the evidence. J Affect Disord 113:21–29, 2009

Goldman W, McCulloch J, Cuffel B, et al: Outpatient utilization patterns of integrated and split psychotherapy and pharmacotherapy for depression. Psychiatr Serv 49:477–482, 1998

Goldsmith SK, Pellmar TC, Kleinman AM, et al (eds): Psychiatric and psychological factors, in Reducing Suicide: A National Imperative. Washington, DC, National Academies Press, 2002, pp 69–118

Gunnell D, Miller M: Strategies to prevent suicide. BMJ 341:c3054, 2010

Gutheil TG, Simon RI: Abandonment of patients in split treatment. Harv Rev Psychiatry 11:175–179, 2003

Harris G: Doctors Inc.: Talk doesn't pay, so psychiatry turns instead to drug therapy. The New York Times Magazine, March 3, 2011, A1

Hawton K, van Heeringen: Suicide. Lancet 373:1372–1381, 2009

Katon WJ, Schoenbaum M, Fan MY, et al: Cost-effectiveness of improving primary care treatment of late-life depression. Arch Gen Psychiatry 62:1313–1320, 2005

Katon WJ, Lin EH, Von Korff M, et al: Collaborative care for patients with depression and chronic illnesses. N Engl J Med 363:2611–2620, 2010

Kessler RC, Berglund P, Demler O, et al: The epidemiology of major depressive disorder: results from the National Comorbidity Survey Replication (NCS-R). JAMA 289:3095–3105, 2003

Malone KM, Oquendo MA, Haas GL, et al: Protective factors against suicidal acts in major depression: reasons for living. Am J Psychiatry 157:1084–1088, 2000

Mann JJ, Apter A, Bertolote J, et al: Suicide prevention strategies: a systematic review. JAMA 294:2064–2074, 2005

Merikangas KR, Jin R, He J, et al: Prevalence and correlates of bipolar spectrum disorder in the World Mental Health Survey Initiative. Arch Gen Psychiatry 68:241–251, 2011

Meyer DJ: Split treatment and coordinated care with multiple mental health clinicians: clinical and risk management issues. Prim Psychiatry 9:56–60, 2002

Mojtabai R, Olfson M: National trends in psychotherapy by office-based psychiatrists. Arch Gen Psychiatry 65:962–970, 2008

Osterberg L, Blaschke T: Adherence to medication. N Engl J Med 353:487–497, 2005

Pies RW: Psychotherapy is alive and talking in psychiatry. Psychiatric Times, March 11, 2011

Resnick PJ: Recognizing that the suicidal patient views you as an adversary. Curr Psychiatr 1:8, 2002

Rothschild AJ, Locke CA: Re-exposure to fluoxetine after serious suicide attempts by three patients: the role of akathisia. J Clin Psychiatry 52:491–493, 1991

Sareen J, Cox BJ, Afifi TO, et al: Anxiety disorders and risk for suicidal ideation and suicide attempts: a population-based longitudinal study of adults. Arch Gen Psychiatry 62:1249–1257, 2005

Sederer LI, Ellison J, Keyes C: Guidelines for prescribing psychiatrists in consultative, collaborative and supervisory relationships. Psychiatr Serv 49:1197–1202, 1998

Simon RI: Just a smile and a hello on the Golden Gate Bridge. Am J Psychiatry 164:720–721, 2007

St Germain v Pfeifer, 418 Mass 511–522 (1994)

U.S. Surgeon General Regina Benjamin: CNN. American Morning, May 11, 2011

Vergouwen AC, Bakker A, Katon WJ, et al: Improving adherence to antidepressants: a systematic review of interventions. J Clin Psychiatry 64:1415–1420, 2003

World Health Organization: The World Health Report 2002: Reducing Risks, Promoting Healthy Life. Geneva, World Health Organization, 2002

PART IV

Treatment Settings

Emergency Services

Divy Ravindranath, M.D., M.S.

D. Edward Deneke, M.D.

Michelle Riba, M.D., M.S.

Mr. F is a 54-year-old man with chronic low back pain, depression, and alcohol dependence in remission. He has been brought to the emergency department (ED) by his wife for suicidal ideation. According to his wife, he has been increasingly depressed for the last few months, secondary to conflicts at work. He still has his job, but because of what he calls office politics, he is being assigned to projects that he cannot complete. He thinks he is going to be fired soon. Beginning the day before he was brought to the ED, according to his wife, Mr. F started talking about preferring death to being unemployed and on the brink of homelessness. She thought that it was an unreasonable statement because they have sufficient savings to last for at least a few months, but he would not accept her reassurance. She also notes that he started drinking alcohol again about a month ago. She contacted his primary care doctor, who has been attempting to improve his depression with a selective serotonin reuptake inhibitor for the last 6 weeks. The primary care doctor instructed her to bring him to the ED. On arrival to the ED, the patient reported suicidal ideation to the triage nurse, who had him searched by security for any weapons and then directed him to a secure ED bay in sight of the nursing station to wait for medical and mental health evaluation. Mr. F was not intoxicated on arrival to the ED.

On interview, Mr. F was cooperative and forthcoming. He confirmed worsening depression, increased hopelessness about his work and finances, and thoughts about death for the last week. His back pain has also been worse in this span and is part of the reason why he started drinking again. He only verbalized these thoughts yesterday perhaps because he thinks he and his wife are drifting apart. He endorsed feeling very alone in his depression and did express some concern about what would happen if he were discharged home. His thoughts about death concern him, and he finds it difficult to dismiss them. He has thought about suicide in the last two days but not about how he would try to kill himself. He would definitely not try to overdose as he did when he was depressed in his 20s, because it did not work. He does own a shotgun for hunting. He finds the thoughts of suicide to be simultaneously hypnotic and repulsive. He maintains strong religious prohibitions against suicide.

You contact Mr. F's primary care doctor with Mr. F's permission. This physician tells you that Mr. F's case seemed to start out as an uncomplicated case of depression but that after about 2 months of monitoring and treatment, he seems only to be getting worse. Mr. F's primary care doctor feels out of his depth.

You explain to Mr. F that severe depression can come with overpowering hopelessness, thoughts of death, and even thoughts of suicide. You point out that some of his thoughts might be distorted by the depression. You express concern that his depression has been worsening despite the efforts of his primary care doctor and state that some changes need to be made. He agrees with this assessment. You relate to him that your immediate concern is regarding his safety. He reassures you that he will not commit suicide if discharged home. You accept his reassurance and reflect that not committing suicide keeps him safe but does not improve his depression. You ask him to participate in safety planning with you, but he cannot come up with activities that reliably make him feel better or people with whom he feels comfortable talking about his suicidal ideation. Therefore, you offer him psychiatric hospitalization. He asks if this is the only option. You tell him that it is the best and safest option and explain to him the difference between a voluntary and an involuntary hospitalization. He agrees to psychiatric hospitalization.

The ED can be a very challenging place in which to assess and manage risk of suicide. The evaluating provider usually does not have any prior experience with the patient. Patients often present after business hours, making it difficult to get in contact with their usual providers. Patients are sometimes compelled to have a mental health evaluation in the ED, either because they came there for some other concern and suicidal ideation was detected surreptitiously or because they were brought to the ED against their will. Finally, if the ED is not specialized for psychiatric emergencies (so-called psychiatric emergency services), then first contact with the patient may be made by a generalist, who would be less savvy about mental health concerns.

Despite these challenges, the ED still represents a critical clinical environment for detection and management of suicide risk. Individuals in the community are brought to emergency rooms because EDs are contained environments in which further treatment planning can take place. One retrospective study found that 40% of individuals who died by suicide presented to the ED at least once during the year prior to their death (Da Cruz et al. 2011). Moreover, the federal regulation Emergency Medical Treatment and Active Labor Act (EMTALA) requires that any patient presenting to an ED receive an evaluation for any life-threatening condition and that said condition be satisfactorily stabilized before release from the ED, including mental health conditions such as suicidal ideation (Quinn et al. 2002). Thus, it is in the best interests of any clinician working in an ED to understand the basic principles of suicide risk assessment and management in that clinical setting. That is the objective of this chapter.

Approach to the Patient

Initial Triage

There are many strategies to identify patients at increased risk for suicide. In the simplest circumstance, the patient will present with the chief complaint of suicidal ideation. The patient may have been referred to the ED by a 911 or crisis-line operator or by his or her current outpatient provider. Alternatively, patients who present with mental health complaints (e.g., depression, anxiety, or hallucinations) may confirm suicidal ideation if asked about it. Or patients may present with medical consequences secondary to a suicide attempt (e.g., unconsciousness after an overdose). Finally, there are multiple validated screening tools for patients presenting with general concerns. These instruments vary from simply asking if a patient has been having thoughts of suicide or a persistently depressed mood in the recent past to complex instruments that delve into the characteristics of the patient's thoughts, plans, and intent for suicide. These instruments, some of which are proprietary and therefore expensive to adopt for universal screening, include tools for children/adolescents (Horowitz et al. 2010; King et al. 2009) and adults (Folse and Hahn 2009). These instruments can be administered by triage staff as they decide the level of care the patient will require in the ED.

A patient at increased risk for suicide should not be left alone in the ED even while receiving needed medical care. Such patients may elope, negating the advantage of being in the ED. Unsupervised patients may also find a way to harm themselves in the ED. In the general ED, for example, typically there are numerous medical instruments available that may be used for this purpose. Alternatively, patients may bring weapons with them.

Various strategies have been developed to keep suicidal patients safe in the ED. These include limiting access to instruments that can be used to harm oneself, searching patients at presumed increased risk for weapons, having such patients change into hospital gowns so that they are easily identified if they do abscond, having such patients wear devices that trigger alarms if they cross the ED threshold, and keeping the patient under direct or arm's-length staff supervision. Whether and under what circumstances such a patient can be kept behind a locked door varies from state to state. Placing high-risk patients in restraints would also keep them from harming themselves, although patients in restraints are at higher risk for agitation and accidental self-injury (Mohr et al. 2003). Thus, restraints should be reserved for patients who cannot be kept safe by any other means.

Although some patients may find comfort in the fact that their thoughts of suicide and related distress are being taken seriously by ED staff, these steps may seem unnecessary to or may be unwanted by some patients. As such, staff should expect at least some resistance from the patient.

This resistance may be overcome by explaining the rationale for the steps to the patient, by explaining that this is part of customary procedure for patients at suspected risk for suicide, and by explaining that the steps may be temporary until the patient receives a complete suicide risk assessment. Resistance despite these suggestions may then trigger a call for help to other staff, who may be able to compel the patient with a simple show of force. At times, the patient may become aggressive, and physical management may be required; this should be reserved for staff with specific training in physical management (e.g., security staff). Management of agitation is discussed in more detail later in this chapter.

Medical Evaluation

Patients presenting to the ED need to receive an evaluation to identify any medical conditions that need treatment prior to evaluation for future suicide risk. This should include evaluation for medical conditions present as a consequence of suicidal behavior, evaluation for chronic medical conditions that may be poorly controlled secondary to the patient's mental condition, evaluation for chronic medical conditions that may impact aspects of the patient's psychiatric care, and evaluation for any comorbid medical conditions that may develop into medical calamities if not addressed. Examples include surface wounds due to self-cutting; high blood pressure due to medication nonadherence, itself secondary to crippling depression; obesity and hyperlipidemia that may influence choice of antipsychotic medication; and active daily alcohol misuse that may develop into alcohol withdrawal if the patient is admitted to a psychiatric facility. There are checklists available in the literature to aid the ED physician in conducting a brief but thorough medical clearance (Shah et al. 2010; Sood and Mcstay 2009).

Of note, some patients may require medical hospitalization or other measures before stabilization of their medical condition (Kudo et al. 2010). In this circumstance, the patient's suicide risk should be evaluated in a serial fashion and not be considered definitive until the patient's medical condition has stabilized. The presence of the medical condition may directly affect the patient's suicide risk (e.g., in the case of a delirium or intoxication) or may indirectly influence a patient's will to live (e.g., in the case of a patient whose hope cannot be restored until after receipt of a liver transplant needed secondary to acetaminophen overdose). Moreover, aspects of suicide risk management in an inpatient setting are different from suicide risk management in the outpatient setting. (Suicide risk management in the inpatient setting is discussed in Chapter 18, "Inpatient Psychiatric Treatment," in this volume.)

Patients who are medically stable can be instructed to wait in a safe area of the ED until the mental health evaluation can be completed. This may be in the ED waiting area with family members or in a seclusion room in restraints, depending on the patient's level of risk in the ED, the patient's cooperation with the risk assessment process, and the policies of the specific ED. In some communities, patients will have to be transferred to a different facility, where there are mental health professionals who can perform the risk assessment. In this circumstance, the medical ED and the receiving facility must agree to the transfer, and all needed documentation must accompany the patient from one facility to the other. Transport in this circumstance should be conducted by trained professionals and not by the patient or the

patient's family. The patient is still assumed to be at high risk for suicide until the risk assessment is completed.

The Interview

As mentioned earlier, the ED may be the first and only time the patient and the mental health professional meet. This presents the dual challenge of establishing sufficient rapport with the patient to elicit a thorough history and mental status exam while not expending so much time as to leave the patient fatigued or to neglect the clinician's other duties in the ED. Challenges to rapport include decreased eye contact; decreased spontaneous elaborations; short, uninfomative statements; and requests to discontinue the interview.

The interviewer must first decide the setting in which to interview the patient. Patients may need to be evaluated in a general medical bay, in an intensive care unit in the ED, in the hallway, in a private room with a door that locks, in the room without a locking door, and so on. As a rule of thumb, the environment in which the interview is conducted should be sufficiently private as to make the patient feel comfortable talking about his or her mental state. Moreover, the patient should not have access to any instruments that can be used as a weapon against him- or herself or against the interviewer. Additionally, both the patient and the interviewer should have equal access to egress pathways in case the patient becomes agitated.

Before beginning the interview, the examiner should inform the patient that the purpose of the interview is for the examiner to assess the patient's risk for self-injury and provide recommendations to the patient and perhaps other treatment providers about how to improve any mental suffering discovered. The examiner can inform the patient that it is in the patient's best interest to provide an accurate accounting of his or her current crisis. Depending on the mechanism for involuntary hospitalization in a given state, the examiner may be required to inform the patient that items discussed during the ED encounter may need to be reported during a court hearing. If this step is described to the patient as a requirement and it is pointed out that the patient is not being singled out, the patient may be more willing to continue the interview in a frank and forthright fashion.

In general, and especially for patients who present to the ED voluntarily, being open and friendly is sufficient to establish initial rapport. Starting with open-ended questions to allow the patient to construct his or her own story gives the interviewer an opportunity to develop a framework of the patient's mental state and current crisis that can later be filled in with details, and it simultaneously gives the patient an opportunity to be heard. In this part of the interview, rapport can be strengthened through use of active listening techniques such as nonverbal expressions of support, empathetic statements, and periodic rephrasing. Once the rapport is strengthened, the patient can be challenged with more specific closed-ended questions and more intrusive parts of the examination.

TABLE 16–1. Signs of agitation

More intense eye contact

Angry tone

Sarcastic comments

Talk of capacity for violence to others

Threatening comments

Increased psychomotor activity

No longer cooperating with simple requests

Clenching fists

Advancing on the interviewer

Agitation

If the patient starts to show signs of agitation (listed in Table 16–1), it may be as a result of the interviewer's line of questioning. It may help repair the rapport to switch to a less sensitive topic or take a break altogether. Additionally, making a process comment, such as "It seems like I've touched on a difficult topic," may give the patient space to explore his or her emotions about this topic and receive validation, making it easier to reapproach the topic later if needed. Although it may be important in terms of overall treatment planning, some topics are sensitive and low yield in terms of establishing suicide risk (e.g., details of childhood sexual abuse) and therefore need not be discussed in the ED setting.

A patient who is losing connection with the interviewer for uncertain reasons may be experiencing a deficiency in a lower-rank need (e.g., need for food/hydration or need for the restroom). A chance to address such a need should be offered to patients, even those who do not identify it as the reason for their lack of complete participation in the interview.

Agitated patients who cannot be calmed down with these simple interventions present a greater challenge. These patients are at increased risk of intentional or unintentional self-injury and injury to others in the ED. It is critical that all staff in the ED, including clerks and other nonclinical staff, be trained in the recognition and initial management of agitation and that each ED have a strategy for addressing agitation in a safe and effective manner. A patient who cannot be calmed down with simple verbal interventions should not be spoken to alone. The first priority of the interviewer, as noted earlier, is to conduct the interview in a safe manner. If the patient is becoming agitated, it may be safest for the interviewer to flee, gather more help, and then return to the patient. Alternatively, the agitated patient may choose to flee and should be allowed to do so as long as he or she can be brought back to the ED with sufficient staff support.

A show of force may be enough to corral and calm down the agitated patient. However, patients who cannot be kept this way without having numerous staff present should be offered medications to help them maintain calm. Most medications used for this purpose fall into the benzodiazepine or antipsychotic category. The specific medication and dose selected should depend on the patient's medical profile. For example, an elderly patient or a child, compared with an adult patient, will need or tolerate only a lower dose of either medication. Also, a severely agitated patient will require a medication with a nonparenteral route of administration for ease of delivery and rapidity of action. Some medications used for management of agitation are listed in Table 16–2.

Restraints and transition to a seclusion room are interventions administered to patients who cannot refrain from being a persistent risk of danger to themselves or others. Such interventions should only be done by trained staff in accordance with local ED policy.

Critical Data

Risk factors for suicide attempts are well known and discussed elsewhere in this text (see, e.g., Chapter 1, "Suicide Risk Assessment: Gateway to Treatment and Management"). However, in the ED, the evaluation focuses on prevention of future suicide attempts. Thus, it is useful to conceptualize the patient as having a baseline risk for suicide—secondary to hereditary, develop-

mental, and historical events—and now experiencing a crisis that elevates the risk above the customary baseline. Table 16–3 outlines some common suicide risk factors with this conceptualization in mind. Given that the patient's experiences cannot be changed, any treatment plan to reduce risk of suicide will focus on modifiable factors in the current crisis.

A thorough evaluation will contain all elements of a standard medical history and physical examination. The history of present illness should begin with the details of the current crisis and should also include a psychiatric review of systems detailing any depressive, manic, anxiety, psychotic, and cognitive symptoms present during the current crisis. The past psychiatric history should provide some details about the patient's recent treatment, including current treatment providers, a very detailed history of any suicide/parasuicide attempts, and history of psychiatric hospitalizations. The substance use history should detail recent alcohol and drug use patterns, history of substance withdrawal, history of legal and social consequences to substance use, and history of self-injury when intoxicated. The patient's medical history should be detailed and a medical review of systems obtained to facilitate medical clearance, with special attention paid to any chronic medical conditions or pain about which the patient feels hopeless. The patient's list of current medications, including adherence patterns, should be obtained. Any family history of self-injury or mental illness should be identified. The social history should include any current stressors or sources of support and any access to means for lethal self-injury. The mental status exam should focus on any factors that help the evaluating physician to grade severity of mental illness (e.g., evidence of poor self-care, the patient's degree of comprehension of ele-

TABLE 16–2. Medications used for agitation management

Medication	Adult dose	Pediatric dose	Indications other than agitation	Side effects
Aripiprazole	9.75 mg im (up to 30 mg/day)		Psychosis	Akathisia Paradoxical activation Expensive
Benztropine	0.5–2 mg po/im	0.25–2 mg po/im	EPS/akathisia	Anticholinergic side effects, including delirium in elderly
Chlorpromazine	25–50 mg im 25–100 mg po	12.5–25 mg im 10–50 mg po	Psychosis	Orthostatic hypotension
Diazepam	5–10 mg po/im		Anxiety Alcohol withdrawal	Oversedation Respiratory depression
Diphenhydramine	25–50 mg po/im	12.5–50 mg po/im	EPS/akathisia	Delirium in elderly Paradoxical activation
Fluphenazine	5–10 mg po/im		Psychosis	EPS QTc prolongation
Haloperidol	0.5–5 mg po/iv/im (up to 15 mg)	0.25–5 mg po/im	Psychosis	EPS QTc prolongation
Lorazepam	0.5–4 mg po/iv/im	0.25–2 mg	Anxiety Alcohol withdrawal EPS/akathisia	Oversedation Respiratory depression
Olanzapine	5–10 mg (up to 20 mg/day)		Psychosis	Maximum dosage achieved quickly Expensive
Risperidone	0.5–2 mg po	0.125–2 mg po	Psychosis	EPS at higher doses
Ziprasidone	10 mg im (up to 40 mg/day)		Psychosis	QTc prolongation Expensive

Note. EPS=extrapyramidal symptoms, including dystonic reactions.
Source. Adapted from three tables in Riba and Ravindranath 2010.

TABLE 16–3. Historical and modifiable risk factors for suicide

Historical risk factors	Modifiable risk factors
Male gender	Substance abuse
Older age	Substance intoxication
Prior suicide attempts	Depressive episode
Chronic physical symptoms and/or pain	Manic/mixed state
Family history of suicide	Psychosis
	Panic attacks/anxiety
	Irritability
	Restlessness/akathisia
	Insomnia
	Diminished concentration
	Hopelessness
	Perceived social isolation
	Access to means

Source. Adapted from Simon 2008.

ments discussed, the patient's response to interventions in the ED).

Patients may be brought to the ED against their will and therefore have an incentive to underreport their degree of suicidal ideation. Alternatively, patients may trump up their suicide risk in order to garner resolution of other needs (e.g., food and shelter) through hospitalization. As such, histories elicited from the patient should be treated as provisional, pending confirmation from independent sources. This treatment is especially true for patients in whom there is obvious motivation for misrepresenting themselves and for patients who seem to have discrepancies in their reporting. A more accurate impression of suicide risk can be constructed on how the patient behaves rather than on what the patient says (Simon 2008). Collateral information can be obtained from the medical record, the patient's outpatient providers, family and friends of the patient, police officers who encountered the patient in the field, and so on.

Privacy concerns should be taken into account when seeking collateral information. Medical records, including the details of an ED visit, are protected by the federal Health Insurance Portability and Accountability Act (HIPAA) and, at times, state or local statutes. However, HIPAA makes exceptions for key information needed to resolve emergency situations, for contacting guardians and other surrogate decision makers for patients who lack capacity for medical decision making, and for continuity of care (Mermelstein and Wallack 2008). Even if it is not illegal to seek information without the patient's consent, the patient's permission should be sought and documented prior to contacting collateral informants. If the patient refuses, the consequence of seeking the information is diminished rapport, although rapport may need to be sacrificed in pursuit of the overall goal. To minimize the consequences to rapport and maintain morality in treatment, the examiner should reveal as little information about the patient and the current visit as possible while getting the needed information from the collateral informant.

The literature describes standardized instruments, such as the Scale for Suicide Ideation (Beck et al. 1988) and the Suicide Assessment Scale (Waern et al. 2010) and structured interviews such as the Columbia Suicide Severity Rating Scale (Mundt et al. 2010), that help determine acute risk for suicide. An ED examiner may decide to incorporate one or more of these tools into his or her approach to suicidal patients, either at the initial triage or at the time when increased suicide risk is suspected. However, these instruments should be considered decision-making aids and sources of augmenting information and not an alternative to a patient interview by an empathetic individual. The rapport generated in the evaluation of the patient can be central to developing a plan to diminish suicide risk, making discharge to the community safe. When the patient reports information to the interviewer that contradicts information reported on a standardized instrument, the examiner then needs to determine which report to believe. The examiner needs to decide whether this is the type of patient who has difficulty feeling comfortable with people and therefore underreports in face-to-face interviews or the type of patient who overreports in face-to-face interviews because of the validation received from another person. This is a challenging decision and one made based on clinical experience. Collateral information, of course, can help in making this decision.

Assessment and Disposition

High-risk patients are those who in the midst of the present crisis cannot resist action on suicidal ideation despite all attempted interventions. These patients generally have a number of other high-risk historical ele-

ments, such as history of serious suicide attempt or multiple suicide attempts, family history of suicide attempts, childhood trauma, chronic medical conditions with no hope for their resolution, and so on.

Low-risk patients are those who have intermittent thoughts of death or suicide but find that these thoughts do not persist for long. These patients can provide multiple reasons as to why they would not want to kill themselves and are also hopeful for improvement in their current state of affairs. They are committed to working with professionals to effect that improvement. These patients also typically lack the historical elements listed earlier that correlate with suicide attempts.

Moderate-risk patients (which could constitute the majority of patients seen in any given ED) are patients who fall in between these two categories. Moreover, because each suicide attempt is potentially lethal, the ED clinician should have a low threshold for declaring a patient moderate or high risk, rather than low risk. As implied earlier, because of efforts in the ED, the patient who was at high risk for suicide on entry to the ED may be at moderate or low risk by the end of the ED encounter. The final declaration of the patient's risk should be made after available efforts are exhausted.

The default disposition for patients at high risk for suicide in the ED is transfer to an inpatient psychiatric facility. This disposition provides access to a safe environment in which to address modifiable risk factors and access to mental health professionals who can help in this process. Hospitalization has the negative consequences of high financial cost and, typically, restriction of the patient's right to free movement. Moreover, the time spent in intensive psychiatric treatment has the opportunity cost of not spending time on other patient life activities such as work and child care. Not attending to these life activities may have its own consequences (e.g., job loss). Because of the high monetary cost of inpatient psychiatric treatment and the ever-expanding patient base, acute inpatient psychiatric beds are a very limited resource in many localities (Sharfstein and Dickerson 2009). This may result in an extended waiting period in the ED, using resources that should go to other emergencies.

Because of these costs and practical considerations, the ED evaluator should do his or her best to modify risk factors in patients with the time and resources available in the ED to reduce the patient's risk for suicide to moderate before determining disposition. For many patients, however, the resources and time available in an inpatient unit will be needed to reduce the risk sufficiently so as to ensure no attempts at suicide are made before entry or reentry into the outpatient mental health system of treatment.

Outpatient Treatment

Every patient who presents to the ED is in the midst of a crisis, even if he or she is presenting to the ED at the wishes of someone else. The crisis may be as simple as the patient being out of his or her medications. The crisis may also be very complicated, such as depression secondary to ongoing family conflicts and stress of multiple chronic and poorly controlled medical problems leading to a suicide attempt and parasuicidal behavior.

Each crisis warrants its own specifically tailored intervention that calls upon the creativity of the ED provider. Common elements of any intervention may include psychopharmacology, psychoeducation for the patient, psychoeducation for the patient's supportive individuals, helping the

patient boost coping skills, helping the patient's supports boost tolerance for the patient, social resources such as access to food and shelter, restriction of access to means for lethal self-injury such as guns or excess medications, and referral for additional professional supports. If at all possible, the patient should also have access to a safe and supportive environment to go to after being discharged from the ED.

It is critical that the patient understand the elements of the intervention designed and have the wherewithal to implement the needed steps. If the patient does not have this capacity or lacks insight into the nature of the crisis and need for the intervention, as is often the case for patients brought to the ED against their will, the bulk of the intervention will need to be performed with the patient's supports. Some risk-reduction steps may need to be completed at home while the patient is still in the ED, such as removal of any alcohol or firearms from the residence. Patient supports will need to assist with this. If this risk reduction cannot be done—for example, the supports are not present, the supports do not feel comfortable taking care of the patient in the manner requested, or the patient does not feel comfortable including supports in the treatment plan in this way—then there is no alternative to inpatient treatment.

Safety plans are quickly becoming the standard of care in many medical environments, such as Veterans Affairs medical facilities, for patients with an intermittent wish for death or suicidal ideation (Worchel and Gearing 2010). Elements of the VA safety plan are listed in Table 16–4. Although there are no randomized controlled trials to support the use of safety plans as of yet, every patient at moderate risk for suicide should complete a safety plan in the ED. The safety plan provides tools to help the patient recognize descent into suicidal thoughts, elucidates tools to slow or reverse the descent, and catalogs phone numbers for personal and professional supports for use in an emergency. The last element, at least, does have research to support a trend in terms of reducing suicide attempts after discharge from an inpatient psychiatric unit (Morgan et al. 1993). The elements of the safety plan should be collected in a single document using the patient's own words. The safety plan document should be given to the patient at the time of discharge from the ED as a tangible reminder of ways to keep safe and improve his or her mood state as well as a tangible reminder of the positive relationships formed in the ED visit. The patient should be instructed to keep the safety plan handy so that he or she can refer to it at times of increased stress.

If the patient already has a safety plan on arrival to the ED, he or she should be asked whether the safety plan was used before coming to the ED. If the safety plan was not used, barriers to its use should be explored and mitigated. If the safety plan was used, then it should be amended to make it more effective. If the patient cannot be motivated to use the safety plan or if the safety plan cannot be amended, then there may be no alternative to hospitalization.

Before the end of the ED encounter, the patient should agree not to attempt suicide without enacting elements of his or her safety plan. Medical systems used to demand that this agreement be documented in a "no-suicide contract." However, subsequent research demonstrated that having a no-suicide contract alone is of very little value (Lewis 2007). Instead, the manner by which the patient engaged in safety planning and committed to refraining from suicide is much more informative, because it speaks to the patient's commitment to continued living and hope for improvement.

TABLE 16–4. Elements of a suicide safety plan

1. *Triggers for thoughts of suicide:* These are emotions, thoughts, or experiences that tend to make the patient feel worse and start the spiral toward thoughts of suicide.

2. *Coping skills:* These are thoughts or behaviors in which the patient can engage in order to feel better and reverse the spiral toward thoughts of suicide or distract him or her from thoughts of suicide if they are there.

3. *Supportive individuals:* These are close friends and family whom the patient can contact if he or she cannot shake thoughts of suicide with Part 2 of the suicide safety plan, if only to ask for help getting to a local ED. List names, relationships, and contact information if available.

4. *Professional supports:* List names and contact information for any supportive medical professionals (e.g., primary care doctors, therapists, psychiatrists, contact information for the local ED, crisis telephone lines available to the patient, and 911).

5. *Ways to keep the environment safe:* List any steps needed to keep the patient from gaining access to lethal means for suicide. This includes putting barriers between the patient and any guns, excess supplies of medications, vehicles, etc. Specific elements will depend on the plans for suicide considered by the patient.

Note. ED=emergency department.
Source. Adapted from Stanley and Brown 2008.

Every patient considered for outpatient treatment from the ED should be able to connect with an outpatient treatment provider within a short while after the date of the ED visit. Different localities have different standards of care, but time to appointment with an outpatient treatment provider may be as short as the next day, a few days, a week, or 2 weeks. The longer the patient has to wait for this appointment, the more likely it is that his or her state will decline and that suicidal ideation or behavior will return (Cedereke et al. 2002). The patient's follow-up appointment may be with a new care provider or an existing care provider. The patient should be told that this provider will help the patient address the current crisis further and hopefully help him or her prevent future crises. As such, the patient should not be given the option of declining a follow-up appointment. Doing so ensures ongoing use of the ED for the patient's mental health needs and risks appearance of a crisis that cannot be managed with available resources and perhaps a resultant suicide attempt (Knesper 2011). Ideally, the patient would have the name of his or her provider and the date and time of the future appointment before discharge from the ED. This may not be possible after business hours, and daytime ED staff may need to follow up with the patient to ensure that this critical element is completed. Other interventions after discharge from the ED have been tested; all seem to boost attendance at the first visit but may not reduce future return to the ED. These interventions include discharge to a mobile crisis unit (Currier et al. 2010), supportive contact from ED staff by text message (Chen et al. 2010) or postcard (Carter et al. 2007), and scheduled telephonic or face-to-face clinical contact with ED staff (Lizardi and Stanley 2010; Newton et al. 2010).

Given the fluctuating nature of suicidal ideation, maintaining continuity of care is a cornerstone for preventing suicide attempts after the ED visit. The patient may have had elevated suicidal ideation before the ED visit, which prompted the visit and disruption of the potentially toxic daily routine. The patient may then feel better after the ED visit, allowing for return to the home environment with recommendations to manage the immediate crisis and a safety plan to assist with future crises. However, the longer the patient stays in his or her potentially toxic daily routine, the more likely it is that a crisis will arise that cannot be managed with the safety plan and that results in a potentially lethal suicide attempt. The fragmented health care system, however, grown in an environment that stigmatizes mental illness, contains many barriers to ensuring rapid follow-up. Thus, systems level interventions are needed to prevent suicide adequately after an ED visit. (For more discussion of these points, see Knesper 2011.)

Inpatient Treatment

As mentioned earlier in this chapter, hospitalization should be reserved for patients who cannot be made less than high risk within the resource confines of the ED. At some point in the encounter, the examiner will have to make a decision as to whether the patient meets these criteria for hospitalization. In one study, factors that correlated with hospitalization from the ED included older age, symptomatic psychotic disorder, symptomatic affective disorder, lack of alcohol intoxication at the time of the attempt, somatic illness, suicide attempt on a weekday, and prior psychiatric treatment (Suominen and Lönnqvist 2006). Acuity of any attempt at self-injury before presentation to the ED also correlates with hospitalization (Kudo et al. 2010).

Once the decision for hospitalization is made, the tone of the ED encounter changes. The ED provider is no longer only concerned about making the patient safe for the community but is concerned about keeping the patient safe until transfer to an inpatient facility can be made.

The decision for hospitalization should be communicated to the patient first. This may elicit either relief and comfort or anger and opposition from the patient. In the former case, the patient will likely remain cooperative and will be willing to complete any paperwork required by the state or by the inpatient facility in order to hasten transfer from the ED. In the latter case, the patient may become uncooperative. Fortunately, every state has a mechanism by which psychiatric patients can be hospitalized against their wishes. Each practitioner should be familiar with local regulations and practice patterns. Of note, involuntary admission typically means that the patient cannot cross state lines; this becomes an important factor when deciding where to send the patient.

Depending on the availability of psychiatric inpatient beds in a given community, the patient may have to wait for a long time (hours to days) before transfer can be made. As such, it is incumbent on the ED provider to anticipate needs to maintain health and safety while the patient remains in the ED. This includes scheduled medications, medications for use as needed, meals, access to grooming facilities, contact from family members, and so on. In some communities, the wait for an inpatient bed is so long that the local psychiatric emergency service turns into a central short-stay psychiatric hospital, where treatment planning also includes strategies that will improve the mental health of the patient, such as new medications and psychotherapeutic interventions.

While the patient is waiting, a designated ED staff person should be looking for an inpatient bed for the patient. This search usually requires calling different facilities to inquire whether there are beds and whether the available space and staff can help the patient improve his or her mental state. Each patient will have different requirements when in the inpatient setting. The patient may be involuntarily admitted and therefore cannot cross state lines. Some patients may be fully cooperative and would do fine

in an unlocked ward, whereas other patients are very combative and may require seclusion and/or restraints, then one-on-one observation by staff immediately on arrival. Some patients may be very medically ill, such that transfer to a psychiatric bed associated with a general hospital would be best. Other patients may have specialized psychiatric needs, such as the need for electroconvulsive treatment. Patients may have health insurance restrictions that would make transfer to one hospital financially feasible but transfer to a neighboring hospital financially prohibitive. Insurance companies may also require preauthorization for treatment, meaning that the case for admission for any given patient will have to be made to both the insurance provider and the hospital. The patient and the patient's family may also have preferences that will need to be taken into consideration. This dizzying array of variables and the barriers these variables pose to timely disposition from the ED is the main reason why some medical centers hire specialists to facilitate transfer of psychiatric patients from the ED. Other medical centers do not have the resources for such specialists, and thus the task falls to the mental health professional recommending hospitalization.

The receiving hospital may request records from the ED visit to detail the process for medical clearance, the suicide risk assessment, confirmation of health insurance coverage, and documentation of any anticipated needs during hospitalization. Thus, timely documentation by all ED clinical staff is critical to timely disposition. After receiving documentation, the receiving hospital may request to speak to the provider recommending hospitalization in order to clarify key points.

Assuming that each of these steps goes well, the patient will then be accepted to a hospital. The sending ED should document the name of the accepting hospital, the physician approving the admission, and the destination of the patient from the ED. ED staff can then arrange for transport to the hospital. This may be as simple as walking the patient from the ED to the psychiatry ward or as complex as arranging for transportation across the state. As noted earlier, transportation should be facilitated by professional staff—an ED staff person in the former case and an ambulance in the latter case—and not by the patient or by the patient's family.

Special Cases

Crisis Calls

At times the ED provider will be asked to field a call from a patient in the community who is concerned about thoughts of suicide. In this circumstance, the same principles for assessment of suicide risk apply, although management becomes much more difficult. The patient is, by definition, in an unsafe space if he or she is determined to be at moderate to high risk for suicide. Thus, in addition to the content discussed earlier, the ED provider should also determine the patient's name and location and who and/or what is around him or her (e.g., weapons, pills with which to overdose, supportive individuals). If possible, the ED provider should speak to any available supportive individuals to collect collateral information and direct them in the treatment plan.

If the patient is judged to be at moderate to high risk, he or she should be referred to an ED for further evaluation and management. The patient may be cooperative with this recommendation, and the cooperation can be reconfirmed with another person who can help in getting the patient to the ED. In that case, the name of the local ED can

be obtained and a report called, as needed. The patient may be hesitant, perhaps because of a concern about forced hospitalization. These patients can be reassured that the reason for further evaluation in the ED is just that, and that it is not guaranteed that they will be hospitalized from the ED. Other patients will be frankly resistant. These patients may need to be compelled by the supportive individuals with whom the ED provider has had contact. If there are no supportive individuals to draw upon or if the patient discontinues the phone conversation, then local authorities should be contacted and asked to perform an immediate face-to-face safety check.

Children and Adolescents

Suicide risk assessment in children and adolescents can be challenging, given that these patients have unique mental health needs. An age-appropriate approach to the interview has the greatest chance for eliciting truthful information. As with any patient, the patient's risk for self-injurious behavior in the present crisis should be determined and compared with the patient's baseline risk for self-injurious behavior. If the risk is significantly elevated and cannot be modified, the patient should then be psychiatrically hospitalized.

In this population, information from parents or guardians is required. These individuals are responsible for the patient's care and may provide the most useful collateral information in determining the patient's risk for suicidal behavior. In many states, children and adolescents can only be psychiatrically admitted or receive outpatient treatment with the permission of a parent or guardian. This is true even if the patient clinically has the mental capacity to consent to the planned intervention. If the parent or guardian disagrees with the

ED provider's treatment recommendations, he or she may be intentionally or unintentionally endangering the child and a child protective services report may need to be filed.

Patients Who Frequently Attempt Suicide

Patients who frequently attempt suicide are particularly challenging for the mental health provider in the ED, in that it can be difficult to tell when the patient is serious about wanting to kill him- or herself when so many prior attempts have been unsuccessful and, at times, triggered by seemingly trivial stressors. On the one hand, the current crisis may be the time when the suicide attempt succeeds. On the other hand, in the setting of limited resources, there are many pressures to keep this patient out of the hospital. Moreover, hospitalization can unintentionally "reward" provocative behavior, as in patients with borderline personality disorder, and thereby exacerbate the underlying mental illness. These patients, regardless of these scenarios, are much more ill than equivalent patients who do not attempt suicide frequently. Presence of long-standing affective disorders, drug/alcohol misuse disorders, anxiety, and a young age at first attempt all correlate with repeated attempts (Lopez-Castroman et al. 2010). Moreover, multiple attempters have a more severe clinical profile, such as deleterious childhood background, increased psychopathology, more suicidal ideation, and poorer interpersonal functioning, even when controlling for comorbid borderline personality disorder (Forman et al. 2004).

With these patients, trying to discern the details of the current psychosocial crisis is absolutely essential in determining risk of suicide after departure from the ED. The thoughts of suicide are the end result of a psychosocial spiral. Although the patient presents to the ED with talk of suicidal ideation, getting the patient to talk about why he or she might be having thoughts of suicide provides more targets for creative intervention, thereby addressing the "real" reason for presenting to the ED. This can be very challenging and the examiner will likely have to try numerous different strategies to get the patient to talk about an experience that is undoubtedly emotionally challenging. As with all ED patients, contact with current providers or other collateral informants can be essential for determining the details of the current crisis. This process may be easier with patients who are currently being trained in dialectical behavior therapy, a treatment shown to decrease suicide attempts and hospitalizations for suicidal ideation in patients with borderline personality disorder (Linehan et al. 2006).

Even with patients who repeatedly attempt suicide, each presentation to the ED must be evaluated in a vacuum, and each corresponding crisis needs to be addressed and the resultant risk of suicide decreased before the patient can be discharged to the community. As such, if the patient is too emotionally overwrought to be able to reasonably discuss the details of the crisis that precipitated the suicidal ideation, then there is no alternative to hospitalization.

Homeless Patients

Homeless patients present another type of challenge in that there is a higher index of suspicion that hospitalization for suicidal ideation is being sought to avoid being on the street or going to a shelter. As discussed earlier, assessing the patient's behavior, rather than taking his or her words at face value, will provide a more accurate evaluation of the patient's risk. Even if the patient is judged to be at sufficiently low risk to be discharged to the community, the patient may refuse to participate in safety planning or other treatment planning attempting to improve his or her mental state. For these patients, keeping from being homeless even for one night is worth sabotaging the help being offered. Some communities have homeless outreach programs to which homeless patients can be referred. Knowing that there may be additional resources available to them may improve the patient's engagement with treatment planning.

Patients With Substance Use Disorders

As discussed earlier, substance use disorders increase the risk for suicide attempt. Patients with substance use disorders who are not actively intoxicated have the additional mental health problem of the use disorder itself. This represents an independent and perhaps primary target for treatment on follow-up from the ED, and a separate treatment plan from that for the patient's primary mental illness (e.g., major depression, bipolar disorder) should be developed.

Many patients will be precontemplative with regard to readiness to cut back or discontinue substance use. For these patients, a motivational interviewing approach, as described by Miller and Rollnick (2002), may be helpful.

Actively intoxicated patients provide a greater challenge. Patients who are actively intoxicated may be at higher risk for intentional self-injury than when they are sober. For example, patients who are intoxicated with alcohol can be both emotionally labile and behaviorally disinhibited. Then, as they are approaching sobriety, some patients may manifest features of withdrawal that again may elevate their risk for suicide. For

example, a patient in cocaine withdrawal may manifest a profound depression. Thus, both intoxication and withdrawal represent states in which identifying and modifying risk for suicide would be difficult or impossible. Some knowledge of the patient's typical behavior when intoxicated or in withdrawal may help inform how he or she will behave in the current crisis, although the examiner must acknowledge that his or her capacity to predict the future accurately in this circumstance is diminished.

As always, psychiatric hospitalization, or at least holding the patient in a safe space until the intoxication and/or withdrawal has cleared, may provide the safest means for assuring no suicide after the patient's discharge to the community.

Documentation

As with any encounter, the ED visit and suicide risk assessment will need to be documented. As noted earlier, the documentation will need to be completed quickly, sometimes while the patient is still in the ED. The ED examiner should keep in mind that suicide attempts and ED visits can be targets for malpractice lawsuits. Documentation should be brief and focused, such that only the pertinent information is documented. The suicide risk assessment, however, should be systematic and comprehensive. Beyond the typical elements of a medical history and mental status exam, one should get into the habit of listing sources of information, patient's consent (or lack thereof with justification) for contacting collateral informants, the patient's historical and dynamic suicide risk factors, risk assessment weighing the pros and cons of inpatient versus outpatient treatment, any interventions to mitigate dynamic risk factors, elements of any safety plan developed, medication instructions at the time of ED discharge, and the plans for follow-up. Patients should also be given copies of the safety plan, medication instructions resultant from their time in the ED with any needed prescription slips, and detailed plans for follow-up.

Copies of the ED documentation should be made available to the patient's outpatient providers, especially those who will be seeing the patient next. This should be done with the patient's written permission if at all possible. This keeps the patient from having to experience the trauma of recounting his or her crisis and also advises the outpatient provider to contact the patient if he or she does not present for the appointment as scheduled.

Key Clinical Concepts

- The emergency department (ED) is a critical juncture between outpatient and inpatient care as well as a contained environment in which acute risk for suicide can be assessed and relevant treatment decisions made.

- Patients should be screened for suicidal ideation as early as possible in the ED visit because there is a chance that they will attempt to abscond or harm themselves while in the ED, defeating the purpose of being there.

- Conducting an interview in the ED can be challenging because of lack of history with the patient and because of patient opposition or agitation. These circumstances can be remedied with techniques to build rapport and manage agitation.

- A suicide risk assessment based on patient behavior and collateral information rather than on patient report may be more accurate.

- ED providers should attempt interventions to decrease risk of suicide and allow for outpatient management before deciding that a patient needs to be in a psychiatric hospital. These interventions may include recommendations for crisis resolution, working with the patient's supportive individuals, and developing a safety plan for the patient.

- Rapid outpatient follow-up is critical to prevention of suicide after discharge from the ED.

- If a patient is to be admitted, the ED provider is then responsible for maintaining, and perhaps improving, the patient's mental and physical health until transfer to the hospital can be accomplished.

References

Beck AT, Steer RA, Ranieri W: Scale for Suicide Ideation: psychometric properties of a self-report version. J Consult Clin Psychol 44:499–505, 1988

Carter GL, Clover K, Whyte IM, et al: Postcards from the EDge: 24-month outcomes of a randomised controlled trial for hospital-treated self-poisoning. Br J Psychiatry 191:548–553, 2007

Cedereke M, Monti K, Ojehagen A: Telephone contact with patients in the year after a suicide attempt: does it affect treatment attendance and outcome? A randomised controlled study. Eur Psychiatry 17:82–91, 2002

Chen H, Mishara BL, Liu XX: A pilot study of mobile telephone message interventions with suicide attempters in China. Crisis 31:109–112, 2010

Currier GW, Fisher SG, Caine ED: Mobile crisis team intervention to enhance linkage of discharged suicidal emergency department patients to outpatient psychiatric services: a randomized controlled trial. Acad Emerg Med 17:36–43, 2010

Da Cruz D, Pearson A, Saini P, et al: Emergency department contact prior to suicide in mental health patients. Emerg Med J 28:467–471, 2011

Folse VN, Hahn RL: Suicide risk screening in an emergency department. Clin Nurs Res 18:253–271, 2009

Forman EM, Berk MS, Henriques GR, et al: History of multiple suicide attempts as a behavioral marker of severe psychopathology. Am J Psychiatry 161:437–443, 2004

Horowitz L, Ballard E, Teach SJ, et al: Feasibility of screening patients with nonpsychiatric complaints for suicide risk in a pediatric emergency department. Pediatr Emerg Care 26:787–792, 2010

King CA, O'Mara RM, Hayward CN, et al: Adolescent suicide risk screening in the emergency department. Acad Emerg Med 16:1234–1241, 2009

Knesper DJ: Continuity of care for suicide prevention and research: suicide attempts and suicide deaths subsequent to discharge from an emergency department or inpatient psychiatry unit. 2011. Available at: http://www.suicidology.org/c/document_library/get_file?folderId=236&name=DLFE-331.pdf. Accessed June 25, 2011.

Kudo K, Otsuka K, Endo J, et al: Study of the outcome of suicide attempts: characteristics of hospitalization in a psychiatric ward group, critical care center group, and non-hospitalized group. BMC Psychiatry 10:4, 2010

Lewis LM: No-harm contracts: a review of what we know. Suicide Life Threat Behav 37:50–57, 2007

Linehan MM, Comtois KA, Murray AM, et al: Two-year randomized controlled trial and follow-up of dialectical behavior therapy vs therapy by experts for suicidal behaviors and borderline personality disorder. Arch Gen Psychiatry 63:757–766, 2006

Lizardi D, Stanley B: Treatment engagement: a neglected aspect in the psychiatric care of suicidal patients. Psychiatr Serv 61:1183–1191, 2010

Lopez-Castroman J, Perez-Rodriguez Mde L, Jaussent I, et al: Distinguishing the relevant features of frequent suicide attempters. J Psychiatr Res 45:619–625, 2010

Mermelstein HT, Wallack JJ: Confidentiality in the age of HIPAA: a challenge for psychosomatic medicine. Psychosomatics 49:97–103, 2008

Miller WR, Rollnick S: Motivational Interviewing: Preparing People for Change, 2nd Edition. New York, Guilford, 2002

Mohr WK, Pett TA, Mohr BD: Adverse effects associated with physical restraint. Can J Psychiatry 48:330–337, 2003

Morgan HG, Jones EM, Owen JH: Secondary prevention of non-fatal deliberate self-harm: the green card study. Br J Psychiatry 163:111–112, 1993

Mundt JC, Greist JH, Gelenberg AJ, et al: Feasibility and validation of a computer-automated Columbia-Suicide Severity Rating Scale using interactive voice response technology. J Psychiatr Res 44:1224–1228, 2010

Newton AS, Hamm MP, Bethell J, et al: Pediatric suicide-related presentations: a systematic review of mental health care in the emergency department. Ann Emerg Med 56:649–659, 2010

Quinn DK, Geppert CM, Maggiore WA: The Emergency Medical Treatment and Active Labor Act of 1985 and the practice of psychiatry. Psychiatr Serv 53:1301–1307, 2002

Riba MB, Ravindranath D: Clinical Manual of Emergency Psychiatry. Washington, DC, American Psychiatric Publishing, 2010, pp 10, 224, 244

Shah SJ, Fiorito M, McNamara RM: A screening tool to medically clear psychiatric patients in the emergency department. J Emerg Med Mar 26, 2010 [Epub ahead of print]

Sharfstein SS, Dickerson FB: Hospital psychiatry for the twenty-first century. Health Aff (Millwood) 28:685–688, 2009

Simon RI: Behavioral risk assessment of the guarded suicidal patient. Suicide Life Threat Behav 38:517–522, 2008

Sood TR, Mcstay CM: Evaluation of the psychiatric patient. Emerg Med Clin North Am 27:669–683, ix, 2009

Stanley B, Brown GK: Safety plan treatment manual to reduce suicide risk: veteran version. Department of Veterans Affairs. August 20, 2008. Available at: http://www.mentalhealth.va.gov/docs/VA_Safety_planning_manual.doc. Accessed July 6, 2011.

Suominen K, Lönnqvist J: Determinants of psychiatric hospitalization after attempted suicide. Gen Hosp Psychiatry 28:424–430, 2006

Waern M, Sjöström N, Marlow T, et al: Does the Suicide Assessment Scale predict risk of repetition? A prospective study of suicide attempters at a hospital emergency department. Eur Psychiatry 25:421–426, 2010

Worchel D, Gearing RE: Suicide Assessment and Treatment: Empirical and Evidence-Based Practices. New York, Springer, 2010, pp 107–117

Outpatient Treatment

John T. Maltsberger, M.D.

Joseph B. Stoklosa, M.D.

Outpatient treatment of patients at risk for suicide rests on the use of core principles of psychiatry and psychotherapy specialized for and adapted to this high-risk population. Given that modern society focuses on shorter-term inpatient hospitalizations and in-community psychiatric rehabilitation, there is now a premium placed on informed, careful outpatient treatment of the suicidal patient.

Alliance: The Heart of the Matter

Treating outpatients at risk for suicide is a dicey undertaking for clinicians in more ways than one. In the first place, not everybody who refers such patients for treatment is likely to have the same agenda. Hospitals want to shorten lengths of stay and move patients into outpatient care quickly. Clinics, institutions, and families want the patient to "get better" and give up the suicide option. Insurance companies want that as well, but fast and on the cheap. Psychiatrists want to see the patients

get better, but the patients themselves are often not so sure. In fact, many of them are uncertain as to whether they would be better off alive or dead.

The first task of the therapist must be to establish a treatment alliance, however fragile, sometimes in the face of near hopelessness. The keystone of the alliance must be mutual intent to build up reasons for living, with patients' commitment to set aside the suicide option and participate in the treatment, at least for the time being. Viktor Frankl recognized this (1959) as core to his logotherapy, aiming to build up meaning in life "1) by creating a work or deed; 2) by experiencing something or encountering someone; and 3) by the attitude we take toward unavoidable suffering" (p. 111). Because these patients' mental states may alter quickly and unexpectedly, the alliance usually fluctuates episodically, sometimes weakening or even breaking down. With other patients for whom life is not at stake, broken alliances are less critical. With suicidal patients, however, everything depends on alliance, and for that reason it must be explicitly addressed from the beginning and systematically monitored as treatment progresses.

Linehan (1993) grasped this principle and centrally integrated it into dialectical behavior treatment. Following her practice, practitioners of all kinds are well advised to take up patients' commitment to living at the very beginning, vigorously and supportively negotiating an agreement to keep alive while pledging the best help with it they can, before embarking on treatment. Plakun's (2009) psychodynamic "Alliance-Based Intervention for Suicide" similarly states how the alliance is predicated on this mutual agreement, because "the work cannot proceed from the perspective that it is the therapist's job to keep the patient alive" (pp. 545–546). This is the first order of business, just as the second is systematically monitoring the state of the alliance throughout the treatment.

"No-suicide contracts" have little use as suicide preventives (Miller 1999), but the patient must understand that the purpose of the treatment is to prevent suicide and, accordingly, must make a serious commitment to the treatment team to work hard to that end. Patients must be persuaded to agree that suicide is "off the table" as a choice, understanding that if they feel they cannot keep this commitment as the treatment goes forward, they will call for help. Clinicians should be well aware that commitments of this kind cannot be relied on to prevent suicides, but patients' commitment to staying alive and working with the treatment team is indispensable from the beginning. It is the heart of the alliance.

When Does Outpatient Treatment Make Sense?

Outpatient treatment is not suitable for patients clearly unwilling to commit themselves to staying alive, but ambivalent or fragile commitment is usually inevitable at first. The clinician should, of course, acknowledge that the commitment is difficult to make and offer the patient reasonable and possible help to keep it, but absent sincere (even if frail) patient commitment, the clinician who begins outpatient treatment of a suicidal patient will be living out the Zen koan: "What is the sound of one hand clapping?"

Negotiating this agreement may not be achievable in one session, but no suicidal person, inpatient or outpatient, can really be "in treatment" until the commitment is made. Outpatient care should not begin before a good suicide risk assessment has been carried out, justifying the conclusion that the patient has a reasonable likelihood of entering and participating in treatment without committing suicide before a therapeutic alliance has a chance to form and begin consolidating. Making a suicide risk assessment is discussed elsewhere in this book (see, e.g., Chapter 1, "Suicide Risk Assessment: Gateway to Treatment and Management") as well as in a practice guideline of the American Psychiatric Association (2003).

One should make sure that the patient is competent to understand and give consent to the treatment offered after its risks and benefits have been explained. A written record of mental capacity, explanation, and consent should be preserved. When circumstances permit, it is generally desirable for the next of kin to sign the consent form as well. When patients are minors, parental consent is of course necessary before undertaking any treatment. Patients and families should understand that outpatient treatment of suicidal patients has its hazards.

Before outpatient treatment is undertaken, the therapist should make sure reasonable backup will be available in the event of a future suicide crisis. What available exterior sustaining resources does the patient have? Who are the people on whom the patient relies for support and validation? The therapist should make a record of their names, whereabouts, and telephone numbers to be prepared if the patient worsens. Unless the clinician is confident that brisk admission to a psychiatric unit will be possible should a suicide crisis evolve, outpatient management may be unwise, and perhaps the patient should be referred to someone else with a hospital-based practice.

Establishing the Treatment Team

Much of the time, recently suicidal patients, or those who are vulnerable to suicide, need more structure for their treatment than occasional office visits can provide. At least in the beginning of their treatment, a partial hospital or day program may be advisable, with continuing group therapy as the patient moves toward greater independence in the community. When substance abuse has been a part of the problem, the therapist should insist the patient participate in Alcoholics Anonymous or some other rehabilitation program.

Enrollment of family and friends in support groups is often very desirable, but in any case there should be some regular avenues for communication to the therapist from those on whom the patient relies for support. Although the patient and the involved, supportive others should all understand that except in an emergency, what the patient says to the treatment team is confidential, those close to the patient must have a reliable means for getting any information they may think important through to the team in general and to the patient's

therapist in particular. This may involve calling a predesignated member of the treatment team from time to time. The family and friends involved in the patient's treatment should be educated at the outset about danger signs that might point to a developing suicide crisis.

In contemporary practice it is common to split the treatment between a psychotherapist and a psychopharmacologist (see Chapter 15, "Split Treatment: Coming of Age," in this volume). Whatever advantages such a division affords, perils are implicit in it: What a patient tells one member of a treatment team he may represent differently to others. This is especially true with a suicidal patient and truer yet if the patient has borderline personality disorder. A patient may report developing suicide plans to the therapist while smoothly assuring the psychopharmacologist that all is well. Another may discuss funeral arrangements with family but deny hopelessness to the therapist. The first principle of team treatment is that communication between all participants should be open, frequent, and regular. Hendin et al. (2006) found that in 9 of 36 suicides that occurred while patients were in treatment, poor communication between treating clinicians was a major factor in the fatal outcome. In one treatment of many months, the psychotherapist and psychopharmacologist never spoke with each other before the patient's death, although both worked in the same clinic. Avena and Kalman's (2010) survey of clinicians unfortunately suggests this trend has continued, with 24 of 53 respondents reporting seeing patients in psychotherapy who are taking medication prescribed by separate psychiatrists with whom the respondents have never communicated.

A final, if occasional, member of the treatment team might well be a consultant colleague with whom the treatment is reviewed either regularly or from time to time as the need arises. Suicidal patients make extraordinary demands on clinicians' stamina and emotional balance. Consultation can serve as a helpful check to make sure nothing is overlooked and as a helpful validation of ongoing clinical judgment.

Before the treatment begins, all clinicians involved should understand who the team leader, or captain, is. Usually this will be the person who sees the patient most intensively, presumably the psychotherapist, who optimally may also be the psychopharmacologist. Responsibility for keeping the team together and in good communication with each other rests with the captain. This is often no small task. The captain needs to be as vigilant as a good sheepdog in tending to this task, keeping tabs on everyone and rounding up strays.

Although to some, such an arrangement may seem anticollaborative and too authoritarian, the designation of a team captain is essential because the responsibility for keeping the treatment on track and the team working together must lie somewhere. The crews of sailboats well understand that smooth and safe operation of the ship requires clear delineation of responsibility with a captain in charge of the enterprise. Under the law, physicians must answer for the conduct of others who collaborate in the treatment of patients under their care, and when suicides occur, it is generally the physician whom families want to hold accountable, whether the doctor considers himself captain of the team or not. Physicians cannot abdicate final responsibility for any patients for whom they prescribe.

Beginning the Treatment

Suicidal patients are currently treated according to a variety of different psychotherapeutic methods. Empirical study has shown a number of them to be effective, some more so than others. The empirically supported treatments include interpersonal psychotherapy (Neu et al. 1978; Tang et al. 2009; Weissman et al. 1981), cognitive therapy (Beck et al. 1979), dialectical behavior therapy (Linehan 1993), mentalization-based therapy (Bateman and Fonagy 2004), transference-based psychotherapy (Clarkin et al. 1999), and psychoanalytic (psychodynamic) psychotherapy (Maltsberger and Weinberg 2006). Currently there is much discussion and debate as to what makes these treatments work and what they have in common. From the clinical perspective, an active, empathically engaged therapist who is supportive and validating is common to all. The therapist concentrates on patients' affective experiences and encourages verbalization and mental exploration of feelings in the context in which they arise. Interpretation, clarification, and education are common to most of these treatments. Most stress the importance of confronting self-defeating behavior, and most attend seriously to the realities of the therapeutic relationship and patients' distortions of it.

Suicide is statistically most likely in the first weeks after hospital discharge (Qin and Nordentoft 2005), a period when mental state is likely to fluctuate. For this reason, patients should be seen frequently to consolidate the therapeutic alliance and monitor progress. Attention to a suicide risk assessment during these visits is crucial, because studies looking at increased "routine visits" alone have yet to show decreased suicide risk (Kim et al. 2010). The frequency of visits will depend on the individual patient, but once weekly is not too often just after discharge. Psychopharmacological follow-up at infrequent intervals and nothing more is hard to justify (Hollon et al. 2005); best care requires relatively frequent visits for combined psychotherapy and medication.

Tracking the Treatment

The patient's progress (or lack thereof) should be systematically monitored, and the team leader is responsible for correlating, recording, and communicating significant observations to all members of the treatment team. Patients' level of commitment to the treatment may be gauged not only by what they say about it but also by the appearance of treatment-interfering behaviors—these would include not keeping appointments, coming late, failing to pay the bill, not complying with medication regimens, substance abuse, and dropping out of substance abuse programs. These behaviors should be supportively confronted in the psychotherapy as departures from the commitment to work at staying alive (Linehan 1993).

In the course of suicide risk assessment, the exterior resources patients need to keep in balance should be identified. An exterior sustaining resource is someone or something else (perhaps a work position or maybe a pet) that the patient relies on to maintain affective regulation and self-integrity (Maltsberger 1988). Suicide crises can be precipitated by losses, or threatened losses, of such resources, and the history may reflect that previous attempts fast followed on an affective storm that blew up when an important someone or something fell away from, or was driven away by, the patient (Maltsberger et al. 2003). The therapist should keep a sharp lookout for these resources.

If the treatment team watches for the evolution of suicidal crises, suicide attempts can often be avoided. The herald of such a crisis is often (not always) a precipitating event (Foster 2011) that triggers a flood of intense, painful, unendurable affect *other than depression*. Sometimes the appearance or the worsening of a sleep disturbance hints at the emergence of a suicide crisis or an incipient mixed-state episode in an affective disorder. A deterioration of the patient's connection to and integration with his social, family, and work situations follows. As the crisis worsens, there will be suicidal hints, communications, or behaviors, coupled with increasing substance abuse or loss of self-control (Hendin et al. 2001).

The affects to watch for, especially as they worsen, are intense anxiety, hopelessness, desperation, rage, abandonment, and self-hate. Desperation is an experience of anguish so intolerable it cries out for immediate relief (Hendin et al. 2004). Combinations of despair (total hopelessness), severe self-hate, and desperation are very dangerous and require immediate attention. Fawcett et al. (1990) have shown that severe anhedonia and intense anxiety are markers of suicide. Combinations of these intense feelings can lead to a sense of entrapment from which patients think suicide is the only escape.

Bear in mind that the subjective experiences described here may not be evident on casual inspection of patients' general appearance and behavior—they must be inquired after and are perhaps even more important than what the patient says about current suicidal intent. Of course, increasing suicidal preoccupation and the appearance and strengthening of impulses are important and should be tracked, but suicide does not occur for most patients until they are overwhelmed by mental pain (Shneidman 1993). Suicidal ideation is therefore secondary; suicide comes to mind as a way out of a trap. Intolerable affect drives the ideation most of the time. As suicide looms, dissociative experiences may appear, signaling incipient self-breakup. Patients can then experience their bodies as something apart from their essential selves, as things to be jettisoned (Maltsberger 2004). Frank delusional thinking can appear.

There is much to be said for keeping a tabular record, and a form for doing so is shown in Figure 17–1. Regular tabulation of this kind not only reminds one of what to monitor, but it lends itself to ready sharing by the treatment team, even by e-mail. This can enhance collaboration and consultation and concentrate collective attention.

Of course, written communications, although helpful, can never take the place of regular oral conferences. Conferences are difficult to arrange in busy clinic settings, but they need not take long and can be scheduled regularly in advance.

Addressing Problems and Difficulties

Many problems in the outpatient care of suicidal patients can be avoided if the treatment team sees them coming ahead of time.

Relying on what patients say about present suicidal intent instead of following the mental state as the primary guide is always tempting, especially when the clinical picture is cloudy. Bear in mind that many patients tell the doctor they do not intend to kill themselves but soon do it anyway. Many patients who have made no-suicide contracts die of suicide regardless (Busch et al. 2003). Let the clinician be skeptical whenever a patient denies suicidal intent or promises no self-harm while experiencing agitation or any combination of the intense painful affects that suggest desperation.

Anguish as a subjective experience has some component of anxiety. Some patients refer to horror or terror in describing it. Clinicians are often reluctant to treat this symptom aggressively with benzodiazepines, especially if there is a history of substance abuse. It remains necessary, however, to get patients out of the desperation zone to prevent suicide attempts. Selective serotonin reuptake inhibitors are currently much favored as anxiolytic agents, but these drugs may take many days to act, and in the face of hypomanic potential, they may increase distress instead of relieving it. Intense affective distress needs immediate relief, if not with a benzodiazepine prescription, then perhaps with one of the anxiolytic antipsychotic agents, such as quetiapine (Depping et al. 2010). Antipsychotics may alleviate psychosis and anxiety, although attention to akathisia as a very distressing potential side effect is important. In urgent states electroconvulsive treatment may be lifesaving. Those suicidal patients vulnerable to fluctuations of mood and prone to fall into very painful mixed states are much helped by the prescription of mood stabilizers, especially lithium salts (Tondo et al. 2003).

Case Example 1

Anthony, a 20-year-old college student, falls into an agitated depression after his estranged parents both blame him for a fracas they set going over a holiday vacation. A month later Anthony is overwhelmed with anguish and talking about suicide to his roommates. On several occasions he goes out onto the roof of his dormitory "just to see what it would be like" if he decides to jump. The nurse practitioner at the health service where his friends take him gives him a prescription for sertraline, even though he has an unrecognized family history of bipolar disorder. (The responsible clinic psychiatrist never meets Anthony, and nobody ever records a suicide risk assessment.) He grows much worse. Within a week, while preparing for a dangerous jump, he luckily is interrupted. Finally another psychiatrist examines him, discovers how suicidal and depersonal-

FIGURE 17–1. Elements for systematic monitoring

Rate level of disturbance as none (0), mild (1), moderate (2), or severe (3).

Enter date:	Date 1	Date 2	Date 3	Date N
Therapeutic alliance				
Exterior sustaining resources				
Interpersonal stability (people, work)				
Suicide hints/communications				
Sleep quality				
Substance/alcohol abuse				
Mental state				
Hopelessness				
Anguish				
Rage				
Aloneness/abandonment				
Anxiety				
Self-hate				
Dissociative experiences				
Entrapment				
Anhedonia				
Suicidal ideation/preoccupation				
Impulses to self-harm				

ized Anthony is, and admits him, in spite of protestations, to a psychiatric unit. The sertraline is stopped, and olanzapine is prescribed. Anthony's recovery is rapid. He readily agrees to outpatient psychotherapy, accepts a prescription for a mood stabilizer, and is treated quite successfully, managing after a time to disentangle himself from his parents' long-standing quarrel.

In the absence of close monitoring, therapists sometimes overlook or forget about troublesome symptoms that the patient may not mention. Certainly the management of anxiety and agitation is of paramount importance, but so indeed is the treatment of psychotic symptoms. Antidepressant drugs can be very helpful, but they are often prescribed in insufficient dosages. Substance abuse, a frequently neglected problem, should not be allowed to continue without supportive but systematic confrontation. Getting substance abuse under control and under treatment is vital.

Sometimes inadequate prescription of appropriate medicines occurs because patients object to side effects or simply do not want to take medicine. Psychiatrists should not resign themselves to such situations but instead should work with these patients to find some acceptable compromise regimen.

Letting the patient control the psychopharmacology is but one example of a common problem. When the patient or the patient's family takes charge of the treatment in whatever sector, matters can get out of hand. In one instance, at the insistence of a patient's relative, an important community leader, the patient was allowed to leave the ward to go out to lunch, against the psychiatrist's better judgment. He eloped from the restaurant and died by suicide.

Outpatients should not have the last word about going into the hospital. When a well-conducted risk assessment shows a suicide attempt is in the offing, the psychiatrist must insist on admission and not agree to let the patient go home and "think it over." Psychiatrists must sometimes find the courage to act decisively and sign an involuntary petition. Remember, he who hesitates not only is lost but can find himself several miles from the next freeway exit. Impending suicide is a medical emergency, and like the surgeon who knows appendicitis requires immediate intervention, the psychiatrist should stand by the diagnosis. Every clinician wants to avoid signing unnecessary involuntary petitions, but when mistakes are made, they are almost always in the other direction—not signing them. A few days in an inpatient unit are much preferable to a few in a medical or surgical intensive care unit or to death.

Sometimes clinicians do not understand that the patient does not have to acknowledge immediate suicidal intent to qualify for involuntary admission, although ignorant insurance company representatives may claim this is so. Admissibility on an involuntary paper in virtually every jurisdiction in the United States requires no more than a physician's informed judgment that an attempt is imminent (more probable than not, and soon) in a patient with mental illness.

Patients are lost to suicide from time to time because clinicians lack confidence in their own assessment of risk. Outpatient treatment of suicidal patients requires familiarity with the principles of risk assessment, and sufficient tolerance for the implicit ambiguities thereof, if one is not to be frozen by indecision at critical moments. Working with a mutually supportive team and keeping a clear clinical assessment in mind at all times are the best protections against therapeutic paralysis.

Finally, therapists' anxiety can cause them to stumble. Suicidal patients often struggle to control their environments, insisting on control of one or another aspect of their treatment. Few patients will agree out of hand when the clinician recommends hospitalization. That is why, in first broaching the subject, one recommends the hospital as a temporary step for the relief of a transient crisis, an occasion for respite, consultation, and regrouping. Only as a last resort should the psychiatrist take an opposing point of view about going into inpatient care. When necessary, however, the psychiatrist should insist on hospitalization as a nonnegotiable step and not back down. After all, just as the physician bears the final responsibility for the patient's safety, it is the physician who must have the last word; the final authority over hospitalization is the physician's.

Case Example 2

Professor S, a 55-year-old classicist and internationally recognized scholar, is being treated as an outpatient in a university clinic by Dr. C, a psychiatrist who provides both psychotherapy and psychopharmacology. The patient is very depressed and appears to be worsening. Several years previously he attempted suicide. His wife is also depressed and has been discussing suicide with her therapist, another psychiatrist in the same clinic. One day she reports that Professor S proposed a suicide pact and has been speaking of getting a gun. The wife's therapist passes this information on to Dr. C, who decides that hospitalization will probably be in order and takes some preliminary preparatory measures. When Professor S arrives for his appointment that day, Dr. C gently raises the matter of his hopelessness and brings up the matter of the gun and the suicide pact. Professor S acknowledges that he has given up hope and that he does indeed have a gun, but he claims he will not kill himself unless his wife agrees to die with him. He disagrees with Dr. C's suggestion of a hospital admission and insists that he should go home. He says that maybe he will talk over going into the hospital with his wife. Dr. C refuses to allow Professor S to leave the clinic, whereupon the patient threatens to get him fired from the university. Still insisting, Dr. C calls the security personnel. They have to forcibly restrain Professor S and carry him kicking and screaming through the clinic waiting room, filled with startled members of the university community, out into an ambulance. On an involuntary certificate Professor S is admitted to a psychiatric unit, where after a few days he agrees to receive a course of electroconvulsive treatment and makes a rapid recovery. Professor S resumes treatment with Dr. C on discharge from the hospital. For many years afterward, he writes Dr. C a note on the anniversary of his hospital admission, thanking him for saving his life.

Occasionally therapists find themselves in control struggles about hospitalization, prescription compliance, frequency of visits, fees, or other matters. Control-sensitive patients can prove obdurate once control battles are engaged in. Negotiation should be one's watchword, but not limitless negotiation. If treatment is to succeed, ultimately the patient must cooperate with the essentials of what is laid out in the treatment plan. Most of the time there is room for discussion, temporizing, and, often, compromise. The temptation to get into unnecessary power struggles often arises because therapists, without quite being aware of it, feel helpless and want to flex their muscles, as it were, to reassure themselves that they are in charge (Adler 1972; Gabbard 1999). We must choose our skirmishes wisely and even be prepared to lose a few if treatment is to succeed and prove effective. On the one hand, we must guard against passive surrender, against giving in to what patients want or demand when essentials are at stake. On the other, we must avoid getting into needless struggles in an effort to show patients (and ourselves) who is boss.

Ultimately patients must comply with the essential parts of the treatment plan: psychotherapy, psychopharmacology, substance abuse treatment, and sometimes hospitalization. When patients refuse to cooperate in the essentials, however, the original treatment alliance to live and to build up a life has been compromised and perhaps has failed. If that commitment cannot be reclaimed and patients refuse to commit themselves to it anew, termination may be necessary. Termination can sometimes be managed on an outpatient basis, but sometimes safety concerns necessitate hospital admission and inpatient renegotiation of the treatment commitment, sometimes with another team.

Key Clinical Concepts

- Before starting outpatient care, make a good suicide risk assessment and keep it up-to-date.
- Remember that informed consent and a risk-benefit analysis are essential.
- Do not accept for outpatient management any patient who is unwilling to make a commitment to keep alive and give the treatment a chance.

- Ensure the availability of prompt inpatient admission. Good backup is essential. Treating suicidal patients outside the hospital means that prompt inpatient admission should be possible should the need arise.

- Identify and keep track of the patient's external sustaining resources.

- Choose a captain to hold the treatment team together.

- Keep in good communication as a team. This is one of the team captain's main responsibilities.

- Do not let the patient control the treatment. Keep the essential components of the treatment clearly in mind and under review with the patient and the team. These components are cooperation in psychotherapy, psychopharmacology, substance abuse treatment, and sometimes hospitalization. A compromise of the essentials is not negotiable.

- Monitor the patient's life adaptation and mental state systematically.

- When in doubt, get consultation.

- Keep good records.

References

Adler G: Helplessness in the helpers. Br J Med Psychol 45:315–326, 1972

American Psychiatric Association: Practice guideline for the assessment and treatment of patients with suicidal behaviors. Am J Psychiatry 160(suppl): 1–60, 2003

Avena J, Kalman T: Do psychotherapists speak to psychopharmacologists? A survey of practicing clinicians. J Am Acad Psychoanal Dyn Psychiatry 38:675–683, 2010

Bateman A, Fonagy P: Psychotherapy for Borderline Personality Disorder: Mentalization Based Treatment. Oxford, UK, Oxford University Press, 2004

Beck AT, Rush AJ, Shaw BF, et al: Cognitive Therapy of Depression. New York, Guilford, 1979

Busch KA, Fawcett J, Jacobs DG: Clinical correlates of inpatient suicide. J Clin Psychiatry 64:14–19, 2003

Clarkin JF, Yeomans FE, Kernberg OF: Psychotherapy for Borderline Personality. New York, Wiley, 1999

Depping AM, Komossa K, Kissling W, et al: Second-generation antipsychotics for anxiety disorders. Cochrane Database of Systematic Reviews 2010, Issue 12. Art. No.: CD008120. DOI: 10.1002/14651858. CD008120.pub2.

Fawcett J, Scheftner WA, Fogg L, et al: Time-related predictors of suicide in major affective disorder. Am J Psychiatry 147:1189–1194, 1990

Foster T: Adverse life events proximal to adult suicide: a synthesis of findings from psychological autopsy studies. Arch Suicide Res 15:1–15, 2011

Frankl VE: Man's Search for Meaning. Boston, MA, Beacon Press, 1959

Gabbard GO (ed): Countertransference Issues in Psychiatric Treatment. Washington, DC, American Psychiatric Press, 1999

Hendin H, Maltsberger JT, Lipschitz A, et al: Recognizing and responding to a suicide crisis. Suicide Life Threat Behav 31:115–128, 2001

Hendin H, Maltsberger JT, Haas AP, et al: Desperation and other affective states in suicidal patients. Suicide Life Threat Behav 34:386–394, 2004

Hendin H, Haas AP, Maltsberger JT, et al: Problems in psychotherapy with suicidal patients. Am J Psychiatry 163:67–72, 2006

Hollon SD, Jarrett RB, Nierenberg AA, et al: Psychotherapy and medication in the treatment of adult and geriatric depression: which monotherapy or combined treatment? J Clin Psychiatry 66:455–458, 2005

Kim HM, Eisenberg D, Ganoczy D, et al: Examining the relationship between clinical monitoring and suicide risk among patients with depression: matched case-control study and instrumental variable approaches. Health Serv Res 45:1205–1226, 2010

Linehan MM: Cognitive-Behavioral Treatment of Borderline Personality Disorder. New York, Guilford, 1993

Maltsberger JT: Suicide danger: clinical estimation and decision. Suicide Life Threat Behav 18:47–54, 1988

Maltsberger JT: The descent into suicide. Int J Psychoanal 85:653–668, 2004

Maltsberger JT, Weinberg I: Psychoanalytic perspectives on the treatment of an acute suicidal crisis. J Clin Psychol 62:223–234, 2006

Maltsberger JT, Hendin H, Haas AP, et al: Determination of precipitating events in the suicide of psychiatric patients. Suicide Life Threat Behav 33:111–119, 2003

Miller MM: Suicide-prevention contracts: advantages, disadvantages, and an alternative approach, in The Harvard Medical School Guide to Suicide Assessment and Intervention. Edited by Jacobs DG. San Francisco, CA, Jossey-Bass, 1999, pp 463–481

Neu C, Prusoff BA, Klerman GL: Measuring the interventions used in the short-term interpersonal psychotherapy of depression. Am J Orthopsychiatry 48:629–636, 1978

Plakun EM: A view from Riggs: treatment resistance and patient authority-XI. An alliance based intervention for suicide. J Am Acad Psychoanal Dyn Psychiatry 37:539–560, 2009

Qin P, Nordentoft M: Suicide risk in relation to psychiatric hospitalization: evidence based on longitudinal registers. Arch Gen Psychiatry 62:427–432, 2005

Shneidman ES: Suicide as psychache. J Nerv Ment Dis 181:145–147, 1993

Tang TC, Jou SH, Ko CH, et al: Randomized study of school-based intensive interpersonal psychotherapy for depressed adolescents with suicidal risk and parasuicide behaviors. Psychiatry Clin Neurosci 63:463–470, 2009

Tondo L, Isacsson G, Baldessarini R: Suicidal behaviour in bipolar disorder: risk and prevention. CNS Drugs 17:491–511, 2003

Weissman MM, Klerman GL, Prusoff BA, et al: Depressed outpatients: results one year after treatment with drugs and/or interpersonal psychotherapy. Arch Gen Psychiatry 38:51–55, 1981

CHAPTER 18

Inpatient Psychiatric Treatment

Glen L. Xiong, M.D.

Amy Barnhorst, M.D.

Donald Hilty, M.D.

When a patient is at acute risk for self-harm and outpatient intervention is insufficient (usually because of time urgency, illness severity, or lack of insight into the need for treatment), inpatient psychiatric treatment is the standard of care (American Psychiatric Association 2003). Inpatient psychiatric treatment options include acute psychiatric hospitals and crisis residential or crisis respite programs, where admission is voluntary but the facility is unlocked. Partial day programs offer another option for patients who are motivated for treatment and able to maintain their safety independently . In this chapter, we review the assessment and management considerations for suicidal patients from inpatient admission to discharge, both at the individual patient level and at the systems level. Forensic inpatient treatment is beyond the scope of this chapter and is covered in Chapter 22 ("Suicide Prevention in Jails and Prisons") of this book.

Epidemiology

Although inpatient psychiatric hospitals are the treatment setting for patients at the highest risk of suicide, completed inpatient suicides are relatively infrequent events. Based on a review of international studies published in 1987–2002, suicides occur in about 100–400 per 100,000 (0.1%–0.4%) of all inpatient admissions (Dong et al. 2005). In the United States, approximately 1,500 deaths occurred on inpatient psychiatric units in 2002 (Mills et al. 2008). This constitutes roughly 4.7% of all suicides deaths, based on reported suicides of 31,655 for 2002 in the United States (American Foundation for Suicide Prevention 2011).

Inpatient suicide declined in Great Britain from 221 cases in 1997 to 144 in 2006. Only 30% of inpatient suicides from 1997 through 2006 took place on the ward itself (Hunt et al. 2010). In a root cause analysis report from New York State, 122 incidents of reported suicides occurred from 2002 through 2008 during and after inpatient psychiatric treatment. This is equivalent to approximately 17 suicides per year, out of 3.7 million bed days each year (New York State Office of Mental Health 2009). Of the 122 deaths, 85 (70%) occurred outside of the hospital postdischarge, on a pass, or while absent without leave, whereas 37 (30%) occurred on inpatient units. The steady decline in the total number of inpatient suicides is due both to institutional quality improvement measures that have reduced environmental hazards and to continued reductions in inpatient lengths of stay.

Despite the relatively low incidence of inpatient suicide, when a suicide event occurs, its emotional toll can be powerful. Loved ones, clinical providers, administrators, and regulators often experience mixed feelings of guilt, anguish, and a universal wish that perhaps such an event could have been prevented.

Suicide Method

Suicide methods in an inpatient setting are necessarily limited to the means available. Despite reasonable efforts to maintain a patient environment free of suicide hazards, it is impossible to completely remove every potential peril. The most commonly reported method of inpatient suicide is hanging, which accounted for 73% of 236 inpatient suicides in one study (Meehan et al. 2006). Most frequently, a door corner in a private area was used to anchor the noose (Meehan et al. 2006), although use of doorknobs has also been reported. Large expanses of fabric have also been tied tightly around patients' necks and can be especially lethal if there is some degree of stretchiness and rebound, allowing for airway restriction without necessitating an anchor point.

Jumping from heights is the second most commonly reported method, accounting for 20% of inpatient suicides (Combs and Romm 2007; Meehan et al. 2006). Cutting or stabbing is common as well, either as suicidal or as parasuicidal behavior. Sharp items can be fashioned from available dining utensils, parts of furniture, or other items available in the hospital. Patients have also been reported to tear trim from the walls or tacking from the carpeting to fashion sharp blades. In addition, razor blades or knives have been smuggled into facilities and hidden inside toilets or other fixtures for future use, even at later admissions.

Less common but still reported methods include drowning, asphyxiation, burning, and overdose. Pills can be "cheeked" and stored in a mattress or other secret location for later overdose. One patient was even reported to have ingested large quantities of a potentially toxic mushroom he found growing on the hospital grounds.

As expected, the most common locations for attempts to occur are the few places that offer some degree of privacy in an otherwise busy inpatient setting. Bathrooms and bedrooms were the most common in the root-cause analysis, accounting for 54% and 30%, respectively, of completed inpatient suicides (New York State Office of Mental Health 2009).

Temporal Characteristics of Inpatient Suicides

The sharpest peaks in suicides of psychiatric inpatients occur in the week after admission and the week after discharge (Hunt et al. 2010; Qin and Nordentoft 2005). Three European studies found that 23%–28% of all inpatient suicides occurred within 7 days of admission (Erlangsen et al. 2006; Hunt et al. 2007; Qin and Nordentoft 2005). In one of the largest studies, which examined 1,100 incidents of suicide, 337 (32%) occurred within the first 2 weeks of discharge and 397 (40%) were before the first outpatient follow-up appointment (Meehan et al. 2006). Deisenhammer et al. (2007) in Austria found that of 665 inpatients who completed suicide postdischarge, 28% ended their lives within 7 days of discharge and 48% died by suicide within 1 month of discharge. In a Great Britain study, 32% of suicides occurred within 30 days after discharge (Hunt et al. 2010).

Psychiatric Diagnosis

Mood and psychotic disorders have been consistently shown as the diagnoses most commonly associated with inpatient suicide (Combs and Romm 2007; Tidemalm et al. 2008), which is consistent with outpatient correlations of diagnosis and suicide rate. In the New York State Office of Mental Health report (2009), 19% of inpatients who completed suicide had been diagnosed with schizophrenia, whereas 67% had been diagnosed with mood disorders. Commonly comorbid diagnoses in patients who complete suicide in inpatient settings include chronic pain, anxiety, and alcohol and polysubstance dependence (Hunt et al. 2010).

Suicide Risk Assessment: From Admission to Discharge

Demographic risk factors for suicide such as age, gender, and race are similar for inpatients when compared with outpatients. As discussed earlier, the initial admission period (within 7 days of admission) and immediate postdischarge period (within 7 and up to 30 days of discharge) are times of high risk for suicide attempts for psychiatric patients. Thus, inpatient treatment necessitates suicide risk assessment and management at three distinct stages: admission, treatment, and discharge (Figure 18–1). Although for clarity the stages are discussed in the following subsections as if they are

distinct, in practice they may overlap temporally or may in fact all occur in the same time period.

Admission Phase

During the admission phase, suicide risk assessment is of paramount importance. Suicidal patients may attempt suicide for the first time or may reattempt after a botched recent attempt. Because the best predictor of future behavior is past behavior, people with a history of suicide attempts are more likely to attempt suicide than those without such a history. Combs and Romm (2007) reported in their literature review that multiple studies demonstrated that previous self-harm (10 studies) and previous suicide attempts (8 studies) are associated with increased risk of inpatient suicide. Other risk factors include chronic mental illness, including affective and psychotic disorders (12 studies), male gender (6 studies), and multiple previous admissions (3 studies). Although retrospective studies are able to identify risk factors, studies of various predictive models have not found these models to have adequate sensitivity and specificity to be used as clinical prognostic tools for future risks (Busch et al. 2003; Powell et al. 2000; Spiessl et al. 2002).

Other risk factors for suicide include a history of impulsive behavior (including violence), severe anxiety, substance dependence, and pain. Paradoxically, many of these symptoms may increase in the more restrictive and seemingly impersonal environment of an inpatient treatment setting. Additionally, patients with poor social support and who are unengaged in inpatient treatment may experience further isolation in the inpatient setting (Hunt et al. 2010); they may feel even more hopelessness and helplessness after being confined to a hos-

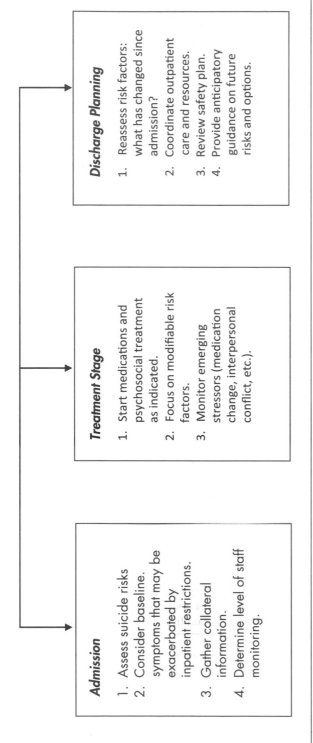

Admission

1. Assess suicide risks
2. Consider baseline. symptoms that may be exacerbated by inpatient restrictions.
3. Gather collateral information.
4. Determine level of staff monitoring.

Treatment Stage

1. Start medications and psychosocial treatment as indicated.
2. Focus on modifiable risk factors.
3. Monitor emerging stressors (medication change, interpersonal conflict, etc.).

Discharge Planning

1. Reassess risk factors: what has changed since admission?
2. Coordinate outpatient care and resources.
3. Review safety plan.
4. Provide anticipatory guidance on future risks and options.

FIGURE 18–1. Inpatient suicide assessment and management.

pital. These individuals require immediate detection and attention.

Therefore, suicide risk assessment at admission must extend beyond traditional risk assessment and also take into account the influence of the more restrictive nature of inpatient treatment on the patients' baseline symptoms and risk factors. This iatrogenic, situational exacerbation of baseline symptoms may place these patients at a higher suicide risk upon admission, and this risk should be managed and weighed against the benefits of hospitalization during the admission period.

Gathering sufficient and accurate clinical information during the admission period is critical (Shea 2004). Understanding the stressors and risk factors particular to each patient will help the treatment team individualize the safety plan on the inpatient unit. Questions should be asked about long-term and more chronic contributors, acute stressors that led up to the current crisis, and ways in which hospitalization may worsen or ameliorate the risks for a given patient (Cassells et al. 2005). For example, a patient facing housing or employment problems may not be able to attend job interviews, pay bills on time, or attend work if hospitalized for a long period.

The treatment team should evaluate which contributors can potentially change and improve during hospitalization; this kind of evaluation provides a basis from which to assess whether or not there has been a reduction in stressors or risks during treatment and prior to discharge. A discharge is harder to justify if there is no significant improvement in one or more risk factors or stressors from the initial admission. Table 18–1 details patient information to consider during the admission stage.

In addition, protective factors should be considered and weighed against the risk factors for suicide to gain a more holistic

TABLE 18–1. Inpatient admission suicide risk assessment

Analysis of current episode

Duration of preceding suicidality

Amount of planning and forethought for attempt

Patient's hope for outcome or attempt

Manner (if any) by which attempt came to attention of others

How patient feels about attempt now

Dynamic risk factors

Housing

Recent breakup

Unemployment

Anniversary of death or loss

Relapse into substance use

Static risk factors

Age

Race

Marital status

Gender

Cultural factors

Religious prohibitions against suicide

Cultural view on suicide

Cultural understanding of mental illness

Belief in afterlife or punishment

Modifiable factors that led to attempt

Alcohol use

Drug use

Lapse in medication

Relationship stressors

New stressors due to inpatient treatment

Anxiety

Insomnia

Inability to attend job or school

Loss of housing

Isolation from social support

sense of an individual patient's potential to take lethal action. One study of 84 inpatients with major depressive disorder compared those who had attempted suicide with those who had not in order to elicit protective factors. Those who had not attempted suicide expressed more feelings of responsibility toward family, more fear of social disapproval, and more moral objections to suicide than those who had attempted suicide (Malone et al. 2000). This finding corroborates the commonly held belief that subscribing to a religious, moral, or social system that holds a negative view of suicide is a protective factor.

Numerous other studies have found correlations between partner or relational problems and suicide risk, as well as lack of employment and suicide risk (Hall et al. 1999; Qin et al. 2003). In women, having a young child conferred a lower risk (Qin et al. 2003). Stable relationships, children, and employment may give the patient the sense of responsibility and contribution that was affirmed by those who did not attempt suicide in the inpatient comparison study. In addition, hopelessness has been shown to be a strong risk factor for suicide attempts (Hall et al. 1999). Patients who have hope that their situation or their symptoms will improve, regardless of current severity, may be at lower risk than those with less drastic situations who feel there is no hope of change.

Case Example 1: A Woman Who Was Concerned That Inpatient Admission Could Worsen Depression and Put Her at Risk for Suicide

A 45-year-old woman was brought to the emergency department (ED) by her mother for an evaluation. The patient had no prior psychiatric history, although both the mother and the patient agreed that she had been depressed for many years. She had previously worked as a flight attendant for 25 years but had to stop because of a back injury. Since then she had struggled on and off with back pain, and she felt her family was very judgmental about her lack of employment and use of pain medications. She was single and lived alone with her cat and had a small network of friends for support. How-

ever, in the last few weeks, one of her best friends had moved away, and she had had to put her cat to sleep because she was not able to pay for its ongoing veterinary care. In addition, she had received a notice 2 weeks previously that the bank would be repossessing her home. Over the course of the week prior to admission, she had cashed out her 401(k) and had begun distributing the money to various creditors whom she owed, paying off all of her outstanding bills. In addition, she had taken multiple loads of clothing and personal items to the thrift store and had started cleaning out her house.

The patient said she had not been sleeping well for months, tossing and turning at night with worries about her finances and her future. Because of her anxiety she had lost her appetite and had lost about 15 pounds. She described a "volcano of anxiety and fear" inside her that was welling up and about to burst. She paced frequently to avoid this sensation. She stated that there was no reason for her to be around anymore and that clearly her family agreed. Her primary concern was that when she took her own life, she did not want to leave any unpaid bills or mess behind for her family to deal with. She did not have a suicide plan. Despite this, because of her multiple chronic and acute precipitating risk factors, the psychiatrist informed her that she would be admitted to a psychiatric inpatient unit. The patient vehemently pled that she was fearful of being "locked up" and that this may in fact worsen her depression and suicidal thoughts.

Safety First!

Although the risk of inpatient treatment (and its corresponding restrictions) should be considered in the overall risk assessment, the benefits of inpatient treatment often outweigh its risks, especially in patients with limited insight regarding the need for treatment (as illustrated in Case Example 1). For example, patients with elevated suicide risks and poor insight often cite that inpatient treatment may worsen their symptoms or exacerbate their social stressors and therefore they do not need inpatient treatment. In many cases, inpatient treatment will reduce their overall symptoms or their acute suicide risks so that the cumulative benefits outweigh the risks. Often these are the same patients whose safety warrants the highest monitoring during the initial admission period.

Once it has been decided that inpatient admission is necessary, other decisions about the level of restriction must be addressed. The clinician must decide whether the admission should be voluntary or involuntary, whether it should be to an open unit or a locked unit, and how frequently the staff needs to monitor the patient. During the admission phase, safety comes first! For patients at highest acute risk for suicide, safety is achieved by providing one-to-one staff monitoring and an environment in which self-harm paraphernalia are removed, usually by involuntary admission to a locked unit. For patients with a slightly lower level of risk, a staff check-in may occur every 15 minutes. Most locked inpatient units have staff checks every 30 minutes as a standard.

Partial Hospitalization Programs

For patients at even lower acute risk for suicide, an open inpatient unit or a crisis residential program is generally the least restrictive. Although the availability of such services may be increasingly limited, partial hospitalization programs are one way of providing intensive daily services in an unlocked environment that allows patients to preserve a connection with their homes, employment, and social support networks. Because patients are not under as close a supervision and restriction as patients in a locked inpatient unit, these programs are appropriate for patients whose suicidality does not put them at acute risk of self-harm and who are motivated for and engaged in treatment.

Multiple studies have compared the efficacy of partial hospitalization programs or day programs to outpatient treatment, especially in patients with borderline personality disorder. One study found that partial hospitalization in this patient population resulted in better improvement in interpersonal and social functioning than standard psychiatric care (Bateman and Fonagy 1999). The study concluded that partial hospitalization may be a viable alternative to hospitalization for patients with borderline personality disorder (Bateman and Fonagy 2001). A large literature review of 18 studies analyzed the efficacy of partial versus inpatient hospitalization for mentally ill adults with other disorders and found no differences on measures of psychopathology, social functioning, family burden, and service utilization between the two groups (Horvitz-Lennon et al. 2001).

Case Example 2: A Patient With a Razor Blade Who Attempts to Hang Herself

A 25-year-old woman with borderline personality disorder was brought to the ED by the police after calling 911 because she was thinking about overdosing on her medications. She had recently had a fight with her boyfriend, who had kicked her out of the house, and her mother had refused to let her return to the mother's house. She felt abandoned and angry, and worried she would not be able to control her impulses.

Upon arrival to the inpatient facility, she was wanded with a metal detector and searched, and her personal items were confiscated. She was upset and labile, becoming belligerent with staff who attempted to set limits with her. After an interaction with one of the staff who had redirected her, she came to the nursing counter with multiple superficial cuts across her wrist that she had made with a razor blade. She confessed that she had smuggled the razor blades in and then taped them to the inside of the toilet with medical tape she had taken from the nursing station. A more thorough search was done, and the razor blades were removed. The following day, after an altercation with a peer during mealtime, she presented with further lacerations on her arms and legs, having sharpened a plastic piece of cutlery from the dining hall into a weapon. She was placed on close dining supervision and prohibited from using utensils at mealtimes. This caused her to become more upset.

Later that afternoon, she was noticed to have been in the bathroom for an extended period of time. When the staff went to check on her, she was found to have wrapped her pant leg around her neck and was having difficulty breathing. She was resuscitated quickly and medically cleared.

At this point, the treatment team agreed that she needed to be placed on 24-hour, one-to-one staff supervision and to not be allowed to wear her own clothes or have access to any personal items. The team involved the patient in a discussion of their reasons for this. In addition, they discussed with her the behaviors that she could change in order to have the supervision and the restrictions reduced or lifted. After a few days of working on these behavioral techniques, the patient was able to demonstrate that she could keep from harming herself despite the availability of means to do so.

Treatment Phase

The previous case demonstrates a rapid evolution of events that culminated in a near-lethal attempt, a situation that fortunately was stabilized with 24-hour, one-to-one staff supervision. After the provision of safety, inpatient treatment then focuses on biological and psychosocial therapeutic interventions, and mobilization of community resources. The person-centered biopsychosocial treatment plan aims to reduce modifiable suicide risk factors (such as depression and anxiety symptoms), provide a supportive environment, reduce acute stressors (often with "a tincture of time"), strengthen existing coping skills, and instill hope.

During the treatment period, emergence of new stressors may acutely renew a patient's suicidal ideation. New stressors may include a relationship breakdown with a loved one (e.g., a mother who decides that she no longer wants her son to live with her), an interpersonal conflict with a peer or staff member, a sudden medication change, an anniversary reaction, an impending court date, and unexpected news. Sudden changes in affect (overt anger or covert withdrawal) or interruption in medication adherence or program attendance should raise suspicion of new emergent stressors.

Case Example 3: An Older Woman Who Felt Ashamed and Abandoned

A 71-year-old Cantonese-speaking woman was brought to the ED from her nursing home after attempting to jump out the window in a suicide attempt. She had emigrated from China with her husband 30 years previously and had three children in the United States. Previously, she had been living at home with her husband and with the assistance of her children. More recently, her husband's health had declined and she had started to have memory problems, requiring more attention than her children were able to provide her. After much deliberation, her family had decided she would be best off in a nursing home, despite the patient's protestation.

On her third day at the nursing home, she attempted suicide by trying to jump from a third-story window. A staff member who happened to be walking by intervened, and the patient was sent to a psychiatric hospital. Upon interview, she expressed disappointment and anger at her family for having abandoned her and for not taking care of her. She also felt ashamed of being a burden and for being emotional and upset about her situation. These feelings were now exacerbated by her recent suicide attempt and her perception that she had brought shame and unnecessary attention to her family and involved outsiders in her family's business. She was adamant that she felt better and wanted to go back to the nursing home and insisted that what she had done was stupid and embarrassing and would not be repeated. She presented with a bright and cheery affect and denied symptoms of depression or family conflict. She was discharged to the nursing home and attempted suicide by the same method 2 days later.

She was readmitted to the psychiatric facility, and this time her family was closely involved in her care and discharge planning. More regular family visits were encouraged, and some of the family's guilt at having put her in an outside facility abated. The family members were congratulated for their utilization of experts in the field to provide the best care for their loved one. In addition, they were encouraged to continue to maintain a role for the patient in the family structure so she did not feel abandoned and disrespected. The Cantonese-speaking staff was encouraged to work with the patient both at the psychiatric facility and at her nursing home after discharge to maintain her ties with her language and her culture. The treatment team worked with the dining staff so they could offer some meals that were more familiar to her, and her family was encouraged to bring in decorations and readings from her country. She slowly reconnected with her family and was able to feel that she had reestablished her place as matriarch, although in a new iteration. This time her suicidal ideation really did remit, and she was able to return safely to the nursing home.

With patients who are unengaged in treatment but whose safety is maintained, the focus is on treatment engagement and establishing a collaborative therapeutic relationship (Ilgen et al. 2009). Often cultural and linguistic differences between the inpatient treatment team and patient pose significant barriers to treatment success, and root cause analyses have found that such barriers may contribute to inpatient suicide (New York State Office of Mental Health 2009). Although family members and significant others are not formally part of the treatment team, it is crucial to engage them in person during inpatient treatment and discharge planning. Language, transportation, and scheduling conflicts can create barriers to meeting face-to-face; however, subtle family dynamics are often missed in phone conversations.

In long-term inpatient psychiatric care settings where the length of stay is months to years, the treatment phase confers a significant risk of suicide. Suicides may occur on the inpatient unit, during passes off the unit, or during absences without leave. In a 10-year retrospective British study, Hunt et al. (2010) found that out of 1,230 off-unit suicides, 761 patients (62%) had been on authorized leave and 469 (38%) had gone absent without leave. The majority of unauthorized departures (termed "absconding" in the study) were from open general psychiatric units (86%). Although on-unit suicides have been declining statistically (due to environmental safeguards against hanging and removal of contraband by searches), it is often difficult to prevent off-unit suicides. Jumping off an elevation and running in front of traffic were the most common suicide methods of patients on leave from psychiatric facilities. Thus, in long-term-care settings, a pass should be treated similarly to a discharge, in which suicide risks are reassessed prior to the pass as if the patient is being discharged.

Pharmacotherapy

There is a dearth of systematic studies that have specifically examined medication and inpatient suicide (Combs and Romm 2007). However, it is reasonable to extrapolate findings from outpatient settings. Clozapine and lithium have been shown to specifically reduce suicide rates. Clozapine has been shown to reduce suicide in patients with schizophrenia in the International Suicide Prevention Trial (InterSePT), perhaps by causing a reduction in psychotic symptoms, conferring fewer extrapyramidal symptoms on patients, and increasing quality of life and hope for the future (Meltzer et al. 2003). A meta-analysis showed suicide to be 82% less frequent while patients were on lithium therapy than while they were receiving other treatments for major affective disorders (Tondo et al. 2001).

One small study of 61 patients who died by suicide in an inpatient hospital showed some significant associations with medication use (Gaertner et al. 2002). Lorazepam reduction or withdrawal was associated with increased risk of suicide. Patients with schizophrenia who had been off medications for 10 days or more had a higher risk than those who were continuing their antipsychotic. Although akathisia has been hypothetically linked to suicide, there is a lack of evidence supporting this theory (Combs and Romm 2007; Dong et al. 2005). In addition, in the Gaertner et al. study, far fewer patients who completed suicide had been taking a mood stabilizer when compared with control subjects. This study suggests that using benzodiazepines and mood stabilizers, as well as avoiding lapses in antipsychotic treatment, may contribute to reduction of risk for suicide in an inpatient setting.

Because medication nonadherence has been shown to be a risk factor for inpatient suicide (Bowers et al. 2000; Hunt et al. 2010), reasons for medication adherence should be addressed. The inpatient treatment setting offers the advantages of having nursing staff available to monitor patients to prevent "cheeking" of medications and of more frequent blood monitoring of serum drug levels. Involuntary medication treatment should be considered early in the inpatient treatment course in patients who lack insight into their need for medications or who are unmotivated for or unengaged in treatment.

Psychosocial Treatment

Dialectical behavior therapy (DBT) is the only psychotherapy treatment that has been shown to reduce suicidal behavior and attempts in patients with borderline personality disorder (Linehan et al. 1991). This treatment modality is an intensive outpatient program in which inpatient treatment is used as an adjunct to manage acute suicide risks. Brief inpatient stabilization and the return of the patient to the outpatient community is optimal so that "therapy-interfering" suicidal behavior is minimized. This enables the patient to continue outpatient skills training in interpersonal effectiveness, emotional regulation, and problem solving. These principles of DBT, as well as DBT groups, can also be used during hospitalization to promote coping skills, increase distress tolerance, and reinforce the outpatient DBT curriculum.

Other psychosocial modalities have not been specifically studied to target suicide as an outcome measure. Supportive psychotherapy, recreation therapy, and social services are the mainstay of inpatient treatment. They aim to provide psychoeducation, promote treatment engagement, strengthen mature coping skills, instill hope, and connect patients to community resources.

Discharge Planning Phase

In the discharge planning phase, inpatient suicide is no longer the major concern and the patient has received sufficient treatment and is deemed safe for discharge (or to go on a pass in long-term-care settings). However, suicides rates, usually within 7–30 days, are higher than rates of suicides that occur on the inpatient unit. Therefore, reassessment of suicide risk factors is mandatory prior to discharge. In an era where the *average* inpatient length of stay is often 7–10 days and the *median* length of stay may be even shorter, some dynamic preadmission risk factors will remain.

So what has changed so that the patient is ready for discharge? Often there is insufficient time for medications to have taken effect from a biological perspective, so the new ingredient is less likely attributable purely to medication effects, except in cases in which anxiety and agitation are reduced by benzodiazepines, mood stabilizers, and antipsychotics. All in all, the new ingredients most likely include addressing stressors that led to the suicidal event (in which often the treatment is the provision of a "holding environment," giving the stressor time to subside), confirmation of a psychiatric diagnosis (via psychoeducation), safeguarding against self-harm paraphernalia (e.g., removal of guns or lethal medications), providing substance withdrawal treatment, and most importantly mobilizing social support and outpatient services.

Case Example 4: A Man With Delusions Who Hears Voices

A 26-year-old man with schizophrenia was brought to the ED by family members for the fourth time in 6 months. He had been living at home since his last discharge from a psychiatric hospital and had stopped taking his antipsychotic medications. This had also happened after each one of his prior hospitalizations; he rarely took his medications for more than a week or two. In the last few weeks he had become increasingly isolated and paranoid, spending time in his room with the door locked. His mother had tried to enter the day prior to admission and he had become very angry and pushed her against a wall, saying if she came in again he would have to kill himself and her.

On interview, he was focused on a delusional system in which demons inhabited his body and those of his family members. In addition, he was having overwhelming auditory hallucinations telling him that death was the only way he could free himself of the demons and telling him to kill himself and his family. He was finding these hallucinations harder and harder to resist. He was treated with an atypical antipsychotic and valproate, and over the course of the next three weeks his auditory hallucinations resolved and his delusions diminished. He no longer had urges to harm himself or his family and was able to articulate with some insight that his delusional thoughts were not real. However, once the team agreed he was ready for discharge and contacted his family, his family refused to allow him to return home, citing his propensity for violence when off medications and his frequent refusals to continue his inpatient medication regimens.

The inpatient team engaged the family in two face-to-face meetings and incorporated family members into the treatment planning. The patient's parents were able to assist the patient, reminding him to take his medications at home and accompanying him to his outpatient appointments. Furthermore, they received education about schizophrenia and were introduced to the mental health system and local family support groups.

Outpatient Care Coordination

During the discharge phase, much anticipation of new and continued outpatient stressors on top of static and dynamic suicide risk assessment should be done and documented. Guidance on discharge medications should be provided, as should education on how to access emergency and outpatient services. Some patients may require an earlier appointment than the standard follow-up appointment of 30 days after discharge. In addition to inquiries about passive and active suicidal ideation, violence risks should also be assessed. Most patients at the discharge phase will not endorse suicidal or homicidal ideation. However, it is important that the clinician provide anticipatory guidance, inquiring about plans if the same stressors that led to the index admission were to reoccur or if conditions worsen (i.e., "What would you do if you were to feel suicidal again?"). Role-play exercises with reenactment of interpersonal conflicts that will likely arise may be helpful.

Further discussion of a safety plan should include removal of firearms, having the patient stay with family members, discussions about alcohol use and prescription pain medication (including limiting supply of medications that could be fatal if overdosed), outpatient appointment schedules, and emergency contact information. A "warm handoff," in which outpatient team members come into the inpatient setting to facilitate follow-up care plans, is ideal for patients eligible for intensive services. For patients with cognitive impairment or limited insight, the provider should have a discharge planning meeting with outpatient caretakers and especially family members.

In terms of documentation, although static factors are unlikely to change and should be recorded in the discharge summary, it is imperative to consider dynamic risk factors. For example, what would happen if the patient could not or refused to adhere to treatment, if he or she were to continue to use substances, of if social support were to diminish? Although it is impossible to predict future suicide, it is important to thoroughly consider and document potential adverse events and attempts to mitigate a bad outcome. Risk levels (low, moderate, high) should be documented based on acute (7 days), short-term (30 days), and long-term (longer than 30 days) risks. It is important to note that there are no standardized suicide rates when referring to the terms "low," "moderate," or "high" risks and no uniform agreement on time periods for "acute," "short-term," and "long-term" categories.

For patients who have benefited from inpatient treatment, it is equally important to document the benefits and lessons learned and how the patient is now more equipped to handle external stressors, and what role family members and outpatient providers may play. Ultimately, the final assessment is a prognostic statement balancing the benefit versus risk of further inpatient treatment. At the time of discharge, the benefits and risks of discharge outweigh further inpatient treatment.

There are a number of factors that influence discharge decisions that are beyond the therapeutic relationship between the inpatient treatment team and the patient. For patients on involuntary psychiatric commitment, the legal system may decertify the involuntary treatment after reviewing the records and hearing testimonies from the patient and treating psychiatrist. In such cases, it is incumbent on the psychiatrist to justify reasons for further inpatient treatment (Brook et al. 2006). If the judge orders discharge, the psychiatrist should nevertheless document suicide risks as well as attempt to arrange for outpatient treatment. For patients with private medical insurance and managed care health plans, utilization reviewers often request justification for further treatment. Often the reviewers are interested in statements of active suicide rather than intensity and severity of suicidal statements. The most challenging cases are where the psychiatrist believes that the patient is at elevated risk, is not actively participating in treatment, and is minimizing his or her suicidal ideation. In such a case, a request to repeal the utilization reviewer's decision often is needed to obtain insurance coverage for further inpatient treatment.

Systems Issues

As discussed previously, inpatient suicides that occur on the unit are declining, and the decline is largely attributable to systemic measures (Tishler and Reiss 2009) that focus on environmental hazards, human errors, and quality improvement (Table 18–2). Systemwide and public health improvements are much more likely to be effective in reducing inpatient suicides than targeting individual treatment providers (Janofsky 2009; Mann et al. 2005).

Environmental Safeguards

Most inpatient units have taken measures to remove common means by which patients can die by suicide. Facility design and furnishings should ensure that anchor points for potential hanging are eliminated

TABLE 18–2. Systems approach to reducing inpatient suicides

Intervention	Example
Periodic review of environmental hazards	Use the Veterans Affairs Mental Health Environment of Care Checklist (www.patientsafety.gov/SafetyTopics.html mheocc).
Reducing communication breakdowns	Review patients at high risk of suicide and violence, and those on special monitoring, during team meetings and in nursing reports. Respect individual staff input at all levels and improve staff morale. Increase staff-to-patient ratio during periods of shift change and when units have highly acute patients.
Quality improvement program	Hold debriefing sessions on minor and major staff errors. Schedule morbidity and mortality case conferences.

and that patients cannot jump from elevations. Other environmental safeguards may include removing plastic bags, locking up bathrooms when not in use, using shelves rather than closets with doors, and avoiding use of glassware or other sharp objects.

The Mental Health Environment of Care Checklist, a toolkit developed by the U.S. Department of Veterans Affairs in 2007 and updated on March 30, 2011, includes a checklist to identify potential environmental hazards by severity (catastrophic, critical, marginal, and negligible), including patient care areas and storage areas, and covers items such as having panic alarms available to staff and securing cleaning chemicals.

Human Errors

Although human errors are much more variable and thus more difficult to address, a systems approach can nevertheless be highly effective. Various analyses indicate that miscommunication and lack of communication among providers, staff, and pa-

tients' social supports tend to be a common theme in completed patient suicides. Communication deficiencies include failure to obtain complete collateral information from outpatient and ED providers and from family members, untimely filing of notes, failure to carry out physician orders in a timely fashion, and poor attendance at inpatient team meetings (Janofsky 2009; Joint Commission 1998; New York State Office of Mental Health 2009). One decisive way to improve communication at team meetings is to add to the agenda a specific discussion of patients who are at high risk of suicide and violence (including patients who are on special observation) and their relevant management plans and progress.

Other unspoken human factors that may contribute to patient recovery include staff morale, their respect for patients and each other, and the value they find in their job duties. Efforts to transform the inpatient psychiatric unit into a less "oppressive and nonstigmatizing" (Hunt et al. 2007) experience will likely improve treatment adherence and patient-staff interactions. These systems improvements may include reducing the staff-to-patient ratio during periods of high acuity and shift change, and providing external staff counseling.

Quality Improvement Programming

It is important to recognize that deaths do occur in most medical specialties and suicide deaths occur in psychiatry. Nevertheless, both mental health professionals and society seem to forget the adage "To err is human" (Mossman 2009) and seemingly take on an all-or-none expectation that inpatient treatment should be error-free, in that no suicide events should ever occur. One common way to acknowledge that errors do occur is to work on continuous quality improvement of even minor errors rather than waiting for major sentinel events to occur. Morbidity and mortality conferences may serve to improve the quality of patient care, expand staff knowledge, and prevent major adverse outcomes. Legal consultation may be indicated in some jurisdictions to ensure that the information discussed is protected by law. The conferences will ideally provide multidisciplinary staff education, build team cohesion, address possible complacency or negligence, and identify individual and systems improvements. They should balance the aim of being supportive for staff members with the ultimate goal of providing better patient care.

Given that inpatient suicides rarely occur, case conferences should also include topics such as suicide attempts, patient-patient violence, patient-staff violence, post-discharge suicides, and discharge planning for high-risk patients. In addition to meeting the needs of the inpatient team members, the conferences should address communication between patients, family members, and hospital administrators.

Key Clinical Concepts

- The most common methods of suicide on inpatient units are hanging on anchor points such as door corners and doorknobs, jumping from elevations, and stabbing.

- The sharpest peaks in suicide risk of hospitalized patients occur in the week after admission and the week after discharge.

- As a conceptual framework, inpatient treatment necessitates suicide risk assessment and management at three distinct yet overlapping stages: admission, treatment, and discharge planning.

- Systems issues to reduce inpatient suicide should focus on reducing environmental hazards, bridging communication gaps, and promoting continuous quality improvement efforts.

References

American Foundation for Suicide Prevention: Facts and figures. 2011. Available at: http://www.afsp.org/index.cfm?fuseaction=home.viewPage&page_ID=04EA1254-BD31-1FA3-C549D77E6CA6AA37. Accessed August 10, 2011.

American Psychiatric Association: Practice Guideline on Suicidal Behaviors. Washington, DC, American Psychiatric Publishing, 2003

Bateman A, Fonagy P: Effectiveness of partial hospitalization in the treatment of borderline personality disorder: a randomized controlled trial. Am J Psychiatry 156:1563–1569, 1999

Bateman A, Fonagy P: Treatment of borderline personality disorder with psychoanalytically oriented partial hospitalization: an 18-month follow-up. Am J Psychiatry 158:36–42, 2001

Bowers L, Jarrett M, Clark N, et al: Determinants of absconding by patients on acute psychiatric wards. J Adv Nurs 32:644–649, 2000

Brook M, Hilty DM, Liu W, et al: Discharge against medical advice from inpatient psychiatric treatment: a literature review. Psychiatr Serv 57:1192–1198, 2006

Busch KA Fawcett J, Jacobs DG: Clinical correlates of inpatient suicide. J Clin Psychiatry 64:14–19, 2003

Cassells C, Paterson B, Dowding D, et al: Long- and short-term risk factors in the prediction of inpatient suicide: a review of the literature. Crisis 26:53–63, 2005

Combs H, Romm S: Psychiatric inpatient suicide: a literature review. Prim Psychiatry 14:67–74, 2007

Deisenhammer EA, Huber M, Kemmler G, et al: Psychiatric hospitalizations during the last 12 months before suicide. Gen Hosp Psychiatry 29:63–65, 2007

Dong JY, Ho TP, Kan CK: A case-control study of 92 cases of in-patient suicides. J Affect Disord 87:91–99, 2005

Erlangsen A, Zarit SH, Tu X, et al: Suicide among older psychiatric inpatients: an evidence-based study of a high-risk group. Am J Geriatr Psychiatry 14:734–741, 2006

Gaertner I, Gilot C, Heidrich P, et al: A case control study on psychopharmacotherapy before suicide committed by 61 psychiatric inpatients. Pharmacopsychiatry 35:37–43, 2002

Hall R, Platt D, Hall R: Suicide risk assessment: a review of risk factors for suicide in 100 patients who made severe suicide attempts. Psychosomatics 40:18–27, 1999

Horvitz-Lennon M, Normand S, Gaccione P, et al: Partial versus full hospitalization for adults in psychiatric distress: a systematic review of the published literature (1957–1997). Am J Psychiatry 158:676–685, 2001

Hunt IM, Kapur N, Webb R, et al: Suicide in current psychiatric in-patients: a case-control study. Psychol Med 37:831–837, 2007

Hunt IM, Windfurh K, Swinson N, et al: Suicide amongst psychiatric in-patients who abscond from the ward: a national clinical survey. BMC Psychiatry 10:1–6, 2010

Ilgen MA, Czyz EK, Welsh DE, et al: A collaborative therapeutic relationship and risk of suicidal ideation in patients with bipolar disorder. J Affect Disord 115:246–251, 2009

Janofsky JS: Reducing inpatient suicide risk: using human factors analysis to improve observation practices. J Am Acad Psychiatry Law 37:15–24, 2009

Joint Commission: Inpatient suicide: recommendations for prevention. Sentinel Event Alert, Nov 6, 1998

Linehan MM, Armstrong HE, Suarez A, et al: Cognitive-behavioral treatment of chronically parasuicidal borderline patients. Arch Gen Psychiatry 48:1060–1064, 1991

Malone K, Oquendo M, Haas G, et al: Protective factors against suicidal acts in major depression: reasons for living. Am J Psychiatry 157:1084–1088, 2000

Mann JJ, Apter A, Bertolote J, et al: Suicide prevention strategies: a systematic review. JAMA 294:2064–2074, 2005

Meehan J, Kapur N, Hunt IM, et al: Suicide in mental health in-patients and within 3 months of discharge: national clinical survey. Br J Psychiatry 188:129–134, 2006

Meltzer HY, Alphs L, Green AI, et al: Clozapine treatment for suicidality in schizophrenia: International Suicide Prevention Trial (InterSePT). Arch Gen Psychiatry 60:82–91, 2003

Mills PD, DeRosier JM, Ballot BA, et al: Inpatient suicide and suicide attempts in Veterans Affairs hospitals. Jt Comm J Qual Patient Saf 34:482–488, 2008

Mossman D: Let's think about human factors, not human failings. J Am Acad Psychiatry Law 37:25–27, 2009

New York State Office of Mental Health: Incident reports and root cause analyses 2002–2008: what they reveal about suicides. June 2009. Available at: http://www.omh.state.ny.us/omhweb/statistics/suicide_incident_rpt/. Accessed August 10, 2011.

Powell J, Geddes J, Deeks J, et al: Suicide in psychiatric hospital in-patients: risk factors and their predictive power. Br J Psychiatry 176:266–272, 2000

Qin P, Nordentoft M: Suicide risk in relation to psychiatric hospitalization: evidence based on longitudinal registers. Arch Gen Psychiatry 62:427–432, 2005

Qin P, Agerbo E, Mortensen P: Suicide risk in relation to socioeconomic, demographic, psychiatric and familial factors: a national register–based study of all suicides in Denmark, 1981–1997. Am J Psychiatry 160:765–772, 2003

Shea S: The delicate art of eliciting suicidal ideation. Psychiatr Ann 34:374–400, 2004

Spiessl H, Hübner-Liebermann B, Cording C: Suicidal behaviour of psychiatric in-patients. Acta Psychiatr Scand 106:134–138, 2002

Tidemalm D, Långström N, Lichtenstein P, et al: Risk of suicide after suicide attempt according to coexisting psychiatric disorder: Swedish cohort study with long term follow-up. BMJ 337:1–6, 2008

Tishler CL, Reiss NS: Inpatient suicide: preventing a common sentinel event. Gen Hosp Psychiatry 31:103–109, 2009

Tondo L, Hennen J, Baldessarini RJ: Lower suicide risk with long-term lithium treatment in major affective illness: a meta-analysis. Acta Psychiatr Scand 104:163–172, 2001

U.S. Department of Veterans Affairs, VHA National Center for Patient Safety: Mental health environment of care checklist. 2009. Available at: http://www.patientsafety.gov/SafetyTopics.html#mheocc. Accessed August 10, 2011.

CHAPTER 19

Patient Safety and Freedom of Movement

Coping With Uncertainty

Robert I. Simon, M.D.

For decades the least restrictive alternative in the mental health field has been an operative principle (*Lake v. Cameron* 1966). In the safety management of suicidal patients, the tension between providing safety and allowing freedom of movement creates uncertainty. Clinicians also experience dissonance between the need to provide adequate supervision for patients at risk for suicide and the denial of insurance coverage by third-party payers for these services. The only certainty is that effective treatment and safety management of the suicidal patient require the clinician's full commitment of time and effort.

After careful assessment, the safety management of the suicidal patient is an informed clinical judgment call. The provision of absolute safety is obviously an impossible task. Patients who are determined to die by suicide will find a way. They view the clinician as their enemy (Resnick 2002). Deception and lack of patient cooperation complicate safety assessments.

As in all medical specialties, psychiatrists will have patients die. This adverse outcome is inherent in the practice of medicine. A patient's death is a tragedy; however, it is not evidence per se of professional negligence. Nonetheless, malpractice suits against psychiatrists remain an occupational hazard. The treatment and safety management of suicidal patients can be anxiety provoking and fatiguing. Some clinicians limit the number of patients at risk of suicide under their care. Others try to avoid treating suicidal patients altogether. Clinicians should realistically assess their ability to tolerate the uncertainty inherent in the treatment of suicidal patients.

Outpatients

The ability to exercise control over outpatients at risk for suicide, including those attending partial hospitalization programs, is limited. In outpatient settings, patient safety is usually managed by clinical interventions such as increasing the frequency and length of visits, providing or adjusting medication, and involving family or other concerned persons, if the patient permits. Appropriate treatment of the patient is an integral aspect of safety management. Voluntary or, if necessary, involuntary hospitalization remains an option for suicidal patients at high suicide risk who can no longer be safely treated as outpatients. Most suicidal patients at moderate suicide risk and even some patients at high risk are treated in outpatient settings.

When to hospitalize a patient can be a trying decision for the clinician. The decision is considerably more complicated when the need for hospitalization is clear but the patient refuses. The action that the clinician takes at this point is critical for the patient's treatment and for risk management.

Hospitalization

The clinician, after systematic suicide risk assessment, determines that the suicidal patient requires hospitalization (see Chapter 1, "Suicide Risk Assessment: Gateway to Treatment and Management," this volume). The risks and benefits of continuing outpatient treatment are weighed against the risks and benefits of hospitalization and shared with the patient. If the patient agrees, arrangements for immediate hospitalization are made. The patient must go *directly* to the hospital, accompanied by a responsible person. The patient should not stop to do errands, get clothing, or make last-minute arrangements. A detour may provide the patient with the opportunity to attempt or to complete suicide. If the patient is driven to the hospital, a safety locking mechanism under the sole control of the driver, if available, may help prevent the patient from jumping out of the car. An

additional passenger may be needed to accompany the patient. In some instances, clinicians have accompanied the patient to the hospital. The clinician, however, has no legal duty to assume physical custody of the patient (*Farwell v. Un* 1990).

If the patient rejects the clinician's recommendation for hospitalization, the matter is immediately addressed as a treatment issue. Because the need for hospitalization is acute, a prolonged inquiry into the patient's reasons for rejecting the recommendation for hospitalization may not be feasible. Furthermore, the therapeutic alliance may be strained. Consultation and referral are options for the clinician to consider, if time and the patient's condition permit. It is this situation that tries the professional and personal mettle of the clinician.

The failure to involuntarily hospitalize a suicidal patient who subsequently attempts or commits suicide is a source of malpractice suits against outpatient clinicians. When an acute, high-risk suicidal patient refuses treatment, the psychiatrist's duty of care to the patient supersedes the patient's refusal. The uncompensated time required, the inconvenience, the disruption of the clinician's schedule, the possibility of a court appearance, and the fear of a lawsuit by the patient may dissuade the clinician from initiating involuntary hospitalization. State commitment statutes grant clinicians immunity from liability when they use reasonable judgment, follow statutory commitment procedures, and act in good faith.

Documenting the suicide risk assessment and the rationale for involuntary hospitalization represents good clinical care as well as sound risk management. When involuntary hospitalization is sought, psychiatrists should leave it to the courts to resolve uncertainty about commitment. The clinician's proper focus is the patient's safety.

Split Treatment

Collaboration and communication between psychiatrist and psychotherapist in split-treatment settings are essential in assessing and managing the patient at risk for suicide. The essence of collaborative treatment is effective communication. The operative principle should be "We are in it together" (Meyer and Simon 1999a, 1999b).

Psychiatrists and psychotherapists with split-treatment practices may not take the time or have the time to adequately collaborate. For example, a psychiatrist who sees 4 patients for medication management every hour, 8 hours a day for 5 days a week, will treat 160 patients a week. Assuming the psychiatrist receives 20 patient telephone calls a day from a patient base of 500, the psychiatrist will receive 100 telephone calls a week, not including weekend calls. Extremely busy, high-volume medication management practices are common. How will the psychiatrist find the time to collaborate?

Collaboration takes time and effort. Communication is necessary to prevent the suicidal patient from falling between the cracks of split treatment (Gutheil and Simon 2003). Clinical responsibilities should be clearly demarcated to prevent role confusion and uncertainty, potentially increasing the patient's risk for suicide. Adequate communication and collaboration between psychiatrist and psychotherapist are standard practice, especially for patients at risk for suicide (see Chapter 15, "Split Treatment: Coming of Age," this volume).

Inpatients

In the managed care era, only the severely mentally ill are admitted to acute-care psychiatric facilities (Simon 1997). The criteria for voluntary admission often exceed the substantive standards required for involuntary hospitalization. Most patients are acutely suicidal or violent toward others or both. Hospitalization is usually brief; the average stay in most short-term psychiatric facilities is between 3 and 5 days. The purpose of hospitalization is crisis intervention, patient safety, and stabilization (Simon 1998).

Patients who are potentially dangerous to themselves and others may be prematurely discharged (Simon 1998). The rapid admission, crisis management, and discharge of severely ill patients may not allow an overburdened staff enough time to evaluate the new patient thoroughly. Brief safety checks made by a succession of mental health personnel are usually insufficient to know and develop a relationship with the patient. Relying solely on a "promise" or "no-harm contract" that the patient will not attempt suicide constitutes inadequate safety management.

The level of supervision of suicidal patients is determined after systematic assessment of suicide risk (Simon 1998). Suicide risk assessment is a process, not a single event that reduces the uncertainty surrounding patient treatment and safety management. Suicide prevention contracts should not be used in lieu of adequate suicide risk assessment.

The treatment team has emerged as an important provider of care for psychiatric inpatients. Among its many advantages, the treatment team has "a thousand eyes" to focus on the safety supervision of suicidal patients. Nonetheless, the treatment team can develop blind spots when communication among team members is faulty, thus increasing the patient's risk for suicide (Table 19–1).

A newly admitted, severely mentally ill patient at significant risk for suicide who is

TABLE 19–1. Inpatient suicides: occurrences

Shortly after admission
During staff shift changes
Shortly after discharge[a]
During mealtime distractions
At changes in psychiatric residents' rotations

[a]A few hours, days, or weeks later (Qin and Nordentoft 2005).

untreated and unknown to the clinical staff should be placed on suicide precautions. Nurses can exercise their discretion to place patients on suicide precautions or increase the precaution level, if the psychiatrist cannot be reached or until the psychiatrist has an opportunity to call or to examine the patient. If suicide precautions are imposed by the nursing staff, the psychiatrist should assess the patient before discontinuing the precautions and document the rationale for discontinuance or write an order to continue the precautions. Nurses cannot lower or discontinue suicide precautions.

Psychiatrists frequently receive phone calls from the nursing staff requesting a change or discontinuation of safety precautions regarding patients previously examined. Psychiatrists routinely make safety management decisions by phone based on adequate on-the-spot suicide risk assessments performed by the clinical staff.

Observation Levels

Systematic suicide risk assessment of the patient at admission informs the level of suicide precautions. For example, does the patient require one-to-one, arm's-length, or close visual observation? Are safety checks every 15 or 30 minutes necessary, or is routine unit observation (usually every 30 minutes or hourly) sufficient? Psychiatrists should know the definition of *close observation*. Definitions of close observation often

differ among hospitals. It is usually easier to place a patient on suicide safety precautions than it is to reduce or discontinue precautions. Patients who are still on one-to-one or 15-minute safety observations should not be immediately discharged. Depending on the patient's safety requirements, a period of observation of the patient off safety precautions that precedes discharge is sound clinical practice.

The usual practice is to initiate 15-minute checks on admission, with adjustment of the safety management as necessary. However, automatic 15-minute checks may not correspond to the patient's safety requirements. Patients can and do kill themselves between 15-minute checks. A patient who has made a near-lethal suicide attempt just prior to admission may require one-to-one supervision.

High-volume admissions of acutely suicidal patients place a heavy burden on inpatient staffs. Limitation of services is a reality in the current managed care environment. Moreover, a patient determined to die by suicide can do it on one-to-one safety precautions. Busch et al. (2003), in a review of 76 inpatient suicides, found that 42 of these patients were on 15-minute suicide checks. Nine percent of patients were on one-to-one observation with a staff member at the time of suicide. Busch et al. concluded that no specific suicide precautions are 100% effective.

When a patient at high risk for suicide is identified, one-to-one supervision may not be ordered because insurance coverage for such services is not available. Moreover, the hospital staff, stretched thin, may not be able to provide one-to-one patient supervision. The patient or family may be unable or unwilling to pay out of pocket for a "sitter." The psychiatrist or clinical staff should not place a high-risk patient in seclusion or restraints merely to obtain insurance coverage for one-to-one supervision. The use of seclusion and restraint is governed by strict clinical and procedural criteria. An acutely suicidal patient placed in seclusion and/or restraints requires one-to-one supervision. The temptation to obtain insurance coverage for such supervision by resorting to the questionable use of seclusion and restraint should be resisted.

Constant observation should be discontinued as soon as possible, consistent with the patient's safety requirement. The psychiatric unit is not a jail. Although safety is a primary concern, the decision to employ close observation must be balanced against the psychological distress it can cause the patient. For example, privacy in the performance of natural functions is lost. The patient cannot go to the bathroom or shower without the presence of an observer. Patients often experience intense embarrassment and humiliation that can increase hopelessness, depression, and suicide risk. Also, constant observation by a stranger is unnerving and intimidating, especially to a paranoid patient.

During periods of peak activity on the psychiatric unit, sufficient staff may not be available to provide one-to-one close observation. The staff can decide to "zone" the patient to an area in front of the nurses' station or to a specific location on the psychiatric unit where the patient can be kept under visual observation. Moreover, the clinical staff may not be able to provide time- and labor-intensive monitored safety precautions at 5- or 10-minute intervals. Other patients are also on suicide precautions. Five- or 10-minute safety checks and documentation may be overlooked, with potential liability consequences. If 5- to 10-minute checks are required, it may be better to place the patient on constant visual observation or on one-to-one arm's-length obser-

vation, monitored by either a staff member or a responsible, trained "sitter." Video observation can be inconsistent. The monitor is usually placed in the busy nurses' station, where distractions frequently occur.

After adequate initial assessment and observation, the newly admitted patient at risk for suicide who attends group meetings, socializes with other patients, and is visible on the unit usually has 15-minute checks discontinued. The patient is placed on standard ward supervision. In contrast, patients who are at high risk for suicide, withdrawn, and isolative may require one-to-one close observation. The persistently withdrawn, nonparticipating patient needs to be distinguished from a newly admitted patient who is initially isolated and withdrawn but after a day or so feels more comfortable about being on a psychiatric unit. This adjustment occurs as the patient gradually establishes a relationship with staff members and peers. The observation level needs to be flexible. For example, a patient with melancholic depression may need closer supervision in the morning, when depressive symptoms are often worse.

Patients who have decided to die by suicide may actually feel better or feign improvement. These patients usually "improve" suddenly, often dramatically, in contrast to patients who improve gradually but haltingly. Core symptoms of psychiatric disorder (e.g., insomnia, anorexia, restlessness, and other symptoms of anxiety and depression) often persist. Distinguishing suicidal patients whose improvement is illusory from patients who are actually improving is one of the most difficult evaluations that psychiatrists must make (Simon and Gutheil 2009). Psychiatrists' expectations that patients will improve while under their care can create a blind spot in safety assessment and management.

During peak periods of activity or shift changes on the unit, a suicidal patient may take advantage of the staff's distraction to attempt or die by suicide. The multidisciplinary team must be able to maintain consistent safety vigilance, even though it is stretched. If the psychiatric unit is understaffed or the staff is overwhelmed by an influx of suicidal patients, temporary closure of the psychiatric unit to new admissions may be necessary. Just a few agitated, high-risk suicidal patients can fully occupy and quickly exhaust the clinical staff.

Imminent Suicide

Psychiatrists have difficulty gauging the imminence of suicide. Imminence is not a psychiatric diagnosis. No risk factor or risk factors identify imminence of suicide (Simon 2006). Suicide risk can vary by the minute, by the hour, or by the day. Patients are often considered to be at "imminent" risk for suicide when found hiding lethal instruments or when vocal about committing suicide at their first opportunity. Nonetheless, suicidal individuals perched on bridges or with guns placed to their heads have been dissuaded from committing an intended lethal act. Some of the two dozen or so survivors who jumped from the Golden Gate Bridge changed their minds after they stepped off the bridge. Of 515 individuals restrained from jumping, 94% were still alive many years later (Seiden 1978). It is imperative to carefully assess, treat, and manage acute high-risk factors that are driving a suicide crisis, rather than to attempt the impossible task of predicting when or whether a patient will attempt suicide. "Imminent" suicide is unfortunately a common usage in clinical practice.

Intensive Care Unit (Critical Care Unit)

The patient admitted to an intensive care unit (ICU) after a suicide attempt may be awaiting transfer to a psychiatric unit. In many hospitals, "sitters" are required to constantly attend the patient. A patient may seize an opportune moment to jump through an unsecured window of an ICU or a medical/surgical unit or to walk off the ICU. Untrained "sitters" or family members rarely provide constant safety supervision. They often assume that the patient is compliant rather than devious in finding a way to die by suicide. They are reluctant to follow the suicidal patient into the bathroom. The patient may be able to die by suicide, usually by strangulation, while in the bathroom.

Medical/surgical units provide many opportunities for the patient to die by suicide with unsecured equipment and other safety hazards. ICUs are not designed for the safety management of the psychiatric patient at risk for suicide. Transfer of the patient to the psychiatric unit should be a priority.

Seclusion and Restraint

The federal government's Center for Medicare and Medicaid Services (CMS)—formerly the Health Care Financing Administration (42 Code of Federal Regulations 1999)—the Joint Commission on Accreditation of Healthcare Organizations (JCAHO) (2001), and most states have developed requirements designed to minimize and avoid the use of seclusion and restraint wherever possible (Simon 2001). Federal requirements may be superseded by more restrictive state laws. *Seclusion* is the involuntary confinement of a person alone in a room where the person is physically prevented from leaving, or the separation of the patient from others in a safe, contained, controlled environment. *Restraint* is the direct application of physical force to an individual, with or without the individual's permission, to restrict his or her freedom of movement. Physical force may involve human touch, mechanical devices, or a combination thereof. Use of these interventions presents an inherent risk to the patient's physical safety and well-being and therefore must occur only when there is "imminent risk" that the patient may inflict harm to self or others. Statutory language may include the use of drugs in the definition of restraint (Simon 2001). Seclusion and restraint should be used only as a last resort and never for the convenience of staff. The overarching therapeutic goal is to protect the patient's safety and dignity.

Qualified staff members may initiate seclusion or restraint for the safety and protection of the patient and staff; however, they must obtain an order from the licensed independent practitioner as soon as possible, within 1 hour of initiation. CMS and JCAHO define stringent requirements for face-to-face evaluation of the patient within 1 hour of initiation and for assessment, frequency of reassessment, monitoring, time-limited orders, notification of family members, discontinuation at the earliest possible opportunity, and debriefing with patient and staff members.

The treatment of psychiatric inpatients has changed in the managed care era. Most psychiatric units, particularly those in general hospitals, have become short-stay, acute-care psychiatric facilities. Generally, only suicidal, homicidal, and gravely disabled patients with major psychiatric disorders pass strict precertification review for hospitalization. Approximately half of these patients have comorbid substance-related disorders. The purpose of hospital-ization is crisis intervention and management to stabilize patients and ensure their safety as soon as possible (Simon and Shuman 2007).

The clinical staff can become temporarily overwhelmed by the rapid admission of very sick patients. The psychiatric unit may need to briefly restrict or curtail new admissions. Patients should not be placed in seclusion or restraint for the convenience of the staff or because of insufficient staffing. The indications and safety precautions for seclusion and restraint should be thoroughly documented. Seclusion and restraint should be used only when all other treatment and safety measures have failed.

The indications and contraindications for seclusion and restraint are discussed elsewhere (see American Psychiatric Association 1985). Seclusion and restraint may be necessary for the patient assessed at high risk for suicide in order to prevent self-harm. If the patient can be engaged by the staff upon admission, a nascent therapeutic alliance may develop. Appropriate medications given at therapeutic levels can rapidly stabilize the high-risk patient. If the suicidal patient is placed in seclusion and restraint, direct observation is required, according to regulatory and hospital policies. Seclusion rooms should have windows or audiovisual surveillance capability (Lieberman et al. 2004). Open-door seclusion is preferable when clinically appropriate.

Freedom of Movement

There must be a rational nexus between patient autonomy in the hospital setting and the patient's diagnosis, treatment, and safety needs. With patients at risk for suicide, standard safety precautions must be observed, such as removal of shoelaces, belts, sharps, glass products, and even pillowcases that can be used for suffocation. A thorough search for contraband on admission is standard procedure. Psychiatric units are usually fitted, at a minimum, with non-weight-bearing fixtures and shower curtain rods, very short cords for electrical beds (properly insulated), cordless telephones or telephones with safety cords, jump-proof windows, barricade-proof doors, and closed-circuit video cameras. The most common and available method of committing suicide by inpatients is strangulation, usually accomplished by a bedsheet hooked up to the patient's bed, door, or bathroom fixtures. Breakaway bedsheets and towels are available. Building safety features such as a stainless steel box around plumbing fixtures, adding "plates" to grab bars to minimize the risk of hanging, and use of solid ceilings are necessary to diminish the risk of hanging. The most dangerous place on the psychiatric unit is the patient's room, especially the bathroom.

Determining safety precautions is complicated by court directives that require highly disturbed patients to be treated by the least restrictive means (Simon 2000). In *Johnson v. United States* (1976/1978/1981), the court noted that an "open-door" policy creates a higher potential for danger. The court went on to say the following:

> Modern psychiatry has recognized the importance of making every effort to return a patient to an active and productive life. Thus, the patient is encouraged to develop his self-confidence by adjusting to the demands of everyday existence. Particularly because the prediction of danger is difficult, undue reliance on hospitalization might lead to prolonged incarceration of potentially useful members of society.

The tension between promoting individual freedom and preventing self-injury introduces an inherent uncertainty in the safety management of suicidal patients (Amchin et al. 1990). In malpractice suits, the individual facts of the case and the reasonableness of the staff's application of the open-door policy are determinative.

Policies and Procedures

Hospital policies and procedures require the patient to be evaluated by the psychiatrist within a specified period of time after admission. Departures from policies and procedures by the psychiatrist deserve a documented explanation. If the psychiatrist departs from the policies and procedures and the patient is harmed, a malpractice suit filed against the psychiatrist may be difficult to defend (*Eaglin v. Cook County Hospital* 1992). Official policies and procedures are consensus statements that often reflect the standard of care. However, they may propound "best practices" rather than the "ordinarily employed" standard care.

Departmental policy may require that a newly admitted patient remain on the psychiatric unit for a specified period of time, usually 24 hours. It is prudent not to issue off-ward privileges to new patients until their psychiatric evaluations are completed and safety needs determined. Emergency admissions of patients often occur late at night or in the early hours of the morning. Severely ill patients at high risk for suicide should be examined by the psychiatrist within a reasonable time after admission. The nursing staff has a duty to contact the psychiatrist in a timely manner after a patient is admitted.

In the managed care era, unaccompanied off-ward privileges or overnight passes for patients are a rarity. Staff-accompanied off-ward passes for in-hospital diagnostic procedures occur frequently. Depending on the urgency of medical problems and the level of assessed suicide risk, adequate supervision must be provided. For example, more than one staff member may be required to accompany the patient.

Newly admitted patients who smoke will often pressure the staff for a pass to go off ward individually or with a smokers' group. A nicotine patch or inhaler may be rejected. No off-ward pass should be issued unless the patient is cleared for the pass after adequate assessment of suicide risk.

Premature Discharge

Patients leave the psychiatric unit against medical advice (AMA) for a variety of reasons. Some smokers leave if they are not allowed to smoke on the unit. Patients with substance abuse disorders often sign out AMA, sometimes in the middle of the night. Informal (purely voluntary) and formal (conditionally voluntary) admission policies determine whether the suicidal patient who demands to leave can be held for a period of evaluation. Purely voluntary patients cannot be held against their will. Only moral suasion can be used to encourage continued hospitalization. Only a few states continue to use informal admission procedures. In some hospitals, both psychiatric and addicted patients are admitted to the psychiatric unit. Patients admitted for substance detoxification may be informal admissions, whereas psychiatric patients on the same unit are formal admissions. Generally, substance-abusing patients without a comorbid psychiatric disorder cannot be held against their will, whereas substance-using patients with comorbid psychiatric disorders usually can be held against their will.

The psychiatrist may not have had the opportunity to examine the patient and perform a suicide risk assessment before the patient decides to leave AMA. Reliance is placed on clinical staff members to conduct an adequate suicide risk assessment and to inform the psychiatrist of their evaluation. Conditionally voluntary patients at significant risk for suicide can be held for a specified period of time for further evaluation. During the holding period, some patients withdraw their requests to leave and decide to stay. Other patients at low risk for suicide may be allowed to leave AMA or may be involuntarily hospitalized if they remain at significant risk for suicide. The decision to release or retain a suicidal patient who signs out AMA depends on the assessed level of risk (Gerbasi and Simon 2003). Some patients at moderate to high suicide risk are currently treated as outpatients, especially when a working therapeutic alliance with an outpatient treater exists and other substantial protective factors are present.

Acutely suicidal patients seen in the emergency department who refuse hospitalization are usually confronted with making a choice between voluntary or involuntary hospitalization. Some patients opt for voluntary hospitalization, only to seek discharge after a brief stay on the psychiatric unit. If the "revolving door" patient is a conditional (formal) voluntary admission, he or she can be held for further evaluation as prescribed by state statute.

Suicide Warnings

The clinician has no legal duty to inform others that a patient is at risk for suicide (*Bellah v. Greenson* 1978). The *Tarasoff* duty to warn and protect endangered third parties, which exists in a number of jurisdictions, applies only if the threats of physical harm are directed toward others, not toward patients themselves (*Tarasoff v. Regents of the University of California* 1976). In *Gross v. Allen* (1994), however, a 1994 California appellate court case, the court held that if a patient has a history of dangerousness to self, the original caretaker is legally responsible for informing the new caretaker of this history. The court applied a *Tarasoff* analysis, extending the duty to warn and protect to threats of suicide.

Gross v. Allen does not appear to create a new duty for psychiatrists in the safety management of patients at risk for suicide. Clinicians often communicate with new treaters after obtaining patients' permission. Standard safety measures include communicating with significant others about the patient's condition, attempting to modify pathological interactions between the patient and family members, and mobilizing family support (e.g., removing lethal weapons, poisons, and drugs; administering and monitoring prescribed medications). Good clinical practice may require that significant others be apprised of the patient's risk of suicide or even be included in the treatment, provided the patient agrees to such interventions. The patient, however, may not grant permission for disclosure. Just listening to others does not violate the patient's confidentiality. The patient should be informed of the contact. *The Principles of Medical Ethics With Annotations Especially Applicable to Psychiatry* (American Psychiatric Association 2009) states, "Psychiatrists at times may find it necessary, in order to protect the patient or the community from imminent danger, to reveal confidential information disclosed by the patient" (Section 4, Annotation 8). Some states provide for statutory waiver of confidential information when a patient threatens self-harm (Simon 1992).

Significant Others

Cooperation and support of significant others in the patient's care are essential. Significant others include family members (spouse, mother, father, sibling, offspring, grandparent, other relatives) and nonfamily members (roommate, friend, fiancé[e], other) (Dervic et al. 2004). The family is often the patient's main support and protective factor against suicide. Often, nonfamily members also play a supportive role. Postdischarge planning addresses the stability of the patient, the stability of the family, and the nature of the interaction between patient and family as important parts of the discharge risk-benefit assessment.

There are potential problems with families providing patient supervision. First, the interaction between the patient and the family may be seriously impaired. Mentally ill patients frequently come from families that display significant psychological impairment. Moreover, some members of the patient's family may be more unstable than the patient. Family members may dissuade the patient from taking necessary medication because of their denial of the patient's mental illness. Disturbed families can become a risk factor for patient suicide. Educating the family about the patient's illness may help decrease destructive attitudes and behaviors that undermine the patient's stability and safety. Psychoeducation is important in postdischarge safety planning.

Family members are not trained to manage suicidal patients. Patients who are intent on killing themselves are ingenious in finding ways to attempt or die by suicide. Asking family members to keep a constant watch on the patient usually fails. Most family members will not follow the patient into the bathroom or be able to stay up all night to observe the patient. Moreover, family members find reasons to make exceptions to constant surveillance due to denial, fatigue, or the need to attend to other pressing matters. For example, one family who was told to keep the patient under constant watch allowed her to drive to church alone. She drove 30 miles to a bridge and jumped to her death. If the patient needs constant supervision to maintain safety, he or she should not be discharged until stabilized.

There is an important role for the family, but it is not as a substitute for the constant safety management provided by trained mental health professionals on an inpatient psychiatric unit. Early discharge of an inpatient based on reliance on family supervision can be precarious. If an outpatient at suicide risk requires constant family supervision, then psychiatric hospitalization may be indicated. Families, however, should be instructed to observe and report specific symptoms and behaviors displayed by the patient that often precede suicide attempts. Family support of the patient and feedback about the patient's thoughts and behaviors are appropriate, helpful roles. Family members who have a supportive relationship with the patient are often sensitive to important reportable changes in the patient's mental condition.

Gun Safety Management

Gun safety management is first and foremost a treatment issue, but the clinician must do more if the patient is at risk for suicide (Table 19–2). Suicidal patients must be asked if they have access to guns. Some patients will volunteer that they have guns at home. Other patients will deny that there are guns at home when there are or if they know that guns are easily accessible elsewhere. Thus, it is necessary to ask the patient, "Do you have guns at home or at any other place?" "Can you get one easily?" Additionally, the patient should be asked, "Do you intend to obtain or purchase a gun?" In the first week following the purchase of a handgun, suicide by firearms among pur-

TABLE 19–2. Principles of gun safety management with patients at risk for suicide

Inquire about guns at home or located outside the home (e.g., car, office). Also inquire if patient intends to obtain or purchase a gun.

Designate a willing, responsible person to remove and safely secure guns and ammunition outside the home at a location unknown to the patient.

Have direct contact with or receive a phone call from the designated person that guns and ammunition are properly removed from the home or from outside the home and safely secured according to the prearranged gun safety management plan. E-mail should not be used to communicate.

Delay discharging inpatients or patients in the emergency department assessed at risk for suicide until guns and ammunition are properly removed and secured.[a]

[a]Outpatients case by case.

chasers was found to be 57 times higher than the adjusted rate for the general population (Wintemute et al. 1999).

Patients who have a gun at home usually have more than one gun. Guns that are described as locked up and safely stored can still be accessible if the patient has a duplicate key or is able to break into where the guns are stored. The clinician should not rely on "no-suicide contracts" given orally or in writing by the patient as part of gun safety management. No evidence exists that such suicide prevention contracts reduce or eliminate suicide risk (Simon 2004; Stanford et al. 1994).

All handguns and long guns must be removed, including ammunition, and stored in a place not accessible to the patient. The patient may want to give the guns to a family member or other persons for safekeeping. This option is risky because it places the patient in direct contact with guns. In some instances, patients have brought guns to the clinician for safekeeping. The risk to the clinician is obvious. The danger of harm persists when the patient requests that the guns be returned. If the clinician disagrees, a counter-therapeutic power struggle may develop that undermines the treatment. It is not the responsibility of the clinician to provide safe storage of patients' firearms.

The optimal situation exists when the patient at risk for suicide acknowledges that guns are at home and agrees to have the guns removed by a designated, responsible person, usually a family member, partner, or neighbor. The treatment boundaries are readjusted to accommodate the designated person. The designated individual must be able to remove the gun(s) without self-injury, and if unable, must contact a capable person or the police to perform the task. The designated person may require competent assistance in disarming the gun(s). Many individuals do not know how to handle firearms or are fearful when around guns.

By a prearranged plan, the designated individual will report back to the clinician that all guns have been removed from the home or from outside the home and safely secured, so that the guns and ammunition cannot be found by the patient. As tragic events demonstrate, simply hiding guns does not suffice. Patients intent on completing suicide are ingenious in finding guns supposedly secured in the home. Even in the case of guns with trigger locks, or guns stored in lockboxes or gun safes, the suicidal patient may have a duplicate key, have the combination written down, or find some other way of defeating these locking devices. The negotiation between clinician, patient, and the designated individual must be fully documented.

The clinician cannot rely upon a task-specific therapeutic alliance with the person designated to implement the gun safety plan unless that individual is in conjoint treatment with the patient at risk for suicide. The clinician's task is to determine whether the designated person understands the gun safety plan and is responsible enough to carry it out. This determination is a clinical judgment call. All the clinician can do is to trust his or her assessment but *verify* by receiving a return call from the designated person that the safety plan was executed in the manner agreed on.

Instructions on gun safety management must be kept as simple and straightforward as possible. The patient's family or partner is often frightened and easily confused. For example, asking the designated person to remove the firing pin of a gun or secure the gun in a combination locking safe, with the combination reset, may overwhelm the designated person and scuttle the safety plan.

A meeting with the patient, the designated responsible person, and the clinician should be arranged, if possible. All participants are encouraged to ask and answer questions. A collaborative team approach helps to preserve the therapeutic alliance and gives the clinician the opportunity to meet the designated person. It should be explained that guns in the home increase the risk of suicide. The designated person is instructed to go directly home and immediately remove the guns and ammunition from the home to safe storage outside the home at a location unknown to the patient. Guns must be unloaded of ammunition. The designated person agrees to call back once the task is performed expeditiously. All other daily tasks and activities are deferred. If no call back is received or the call is not received in a prearranged timely manner, the patient's gun safety plan is no longer viable. A fallback plan should be implemented, if possible. There are limitations on the ability of the clinician to ensure that the patient and designated person comply with a gun safety management plan.

Therapeutic Risk Management

The fear of being sued can undermine patient safety management when clinically indicated interventions are compromised by avoidant defensive practices. The diffident, fearful clinician attempts to avoid the inherent uncertainties in the safety management of suicidal patients by adopting unduly defensive practices (Simon 1985, 1987). An affirmative, full commitment to the patient's care is lost. For example, a clinician who fails to hospitalize involuntarily a litigious, treatment-refusing patient at high risk for suicide because he or she fears being sued increases his or her liability exposure if the patient attempts or commits suicide.

Risk management is a reality of psychiatric practice, especially in the assessment and management of patients at risk for suicide. Risk management guidelines usually recommend *ideal* or *best* practices, whereas the actual standard of care is ordinary or reasonable prudent care. Moreover, suicide cases are challenging, multifaceted, and nuanced, making it difficult to provide precise assessment and management guidelines.

Therapeutic risk management is patient centered (see Chapter 1, "Suicide Risk Assessment," and Chapter 2, "The Interpersonal Art of Suicide Assessment," in this volume); it supports the treatment process and the therapeutic alliance (see Table 19–3). At a minimum, it follows the fundamental ethical principle in medicine to "first do no harm." A working knowledge of the legal regulation of psychiatry enables the practi-

TABLE 19–3. Basic elements of therapeutic risk management

Patient centered

Clinically appropriate

Supportive of treatment and the therapeutic alliance

Working knowledge of legal regulation of psychiatry

Clinical management of psychiatric-legal issues

Wellness, not legal, agenda

"First do no harm" ethic

Source. Reprinted from Simon RI: *Assessing and Managing Suicide Risk: Guidelines for Clinically Based Risk Management.* Washington, DC, American Psychiatric Publishing, 2004, p. 19. Copyright 2004, American Psychiatric Publishing. Used with permission.

tioner to manage psychiatric-legal issues more effectively. Therapeutic risk management also provides the practitioner with a significant measure of practice comfort that supports the clinician's treatment role with patients at risk for suicide. Defensive practices that can undermine patient safety management are reduced.

Conclusion

The clinician's full commitment of time and effort to the care of the suicidal patient is the single most important factor in reducing the clinical uncertainties surrounding safety management. Uncertainty about clinical judgment calls is inevitable. Clinicians should assess their limits in coping with uncertainty and anxiety. The emotional and physical fatigue associated with the care of suicidal patients is considerable. Some clinicians limit the number of suicidal patients under their care or simply do not accept patients known to be at risk for suicide.

Key Clinical Concepts

- Effective treatment and safety management of the suicidal patient require the full commitment of time and effort from the clinician.

- Safety management is part of an overall effective treatment plan.

- Suicide risk assessment is an evolving process, not an event. It is key to determining informed, ongoing treatment and safety management. It is performed with all patients at suicide risk.

- Reliance on suicide prevention contracts with new, unknown patients who are acutely ill is unwarranted. Suicide prevention contracts can create the illusion of safety where none exists.

- Suicide prevention contracts should not be used in the place of adequate suicide risk assessment.

- Good clinical care, not the fear of being sued, directs the clinician's decision making regarding involuntary hospitalization of a suicidal patient.

- Appropriate levels of patient safety management should be provided despite third-party payer denial of coverage for the cost of close supervision.

- Denials of coverage for the supervision requirements of a patient at high suicide risk should be appealed. Rejection of coverage or the appeal by third-party payers must not determine the level of supervision provided to the patient. This is the clinician's responsibility.

- The entire treatment team participates in the supervision of the patient at suicide risk. The proper supervision of patients at risk for suicide in rapid-turnover inpatient settings cannot be the responsibility of only a few people.

- Families and other caretakers play an important role in safety management of the patient, especially when educated about their appropriate role. Significant others should not be asked to provide constant supervision of the patient.

- If constant supervision is required, the treatment team should consider hospitalizing the patient or delaying discharge from the hospital until the patient is stabilized.

- The clinician should not worry alone. Consultation is always an option.

- Therapeutic risk management preserves the clinician's treatment role with the patient. It is patient centered, incorporates an understanding of legal matters affecting clinical practice, and pursues a wellness, not a legal, agenda.

References

42 Code of Federal Regulations 482.13 (f)3 (II) (C) (1999)

Amchin J, Wettstein RM, Roth LH: Suicide, ethics, and the law, in Suicide Over the Life Cycle. Edited by Blumenthal SJ, Kupfer DJ. Washington, DC, American Psychiatric Press, 1990, pp 637–663

American Psychiatric Association: The Psychiatric Uses of Seclusion and Restraint (Task Force Report No 22). Washington, DC, American Psychiatric Association, 1985

American Psychiatric Association: The Principles of Medical Ethics With Annotations Especially Applicable to Psychiatry. Washington, DC, American Psychiatric Association, 2009

Bellah v Greenson, 81 Cal App 3d 614, 146, Cal Rptr 525 (1978)

Busch KA, Fawcett J, Jacobs DG: Clinical correlates of inpatient suicide. J Clin Psychiatry 64:14–19, 2003

Dervic K, Oquendo MA, Grunebaum MF, et al: Religious affiliation and suicide attempt. Am J Psychiatry 161:2303–2308, 2004

Eaglin v Cook County Hospital, 227 Ill App 3d 724, 592 NE2d 205 (1992)

Farwell v Un, 902 F2d 282 (4th Cir. 1990)

Gerbasi JB, Simon RI: Patients' rights and psychiatrists' duties: discharging patients against medical advice. Harv Rev Psychiatry 11:333–343, 2003

Gross v Allen, 22 Cal App 4th 345, 27 Cal Rptr 2d 429 (1994)

Gutheil TG, Simon RI: Abandonment of patients in split treatment. Harv Rev Psychiatry 11:175–179, 2003

Johnson v United States, 409 F Supp 1283 (MD Fla 1976), rev'd 576 F2d 606 (5th Cir 1978), cert denied, 451 US 1019 (1981)

Joint Commission on Accreditation of Healthcare Organizations: Comprehensive Accreditation Manual for Behavioral Health Care: Restraint and Seclusion Standards for Behavioral Health. Chicago, IL, Joint Commission on Accreditation of Healthcare Organizations, 2001, pp TX 7.1.5, TX 7.1.6

Lake v Cameron, 364 F2d 657 (DC Cir), cert denied. 382 US 863 (1966)

Lieberman DZ, Resnik HLP, Holder-Perkins V: Environmental risk factors in hospital suicide. Suicide Life Threat Behav 34:448–453, 2004

Meyer DJ, Simon RI: Split treatment: clarity between psychiatrists and psychotherapists, part I. Psychiatr Ann 29:241–245, 1999a

Meyer DJ, Simon RI: Split treatment: clarity between psychiatrists and psychotherapists, part II. Psychiatr Ann 29:327–332, 1999b

Qin P, Nordentoft M: Suicide risk in relation to psychiatric hospitalization: evidence based on longitudinal registers. Arch Gen Psychiatry 62:427–432, 2005

Resnick PJ: Recognizing that the suicidal patient views you as an adversary. Curr Psychiatr 1:8, 2002

Seiden RH: Where are they now? A follow-up study of suicide attempters from the Golden Gate Bridge. Suicide Life Threat Behav 8:203–216, 1978

Simon RI: Coping strategies for the defensive psychiatrist. Med Law 4:551–561, 1985

Simon RI: A clinical philosophy for the (unduly) defensive psychiatrist. Psychiatr Ann 17:197–200, 1987

Simon RI: Clinical Psychiatry and the Law, 2nd Edition. Washington, DC, American Psychiatric Press, 1992

Simon RI: Discharging sicker, potentially violent psychiatric inpatients in the managed care era: standard of care and risk management. Psychiatr Ann 17:726–733, 1997

Simon RI: Psychiatrists' duties in discharging sicker and potentially violent inpatients in the managed care era. Psychiatr Serv 49:62–67, 1998

Simon RI: Taking the "sue" out of suicide: a forensic psychiatrist's perspective. Psychiatr Ann 30:399–407, 2000

Simon RI: Psychiatry and Law for Clinicians, 3rd Edition. Washington, DC, American Psychiatric Publishing, 2001

Simon RI: Assessing and Managing Suicide Risk: Guidelines for Clinically Based Risk Management. Washington, DC, American Psychiatric Publishing, 2004

Simon RI: Imminent suicide: the illusion of short-term prediction. Suicide Life Threat Behav 36:296–301, 2006

Simon RI, Gutheil TG: Sudden improvement in high risk suicidal patients: should it be trusted? Psychiatr Serv 60:387–389, 2009

Simon RI, Shuman DW: Clinical Manual of Psychiatry and Law. Washington, DC, American Psychiatric Publishing, 2007

Stanford EJ, Goetz RR, Bloom JD: The no harm contract in the emergency assessment of suicidal risk. Clin Psychiatry 55:344–348, 1994

Tarasoff v Regents of the University of California, 17 Cal 3d 425, 551 P2d 334, 131 Cal Rptr 14 (1976)

Wintemute GJ, Parham CA, Beaumont JJ, et al: Mortality among recent purchasers of handguns. N Engl J Med 341:1583–1589, 1999

PART V

Special Populations

Children, Adolescents, and College Students

Peter Ash, M.D.

Suicide is the third leading cause of death in 15- to 19-year-olds, after accidents and homicide, and accounts for approximately 1,500 deaths in the United States per year (6.87 per 100,000 in 2007; National Center for Injury Prevention and Control 2011). In early adolescents, suicide is much less common (0.89 per 100,000 in 2007 in 10- to 14-year-olds) and rare in prepubertal children. Many of the principles pertinent to the assessment and treatment of adults detailed elsewhere in this volume are relevant to the assessment and treatment of suicidal adolescents, but because of developmental differences, different living circumstances, and different legal status, approaches to younger patients are somewhat different from those utilized with adults. Key differences are shown in Table 20–1.

College students are typically legally adults but present special issues because they are often not self-supporting, and colleges have some responsibility for them and for the well-being of other students. A number of highly publicized suicides of college students have led to concern that there is an epidemic of college suicides. This perception is false. Although there are few good data on completed suicides by college students, the available data suggest that the rate is about 7 per 100,000, similar to that of 15- to 19-year-olds, and about half that of an age-matched community sample; the rate has not increased markedly over the past 10 years (Schwartz 2006; Silverman et al. 1997).

Epidemiology and Demographics

Adolescent suicide rates have been quite variable: rates for white males tripled from 1964 to 1991 and then over the next 10 years fell back to rates comparable to those in the 1970s (National Center for Health Statistics 2004). The changes in youth suicide rates roughly parallel the directions of changes in youth homicide rates (National Center for Health Statistics 2004). The National Center for Injury Prevention and Control

TABLE 20–1. Suicidal adolescents: key differences from suicidal adults

Category	Difference(s) from suicidal adults
Risk factors	Suicide accounts for a higher proportion of all deaths. Suicidal ideation is more common. Suicide attempts are more common. Disruptive behavior disorders increase risk. Contagion effects are more powerful.
Diagnostic differences	Psychotic disorder is much less common.
Symptoms	Although more common, suicidal ideation is more likely to be denied when asked about. Lethality of means is more commonly misjudged.
Treatment	Selective serotonin reuptake inhibitors require more monitoring. Family involvement in treatment is more important.
Legal status	Legal consent for treatment needs to be provided by someone other than patient. Hospitalization over patient's objection can often be accomplished without resorting to civil commitment. Patient's responsibility for treatment compliance is reduced.
Aftermath of completed suicide	Full discussion with parents is less constrained by confidentiality limitations because parents control record release.

has created the Web-based Injury Statistics Query and Reporting System (WISQARS, at www.cdc.gov/injury/wisqars), which is an interactive database that allows any user to generate reports of injury data, including suicide data, that can be broken down by a variety of variables.

Suicide rates increase with age from childhood through adolescence, and continue to increase through early adulthood. Boys are about five times more likely to die by suicide than girls (National Center for Injury Prevention and Control 2011), although girls are considerably more likely to make nonlethal suicide attempts (Eaton et al. 2010). Although sex differences are explained in part by the means employed— teenage males tend to use more lethal methods, such as firearms and hanging, rather than the less dangerous methods often used by females, such as poisoning (e.g., carbon monoxide or pill overdose) or wrist cutting—the difference more clearly reflects the nature of suicidal intent. There are significant racial differences as well: Native Americans have the highest rates of completed suicide, followed by whites, and African Americans have the lowest rates (National Center for Injury Prevention and Control 2011), although the gap has narrowed following a large jump in the rates among African American youth in the 1980s (Gould et al. 2003).

Although firearms are still the most common means of adolescent suicide, suicides with firearms have been decreasing, currently accounting for less than half of completed suicides (National Center for Injury Prevention and Control 2011). Increased prescribing of antidepressant medication may have contributed to the decreasing suicide rates (Olfson et al. 2003).

Suicidal thinking and attempts are fairly common in late adolescence. The Youth Risk Behavior Survey (YRBS), conducted annually by the Centers for Disease Control and Prevention, surveys U.S. high school students regarding a variety of risky behaviors. In 2009, the YRBS found that 13.8% of high school students had seriously considered suicide in the previous 12 months, 10.9% had made a plan, 6.3% had attempted suicide, and 12.9% had made an attempt that required medical attention (Eaton et al. 2010). When these rates are compared with the completed suicide rate of approximately 0.007%, it is clear that the ratio of suicidal ideation to completed suicide is very high (about 2,000:1). This high ratio contributes to low specificity when ideation is used as a risk factor, and this complicates clinical risk assessment. The YRBS found that girls are more likely than boys to have suicidal ideation, make plans, and carry out attempts.

Rates of suicidal ideation among college students are also high. A 2008 survey found that 9%–10% of college students had seriously considered suicide in the previous year and a little over 1% had made an attempt (American College Health Association 2009).

Although completed suicide is rare in prepubertal children, self-destructive thoughts and behavior are frequent in this young age group, and those children who express suicidal ideation are more likely to have symptoms of psychiatric illness and are more likely to evidence suicidal behavior later in adolescence (Pfeffer et al. 1997). As with rates for completed suicide, rates for suicide attempts increase through adolescence (Gould et al. 2003). Of concern, about one-third of suicidal youth think they should be able to handle problems on their own and avoid seeking help, and one-quarter think they should keep their suicidality a secret (Gould et al. 2004).

Case Examples

Case 1: Girl in the Emergency Department

Fifteen-year-old Stephanie is brought to the emergency department (ED) after an overdose on an undetermined number of aspirin tablets. She has no history of psychiatric treatment, and her parents say that she has been functioning fairly well, although she has sometimes been moody, which they put down to "being a teenager." She was found difficult to arouse in her room around 9 P.M., when her parents went to tell her that two girlfriends had stopped by to pick her up to go to a party.

After being medically stabilized in the ED, she tells the examining psychiatrist that earlier that evening her boyfriend of 8 months broke up with her over the phone, and she "couldn't bear to face anyone" that night but just "wanted to get some sleep" and "didn't want to die." She does not recall any plans to go to a party, but her girlfriends told Stephanie's parents that the plan to attend the party together had been made 2 days earlier.

Case 2: Indirect Threat by an Outpatient

John, a 16-year-old boy, was removed from his biological mother at age 6 for neglect and has been in a series of foster homes and group homes since that time. He reports that he gets along well with the family he is currently living with but thinks, "They like me OK, but they know I'll be gone as soon as I turn 18." He has been in and out of outpatient psychiatric treatment at a community mental health center for 3 years for depression. Antidepressant medication has been tried but has done little to relieve his depressive symptoms, which appear to derive from feeling unwanted and vary widely in severity in response to current stressors.

Two years ago, after he was removed from a foster placement for disruptive behavior and placed in a group home, he tried to hang himself with a belt tied to the clothes bar in his closet, but his weight broke the bar, and he saw this as "a sign I should go on." He did not tell anyone about this attempt until asked about suicidal thinking at his regular medication check a month later.

John has been associating with a delinquent crowd, engaging in occasional vandalism and some burglary, and regularly gets stoned on marijuana with his friends. After witnessing a nonfatal shooting at a club, John started carrying a handgun he had obtained in a burglary "for protection" when going to the club. Last week, after his girlfriend called him "a loser" and broke up with him, he went out with some friends, got drunk, got into a fight with some other youths on the street, and was arrested for assault. He is now quite upset about the prospect of incarceration, and told his protective services worker, "There's no way I'm going to prison. No way." She relayed this to his therapist.

Case 3: Suicidal College Student

Jennifer, a 19-year-old college freshman, tells her roommate that she is upset that her boyfriend has broken up with her, that she is feeling terribly lonely and thinking about hurting herself, but that "I want to handle it myself." Her worried roommate arranges with several friends to take turns staying with Jennifer day and night to help keep her safe. This arrangement comes to light when the upperclassman residential advisor comments on how tired the roommate looks. When Jennifer is then interviewed by a more senior college administrator, she says that she has been to student health services and declines to release her mental health records to school officials. She also says that she does not want the college to tell her parents. The college administration is considering suspending her from school.

Assessment

The key to effective intervention is a careful assessment of suicide risk. Asking about suicidal ideation and a history of attempts at self-harm, depressive feelings and symptoms, family problems, and recent stressors should be a routine part of the initial evaluation of any adolescent or depressed child. As with adults, there are no studies that identify factors that will allow a clinician to predict accurately which adolescents will die by suicide. Research has therefore focused on risk factors. The literature on

suicide risk factors is complex, because a variety of factors, including age, sex, and race, affect the potency of various risk factors. Risk factors have been reviewed in a practice parameter of the American Academy of Child and Adolescent Psychiatry (AACAP) on the assessment and treatment of suicidal behavior (American Academy of Child and Adolescent Psychiatry 2001) and in other reviews (Brent 2001; Brent and Melhem 2008; Brent et al. 2009; Bridge et al. 2006; Cavanagh et al. 2003; Dervic et al. 2008; Evans et al. 2004; Fergusson et al. 2000; Gould et al. 2003; Waldrop et al. 2007). Risk factors commonly cited in the literature appear in Table 20–2.

Of these factors, a history of a previous attempt is the strongest predictor of completed suicide, an effect that is considerably stronger for boys. Boys with a previous attempt are at 30 times greater risk than boys who have not attempted suicide, while girls with a previous attempt are at 3 times greater risk than nonattempters (Brent et al. 1999; Shaffer et al. 1996). Asking about a history of previous suicidal ideation and suicide attempts should always be a component of an adolescent's or depressed child's assessment.

Intent in a Recent Attempt

Clinically, suicidal ideation or a recent suicide attempt, especially when coupled with a plan involving lethal means, is most often the trigger to a judgment of imminent danger requiring hospitalization. Multiple past attempts increase the risk. Individuals who attempt suicide make further attempts at a rate of 6%–15% per year. The time of greatest risk for another suicide attempt is within the first 3 months to 2 years after an initial attempt. Suicidal intent needs to be differentiated from nonsuicidal self-harm, such as repetitive cutting.

TABLE 20–2. Leading risk factors for completed suicide in adolescents

Individual factors

Explicit suicidality

    Stated intent with or without plan

    Previous suicide attempt

    High intent/lethality of method

Psychopathology

    Diagnoses

        Major depression

        Bipolar disorder

        Substance abuse comorbid with other psychopathology

        Schizophrenia

        Conduct or personality disorder, especially with impulsive characteristics

    Symptoms

        Helplessness and hopelessness

        Impulsivity

        Conflicts over same-sex or bisexual orientation

Demographic factors

Increased risk with age (over age 14)

Male

White

Unwed/unwanted pregnancy

Family and environmental factors

Family history of suicidal behavior

Parental psychopathology

Family pathology/discord

Abuse (physical or sexual)

History of violence

Firearm in the home

Recent stressors

    Interpersonal loss

    Arrest/legal problems

Kingsbury (1993), utilizing the Beck Suicide Intent Scale, identified four factors that are useful to consider in assessing intent in a recent attempt: belief about intent, preparation, prevention of discovery, and communication (see Table 20–3). Because adoles-

cents often minimize their intent following an attempt, it is important to obtain corroborative data about what occurred.

Assessing risk in children and adolescents is complicated by the fact that completed suicide is rare when compared with clinical presentations of suicidal ideation and suicide attempts. Stephanie, the adolescent described in the first case example, presents a common picture. In interviewing Stephanie, it would be important to elucidate what she remembers thinking in the time leading up to taking the pills. Beginning with open-ended questions may obtain more information than beginning with direct questions about whether the adolescent wished to die, especially because adolescents not uncommonly minimize their intent when seen in the ED because of repression, a wish to avoid embarrassment, or a wish to avoid hospitalization. Youth, especially younger adolescents and preadolescents, are more likely than adults to misjudge the lethality of means. The clinician must consider that an attempt involving an overdose that was not pharmacologically dangerous might have seemed likely to the adolescent to cause death and that some potentially lethal attempts (such as an aspirin overdose) might have seemed like a gesture to a youth who thought she was ingesting a fairly benign medication.

Planning and concealment may be revealed by the adolescent after an attempt, but other sources, such as parents or friends who found the victim, are invaluable in achieving a comprehensive picture of what occurred. Information such as whether the attempt was carried out in a way that was likely to be discovered, or whether a note was left, should be given higher weight than a retrospective account of intent provided by the patient. In the case example, Stephanie took the pills at home, and it would be useful to understand whether she

TABLE 20–3. Assessing lethal intent of a recent suicide attempt

Clinical component	Example issues
1 Belief about intent	Purpose of the attempt Expectation of dying Lethality of means
2. Preparation	Saving up pills for overdose Saying good-bye Planning

3. Concealment	Planning attempt to avoid discovery:
	    Timing so no one will find soon
	    Choosing an isolated place

4. Communication	Telling others, directly or indirectly, about suicidal thinking Suicide note

Source.   Adapted from Kingsbury 1993.

might reasonably have expected her parents to check on her at some point in the evening. It would also be important to clarify whether she knew that her friends would be stopping by. Asking others who know the patient about whether the patient has communicated suicidal thinking can also provide important data about the duration of suicidal intent. The initial assessment is also a good time to alert family and others to be on the lookout for suicidal thinking in the future, to urge them to take such communications seriously, and to encourage them to inform treatment providers of their observations. One of the key principles of intervention is to improve the interpersonal surveillance network that surrounds the patient.

Intent in Reported Suicidal Ideation

Brent (2001) suggested that when an outpatient reports suicidal ideation, the severity and pervasiveness of the ideation are key dimensions to assess. *Severity* refers to the continuum from passive thoughts of

wanting to die, through an active wish to die, to an active wish with a plan involving lethal means. *Pervasiveness* refers to the intensity and frequency of the suicidal thinking. In the case example of John, the arrested boy with a history of attempted hanging who makes an indirect threat in saying he will not go to prison, it would be important to obtain a detailed picture of just what his current threat entails, what time (pretrial? postconviction?) he anticipates acting, and the likelihood of incarceration. His history suggests that when stressed, he is at significant risk for making an attempt with lethal means.

Psychopathology

Adolescents who complete suicide have very high rates of psychiatric disorder (around 90%) (Brent et al. 1993b; Shaffer et al. 1996). Affective disorder appears to pose a risk of over 11 times that of the general population (Gould et al. 2003). Major depressive disorder is the most prominent finding and poses the most risk. One follow-up study (Rao et al. 1993) found 4.4% of children diagnosed with major depression committed suicide in the following 10 years. Although the majority of completers had long-standing symptoms, in one study (Brent 1993) about one-third of the depressed group had developed symptoms in the previous 3 months. One epidemiological study found that generalized anxiety disorder significantly elevated risk in depressed adolescents (Foley et al. 2006). Bipolar disorder also elevates risk. Comorbid substance abuse significantly increases the risk of affective illness (Brent et al. 1993b; Giner et al. 2007; Shaffer et al. 1996) and disruptive disorders (Renaud et al. 1999). Conduct disorder appears to be a potent risk factor for boys but not for girls. As with adults, youths with schizophrenia are at increased risk for suicide, but schizophrenia has a low incidence in children and adolescents.

Axis II psychopathology is also found in many suicide completers, particularly Cluster B types (histrionic, borderline, narcissistic, antisocial) (Brent et al. 1990; Low and Andrews 1990; Marttunen et al. 1991) and Cluster C types (avoidant-dependent) (Brent et al. 1994a). High school suicide attempters, both boys and girls, are approximately four times as likely to have been in physical fights in the preceding year (Swahn et al. 2004). Females with learning disabilities have been found to have twice the risk for suicidal behavior and violence in comparison with peers (Svetaz et al. 2000).

In the minority of youth who do not evidence clear psychopathology, suicide is associated with recent legal or discipline problems, interpersonal loss or conflicts, and the presence of firearms (Brent et al. 1993c; Marttunen et al. 1994).

In many respects, the assessment of underlying psychopathology in suicidal youth is very similar to the assessment in non-suicidal youth. The AACAP has developed practice guidelines for the assessment and treatment of many disorders, including suicidal behavior (American Academy of Child and Adolescent Psychiatry 2001), depression (Birmaher et al. 2007), bipolar disorder (McClellan et al. 2007), conduct disorder (American Academy of Child and Adolescent Psychiatry 1997), and substance use disorders (Bukstein et al. 2005). Symptoms that deserve particular emphasis in assessing suicidality include hopelessness, impulsiveness, poor problem solving, social skills deficits, and aggressiveness, because these characteristics play directly into lowering the threshold for suicidal behavior.

Treatment of underlying psychopathology is clearly indicated, but only 30%–50% of adolescent suicide victims have had prior contact with a mental health professional (Blumenthal 1990). Relatively few victims are in active treatment at the time of a suicide, and noncompliance with outpatient treatment is correlated with increased risk for a recurrence of suicidality (Greenhill and Waslick 1997). Worsening suicidal ideation while in ongoing treatment, particularly when not related to identifiable stressors, is a worrisome risk factor.

Family and Social Factors

A number of family stressors have been found to be risk factors for suicide, including family member suicide attempts (Agerbo et al. 2002; Brent et al. 1996), not living with both parents (Groholt et al. 1998), family history of depression and substance abuse (Brent et al. 1994b; Melhem et al. 2007), and parent-child discord (Brent et al. 1994b; Gould et al. 1996). Parental divorce does not appear to be a significant risk factor (Gould et al. 1998). Physical abuse, although associated with suicide, is only a weak factor when other factors are controlled for (Fergusson et al. 1996; Johnson et al. 2002), but sexual abuse appears to increase risk (Brodsky et al. 2008). Children and adolescents also commonly react to the suicide of a family member with posttraumatic stress disorder and suicidal ideation (Pfeffer et al. 1997).

Family cohesion also functions as a crucial protective factor (Rubenstein et al. 1998). Once a family is alerted to a child's or adolescent's difficulties, the family can be of great assistance in supervising and supporting a suicidal youth, making the home safe, monitoring medication, and ensuring treatment compliance. Conversely, families who cannot provide these functions complicate treatment, and will likely need to be a focus of intervention.

There is some evidence that religiosity functions as a protective factor, but the studies have not controlled for possible confounding variables, such as substance abuse (Gould et al. 2003).

In the case examples, the motivation and ability of the families to support and monitor the suicidal adolescent will need to be assessed carefully. The assessment of John, the boy in foster care who is already involved in illegal and secretive behaviors, is likely to be the more problematic, both because the foster family may have less influence with or control over him and because his affective ties to them appear weak. His social support network extends beyond the foster family and includes workers from protective services and the juvenile court who are in a position both to anticipate stressors and affect their nature (through formulating recommendations for disposition of his assault charge).

Environmental Factors

Low socioeconomic status appears to have little effect on adolescent suicidality (Agerbo et al. 2002; Brent et al. 1988). There is considerable evidence that personal contact with a suicide or high media coverage of suicides can lead to increased suicidal behavior in adolescents (Gould et al. 2003). Contagion effects appear to be inversely related to age: they are strongest among younger adolescents (Holinger 1990) and much weaker after age 24 (Gould et al. 1994). Imitation seems most likely to occur among adolescents with preexisting risk factors (Shaffer et al. 1990).

Firearms are the most common method of committing suicide, and firearms, particularly handguns, in the home are associated with a four-fold increase in risk for suicide (Brent et al. 1993a).

Precipitants

Most, but by no means all, suicides and suicide attempts have a clearly identified precipitant. However, a stressor alone, in the absence of preexisting vulnerability, likely does not lead to suicide. Marttunen et al. (1993) found a precipitating stressor in 70% of a series of completed suicides of Finnish adolescents. Half the stressors occurred in the 24 hours preceding the suicide. Thus, it appears that many adolescent suicides are impulsive responses to stressors, which leaves a very brief time window between the time when an adolescent develops suicidal ideation and the time when he or she carries out a suicidal act.

Separation and loss issues are the most common stressors. Parent-child conflict is the more common precipitant for younger adolescents, whereas separation issues among peers (such as romantic difficulties) predominate among older adolescents (Brent et al. 1999; Groholt et al. 1998). Incarcerated adolescents are at particularly high risk for suicide (Penn et al. 2003; Sanislow et al. 2003).

Biological Factors

There are intriguing data regarding the effects of serotonin dysregulation and genetic factors on suicidality, especially involving

FK506 binding protein 5 (also known as FKBP5) polymorphisms (Brent et al. 2010), but at the present time these findings are preliminary and have little impact on clinical practice. Homosexual or bisexual orientation is associated with significantly increased risk, but much of the risk is attributable to other comorbid risk factors, and the independent contribution from sexual orientation appears fairly small (Russell and Joyner 2001).

Questionnaire Assessments

A variety of questionnaires and scales have been developed for the assessment of suicidality in adolescents in clinical samples (Winters et al. 2002) or for screening community samples (Shaffer et al. 2004). The scales suffer either from limited psychometric data or from low specificity. Therefore, at present, such scales may be used either as adjunctive measures or as screening instruments but should not replace a psychiatric interview for high-risk youth.

Treatment

Treatment of children and adolescents at risk for suicide encompasses four major components: protecting the patient, continuing assessment of risk, ameliorating risk factors, and enhancing protective factors (Table 20–4).

Protect the Patient

Protection of the patient is the first consideration. The decision about whether to discharge from the ED a patient who recently made an attempt turns on a careful balancing of the risk and protective factors discussed previously. The AACAP guideline (American Academy of Child and Adolescent Psychiatry 2001) noted that although there have been no randomized studies to

TABLE 20–4. Components of the treatment of suicidal children and adolescents

1. Protect the patient.
2. Continue to assess risk.
3. Ameliorate risk factors.
4. Enhance protective factors.

determine whether hospitalization actually saves lives, attempters who express a persistent wish to die or have a clearly abnormal state, such as major depression with psychotic features or rapid cycling with impulsive behavior and irritability, should be admitted and continued in inpatient treatment until they are stabilized. Further, before discharging the patient, the clinician must be convinced that the living situation to which the patient is returning will provide adequate support, monitoring, and supervision of the patient and that parents or family will eliminate the patient's access to firearms and lethal medications. A plan for follow-up treatment should be devised, preferably with a scheduled appointment. The patient and family should be given information about an available care provider who can be contacted if help is needed prior to the appointment. If the appointment cannot be scheduled in the ED, a follow-up mechanism should be in place for contacting the family to make sure outpatient treatment was sought.

In outpatient treatment, when new or worsening risk is elucidated, the decision similarly turns on whether the protective factors are sufficiently strong to feel confident the patient is safe. As with the decision to discharge, the family must feel comfortable with the outpatient plan and agree to accept some of the responsibility for the patient's safety. In assessing a patient's capacity to be treated as an outpatient, it may be helpful to ask what the patient would do if stressors recurred. As with adults, "no-suicide contracts," in which the patient promises to tell an adult if he or she is feeling suicidal, have not been shown to be effective and should not be relied on to protect the patient, although discussions about these agreements may be useful in assessing and fostering the therapeutic alliance (Simon 2004).

Ameliorate Risk Factors

Treatment should include addressing and diminishing dynamic risk factors. Central to this is the treatment of underlying psychopathology. In the past 10 years, several multisite studies have suggested that a combination of psychotherapy and medication are the preferred approach to suicidal adolescents. The Treatment for Adolescents with Depression Study (TADS) showed that a combination of fluoxetine and cognitive-behavioral therapy (CBT) resulted in significant improvement in 71% of moderately to severely depressed adolescents (March et al. 2004). Drug treatment alone and CBT alone also showed positive, although somewhat weaker, effects. Suicidal thinking was also significantly reduced in all groups, including the placebo group, although treatment effects in comparison with response seen with placebo were weak for this symptom. The Treatment of Adolescent Suicide Attempters (TASA) Study suggested that adolescent suicide attempters treated with psychotherapy and medication improved at about the same rate as nonsuicidal depressed adolescents (Vitiello et al. 2009).

The use of selective serotonin reuptake inhibitors (SSRIs), the mainstay pharmacological treatment for depression, has become more problematic since 2004, when the U.S. Food and Drug Administration (FDA) be-gan requiring a black box warning for SSRIs that includes a notice that antidepressants increase the risk of suicidality in children and adolescents (U.S. Food and Drug Administration 2005). The FDA based its decision on a pooled analysis that found that reports of suicidal thinking increased from 2% on placebo to 4% on active drug (Hammad 2004). While the initial 2005 black-box warning specified weekly patient-clinician contact when an SSRI is being started, the current black-box warning only says that patients should be "monitored appropriately and observed closely" for worsening symptoms (U.S. Food and Drug Administration 2007). Despite these recommendations, there are data showing that most psychiatrists and pediatricians did not increase their level of monitoring (Morrato et al. 2008). The clinician should also consider the possibility that a suicidal adolescent patient might overdose and should either arrange for parental control of the medication or prescribe nonlethal quantities.

Psychotherapy plays an important role in treatment in providing information about continuing risk, delineating how the youth thinks about suicide, addressing underlying psychopathology, correcting cognitive distortions involved in hopelessness, improving social skills, helping the adolescent cope with such stressors as may be present, and enhancing protective factors such as more adaptive defenses or coping strategies. While a number of psychotherapies have been shown to be efficacious for depression and other underlying psychopathology, there are very limited data demonstrating effectiveness in reducing suicide attempts in adolescents when compared with control subjects. In part, the limited data reflect that many treatment studies exclude suicidal patients. Multisystemic therapy (Huey et al. 2004) has been shown to reduce repeat attempts when compared with hospitalization. Most studies of psychosocial treatments have been of fairly brief duration (up to 20 weeks), and it may well be that longer treatments are necessary to improve what is often a chronic condition.

Enhance Protective Factors

Some factors, including ameliorating disruptive or stressful family patterns and eliminating access to firearms, are best dealt with in a family context. Unfortunately, parental compliance with a recommendation to remove firearms is fairly low, even when parents are provided with considerable information about the risks and strong recommendations (Brent et al. 2000). Working to increase family support is an important component of enhancing protective factors, and the family's role in monitoring the youth's condition is very important. Finally, it must be emphasized that any treatment modality employed with suicidal youth should include ongoing, repeated, and documented assessments of suicide risk.

Legal and Risk Management Considerations

Consent to Treatment

In most jurisdictions, children and adolescents are legally incompetent to consent to treatment except under special circumstances. Emancipated minors—those who live separately from their parents, are self-supporting, and have been declared emancipated by a court, and minors who are married or in the military—are able to make health care decisions as if they were adults. Some states provide exceptions for certain actions, such as seeking outpatient treatment, or have "mature minor" rules that allow defined classes of youth to seek health

care as though they are adults. Youth can generally obtain treatment for substance abuse, sexually transmitted diseases, pregnancy, and contraception independently of their parents, although parent notification issues can get complex depending on the type of intervention and laws of the local jurisdiction, especially with abortion. However, for most minors who come to psychiatrists, the parent or guardian needs to provide informed consent for treatment and controls the release of information.

For these reasons, family members are key participants in the treatment in a manner different from the treatment of adults. The U.S. Supreme Court has found that a physician's recommendation and the consent of a parent are sufficient for hospitalizing a minor over the minor's objections (*Parham v. J.R. and J.L.* 1979). State law varies as to the procedures available to a minor who objects to hospitalization, the age at which an adolescent may file a formal objection, and what happens following an objection (usually a court hearing on the question of continuing hospitalization). If the parents are unavailable or refuse to consent to hospitalization, then involuntary hospitalization is available, provided the youth meets the state's involuntary commitment criteria.

Confidentiality

A dilemma that can arise during the treatment of a depressed child or adolescent patient is the clinical need to break the patient's confidentiality without his or her assent and inform parents of the patient's status, such as when an adolescent becomes suicidal and parents need to be involved in management. Adolescents usually prize treatment confidentiality, and breaking it, even when clinically indicated and legally allowable, runs the risk of negatively affecting the treatment alliance. It is therefore important at the outset of the treatment of a suicidal patient to discuss with the minor patient the conditions under which the therapist will communicate information to the parents. When the clinician needs to discuss a management issue with parents— for example, when a youth becomes more depressed and the therapist wishes to advise the parents to remove firearms from the home—it is preferable to raise the need to talk to the parents with the adolescent patient and obtain his or her assent. If the adolescent objects but the therapist has significant concerns about the youth's safety, the therapist generally may discuss these issues with the parents over the adolescent's objections, because in most cases the parents legally speak for the child and control access to information about treatment. In those rare instances when the minor patient legally controls release of information, such as when the minor is an emancipated minor or has "mature minor" status in a state that recognizes such a status, such a breach may not be legal, and the clinician then has fewer options and is in essentially the same dilemma as when treating an adult. If the opportunity to involve the adolescent's support system is limited, the threshold for hospitalization is lowered.

College Students

College students who are 18 years of age or older, and are therefore legally adults, may themselves consent to psychiatric treatment, and they control the release of health information about themselves. College administrators also have an interest in their students obtaining effective treatment. A suicidal student may affect the lives of other students, as exemplified in Case 3, in which a group of friends took on the taxing chore of keeping a fellow student safe. Colleges are concerned that they may have some legal liability for a student's suicide, and they are concerned that a spate of student suicides may bring adverse publicity to the school. There have been instances of universities summarily suspending allegedly suicidal students, a practice that can lead to a worsening of the student's depression, because the student then has to deal not only with the difficulties he or she had as a student but also with separation from college friends and a sense of failing at college. In a number of high publicity cases, discharged students later sued their schools for violations of their civil rights and settled for considerable amounts (Department of the Public Advocate, Division of Mental Health Advocacy, State of New Jersey 2009). College administrators are put in the challenging position of needing to balance the rights and needs of the suicidal student, the needs of other students, and the well-being of the college. Administrators may feel frustrated that school mental health services require a release from the student to provide them with information that they may find helpful in determining whether to allow the student to stay in school. The evolving practice seems to be that it is not possible to have one approach for all suicidal students but that each case needs to be assessed individually. In those cases in which a student does not release mental health information, the school can typically require a mental health assessment, much as an employer might require a fitness for duty evaluation for an employee whose job performance or the safety of others may be adversely affected by psychiatric problems.

Although release of mental health records of adult college students, including records of student mental health services, is controlled by the student, information that is obtained by school administrators is generally considered part of the education record. Information about a student's potential suicidality that is provided to an administrator by other students, teachers, or dorm advisors typically would be considered part of the education record. Release of educational records is governed in large part by a federal law the Family Educational Rights and Privacy Act (FERPA) (1974). Although the general thrust of FERPA is that an adult student who is not dependent on parents controls release of educational records, there is an explicit exception for a health or safety emergency that allows a college to release information to parents and other appropriate parties. Thus, in Case 3, although the suicidal student does not want the administration to contact her parents, the administration may do so if they think it is important in developing a plan to help the student.

Aftermath of a Completed Suicide

The tragic outcome of a completed suicide by a patient in treatment generates strong feelings in family members and friends of the patient and in the treating clinician. It may also give rise to a malpractice action against the treating psychiatrist. The clinician is faced with the tasks of grieving, helping the patient's family with their grief, and limiting legal liability.

An important first step following a suicide is to notify one's malpractice carrier and obtain suggestions from their risk management unit. It is appropriate for the clinician to meet with the family and discuss the patient's condition. Because the parents generally control the release of information, there are not usually the confidentiality problems that may attend discussing the suicide of an adult patient. In such a discussion, it is generally appropriate for the clinician to express his or her own grief and to

be relatively open about the patient's condition. Most risk management units will caution a clinician not to express guilt or fault for the suicide. It is generally appropriate for the clinician to attend the funeral if he or she wishes to, but permission from the family should be obtained beforehand. Although informing the family and participating in the grieving process are humane things to do, there are few data to suggest these actions significantly lessen the likelihood of a malpractice suit.

In a malpractice case involving an outpatient suicide, a threshold question is whether the suicide was reasonably foreseeable. If suicide was reasonably foreseeable, the psychiatrist had a duty to take reasonable steps to protect the patient, most commonly by hospitalizing him or her. If the suicide was not reasonably foreseeable, then the duty to protect the patient is much reduced. Many issues in adolescent suicide cases are similar to those in malpractice cases involving adult suicides (see Chapter 28, "Patient Suicide and Litigation," this volume). Issues that tend to be different from adult malpractice cases include whether informed consent was obtained from the parents for certain components of the treatment, whether the parents were sufficiently informed and involved in managing the patient, and the level of responsibility attributed to the minor patient (Ash 2002). In malpractice litigation involving an adult who committed suicide, the degree to which the adult was responsible for his or her own acts, and thus a contributor to the outcome, is often important. When a minor commits suicide, the presumption that minors are not as competent as adults reduces the responsibility of the minor for his or her actions and tends to increase the blame attributable to responsible adults, such as the clinician or parents.

As in adult malpractice cases, the psychiatrist's documentation of treatment will be carefully scrutinized. It is therefore very important to document carefully the assessment process, noting which risk factors and protective factors for suicide were assessed and how they were weighed. The assessment process is an ongoing one, and subsequent assessments should also be documented.

One of the effects of managed care has been to increase the threshold of severity necessary to justify inpatient hospitalization, so the presence of some suicide risk factors is quite common among inpatient adolescents. Malpractice cases arising out of the tragedy of an adolescent committing

suicide on an inpatient psychiatric unit tend to follow the general pattern of cases involving the suicide of an adult inpatient (see Chapter 18, "Inpatient Psychiatric Treatment," this volume). The two most common issues are the adequacy of the assessment of the patient's suicidality by the doctor and hospital staff and the reasonableness of the measures instituted to protect the patient. The attending psychiatrist needs to be aware of clinical findings by the staff. As in outpatient cases, good documentation is critical. When the level of suicide precautions is decreased, the notes should reflect the basis for making the change.

Key Clinical Concepts

- Completed suicide is rare in preadolescents. Risk increases with age through adolescence, and is highest for boys, while suicide attempts are more common in girls.

- Suicidal ideation is quite common among high school students (1 in 6 per year), as are suicide attempts (1 in 12 per year), although less than 1 in 1,000 attempts result in death. Assessing the lethality of suicidal intent is complex but is nevertheless a key to planning intervention.

- Affective disorder is the most common underlying psychopathology and is frequently responsive to combined medication and psychosocial treatments.

- Use of selective serotonin reuptake inhibitors (SSRIs) remains one of the mainstays of treatment of depressed youth, although the Food and Drug Administration black box warning for SSRIs prescribed to adolescents requires more monitoring of the effects of these medications in early phases of treatment.

- The social and legal status of adolescents as more immature and less competent than adults requires that parents be very involved in treatment and treatment decisions of suicidal children and adolescents.

- The decision regarding whether to suspend a college student on the basis of the student's suicidality requires an individualized weighing of what is in the best interests of the suicidal student, of other students, and of the institution.

References

Agerbo E, Nordentoft M, Mortensen PB: Familial, psychiatric, and socioeconomic risk factors for suicide in young people: nested case-control study. BMJ 325:74–78, 2002

American Academy of Child and Adolescent Psychiatry: Practice parameters for the assessment and treatment of children and adolescents with conduct disorder. J Am Acad Child Adolesc Psychiatry 36:122S–139S, 1997

American Academy of Child and Adolescent Psychiatry: Practice parameter for the assessment and treatment of children and adolescents with suicidal behavior. J Am Acad Child Adolesc Psychiatry 40(suppl):24S–51S, 2001

American College Health Association: American College Health Association–National College Health Assessment Spring 2008 Reference Group Data Report (abridged): the American College Health Association. J Am Coll Health 57:477–488, 2009

Ash P: Malpractice in child and adolescent psychiatry. Child Adolesc Psychiatr Clin N Am 11:869–886, 2002

Birmaher B, Brent D; AACAP Work Group on Quality Issues, et al: Practice parameter for the assessment and treatment of children and adolescents with depressive disorders. J Am Acad Child Adolesc Psychiatry 46:1503–1526, 2007

Blumenthal SJ: Youth suicide: risk factors, assessment, and treatment of adolescent and young adult suicidal patients. Psychiatr Clin North Am 13:511–556, 1990

Brent DA: Depression and suicide in children and adolescents. Pediatr Rev 14:380–388, 1993

Brent DA: Assessment and treatment of the youthful suicidal patient. Ann N Y Acad Sci 932:106–128, 2001

Brent DA, Melhem N: Familial transmission of suicidal behavior. Psychiatr Clin North Am 31:157–177, 2008

Brent DA, Perper JA, Goldstein CE, et al: Risk factors for adolescent suicide: a comparison of adolescent suicide victims with suicidal inpatients. Arch Gen Psychiatry 45:581–588, 1988

Brent DA, Kolko DJ, Allan MJ, et al: Suicidality in affectively disordered adolescent inpatients. J Am Acad Child Adolesc Psychiatry 29:586–593, 1990

Brent DA, Perper JA, Moritz G, et al: Firearms and adolescent suicide: a community case-control study. Am J Dis Child 147:1066–1071, 1993a

Brent DA, Perper JA, Moritz G, et al: Psychiatric risk factors for adolescent suicide: a case-control study. J Am Acad Child Adolesc Psychiatry 32:521–529, 1993b

Brent DA, Perper J, Moritz G, et al: Suicide in adolescents with no apparent psychopathology. J Am Acad Child Adolesc Psychiatry 32:494–500, 1993c

Brent DA, Johnson BA, Perper J, et al: Personality disorder, personality traits, impulsive violence, and completed suicide in adolescents. J Am Acad Child Adolesc Psychiatry 33:1080–1086, 1994a

Brent DA, Perper JA, Moritz G, et al: Suicide in affectively ill adolescents: a case-control study. J Affect Disord 31:193–202, 1994b

Brent DA, Bridge J, Johnson BA, et al: Suicidal behavior runs in families: a controlled family study of adolescent suicide victims. Arch Gen Psychiatry 53:1145–1152, 1996

Brent DA, Baugher M, Bridge J, et al: Age- and sex-related risk factors for adolescent suicide. J Am Acad Child Adolesc Psychiatry 38:1497–1505, 1999

Brent DA, Baugher M, Birmaher B, et al: Compliance with recommendations to remove firearms in families participating in a clinical trial for adolescent depression. J Am Acad Child Adolesc Psychiatry 39:1220–1226, 2000

Brent DA, Greenhill LL, Compton S, et al: The Treatment of Adolescent Suicide Attempters study (TASA): predictors of suicidal events in an open treatment trial. J Am Acad Child Adolesc Psychiatry 48:987–996, 2009

Brent D, Melhem N, Ferrell R, et al: Association of FKBP5 polymorphisms with suicidal events in the Treatment of Resistant Depression in Adolescents (TORDIA) study. Am J Psychiatry 167:190–197, 2010

Bridge JA, Goldstein TR, Brent DA: Adolescent suicide and suicidal behavior. J Child Psychol Psychiatry 47:372–394, 2006

Brodsky BS, Mann JJ, Stanley B, et al: Familial transmission of suicidal behavior: factors mediating the relationship between childhood abuse and offspring suicide attempts. J Clin Psychiatry 69:584–596, 2008

Bukstein OG, Bernet W, Arnold V, et al: Practice parameter for the assessment and treatment of children and adolescents with substance use disorders. J Am Acad Child Adolesc Psychiatry 44:609–621, 2005

Cavanagh JT, Carson AJ, Sharpe M, et al: Psychological autopsy studies of suicide: a systematic review. Psychol Med 33:395–405, 2003

Department of the Public Advocate, Division of Mental Health Advocacy, State of New Jersey: College Students in Crisis: Preventing Campus Suicides and Protecting Civil Rights. Trenton, NJ, Department of the Public Advocate, 2009

Dervic K, Brent DA, Oquendo MA: Completed suicide in childhood. Psychiatr Clin North Am 31:271–291, 2008

Eaton DK, Kann L, Kinchen S, et al: Youth risk behavior surveillance—United States, 2009. MMWR Surveill Summ 59:1–142, 2010

Evans E, Hawton K, Rodham K: Factors associated with suicidal phenomena in adolescents: a systematic review of population-based studies. Clin Psychol Rev 24:957–979, 2004

Family Educational Rights and Privacy Act (FERPA), 20 U.S.C. § 1232g; 34 CFR Part 99 (1974)

Fergusson DM, Horwood LJ, Lynskey MT: Childhood sexual abuse and psychiatric disorder in young adulthood, II: psychiatric outcomes of childhood sexual abuse. J Am Acad Child Adolesc Psychiatry 35:1365–1374, 1996

Fergusson DM, Woodward LJ, Horwood LJ: Risk factors and life processes associated with the onset of suicidal behaviour during adolescence and early adulthood. Psychol Med 30:23–39, 2000

Foley DL, Goldston DB, Costello EJ, et al: Proximal psychiatric risk factors for suicidality in youth: the Great Smoky Mountains Study. Arch Gen Psychiatry 63:1017–1024, 2006

Giner L, Carballo JJ, Guija JA, et al: Psychological autopsy studies: the role of alcohol use in adolescent and young adult suicides. Int J Adolesc Med Health 19:99–113, 2007

Gould MS, Petrie K, Kleinman MH, et al: Clustering of attempted suicide: New Zealand national data. Int J Epidemiol 23:1185–1189, 1994

Gould MS, Fisher P, Parides M, et al: Psychosocial risk factors of child and adolescent completed suicide. Arch Gen Psychiatry 53:1155–1162, 1996

Gould MS, King R, Greenwald S, et al: Psychopathology associated with suicidal ideation and attempts among children and adolescents. J Am Acad Child Adolesc Psychiatry 37:915–923, 1998

Gould MS, Greenberg T, Velting DM, et al: Youth suicide risk and preventive interventions: a review of the past 10 years. J Am Acad Child Adolesc Psychiatry 42:386–405, 2003

Gould MS, Velting D, Kleinman M, et al: Teenagers' attitudes about coping strategies and help-seeking behavior for suicidality. J Am Acad Child Adolesc Psychiatry 43:1124–1133, 2004

Greenhill LL, Waslick B: Management of suicidal behavior in children and adolescents. Psychiatr Clin North Am 20:641–666, 1997

Groholt B, Ekeberg O, Wichstrom L, et al: Suicide among children and younger and older adolescents in Norway: a comparative study. J Am Acad Child Adolesc Psychiatry 37:473–481, 1998

Hammad TA: Results of the analysis of suicidality in pediatric trials of newer antidepressants. Presentation at the FDA Center for Drug Evaluation and Research, Bethesda, MD, September 13, 2004. Available at: http://www.fda.gov/ohrms/dockets/ac/cder04.html#Psychopharmacologic-Drugs. Accessed June 23, 2011.

Holinger PC: The causes, impact, and preventability of childhood injuries in the United States: childhood suicide in the United States. Am J Dis Child 144:670–676, 1990

Huey SJ Jr, Henggeler SW, Rowland MD, et al: Multisystemic therapy effects on attempted suicide by youths presenting psychiatric emergencies. J Am Acad Child Adolesc Psychiatry 43:183–190, 2004

Johnson JG, Cohen P, Gould MS, et al: Childhood adversities, interpersonal difficulties, and risk for suicide attempts during late adolescence and early adulthood. Arch Gen Psychiatry 59:741–749, 2002

Kingsbury SJ: Clinical components of suicidal intent in adolescent overdose. J Am Acad Child Adolesc Psychiatry 32:518–520, 1993

Low BP, Andrews SF: Adolescent suicide. Med Clin North Am 74:1251–1264, 1990

March J, Silva S, Petrycki S, et al: Fluoxetine, cognitive-behavioral therapy, and their combination for adolescents with depression: Treatment for Adolescents With Depression Study (TADS) randomized controlled trial. JAMA 292:807–820, 2004

Marttunen MJ, Aro HM, Henriksson MM, et al: Mental disorders in adolescent suicide: DSM-III-R Axes I and II diagnoses in suicides among 13- to 19-year-olds in Finland. Arch Gen Psychiatry 48:834–839, 1991

Marttunen MJ, Aro HM, Lönnqvist JK: Precipitant stressors in adolescent suicide. J Am Acad Child Adolesc Psychiatry 32:1178–1183, 1993

Marttunen MJ, Aro HM, Henriksson MM, et al: Psychosocial stressors more common in adolescent suicides with alcohol abuse compared with depressive adolescent suicides. J Am Acad Child Adolesc Psychiatry 33:490–497, 1994

McClellan J, Kowatch R, Findling RL, et al: Practice parameter for the assessment and treatment of children and adolescents with bipolar disorder. J Am Acad Child Adolesc Psychiatry 46:107–125, 2007

Melhem NM, Brent DA, Ziegler M, et al: Familial pathways to early onset suicidal behavior: familial and individual antecedents of suicidal behavior. Am J Psychiatry 164:1364–1370, 2007

Morrato EH, Libby AM, Orton HD, et al: Frequency of provider contact after FDA advisory on risk of pediatric suicidality with SSRIs. Am J Psychiatry 165:42–50, 2008

National Center for Health Statistics: Health, United States, 2004 (DHHS Publ No 2005-0152). Hyattsville, MD, National Center for Health Statistics, 2004

National Center for Injury Prevention and Control: Injury Prevention & Control: Data & Statistics (WISQARS). Centers for Disease Control and Prevention, 2011. Online computer database available at: http://www.cdc.gov/injury/wisqars/index.html. Author analysis conducted April 1, 2011

Olfson M, Shaffer D, Marcus SC, et al: Relationship between antidepressant medication treatment and suicide in adolescents. Arch Gen Psychiatry 60:978–982, 2003

Parham v. J.R. and J.L., 442 U.S. 584 (1979)

Penn JV, Esposito CL, Schaeffer LE, et al: Suicide attempts and self-mutilative behavior in a juvenile correctional facility. J Am Acad Child Adolesc Psychiatry 42:762–769, 2003

Pfeffer CR, Martins P, Mann J, et al: Child survivors of suicide: psychosocial characteristics. J Am Acad Child Adolesc Psychiatry 36:65–74, 1997

Rao U, Weissman MM, Martin JA, et al: Childhood depression and risk of suicide: a preliminary report of a longitudinal study. J Am Acad Child Adolesc Psychiatry 32:21–27, 1993

Renaud J, Brent DA, Birmaher B, et al: Suicide in adolescents with disruptive disorders. J Am Acad Child Adolesc Psychiatry 38:846–851, 1999

Rubenstein JL, Halton A, Kasten L, et al: Suicidal behavior in adolescents: stress and protection in different family contexts. Am J Orthopsychiatry 68:274–284, 1998

Russell ST, Joyner K: Adolescent sexual orientation and suicide risk: evidence from a national study. Am J Public Health 91:1276–1281, 2001

Sanislow CA, Grilo CM, Fehon DC, et al: Correlates of suicide risk in juvenile detainees and adolescent inpatients. J Am Acad Child Adolesc Psychiatry 42:234–240, 2003

Schwartz AJ: College student suicide in the United States: 1990–1991 through 2003–2004. J Am Coll Health 54:341–352, 2006

Shaffer D, Vieland V, Garland A, et al: Adolescent suicide attempters: response to suicide-prevention programs. JAMA 264:3151–3155, 1990

Shaffer D, Gould MS, Fisher P, et al: Psychiatric diagnosis in child and adolescent suicide. Arch Gen Psychiatry 53:339–348, 1996

Shaffer D, Scott M, Wilcox H, et al: The Columbia Suicide Screen: validity and reliability of a screen for youth suicide and depression. J Am Acad Child Adolesc Psychiatry 43:71–79, 2004

Silverman MM, Meyer PM, Sloane F, et al: The Big Ten Student Suicide Study: a 10-year study of suicides on midwestern university campuses. Suicide Life Threat Behav 27:285–303, 1997

Simon RI: Assessing and Managing Suicide Risk: Guidelines for Clinically Based Risk Management. Washington, DC, American Psychiatric Publishing, 2004

Svetaz MV, Ireland M, Blum R: Adolescents with learning disabilities: risk and protective factors associated with emotional well-being: findings from the National Longitudinal Study of Adolescent Health. J Adolesc Health 27:340–348, 2000

Swahn MH, Lubell KM, Sinmon TR: Suicide attempts and physical fighting among high school students—United States, 2001. MMWR Morb Mortal Wkly Rep 53:474–476, 2004

U.S. Food and Drug Administration: Class suicidality labeling language for antidepressants. 2005. Available at: http://www.accessdata.fda.gov/drugsatfda_ docs/label/2005/20031s045,20936s020lbl. pdf. Accessed June 23, 2011.

U.S. Food and Drug Administration: Revisions to product labeling, 2007. Available at: http://www.fda.gov/downloads/Drugs/DrugSafety/InformationbyDrugClass/UCM173233.pdf. Accessed January 21, 2012.

Vitiello B, Brent DA, Greenhill LL, et al: Depressive symptoms and clinical status during the Treatment of Adolescent Suicide Attempters (TASA) Study. J Am Acad Child Adolesc Psychiatry 48:997–1004, 2009

Waldrop AE, Hanson RF, Resnick HS, et al: Risk factors for suicidal behavior among a national sample of adolescents: implications for prevention. J Trauma Stress 20:869–879, 2007

Winters NC, Myers K, Proud L: Ten-year review of rating scales, III: scales assessing suicidality, cognitive style, and self-esteem. J Am Acad Child Adolesc Psychiatry 41:1150–1181, 2002

CHAPTER 21

The Elderly

Yeates Conwell, M.D.

Marnin J. Heisel, Ph.D.

In recent years suicide has come to be recognized as a major public health concern and a target for prevention. The Office of the Surgeon General's *National Strategy for Suicide Prevention* (U.S. Public Health Service 2001) and an influential Institute of Medicine (2002) report are illustrative landmarks of the process by which suicide prevention has emerged as a public health priority. The needs of older adults tend to be less apparent than those of younger adults in the United States, where the predominant cultural values are youth, beauty, and a vigorous lifestyle. It often goes unrecognized, therefore, that older adults have among the highest suicide rates of any segment of the population and so warrant special focus in the development and implementation of effective prevention strategies.

In this chapter, we use the case history of an influential older American to illustrate the characteristics of, and risk factors for, suicide in this age group. We then review the evidence base for management of acutely suicidal older adults and recommendations for approaches to suicide prevention in this rapidly growing segment of the population.

Death by Suicide of George Eastman

On March 14, 1932, George Eastman, founder of the Eastman Kodak Company, visited with his organist, his personal secretary, and Kodak executives in his Rochester, New York, mansion and signed an updated copy of his will. After his visitors left, Eastman smoked a final cigarette, put a gun to his chest, and fatally wounded himself. His secretary found a note on his night table that read, "To my friends. My work is done. Why wait? GE." Eastman, a generous philanthropist who had once been considered the wealthiest bachelor in America, was dead at 77 years of age.

Although Eastman's great wealth and success set him apart from most who die by suicide, his death was in many respects understandable because the events and circumstances surrounding it exemplify many common risk factors for late-life suicide—namely, multiple losses, personality vulnerability, physical illness, functional impairment, social isolation, and depression.

Eastman was born on July 12, 1854, in Waterville, New York, into a distinguished family. His ancestors had immigrated to America from Wales in 1635. His father, an industrious self-made man who founded and ran a local business college, died of neurological impairment associated with "inflammatory rheumatism" when George was only 7. Younger brother to two sisters, one of whom died from polio at age 8, Eastman stepped early into the role of young breadwinner, actively contributing to the household income. He was hardworking, serious, and conscientious. As an adolescent, Eastman paid for his sister's body to be transported from Rochester to a cemetery in Waterville; as an adult, he lived with and cared for his ailing mother until her death. Even after his photographic plate company started achieving success, Eastman continued working in a bank during the day to ensure a stable income, dedicating the evenings to painstaking work on his fledgling business.

A robust and self-determined individual, Eastman was a firm believer in eugenics and euthanasia. His philosophy of life and death was likely fueled, in part, by multiple painful losses of close family, friends, acquaintances, and business associates to debilitating physical illnesses. In addition to losing his father and sister at a young age, Eastman witnessed many other examples of once-vibrant individuals slowly succumbing to painful disease processes, including his beloved mother, who spent the final days of her life confined to a wheelchair. After her death in 1907, a dejected Eastman told friends, "I don't want to live that long" (Brayer 1996, p. 515). As his own physical illness, most likely spinal stenosis, made walking and functioning more difficult and painful, Eastman began expressing a longing for death and even for self-destruction. As the once robust and adventuresome entrepreneur grew dependent on others for assistance with even basic bodily functions, Eastman confided to friends of feeling that there was nothing left to live for and occasionally talked of suicide. In one portentous conversation with a personal friend, Eastman spoke in favor of suicide in the case of a hypothetical "man with an incurable disease who has discharged all his obligations and has no one dependent on him," asking, "What is there ethically against his committing suicide?" (p. 516). He had similar conversations with his doctors, once asking his personal physician about the lethality of strychnine and later asking that he outline the precise location of Eastman's heart.

As his physical pain increased and his functioning grew increasingly impaired, Eastman withdrew from society and from the company of all but his closest friends and acquaintances, a self-imposed isolation characterized by painful loneliness and growing dependency on visitors and members of his personal staff. During the final months of his life, Eastman corresponded with close family and friends, expressing his devotion to them and stating that his work was done.

After his death, Eastman's business associates and members of his staff recounted with pity the sadness of his final months, noting that he "shuffled along in great pain, inexplicably weepy and depressed, dragging one foot behind" him (Brayer 1996, p. 517). Eastman began pitying himself as well, once stating, "When a man is alone and hasn't anybody interested in him, there's no reason for getting old" (p. 516). Statements like "There isn't much to live for" (p. 519) further speak to Eastman's growing despair. Only after Eastman revised his will did his demeanor change; he grew more cheerful, his mind apparently made up.

Eastman's legacy consists of making photography accessible to and popular with the public as well as his philanthropic contributions to Rochester and the world. As well, however, he contributed to our understanding of late-life suicide. His is an example of the potentially lethal combination of multiple losses, personality vulnerability, physical illness, functional impairment, social isolation, perceived loss of meaning and hope, and depression. Eastman's story additionally exemplifies the many potential points of entry for suicide intervention, from family and friends whom he longed to be with but was embarrassed to see, to his physician to whom he expressed suicidal despair. Perhaps only after learning from his example how we might intervene to prevent suicide among at-risk older adults can we agree that his work is truly done.

Characteristics of and Risk Factors for Suicide in Older Adults

Scope and Nature of the Problem

Suicide rates increase with age for both men and women in many countries that report death statistics to the World Health Organization (Pearson and Conwell 1995). The United States, however, shows a somewhat different pattern, as illustrated in Figure 21–1. Increased rates among older adults are largely explained by elevated risk for white men over the age of 65. African American men show a bimodal distribution, with peaks in younger adulthood and older age. Rates among women are generally lower, peaking at midlife and declining or remaining stable throughout the remainder of the life course. Reasons for this

apparent interaction between age, race, and sex in determining suicide risk remain speculative.

The prevalence of suicide attempts among older people is less well established than rates of completed suicide. However, it is clear from surveillance data that older adults both report a history of suicide attempts and present for care following nonfatal suicidal acts less often than do their younger counterparts (Moscicki 1997). Suicidal ideation shows a similar pattern, in which older adults consistently report lower rates than middle-aged and younger adults (Gallo et al. 1994). Table 21–1 summarizes the prevalences and correlates of suicidal ideation and/or death ideation (thoughts of death without suicidal intent) from studies in a range of community and clinical samples (Callahan et al. 1996; Corna et al. 2010; Crosby et al. 1999; Forsell et al. 1997; Jorm et al. 1995; Linden and Barnow 1997; Pfaff and Almeida 2004; Rao et al. 1997; Raue et al. 2007; Scocco et al. 2001; Shah et al. 2000; Skoog et al. 1996; Vilhjalmsson et al. 1998; Yip et al. 2003). In addition to the different populations sampled, the wide variation in rates observed is explained by the varying measures (Heisel and Flett 2006) and definitions of death and suicidal ideation used, and by the variable time frames examined.

The presence of a history of either suicidal ideation or behavior increases risk for subsequent suicidal behavior and death by suicide in older adults, just as at earlier points in the life course. However, the lethality of suicide attempts increases with age. Whereas there may be from 8 to 40 or more suicide attempts per death by suicide in the general population, that ratio may be 4:1 or lower in older adults (Crosby et al. 1999; McIntosh et al. 1994). Self-destructive acts are more likely to result in death among

TABLE 21–1. Studies of suicidal ideation (SI) and death ideation (DI) among older adults

Study[a]	Location	Ages, years	Sample	Time frame	Prevalence	Correlates
Callahan et al. 1996	Indiana, U.S.	≥60	301 primary care depressed patients	1 week	SI: 4.6%	Depressive illness, functional impairment
Corna et al. 2010	Canada	≥55	12,793 community-residing	1 year Lifetime	SI: 2.2% SI: 8.7%	Male gender, younger age, widowed, low social support, higher psychological distress
Crosby et al. 1999	United States	≥65	760 telephone survey respondents	1 year	SI: 1.0%	Older age
Forsell et al. 1997	Kungsholmen, Stockholm, Sweden	≥75	969 community survey respondents	2 weeks	SI: 10.1 fleeting, SI: 2.5% frequent	Major depression (50% of those with frequent SI), institutionalization, functional disability, visual problems
Jorm et al. 1995	Canberra, Australia	≥70	923 community survey respondents	2 weeks	SI/DI: 2.3%	Depressive disorder, poor health, disability, vision and hearing impairments, unmarried, in residential care
Linden and Barnow 1997	Berlin, Germany	≥70	516 community-residing	1 week	SI: 1% DI: 21.1%	Major depressive disorder (50%–75%)
Paykel et al. 1974	Connecticut, U.S.	≥60	156 community-residing	1 year	SI/DI: 9%	(Analyzed for all subjects ≥18); psychiatric symptoms, social isolation, more life events
Pfaff and Almeida 2004	Western Australia	≥60	504 primary care patients	Current	SI: 6.3%	Depressive symptoms
Rao et al. 1997	Cambridge, U.K.	≥81	125 community-residing	2 years	SI: 7% DI: 20%	Female gender, depression symptoms and diagnosis, dementia
Raue et al. 2007	New York, U.S.	≥65	539 visiting nurse home care patients	1 month	SI: 11.7%	Depressive symptoms, medical comorbidity, poor subjective social support

TABLE 21–1. Studies of suicidal ideation (SI) and death ideation (DI) among older adults (*continued*)

Study[a]	Location	Ages, years	Sample	Time frame	Prevalence	Correlates
Scocco et al. 2001	Padua, Italy	≥65	611 community-residing	1 month 1 year Lifetime	SI/DI: 6.5% 9.2% 17%	Depression, anxiety, hostility, hypnotic use
Shah et al. 2000	West Middlesex, U.K.	≥65	55 medical inpatients	1 month	SI: 36% DI: 33%	Depressive symptoms and diagnosis, antidepressants
Skoog et al. 1996	Göteborg, Sweden	≥85	345 community-residing	1 month	SI/DI: 15.9%	Major depression, psychotic disorders, heart and peptic ulcer disease, anxiolytics, and neuroleptics
Vihjalmsson et al. 1998	Reykjavik, Iceland	60–70	114 community-residing	1 week	SI: 2.6%	Not specified for older adults
Yip et al. 2003	Hong Kong	≥60	917 community-residing	Lifetime	SI/DI: 5.5%	Depressive symptoms, number of medical illnesses, vision or hearing problems, involved in court case

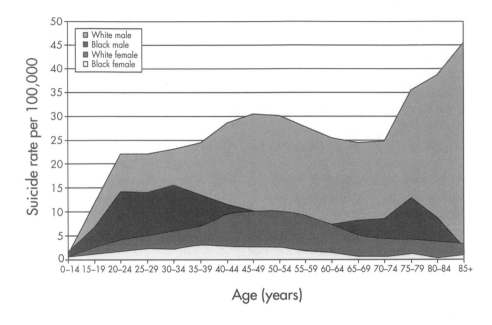

FIGURE 21–1. Suicide rates in the United States, by age, sex, and racial group, 2007.
Source. Data from the Centers for Disease Control and Prevention, National Center for Health Statistics, 2010.

older adults because they have increased physical illness burden and therefore less ability to withstand the physical insult. Furthermore, older people who attempt suicide are more likely to live alone than younger people and thus escape timely detection and rescue. Equally important is another characteristic illustrated so well by Mr. Eastman: older people in suicidal states tend to plan more, are more determined to die, and use more immediately lethal means such as firearms (Conwell et al. 1998). Almost three-quarters of older Americans who take their own lives do so with a gun, compared with approximately 55% of younger people. Like Mr. Eastman, the modal older person who dies by suicide is a man who carefully considers and plans his actions but tends to be indirect with others about his intent before ending his life with a gun.

Psychiatric Illness

Much of our knowledge about the correlates and risk factors for suicide in older people is derived from psychological autopsy studies, in which the mental, physical, and social circumstances are reconstructed from records and interviews with next of kin and other knowledgeable informants. Comparison with similar data from carefully selected control groups enables identification and quantification of risk factors. Such studies have repeatedly and consistently demonstrated that psychiatric illness is present in the great majority of older adults who take their own lives and in proportions far greater than in comparison groups of older adults who do not die by suicide. Table 21–2 shows the distribution of mental disorders in psychological autopsy studies conducted throughout the world (Barraclough 1971; Beautrais 2002; Carney et al. 1994; Chiu et al. 2004; Conwell et al. 1996, 2009; Harwood et al. 2001; Henriksson et al. 1995; McGirr et al. 2008; Waern et al. 2002b), and Table 21–3 lists odds ratios for suicide among older adults with mental disorders as determined in those few case-control studies that included a matched comparison sample (Beautrais 2002; Chiu et al. 2004; Conwell et al. 2009; Harwood et al. 2001; Waern et al. 2002a).

Affective illness—and in particular major depressive disorder—is the predominant mental disorder present in 44%–87% of cases. The data from controlled studies are inconclusive regarding the contribution of substance use disorders, anxiety disorders, and nonaffective psychoses to late-life suicide, and no study has yet shown that a diagnosis of dementia or delirium increases risk for suicide. The lack of association of dementia with increased suicide risk is counterintuitive, given the devastating impact of the illness, its close association in its early phases with mood disorder, and the association of decreased cognitive functioning with elevated suicidal ideation. These findings no doubt reflect the limitations of retrospective and informant report data. The few available prospective cohort studies of suicide in later life, however, reinforce the central role played by mood disorders and hopelessness (Ross et al. 1990; Turvey et al. 2002).

Although psychiatric illness is the rule among older adults who take their own lives, it often goes undiagnosed (Wells et al. 2002). As with George Eastman, the symptoms of depression, demoralization, and hopelessness may be easily masked by comorbid physical illness and a reluctance to acknowledge emotional pain. These characteristics of mood disorders in older adults, and among men in particular, make the detection—and therefore the prevention—of suicide particularly challenging.

Physical Illness

Another domain in which George Eastman's death is typical of older adult suicide is physical health status: he had a painful and debilitating physical condition that greatly impaired his ability to function independently. For a man of such power and authority, such dependency must have been particularly noxious.

Of course, ill health and functional impairments are common in later life, making their specific associations with suicide difficult to prove. Record linkage studies coupling physical illness registries with death registries have shown significantly increased relative risk for suicide associated with disorders of the central nervous system such as multiple sclerosis, Huntington disease, seizure disorders, spinal cord injury, and stroke; systemic lupus erythematosus; HIV/AIDS; and malignant neoplasms (with the exception of skin cancer), among other conditions (Harris and Barraclough 1994; Juurlink et al. 2004; Quan et al. 2002). Results are mixed in case-control psychological autopsy studies of older adult suicides, in which some (Conwell et al. 2009; Duberstein et al. 2004b; Waern et al. 2002a) but not other (Beautrais 2002) investigators report serious physical illness or functional impairment to be an independent risk factor for suicide after controlling for psychiatric illness. This latter point is important because of the close association between so many physical disorders, functional impairments, and affective illnesses.

In many instances, including perhaps that of Mr. Eastman, the older person may become suicidal in the face of physical illness and functional decline only if depression intervenes. Our own group compared physical health and functional status of adults age 60 years or older enrolled in primary care practices who had taken their

TABLE 21–2. Axis I diagnoses made by psychological autopsy in studies of late-life suicide

Study	Location	Age, years	Sample size, N	Major depression	Other mood disorder	Alcohol use disorder	Other substance use disorder	Nonaffective psychosis	Anxiety disorder	No diagnosis
								Diagnosis, %		
Barraclough 1971	West Sussex, U.K.	≥65	30	87		3		0	—	13
Beautrais 2002	New Zealand	≥55	31	86		14		—	—	9
Carney et al. 1994	San Diego, California, U.S.	≥60	49	54		22		—	—	14
Chiu et al. 2004	Hong Kong	≥60	70	53	26	3	—	9	1	14
Clark 1991	Chicago, Illinois, U.S.	≥65	54	54	11	19		0	2	24
Conwell et al. 1996	Monroe County, New York, U.S.	55–74	36	47	17	43	3	6	11	8
		75–92	14	57	21	27	7	0	0	29
Conwell et al. 2009	Western New York, U.S.	50–64	33	29	39	27	18	9	24	3
		65–99	53	51	26	9	2	2	9	23
Harwood et al. 2001	Central England, U.K.	≥60	100	63		5	5	4	—	23
Henriksson et al. 1995	Finland	≥60	43	44	21	25	5	12	—	9
McGirr et al. 2008	Quebec, Canada	50–59	88	60			45	—	15	—
		60–69	31	48			24	—	24	—
		≥70	21	46			39	—	23	—
Waern et al. 2002b	Göteborg, Sweden	≥65	85	46	36	27		8	—	5

TABLE 21–3. Odds ratios for suicide by Axis I diagnosis in case-control studies of older adults

Study[a]	Any Axis I diagnosis	Any mood disorder	Major depressive episode	Substance use disorder	Anxiety disorder	Nonaffective psychosis	Dementia/ delirium
Harwood et al. 2001	—	4.0	—	NS	—	NS	0.2
Beautrais 2002	43.9	184.6	—	4.4	—	—	—
Waern et al. 2002b	113.1	63.1	28.6	43.1	3.6	10.7	NS
Chiu et al. 2004	50.0	59.2	36.3	NS	NS	>1	NS
Conwell et al. 2009	44.6	47.7	12.2	NS	5.9	NS	NS

[a]Comparison groups for samples who died by suicide consisted of living community controls in all studies, except Harwood et al. (2001), who used older adults who died of natural causes. NS=not significant.

own lives with matched primary care older adults who had not (Conwell et al. 2000). Physical health and functional measures significantly distinguished the two groups. However, after adjustment for the presence of mood disorders, the physical health and functional variables were no longer associated with suicide status. Furthermore, studies of individuals with terminal illness have repeatedly demonstrated that suicidal ideation is rare in the absence of depression (Chochinov et al. 1995). The complex relationships between physical health, functional status, and psychiatric disorders, in particular depression, require additional study. It is most prudent at this stage, however, to assume that although real, perceived, or anticipated physical decline may place an older adult at increased risk for suicide, its impact is greatly exacerbated by the advent of comorbid depressive symptomatology.

Stressful Life Events

In the life of George Eastman, physical illness and functional decline may have served as powerful stressors precipitating his demoralized state, and possibly a major depressive episode, preceding his suicide. A range of other life circumstances common to older adulthood have been associated with suicide as well. Although bereavement clearly increases risk for suicide for several years after the loved one's death, the impact may be greater on middle-aged and younger adults who lose a spouse than in later life, when such tragic events are more often expected (Duberstein et al. 1998). Retirement and other forms of life transition have been implicated in late-life suicide, particularly for older men, with George Eastman as one possible example. However, studies to date do not provide empirical support for

retirement itself as a risk factor, and functional decline may be the best approximation for other role changes examined in the literature.

Two case-control psychological autopsy studies examined the associations of other specific stressors with suicide in older adults. Both Beautrais (2002) and Rubenowitz et al. (2001) found that financial and relationship problems distinguished older adults who died by suicide from matched community control subjects. When other factors such as medical and psychiatric illness, age, and sex were taken into account, financial stressors were no longer predictive. However, family discord remained significantly associated with suicide case status. The powerful contribution of interpersonal relationships and social support to suicide risk in older adults is supported by other findings as well. Turvey et al. (2002) found in secondary analyses of data from a prospective cohort study of older adults that those who had more friends and relatives in whom to confide were less likely to take their own lives. Miller (1978) reported in a psychological autopsy study that elderly men who took their own lives were less likely to have had a confidant than were age-matched community control subjects. Finally, our group also found that those over 50 years of age who died by suicide had significantly fewer social contacts than a living comparison sample matched for age, sex, race, community residence, and history of psychiatric illness (Duberstein et al. 2004a). Again, George Eastman is an instructive example. Unmarried, without children, facing the loss of friends and professional colleagues, and increasingly restricted to his home by his functional limitations, Mr. Eastman was isolated from the people and activities that lent meaning to his life.

Other Factors to Consider

Psychiatric illness, physical health problems, and other stressful life circumstances can affect individuals in myriad ways. Because the vast majority of older people with any of these problems do not take their own lives, other factors must be involved that help explain who would have suicidal thoughts under those circumstances and who would act on them.

Personality traits are normally distributed across the older adult population, so none has value as an independent predictor of suicide. However, studies have identified several traits that are associated with suicidal thoughts and behaviors in later life and that help us understand who may be at risk in the face of other "more potent" suicide risk factors (e.g., Heisel et al. 2007). Descriptive studies have linked suicide in older adults with the characteristics of hypochondriasis, hostility, shy seclusiveness, and a rigid, independent style. Harwood et al. (2001) found in a case-control psychological autopsy study that older adults who died by suicide had significantly more anxious and obsessive traits than did control subjects. Duberstein (1995) used reliable and valid measures of personality traits derived from the Five-Factor Model to yield similar findings. Specifically, high levels of Neuroticism and low scores on the Openness to Experience (OTE) factor of the NEO Personality Inventory (Costa and McCrae 1992) distinguished persons age 50 years or older who took their own lives from matched control subjects. Low OTE scores are characteristic of individuals best described as having a constricted range of interests and muted affective and hedonic responses to their environment. They prefer the familiar to the novel. The investigators also found that individuals low in OTE were *less* likely to endorse suicidal ideation, even controlling for presence of an Axis I disorder, hopelessness, and medical illness burden (Heisel et al. 2006). Duberstein (2001) proposed a model in which older adults with low OTE scores are at increased risk both because they are less well equipped socially and psychologically to manage the challenges of aging and because the difficulty they have expressing suicidal ideation makes them more likely to escape detection and lifesaving interventions. At the same time, the low OTE trait may be adaptive for younger and middle-aged men able to exercise power over their environments. It is only when illness-related changes conspire to rob them of that power that these traits may contribute to risk for suicide.

An exciting and expanding body of research involves the role that neurobiological factors may play in the pathogenesis of suicide (Ernst et al. 2009). The associations between measures of central serotonin functioning and impulsive, aggressive behaviors have received the most attention, although many other systems have been implicated as well. The distinctive pattern of suicide rates shown in Figure 21–1 raises the possibility that aging-related changes in neurobiological systems may contribute. However, studies of neurobiological mechanisms in older people are greatly complicated by the high rates of comorbid physical illness and medication prescription in this population. At this stage, theories about neurobiological contributions to late-life suicidal behavior remain largely untested.

Finally, we know from both ecological and case-control studies that access to lethal means increases risk for suicide (Conwell et al. 2002a) and that restriction of that access has been associated with reduction in suicide rates (see, for example, Hawton et al. 2001). As previously noted, firearms are the means used for almost three-quarters of older people who die by suicide in the United States. In a psychological autopsy study of older men in Arizona, Miller (1978) found that older adults who died by suicide were significantly more likely than living control subjects to have acquired a weapon within the past year. Our group, using the same method, found that having access to a firearm in the home was a significant predictor of suicide in men, but not women, older than 50 years. Furthermore, we found that the effect was specific to handguns; having a long gun in the home did not appear to confer additional risk (Conwell et al. 2002b).

Management of Suicide Risk in Late Life

Together with shifting population demographics consistent with the aging of the baby-boom birth cohort, the observation that suicidal behavior in older people is highly malignant and more often results in death than in younger people has important implications for management and prevention.

Assessment and Intervention

Older adults tend to deny or downplay the presence and intensity of depressive symptoms and suicidal ideation, necessitating the establishment of respectful and supportive rapport and use of sensitive and age-specific assessment tools and approaches (Canadian Coalition for Seniors' Mental Health 2006; Heisel and Flett 2006). Validated assessment tools have been developed to assess the presence and/or severity of late-life suicidal ideation and associated risk and resiliency factors (the Geriatric Suicide Ideation Scale; Heisel and Flett 2006),

reasons for living (the Reasons for Living Scale—Older Adult version; Edelstein et al. 2009), and risk for suicidal and other harmful behaviors among nursing home residents (the Harmful Behaviors Scale; Draper et al. 2002).

When an older person is recognized as being suicidal, aggressive action must be taken to intervene. The initial step should be more detailed assessment to determine the extent and specificity of current and past suicidal thoughts, including the degree of planning undertaken, reasons for considering suicide, current and previous history of self-harm behavior, and the physical and interpersonal outcomes of such behavior. One should also assess potential resiliency factors that may decrease suicide risk in the presence of risk factors, including the older patient's reasons for living (Edelstein et al. 2009), perceived sources of meaning in life (Heisel and Flett 2008), and quality of interpersonal relationships (Purcell et al., in press), because these may indicate sources of ambivalence and potential avenues for preventive intervention. If an older suicidal person has lethal intent (e.g., determination to end one's life and specific plans about how to do so) or is unable or unwilling to share his or her thoughts with the evaluator, hospitalization to ensure the person's safety and enable further evaluation may be indicated. Assessment should further include determining whether the individual has access to potentially lethal means, in particular firearms. If so, the most responsible course would be to contact trusted family members, friends, or local law enforcement, with the patient's consent, and ask them to remove the weapons. In emergency situations consent may not be required. Family members may give the firearms to the police for temporary safe keeping. Every effort should be made to provide a safe environment for the person to return to. If the patient refuses to relinquish the gun or to make accommodations to ensure safety from other potential means of self-harm, then hospitalization should again be considered.

Given the integral role played by social supports in late-life suicide prevention, assessment and mobilization of the at-risk older person's formal and informal social networks are critical and may help in detecting the presence of suicidal ideation (Heisel et al. 2011) and in defusing the acute crisis as well. Family members and friends may be invited to provide instrumental support and supervision, but only if their relationship with the patient is a trusted and comfortable one. Education of the involved support system is important with regard to risk assessment and the need for consistent follow-up and sustained treatment.

Beyond assessment and management of the acute suicidal crisis, the treating provider should conduct a thorough multiaxial diagnostic evaluation that incorporates consideration of major psychiatric diagnoses, including personality disorders, as well as pertinent traits and characteristic coping styles, physical health and functional status, sources of stress in the person's life, and resources that he or she has (intra- and interpersonal as well as social and economic) to manage them. On this basis, a treatment plan can then be formulated that addresses not only the intolerable pain driving the acute suicidal crisis but also the underlying factors that promote it.

Prevention of Suicide in Later Life

A second implication of the apparent lethality of late-life suicidality is that high priority should be placed on preventing the development of suicidal states in older people, because once suicidal ideation and behaviors are established, they can be challenging to detect and treat.

A spectrum of prevention efforts—indicated, selective, and universal approaches to intervention—may be necessary to address mental disorders in a comprehensive fashion (Institute of Medicine 1994) (see Table 21–4). Because suicide is a relatively rare outcome (and even more so in a subgroup of the population such as older adults), few studies have examined the impact of specific preventive interventions on late-life suicidal behaviors. However, the few whose results have been reported show promise for further development as elements of a comprehensive late-life suicide prevention strategy.

Indicated Approaches

Indicated approaches for the reduction of late-life suicide are designed to support the detection and effective treatment of suicidal ideation and the associated psychiatric illnesses that place older adults at immediate risk. As prescription rates for antidepressants, and selective serotonin reuptake inhibitors in particular, have risen in recent years, suicide rates have declined, including those among older adults. Although unable to establish a causal relationship between antidepressant prescriptions and suicide prevention, correlational studies support the notion that wider access to effective treatment for depression results in fewer deaths by suicide (Erlangsen et al. 2008; Gibbons et al. 2005). Up to three-quarters of older adults who took their own lives had been in the office of a primary care provider within the previous 30 days; approximately one-third had been in their provider's office within the last week of life (Conwell et al. 2002a). These observations suggest that improved detection and treatment of depression by primary care physicians should be a prime

TABLE 21–4. The language of prevention science applied to suicide in later life

Intervention terminology	Approach	Target	Objectives	Examples of possible prevention efforts

Universal prevention	Population	Entire population, not identified based on individual risk	Implement broadly directed initiatives to prevent suicide-related morbidity and mortality through reducing risk and enhancing protective factors	1. Education of the general public, clergy, the media, and health care providers concerning
				  * Normal aging
				  * Ageism and stigma regarding mental illness
				  * Pain and disability management
				  * Depression
				  * Suicidal behaviors
				2. Restrict access to lethal means, such as handguns

Selective prevention	Population, high risk	Asymptomatic or presymptomatic individuals or subgroups with "distal" risk factors for suicide or who have a higher-than-average risk of developing mental disorders or other more "proximal" risk factors	Prevent suicide-related morbidity and mortality through addressing specific characteristics that place elders at risk	1. Promote church-based and community programs to contact and support isolated elders 2. Focus medical and social services on reducing disability and enhancing independent functioning 3. Increase access to home care and rehabilitation services 4. Improve access to pain management and palliative care services

TABLE 21–4. The language of prevention science applied to suicide in later life *(continued)*

Intervention terminology	Approach	Target	Objectives	Examples of possible prevention efforts
Indicated prevention	High risk	Individuals with detectable symptoms and/or other proximal risk factors for suicide	Treat individuals with precursor signs and symptoms to prevent development of disorder or the expression of suicidal behavior	1. Train gatekeepers in recognition of symptomatic and at-risk elders 2. Link outreach and gatekeeper services to comprehensive evaluation and health management services in a continuum of care 3. Implement strategies to provide more accessible, acceptable, and affordable mental health care to elders 4. Treat elders with chronic pain syndromes more effectively 5. Increase screening/treatment in primary care settings for elders with depression, anxiety, and substance misuse 6. Improve providers' assessment and restriction of access to lethal means

Note. This table was developed in collaboration with Kerry Knox, Ph.D., and Eric D. Caine, M.D.

target for late-life suicide preventive interventions.

One rigorous test of this hypothesis is provided by work from the Prevention of Suicide in Primary Care Elderly: Collaborative Trial (PROSPECT) (Bruce et al. 2004). In this study, 598 older patients with depressive disorders were recruited from primary care practices and randomly assigned to receive either care as usual or a multicomponent intervention based on a collaborative, stepped-care model. The treatment condition included the use of treatment guidelines applied in the primary care setting with support of a depression care specialist who worked in close collaboration with the primary care physician, patient, and family to optimize compliance, tailoring care to the patient's needs and preferences. Treatment may have included medications, interpersonal psychotherapy, and education/family support.

Rates of suicidal ideation declined significantly faster in intervention patients than control subjects (Bruce et al. 2004), with greater reductions sustained over 24 months (Alexopoulos et al. 2009). Intervention patients also had significantly better outcomes over 2 years of follow-up with regard to major depressive symptoms. The incidence of suicide attempts was too small to judge the intervention's impact on that outcome. Nevertheless, the consistent associations observed among depression, suicidal ideation, and death by suicide on the one hand and between treatment of depression and reduced rates of suicidal ideation and suicide on the other provide powerful reinforcement for further study and implementation of preventive approaches targeting depression in late-life primary care (see also Unützer et al. 2006) and treatment of suicidal older adults with focused psychotherapeutic interventions (e.g., Heisel et al. 2009).

Selective Approaches

Selective preventive interventions target groups of older adults at risk for developing suicidal states as a result, in particular, of social isolation and impaired social supports, physical illness and functional impairment, and the presence of mild or subsyndromal depressive symptomatology. Within this framework, many existing medical and social services could be considered selective suicide prevention strategies. For example, comprehensive geriatric assessment clinics that provide thorough multidisciplinary diagnostic and treatment services to older adults may have that additional benefit. Social services that provide outreach to isolated older adults in the community and care management services that address their other social needs may lower suicide risk as well.

Work by De Leo et al. (2002) supports this hypothesis. The Telehelp/Telecheck service in Padua, Italy, provided telephone-based outreach, evaluation, and support services to more than 18,000 frail elders. The authors observed that over 11 years of service delivery, there were significantly fewer than expected suicides among their clients in the elder population of that region. Unfortunately, few social services have the expertise or resources to conduct the rigorous evaluations necessary to show their impact on suicidal ideation and behavior in the populations that they serve.

Universal Approaches

Finally, a comprehensive late-life suicide prevention strategy should include approaches that target the entire population regardless of any individual's risk status. Although not typically the purview of health care providers, universal prevention strategies are becoming increasingly recognized as integral components of public health and population-oriented health care delivery. Such approaches to late-life suicide prevention may include, for example, educational programs to decrease ageism and stigmatization among older adults about receiving mental health care, and educational or legislative approaches to lethal means restriction. An example of the latter was provided in Great Britain when, in 1998, legislation took effect limiting the size of packs of paracetamol (or acetaminophen) and salicylates (aspirin) sold over the counter (Hawton et al. 2001). As the number of tablets per pack decreased, so did the annual number of deaths from overdose by these commonly used medications.

A second example that pertains more directly to older adults is the introduction of gun control through the Brady Handgun Violence Prevention Act of 1994. Known as the Brady Act, it requires licensed firearms dealers to observe a waiting period and initiate a background check prior to each handgun sale. Ludwig and Cook (2000) examined the patterns of change in suicide and homicide rates before and after the act went into effect to determine whether specific changes in rates may have been associated with implementation of its policies. Eighteen states already had equivalent legislation in place, which the investigators called "control states"; 32 states were required to newly implement the Brady Act's procedures (the "intervention states"). The authors found no difference between intervention and control states in patterns of change in *homicide* rates for either the population age 21 years or older or adults age 55 years or older, and no difference for suicide rates among younger adults. However, after implementation of the act, the rate of suicide by firearms among individuals older than 55 years of age declined significantly more in the intervention states than in the control states. This finding is of particular interest

because it appears to suggest that handgun control may be a relatively more effective suicide prevention strategy for older adults and especially for older men.

Comprehensive Approaches

Ultimately the most effective strategy for reducing suicide deaths in the older adult population is one that combines elements of indicated, selective, and universal approaches in a comprehensive and coordinated program of prevention. Oyama et al. (2008) examined variations of such a multifaceted prevention program in a series of five quasi-experimental studies. Although the details differed somewhat between studies, each was conducted in a different Japanese rural region with high suicide rates among older people (greater than 160 per 100,000). Implemented over 5- to 10-year periods, the interventions included systematic community-wide screening, referral to primary care or mental health care as indicated, and, to varying degrees, public education and socialization programs for older adults. The investigators examined changes in the relative risk or incidence risk ratios for suicide in older adults before and after the programs' implementation and relative to neighboring reference regions of similar size and character. Overall, risk was significantly reduced in men and women when those who screened positive for depression were referred to a psychiatrist, but only in women when follow-up was conducted by general practitioners.

Conclusion

Older adults are at higher risk for suicide than any other age group, although in the United States it is older men who particularly bear that risk. The detection and management of suicidal older adults present special challenges to the health care and social services systems. They are less likely than younger adults to endorse suicidal ideation or engage in suicidal behavior, yet they have substantially higher rates of suicide. The self-destructive acts that an older person implements are likely to be far more lethal in planning, implementation, and outcome. Therefore, clinical interventions must be aggressively made when an older patient is recognized to be suicidal. These should include immediate comprehensive assessment of the nature and extent of suicidal thoughts and plans, access to means, and past history of suicidal behavior, as well as a systematic review of risk and resiliency factors. On that basis an acute management plan can be articulated to help maintain the patient's safety while assessing and treating underlying pathology.

Recent case-control psychological autopsy studies, supplemented by prospective cohort and record linkage studies, have helped to identify factors that place older adults at risk for suicide. Chief among them is psychiatric illness, in particular mood disorders. Medical illness and functional impairment, social isolation, and life stressors (especially bereavement and family discord) also are major contributors. Hopelessness and the personality traits of neuroticism and low OTE should also be considered as vulnerabilities to development of suicidal states. Finally, access to lethal means, and in particular handguns, appears to be a factor contributing to suicide in later life.

In addition to aggressive intervention for older adults recognized to be suicidal, we must implement and test strategies designed to prevent those with more "distal" risk factors from deteriorating into a suicidal state. These strategies should include a coordinated combination of indicated (e.g., primary care–based models to improve detection and treatment of late-life depression, use of psychotherapeutic interventions), selective (e.g., outreach and support for socially isolated elders in the community), and universal (e.g., screening for depression and/or suicide risk, education to reduce the stigma of mental illness, and restricted access to lethal means) approaches.

George Eastman's suicide note—"My work is done. Why wait?"—suggests that he had choices to make about how and when his life would end. However, as with most suicidal persons, he most likely saw little alternative to death other than a period of intolerable psychic pain and suffering. The clinician's duty is to recognize that intolerable pain and to help create more desirable alternatives to death by one's own hand. Treatment and prevention strategies provide us with the tools needed to create those alternative solutions and thereby provide elders with the choice to live.

Key Clinical Concepts

- Older adults are at greater risk for suicide than other segments of the population.
- Mental illnesses, in particular affective disorders and a history of attempted suicide, are the most powerful determinants of risk.
- Physical illness and functional impairment, pain, social isolation, family discord, other life stressors, and a rigid coping style also contribute to risk for suicide in later life.

- For older adults with suicidal ideation, especially those with a plan and access to means, intervention must be aggressive and may include acute hospitalization to provide for their safety, evaluation, and treatment.

- Development and implementation of pharmacological and psychotherapeutic interventions designed to prevent onset of the acutely suicidal state are particularly high priorities.

- Specific indicated, selective, and universal interventions have shown promise as means to reduce suicide mortality in later life.

References

Alexopoulos GS, Reynolds CF III, Bruce ML, et al: Reducing suicidal ideation and depression in older primary care patients: 24-month outcomes of the PROSPECT study. Am J Psychiatry 166:882–890, 2009

Barraclough BM: Suicide in the elderly: recent developments in psychogeriatrics. Br J Psychiatry Suppl 6:87–97, 1971

Beautrais AL: A case control study of suicide and attempted suicide in older adults. Suicide Life Threat Behav 32:1–9, 2002

Brayer E: George Eastman: A Biography. Baltimore, MD, Johns Hopkins University Press, 1996

Bruce ML, Ten Have TR, Reynolds CF III, et al: Reducing suicidal ideation and depressive symptoms in depressed older primary care patients: a randomized controlled trial. JAMA 291:1081–1091, 2004

Callahan CM, Hendrie HC, Nienaber NA, et al: Suicidal ideation among older primary care patients. J Am GeriatrSoc 44:1205–1209, 1996

Canadian Coalition for Seniors' Mental Health: National Guidelines for Seniors' Mental Health: The Assessment of Suicide Risk and Prevention of Suicide. Toronto, ON, Canadian Coalition for Seniors' Mental Health, 2006

Carney SS, Rich CL, Burke PA, et al: Suicide over 60: the San Diego study. J Am Geriatr Soc 42:174–180, 1994

Chiu HF, Yip PS, Chi I, et al: Elderly suicide in Hong Kong: a case-controlled psychological autopsy study. Acta Psychiatr Scand 109:299–305, 2004

Chochinov HM, Wilson KG, Enns M, et al: Desire for death in the terminally ill. Am J Psychiatry 152:1185–1191, 1995

Clark DC: Suicide Among the Elderly: Final Report to the AARP Andrus Foundation. Chicago, IL, 1991

Conwell Y, Duberstein PR, Cox C, et al: Relationships of age and Axis I diagnoses in victims of completed suicide: a psychological autopsy study. Am J Psychiatry 153:1001–1008, 1996

Conwell Y, Duberstein PR, Cox C, et al: Age differences in behaviors leading to completed suicide. Am J Geriatr Psychiatry 6:122–126, 1998

Conwell Y, Lyness JM, Duberstein P, et al: Completed suicide among older patients in primary care practices: a controlled study. J Am Geriatr Soc 48:23–29, 2000

Conwell Y, Duberstein PR, Caine ED: Risk factors for suicide in later life. Biol Psychiatry 52:193–204, 2002a

Conwell Y, Duberstein PR, Connor K, et al: Access to firearms and risk for suicide in middle-aged and older adults. Am J Geriatr Psychiatry 10:407–416, 2002b

Conwell Y, Duberstein PR, Hirsch JK, et al: Health status and suicide in the second half of life. Int J Geriatr Psychiatry 25:371–379, 2009

Corna LM, Cairney J, Streiner DL: Suicide ideation in older adults: relationship to mental health problems and service use. Gerontologist 50:785–797, 2010

Costa PT, McCrae RR: Revised NEO Personality Inventory and NEO Five Factor Inventory: Professional Manual. Odessa, FL, Psychological Assessment Resources, 1992

Crosby AE, Cheltenham MP, Sacks JJ: Incidence of suicidal ideation and behavior in the United States, 1994. Suicide Life Threat Behav 29:131–140, 1999

De Leo D, Dello BM, Dwyer J: Suicide among the elderly: the long-term impact of a telephone support and assessment intervention in northern Italy. Br J Psychiatry 181:226–229, 2002

Draper B, Brodaty H, Low LF, et al: Self-destructive behaviors in nursing home residents. J Am Geriatr Soc 50:354–358, 2002

Duberstein PR: Openness to experience and completed suicide across the second half of life. Int Psychogeriatr 7:183–198, 1995

Duberstein PR: Are closed-minded people more open to the idea of killing themselves? Suicide Life Threat Behav 31:9–14, 2001

Duberstein PR, Conwell Y, Cox C: Suicide in widowed persons: a psychological autopsy comparison of recently and remotely bereaved older subjects. Am J Geriatr Psychiatry 6:328–334, 1998

Duberstein PR, Conwell Y, Conner KR, et al: Poor social integration and suicide: fact or artifact? A case-control study. Psychol Med 34:1331–1337, 2004a

Duberstein PR, Conwell Y, Conner KR, et al: Suicide at 50 years of age and older: perceived physical illness, family discord and financial strain. Psychol Med 34:137–146, 2004b

Edelstein BA, Heisel MJ, McKee DR, et al: Development and psychometric evaluation of the Reasons for Living—Older Adults scale: a suicide risk assessment inventory. Gerontologist 49:736–745, 2009

Erlangsen A, Canudas-Romo V, Conwell Y: Increased use of antidepressants and decreasing suicide rates: a population-based study using Danish register data. J Epidemiol Community Health 62:448–454, 2008

Ernst C, Mechawar N, Turecki G: Suicide neurobiology. Prog Neurobiol 89:315–333, 2009

Forsell Y, Jorm AF, Winblad B: Suicidal thoughts and associated factors in an elderly population. Acta Psychiatr Scand 95:108–111, 1997

Gallo JJ, Anthony JC, Muthén BO: Age differences in the symptoms of depression: a latent trait analysis. J Gerontol 49:P251–P264, 1994

Gibbons RD, Hur K, Bhaumik DK, et al: The relationship between antidepressant medication use and rate of suicide. Arch Gen Psychiatry 62:165–172, 2005

Harris EC, Barraclough BM: Suicide as an outcome for medical disorders. Medicine (Baltimore) 73:281–296, 1994

Harwood D, Hawton K, Hope T, et al: Psychiatric disorder and personality factors associated with suicide in older people: a descriptive and case-control study. Int J Geriatr Psychiatry 16:155–165, 2001

Hawton K, Townsend E, Deeks J, et al: Effects of legislation restricting pack sizes of paracetamol and salicylate on self poisoning in the United Kingdom: before and after study. BMJ 322:1203–1207, 2001

Heisel MJ, Flett GL: The development and initial validation of the Geriatric Suicide Ideation Scale. Am J Geriatr Psychiatry 14:742–751, 2006

Heisel MJ, Flett GL: Psychological resilience to suicide ideation among older adults. Clin Gerontol 31:51–70, 2008

Heisel MJ, Duberstein PR, Conner KR: Personality and reports of suicide ideation among depressed adults 50 years of age or older. J Affect Disord 90:175–180, 2006

Heisel MJ, Links PS, Conn D, et al: Narcissistic personality and vulnerability to late-life suicidality. Am J Geriatr Psychiatry 15:734–741, 2007

Heisel MJ, Duberstein PR, Talbot NL, et al: Adapting interpersonal psychotherapy for older adults at risk for suicide: preliminary findings. Prof Psychol Res Pr 40:156–164, 2009

Heisel MJ, Conwell Y, Pisani AR, et al: Concordance of self- and proxy-reported suicide ideation in depressed adults 50 years of age or older. Can J Psychiatry 56:219–226, 2011

Henriksson MM, Marttunen MJ, Isometsä ET, et al: Mental disorders in elderly suicide. Int Psychogeriatr 7:275–286, 1995

Institute of Medicine: Reducing Risks for Mental Disorders: Frontiers for Preventive Intervention Research. Washington, DC, National Academy Press, 1994

Institute of Medicine: Suicide Prevention and Intervention: Summary of a Workshop. Washington, DC, National Academy Press, 2001

Jorm AF, Henderson AS, Scott R, et al: Factors associated with the wish to die in elderly people. Age Ageing 24:389–392, 1995

Juurlink DN, Herrmann N, Szalai JP, et al: Medical illness and the risk of suicide in the elderly. Arch Intern Med 164:1179–1184, 2004

Linden M, Barnow S: 1997 IPA/Bayer Research Awards in Psychogeriatrics: the wish to die in very old persons near the end of life: a psychiatric problem? Results from the Berlin Aging Study. Int Psychogeriatr 9:291–307, 1997

Ludwig J, Cook PJ: Homicide and suicide rates associated with implementation of the Brady Handgun Violence Prevention Act. JAMA 284:585–591, 2000

McGirr A, Renaud J, Bureau A, et al: Impulsive-aggressive behaviours and completed suicide across the life cycle: a predisposition for younger age of suicide. Psychol Med 38:407–417, 2008

McIntosh JL, Santos JF, Hubbard RW, et al: Elder Suicide: Research, Theory, and Treatment. Washington, DC, American Psychological Association, 1994

Miller M: Geriatric suicide: the Arizona study. Gerontologist 18:488–495, 1978

Moscicki EK: Identification of suicide risk factors using epidemiologic studies. Psychiatr Clin North Am 3:499–517, 1997

Oyama H, Sakashita T, Ono Y, et al: Effect of community-based intervention using depression screening on elderly suicide risk: a meta-analysis of the evidence from Japan. Community Ment Health J 44:311–320, 2008

Paykel ES, Myers JK, Lindenthal JJ, et al: Suicidal feelings in the general population: a prevalence study. Br J Psychiatry 124:460–469, 1974

Pearson JL, Conwell Y: Suicide in late life: challenges and opportunities for research. Int Psychogeriatr 7:131–136, 1995

Pfaff JJ, Almeida OP: Identifying suicidal ideation among older adults in a general practice setting. J Affect Disord 83:73–77, 2004

Purcell B, Heisel MJ, Speice J, et al: Family connectedness moderates the association between living alone and suicide ideation in a clinical sample of adults 50 years and older. Am J Geriatr Psychiatry (in press)

Quan H, Arboleda-Flórez J, Fick GH, et al: Association between physical illness and suicide among the elderly. Soc Psychiatry Psychiatr Epidemiol 37:190–197, 2002

Rao R, Dening T, Brayne C, et al: Suicidal thinking in community residents over eighty. Int J Geriatr Psychiatry 12:337–343, 1997

Raue PJ, Meyers BS, Rowe JL, et al: Suicidal ideation among elderly homecare patients. Int J Geriatr Psychiatry 22:32–37, 2007

Ross RK, Bernstein L, Trent L, et al: A prospective study of risk factors for traumatic death in the retirement community. Prev Med 19:323–334, 1990

Rubenowitz E, Waern M, Wilhelmsson K, et al: Life events and psychosocial factors in elderly suicides: a case control study. Psychol Med 31:1193–1202, 2001

Scocco P, Meneghel G, Caon F, et al: Death ideation and its correlates: survey of an over-65-year-old population. J Nerv Ment Dis 189:210–218, 2001

Shah A, Hoxey K, Mayadunne V: Suicidal ideation in acutely medically ill elderly inpatients: prevalence, correlates and longitudinal stability. Int J Geriatr Psychiatry 15:162–169, 2000

Skoog I, Aevarsson O, Beskow J, et al: Suicidal feelings in a population sample of non-demented 85-year-olds. Am J Psychiatry 153:1015–1020, 1996

Turvey CL, Conwell Y, Jones MP, et al: Risk factors for late-life suicide: a prospective, community-based study. Am J Geriatr Psychiatry 10:398–406, 2002

Unützer J, Tang L, Oishi S, et al: Reducing suicidal ideation in depressed older primary care patients. J Am Geriatr Soc 54:1550–1556, 2006

U.S. Public Health Service: National Strategy for Suicide Prevention: Goals and Objectives for Action. Rockville, MD, U.S. Department of Health and Human Services, U.S. Public Health Service, 2001

Vilhjalmsson R, Kristjansdottir G, Sveinbjarnardottir E: Factors associated with suicide ideation in adults. Soc Psychiatry Psychiatr Epidemiol 33:97–103, 1998

Waern M, Rubenowitz E, Runeson B, et al: Burden of illness suicide in elderly people: case-control study. BMJ 324:1355–1358, 2002a

Waern M, Runeson B, Allebeck P, et al: Mental disorder in elderly suicides. Am J Psychiatry 159:450–455, 2002b

Wells KB, Miranda J, Bauer MS, et al: Overcoming barriers to reducing the burden of affective disorders. Biol Psychiatry 52:655–675, 2002

Yip PS, Chi I, Chiu H, et al: A prevalence study of suicide ideation among older adults in Hong Kong SAR. Int J Geriatr Psychiatry 18:1056–1062, 2003

CHAPTER 22

Suicide Prevention in Jails and Prisons

Jeffrey L. Metzner, M.D.

Lindsay M. Hayes, M.S.

L*ocal jails,* which are usually administered by city or county officials, are facilities that hold inmates beyond arraignment, generally for 48 hours but less than a year. *Prisons* are state-operated or federally operated correctional facilities in which persons convicted of major crimes or felonies serve sentences that are usually in excess of 1 year. Six states (Alaska, Connecticut, Delaware, Hawaii, Rhode Island, and Vermont) and the District of Columbia have combined jail and prison systems (Glaze 2010; Metzner 1997). Despite the clear legal status differences between pretrial detainees in jails and inmates in prisons, the term *inmate* is used throughout this chapter to refer to both.

About 2,374,000 persons were incarcerated in prisons and jails combined within the United States at year-end 2009. Inmates in state prisons and the federal prison system accounted for almost two-thirds of the incarcerated population (1,524,513 inmates). These inmates were housed in about 1,670 different facilities. The other third (760,400) were held in over 3,300 county jails. Only

0.94% (7,220) of the total adult jail population was under the age of 18. The total prison population included 113,642 women, which accounted for 7% of all prisoners nationwide, compared with 93,729 women in jail (12.2% of the total jail population), as of June 2009 (Glaze 2010; Metzner 2002; Minton 2010).

Studies and clinical experience have consistently indicated that 8%–19% of prison inmates have psychiatric disorders that result in significant functional disabilities, and another 15%–20% will require some form of psychiatric intervention during their incarceration (Ditton 1999; Metzner 1993; Steadman et al. 2009; Torrey et al. 2010). A very high prevalence rate of substance abuse and substance use disorders among male prisoners has been frequently reported (Beck et al. 1993; Gunter and Antoniak 2010).

Suicide in Jails and Prisons

The National Center on Institutions and Alternatives (NCIA) previously reported that the aggregated suicide rate (107 per 100,000 jail inmates) in jails of all types and sizes (e.g., rural and urban county jails, city jails, and police department lockups) during 1986 was approximately nine times greater than that of the general population (Hayes 1989). Hayes (1995) provided a very useful literature review of prison suicide rates and described the NCIA national survey results pertinent to suicides in prisons during 1993. Based on a total prison population of 889,836 inmates, the national suicide rate for 1993 was reported to be 17.8 per 100,000 inmates.

In 2006, the suicide rate in jails was 38 deaths per 100,000 inmates, which is a significant decrease in the rate of suicide in jails during the preceding 20 years (Hayes 2010), although it remained three times greater than the rate found in the nonincarcerated. The most likely explanations for this significant decrease include increased awareness of the problem, successful implementation of suicide prevention programs within correctional facilities (including better staff training and intake screening inquiry), promulgation of national correctional standards that require such programs, and the impact of successful litigation involving suicides occurring in correctional facilities (Hayes 2010). Although controversy exists about the actual suicide rate in correctional facilities per 100,000 inmates, related to methodological issues in calculating such a rate (Metzner 2002), there is no question that many suicides in jails and prisons are preventable.

Nationwide, suicide accounted for 6.3% of all deaths in prisons from 2001 through 2007, and AIDS, the second leading cause of death in prison, accounted for 3.5% of deaths. Some form of illness accounted for 84% of all deaths. The rate of suicide in prisons was 16 per 100,000 in 2007 (Noonan 2010a). Suicide was the single leading cause of death in local jails (29%), followed by deaths associated with cardiac disease (22%), intoxication (7%), and AIDS-related causes (5%) (Noonan 2010b).

Recent data suggest a changing pattern to jail suicides (Hayes 2010). Jail suicides once typically involved inmates confined for minor offenses but most recently involve those confined for personal and/or violent charges. Intoxication was previously viewed as a leading precipitant to inmate suicide (Hayes 1989), yet recent data indicate that intoxicationit is now found in only a minority of cases. Previously, more than half of all jail suicide victims were dead within the first 24 hours of confinement (Hayes 1989); recent data suggest that less than one-quarter of all victims die by suicide during this time period, with an equal number of deaths occurring between 2 and 14 days of confinement (see Table 22–1). In addition, it appears that inmates who died by suicide in jail were far less likely to have been housed in isolation than previously reported (Hayes 2010).

These recent national findings are similar to those from prior research on suicides in urban jail facilities. Most victims of suicide in urban facilities had been arrested for violent offenses and were dead within 1–4 months of incarceration. Intoxication was normally not the salient factor in urban jails. Suicide victim characteristics such as age, race, sex, method (hanging), and instrument (bedding) remain generally consistent in both urban and nonurban jails (DuRand et al. 1995; Frottier et al. 2002; Hayes 2010; Marcus and Alcabes 1993; Winter 2003).

Findings by Hayes (1995) and Bonner (2000) relevant to common characteristics of prison suicide victims described in the literature are summarized in Table 22–2. These findings are consistent with a New York State Department of Correctional Services review of psychological autopsies of a sample of 40 cases of inmate suicide that

TABLE 22–1. Common characteristics of jail suicides

More likely to occur within first 24 hours or between 2 and 14 days

Incarceration for violent/personal offense

Close proximity to telephone call, visit, and/or legal proceeding

Presence of mental illness and prior suicidal behavior

TABLE 22–2. Common characteristics of prison suicide victims

Presence of serious mental illness

History of suicide attempts

Older age

Lengthy sentences

Institutional problems involving protective custody and immigration status

Segregated and isolated housing

took place between 1993 and 2001. These inmates had all received mental health services during their incarceration. Factors associated with suicide included substance abuse, history of prior suicide attempts, mental health treatment prior to incarceration, recent "bad news," recent disciplinary action, and manifestation of agitation and/or anxiety. A total of 76 inmates died by suicide in New York Department of Correctional Services facilities from 1993 to 1999. Significant demographic differences between the inmates committing suicide and the general prison population were reported. White inmates, inmates convicted for violent offenses, and inmates with schizophrenia were all overrepresented, and African American inmates were underrepresented among the inmates committing suicide (Kovasznay et al. 2004).

He et al. (2001) found a strong association between completed suicides and prior suicide attempts during confinement. They reviewed Texas prison suicides occurring over a 12-month period and found that more than 64% of inmates who died by suicide had made at least one prior suicide attempt while in prison. In addition, almost two-thirds of victims had been diagnosed with a psychiatric disorder, with the most frequent being mood disorders (64%), personality disorders (56%), and psychotic disorders (44%).

Patterson and Hughes (2008) reviewed health care records of all 154 inmates who

died by suicide in the California Department of Corrections and Rehabilitation from 1999 through 2004. Analysis of these cases suggested some notably persistent variables:

- Single-cell housing (73%)
- Segregation (46%); within 3 weeks of lockdown (53%)
- Method: hanging (85%)
- Past history of suicidal behavior (62%)
- Preventable or foreseeable, resulting from inadequate assessment (canceled appointments, referrals not completed, past records not reviewed, unsupported diagnosis, inappropriate level of mental health care assignment) (60%)
- Inadequate (or lack of) emergency medical response (27%)
- Mental health history (73%)
- Current mental health caseload (54%)
- Race (African American, 16%; Asian, 3%; Caucasian, 40%; Hispanic, 36%; and other, 5%)
- Gender (male, 94%)

The finding that a disproportionate number of prison suicides occurred in segregation, with most of these deaths occurring within 3 weeks of lockdown, was significant and consistent with findings from another large state prison system (Way et al. 2007).

In addition to the previously referenced high-risk periods during which an inmate may become suicidal in a correctional facility, an American Psychiatric Association (APA) task force report emphasized that an inmate may become suicidal at any point during his or her incarceration (American Psychiatric Association 2000). There is also a strong association between suicide in correctional facilities and housing assignments. Specifically, an inmate placed in and unable to cope with administrative segregation or other similar specialized housing assignments (especially single-cell) may also be at increased risk of suicide. Such housing units usually involve an inmate being locked in a cell for 23 hours per day for significant periods of time (American Psychiatric Association 2000; Bonner 1992; Kovasznay et al. 2004; Patterson and Hughes 2008; Way et al. 2007; White et al. 2002).

Case Example 1

John Smith is a 21-year-old male who was arrested after randomly shooting at five persons in a large shopping mall and inflicting serious injuries. While in the county jail, he is initially placed on suicide precautions as a result of information obtained from the arresting officers that he appeared to be encouraging them to return gunfire in a "suicide-by-cop" attempt to end his life. During the subsequent 4 months of his incarceration, Mr. Smith is only intermittently compliant with psychotropic medications prescribed to him for treatment of a serious mental disorder associated with periodic auditory hallucinations.

Mr. Smith is later involuntarily hospitalized on the psychiatric unit in the county jail due to increasing depression and suicidal thinking, which is voiced in the context of his almost total certainty that a conviction would result in a life sentence. However, an administrative law judge overturns the petition for involuntary hospitalization, although the written opinion is vague relevant to the rationale for this opinion.

The mental health staff is required to discharge Mr. Smith from the psychiatric ward immediately following this decision. However, they do not clearly convey to the custody staff their concern relevant to Mr. Smith's suicide potential and perceive that the administrative law judge's decision essentially prohibits them

from further suicide prevention efforts related to Mr. Smith. Custody staff determine that Mr. Smith should be housed in a segregation unit for protective custody purposes because of the high-profile nature of his alleged crimes. He is subsequently single-celled in such a unit.

A psychiatrist meets with Mr. Smith 5 days after his discharge from the psychiatric ward. Mr. Smith continues to deny any suicidal thinking, as he did during the involuntary hospitalization hearing, or any need for further mental health intervention. The plan is to follow up with Mr. Smith at his request on an as-needed basis only.

Three weeks later Mr. Smith is found hanging in his cell. Cardiopulmonary resuscitation (CPR) is unsuccessful.

This case demonstrates the need for effective communication between custody and mental health personnel in the context of suicide prevention efforts. The housing placement for Mr. Smith was not appropriate, nor was the lack of timely and consistent mental health follow-up. In addition, mental health staff demonstrated a negative attitude relevant to suicide prevention after the appropriate attempt to involuntarily hospitalize Mr. Smith. In the next section, we provide more detailed discussion relevant to these issues.

Suicide Prevention Programming

Experience has shown that negative attitudes often impede meaningful suicide prevention efforts. Such attitudes are not simply errors in judgment that contributed to an inmate's suicide or a reluctance to thoroughly investigate the death; they reflect a systemic state of mind that implies inmate suicides cannot be prevented. Examples include the following:

- "If someone really wants to kill themselves, there's generally nothing you can do about it."

- "We didn't consider him suicidal; he was simply being manipulative, and I guess it just went too far."
- "If you tell me you're suicidal, we're going to have to strip you of all your clothes and house you in a bare cell."
- "Suicide prevention is a medical problem . . . it's a mental health problem . . . it's not our problem."
- "Statistically speaking, suicide in custody is a rare phenomenon, and rare phenomena are notoriously difficult to forecast due to their low base rate. We cannot predict suicide because social scientists are not fully aware of the causal variables involving suicide."

Comprehensive suicide prevention programming has been advocated nationally by organizations such as the American Correctional Association, APA, and National Commission on Correctional Health Care (NCCHC) and most recently in the U.S. Department of Homeland Security's Immigration and Customs Enforcement (ICE) standards. These groups have promulgated national correctional standards that are adaptable to individual jail and prison facilities (American Correctional Association 2004; American Psychiatric Association 2000; National Commission on Correctional Health Care 2008a, 2008b; U.S. Department of Homeland Security 2008).

The APA, NCCHC, and ICE standards provide the more instructive guidelines and ingredients for a suicide prevention program: identification, training, assessment, monitoring, housing, referral, communication, intervention, notification, reporting, review, and critical incident debriefing (American Psychiatric Association 2000; National Commission on Correctional Health Care 2008a, 2008b; U.S. Department of Homeland Security 2008). Despite these guidelines, recent research has found that although most county jail systems experiencing an inmate suicide in the years 2005–2006 self-reported a written suicide prevention program, the vast majority did not have comprehensive programs that contained most, if not all, of these ingredients (Hayes 2010). Consistent with these national correctional standards, in the following sections we describe eight components of a comprehensive suicide prevention policy as listed in Table 22–3. It is recommended that a suicide prevention committee, consisting of key health care and custody staff, meet on a regular basis to implement and monitor the suicide prevention plan.

Staff Training

The essential component to any suicide prevention program is properly trained correctional staff, who form the backbone of any jail or prison facility. Very few suicides are actually directly prevented by mental health, medical, or other professional staff, because suicides are usually attempted in inmate housing units and often during late evening hours or on weekends, when program staff are not always present. Suicides, therefore, must be prevented by correctional staff who have been trained in suicide prevention and have developed an intuitive sense about the inmates under their care. Correctional officers are often the only staff available 24 hours a day and form the primary line of defense in preventing suicides.

All correctional staff, as well as medical and mental health personnel, should receive at least 8 hours of initial suicide prevention training followed by 2 hours of refresher training each year. Training should include why correctional environments are conducive to suicidal behavior, staff attitudes about suicide, potential predisposing

TABLE 22–3. Components of a comprehensive suicide prevention policy
Staff training
Intake screening and ongoing assessment
Communication
Housing
Levels of observation and management
Intervention
Reporting
Follow-up and mortality review

factors to suicide, high-risk suicide periods, warning signs and symptoms, identification of suicide risk despite the denial of risk, liability issues, inmate suicide research, recent suicides and/or serious suicide attempts within the facility/agency, and details of the facility's/agency's suicide prevention policy (Rowan and Hayes 1995). In addition, all staff who have routine contact with inmates should receive standard first-aid and CPR training. All staff should also be trained in the use of various emergency equipment located in each housing unit. In an effort to ensure an efficient emergency response to suicide attempts, mock drills should be incorporated into both initial and refresher training.

Intake Screening and Ongoing Assessment

Screening of inmates when they enter a facility and ongoing assessment during other high-risk periods are critical to a correctional facility's suicide prevention efforts. Although there is no single set of risk factors that mental health and medical communities agree can be used to predict suicide, there is little disagreement about the value of screening and assessment in preventing suicide (Hughes 1995; Spiers et al. 2006). Screening and assessment are critical

because research consistently reports that two-thirds or more of all suicide victims communicate their intent sometime before death and that any individual with a history of one or more self-harm episodes is at a much greater risk for suicide than those without such episodes (Clark and Horton-Deutsch 1992; Maris 1992). Screening for suicide risk may be contained within the medical screening form or as a separate form and should include inquiry regarding risk factors as summarized in Table 22–4. To increase the likelihood of an inmate's truthful response, staff must ensure that the physical environment provides reasonable privacy. The process should also include procedures for referral to mental health and/or medical personnel for assessment. Following the intake process, if staff hear an inmate verbalize a desire or intent to die by suicide, observe an inmate engaging in any self-harm, or otherwise believe an inmate is at risk for self-harm or suicide, referral procedures should be implemented. Such procedures direct staff to take immediate steps to ensure that the inmate is continuously observed until appropriate medical, mental health, and supervisory assistance are obtained.

Finally, given the strong association between inmate suicide and special-management (e.g., disciplinary and/or administrative segregation) housing unit placement (Bonner 2000; Kovasznay et al. 2004; Patterson and Hughes 2008; Way et al. 2007), any inmate assigned to such a special housing unit should receive a written assessment for suicide risk by mental health staff upon admission.

Communication

Certain behavioral signs exhibited by the inmate may be indicative of suicidal behavior. Detection of these signs and communi-

TABLE 22–4. Key points to inquire about in screening for suicide risk

Past suicidal ideation or suicide attempts

Current ideation

Threat

Plan

Prior mental health treatment and hospitalization

Recent significant loss (e.g., job, relationship, death of family member/close other)

History of suicidal behavior by family member/close other

Lack of forward thinking (expresses hopelessness and/or helplessness)

Suicide risk during prior confinement

Belief of arresting/transporting officer(s) that inmate is currently at risk

cation of them to others may prevent a suicide. There are essentially three levels of communication in preventing inmate suicides: 1) communication between the arresting or transporting officer and correctional staff; 2) communication between and among facility staff, including correctional, medical, and mental health staff; and 3) communication between facility staff and the suicidal inmate.

In many ways, suicide prevention begins at the point of arrest. What an individual says and how he or she behaves during arrest, during transportation to the jail, and at booking are crucial in detecting suicidal behavior. The scene of arrest is often the most volatile and emotional time. Arresting officers should pay close attention to the arrestee during this time; thoughts of suicide or suicidal behavior may be occasioned by the anxiety or hopelessness of the situation, and previous behavior can be confirmed by onlookers such as family and friends. Any pertinent information regarding the arrestee's well-being must be communicated to correctional staff by the arresting or transporting officer. Effective management of sui-

cidal inmates in the facility is based on communication among correctional officers and other professional staff.

Because inmates can become suicidal at any point during incarceration, including following telephone calls, visits, and legal proceedings (Hayes 2010; Marcus and Alcabes 1993), correctional officers must maintain awareness, share information, and make appropriate referrals to mental health and medical staff. Facility staff must use various communication skills with the suicidal inmate, including active listening, physically staying with the inmate if they suspect immediate danger, and maintaining contact through conversation, eye contact, and body language. Correctional staff should trust their own judgment and observation of risk behavior and avoid being misled by others (including mental health staff) into ignoring signs of suicidal behavior.

The communication breakdown between correctional, medical, and mental health personnel is a common factor found in the reviews of many inmate suicides (see Appelbaum et al. 1997; Hayes 1995). In both jail and prison systems, communication problems are often caused by lack of respect, personality conflicts, and other boundary issues. Simply stated, facilities that maintain a multidisciplinary approach generally avoid preventable suicides. As aptly stated by one clinician:

> The key to an effective team approach in suicide prevention and crisis intervention is found in throwing off the cloaks of territoriality and embracing a mutual respect for the detention officer's and mental health clinician's professional abilities, responsibilities and limitations. All of us, regardless of professional affiliation, need to make a dedicated commitment to come forward and acknowledge that suicide prevention and related mental health services are only effective when delivered by professionals acting

in unison with each other. Just as the security officer alone cannot ensure the safety and security of the jail facility, neither can the mental health clinician alone ensure the safety and emotional well-being of the individual inmate. (Severson 1993)

Housing

In determining the most appropriate housing location for a suicidal inmate, correctional officials (with concurrence from medical or mental health staff) often tend to physically isolate (or segregate) and sometimes restrain the individual. These responses might be more convenient for all staff, but they are detrimental to the inmate because the use of isolation escalates the inmate's sense of alienation and further removes the individual from proper staff supervision. To every extent possible, suicidal inmates should be housed with the general population or in the mental health unit or medical infirmary, located close to staff. Furthermore, removal of an inmate's clothing (excluding belts and shoelaces) and the use of physical restraints (e.g., restraint chairs, bunks or boards, leather straps) should be avoided whenever possible. They should be used only as a last resort, when the inmate is physically engaging in self-injurious behavior. Handcuffs should rarely be used to restrain a suicidal inmate. Housing assignments should be based on the ability to maximize staff interaction with the inmate, and assignments that heighten the depersonalizing aspects of incarceration should be avoided.

All cells designated to house suicidal inmates should be as suicide-resistant as is reasonably possible, be free of all obvious protrusions, and provide full visibility. These cells should contain tamperproof light fixtures, smoke detectors, and ceiling/wall air vents that are protrusion-free. In addition, the cells should not contain any live electrical switches or outlets, bunk holes or bunks with open bottoms, any type of clothing hook, towel racks on desks and sinks, radiator vents, or any other object that provides an easy anchoring device for hanging. Each cell door should contain a heavy gauge Lexan (or equivalent-grade) clear panel that is large enough to allow staff a full and unobstructed view of the cell interior (Atlas 1989; Hayes 2006). Finally, each housing unit in the facility should contain various emergency equipment, including a first-aid kit, pocket mask or Ambu bag, and rescue tool (to quickly cut through fibrous material). Correctional staff should ensure that such equipment is in working order on a daily basis.

Levels of Supervision

The promptness of response to suicide attempts in correctional facilities is often driven by the level of supervision afforded the inmate. The planning and preparation for suicide can take several minutes; brain damage from strangulation caused by a suicide attempt can occur within 4 minutes and death often within 5–6 minutes (American Heart Association 1992). Standard correctional practice requires that "special management inmates," including those housed in administrative segregation, disciplinary detention, and protective custody, be observed at intervals not exceeding 30 minutes, with mentally ill inmates observed more frequently (American Correctional Association 2003, 2004). Inmates held in medical restraints and "therapeutic seclusion" should be observed at intervals of not more than 15 minutes (National Commission on Correctional Health Care 2008a, 2008b).

Consistent with national correctional standards and practices, two levels of supervision are generally recommended for suicidal inmates: close observation and constant observation. *Close observation* is reserved for the inmate who is not actively suicidal but expresses suicidal ideation (e.g., expressing a wish to die without a specific threat or plan) or has a recent prior history of self-injurious behavior. In addition, an inmate who denies suicidal ideation or does not threaten suicide but demonstrates other concerning behavior (through actions, current circumstances, or recent history) indicating the potential for self-injury should be placed under close observation. Staff should observe such an inmate at staggered intervals of not more than 10 minutes (e.g., 5, 10, 7 minutes and so forth). *Constant observation* is reserved for the inmate who is actively suicidal, either threatening or engaging in suicidal behavior. Staff should observe such an inmate on a continuous, uninterrupted basis. Other aids (e.g., closed-circuit television, inmate companions or watchers) can be used as a supplement to, but never as a substitute for, these observation levels. Because death from a suicide attempt can occur within a short duration, observation of a suicidal inmate at intervals less frequent than continuous observation can only be successful if the observation is staggered and the cell is suicide-resistant.

In addition, mental health staff should assess and interact with (not just observe) the suicidal inmate on a daily basis. Unless contraindicated by safety/security concerns, cell-front assessments should be avoided, and every effort should be made to conduct suicide risk assessments in a reasonably private and confidential location. The daily assessment should focus on the current behavior as well as changes in thoughts and behavior during the past 24 hours. For example, if suicidal ideation is denied, then the questions become "How have your feelings and thoughts changed over the past 24 hours?" and "What are some of the things you have done or can do to change these thoughts and feelings?" Table 22–5 provides a summary of essential components of such an assessment.

TABLE 22–5. Essential components of a clinical risk assessment for suicide

History of suicidal intent or suicide attempts
  Is there a history of admitted suicidal intent or suicide attempt?
  Severity of ideation or attempt?
  Recent?
Degree of current suicidal ideation
  Has the person thought about how he or she might end his or her life?
  Did or does the person have a plan?
  Does the person have the means to carry out the plan?
  Was or is the plan reasonable?
  Does the person express feelings of peace/ resolution?
  Is the person attending to personal effects?
  Did the person write good-bye letters?
Systematic inquiry into
  Current mood
  Known risk factors—individual and group
  Known protective factors
  Stated intentions about suicide
  What has changed since attempt and/or last assessment?
  Evidence or absence of futuristic thinking
  Evidence of connectedness
Effect of suicide precautions on denial of suicidal ideation
  Is the person's current denial of suicidal ideation being influenced by the restrictive nature of the suicide precautions (e.g., restrictive clothing, shower, food, possessions, out-of-cell time)?
Treatment plan
  If the inmate is removed from suicide precautions, what is the treatment plan?

Source. J. Dvoskin, L. Hayes, personal communication, October 20, 2010.

An individualized treatment plan (to include follow-up services) should be developed for each inmate on suicide precautions longer than 24 hours. The plan should be developed by qualified mental health staff in conjunction with not only the inmate, but with medical and correctional personnel. The treatment plan should describe signs, symptoms, and the circumstances under which the risk for suicide is likely to recur, how recurrence of suicidal thoughts can be avoided, and actions the inmate and staff will take if suicidal ideation reoccurs.

Finally, because of the strong correlation between suicide and prior suicidal behavior, in order to safeguard the continuity of care for suicidal inmates, all inmates discharged from suicide precautions should receive regularly scheduled follow-up assessments by mental health personnel until their release from custody. Although there is not any nationally accepted schedule for follow-up, a suggested assessment schedule following discharge from suicide precautions might be 24 hours, 72 hours, 1 week, and for some inmates, periodically until release from custody.

Intervention

The degree and promptness of staff intervention often determine whether the victim will survive a suicide attempt. National correctional standards and practices generally acknowledge that facility policy regarding intervention should contain three primary components (National Commission on Correctional Health Care 2008a, 2008b). First, all staff who come in contact with inmates should be trained in standard first-aid procedures and CPR. Second, any staff member who discovers an inmate engaging in self-harm should immediately survey the scene to assess the severity of the emergency, alert other staff to call for medical personnel if necessary, and begin standard first aid and/or CPR as necessary. Third, staff should never presume that the inmate is dead but rather should initiate and continue appropriate lifesaving measures until relieved by arriving medical personnel. In addition, medical personnel should ensure, on a daily basis, that all facility emergency response equipment is in working order.

Reporting

In the event of a suicide attempt or suicide, all appropriate correctional officials should be notified through the chain of command. Following the incident, the victim's family should be immediately notified as well as appropriate outside authorities. All staff who came in contact with the victim prior to the incident should be required to submit a statement that includes their full knowledge of the inmate and incident.

Follow-Up and Mortality Review

An inmate suicide is extremely stressful for staff, who may feel angry, guilty, and even ostracized by fellow personnel and administration officials. After a suicide, reasonable guilt is sometimes displayed by the officer who wonders, "What if I had made my cell check earlier?" When suicide or a suicidal crisis occurs, staff affected by such a traumatic event should receive appropriate assistance. One form of assistance is critical incident stress debriefing (CISD). A CISD team, made up of professionals trained in crisis intervention and traumatic stress awareness (e.g., police officers, paramedics, firefighters, clergy, and mental health personnel), provides affected staff with an opportunity to process their feelings about the incident, develop an understanding of critical stress symptoms, and develop ways of dealing with those symptoms (Meehan

1997; Mitchell and Everly 1996). For maximum effectiveness, the CISD process or other appropriate support services should occur within 24–72 hours of the critical incident.

Every completed suicide, as well as each suicide attempt of high lethality (e.g., an attempt requiring hospitalization), should be examined through a mortality review process. If resources permit, clinical review through a psychological autopsy is also recommended (Aufderheide 2000; Sanchez 1999). Ideally, the mortality review should be coordinated by an outside agency to ensure impartiality. The review, separate and apart from other formal investigations that may be needed to determine the cause of death, should include information as summarized in Table 22–6.

Case Example 2

George Baxter enters the reception center at the state department of corrections to serve a 4-year sentence for aggravated robbery. He has a history of mental illness and is taking psychotropic medication for depression. During the intake screening process at the reception center, Mr. Baxter's behavior and responses to questions from the nurse are cause for concern. It is his first prison experience, and the 18-year-old appears anxious, expresses helplessness, and is crying during the interview. He heard stories of violence and intimidation in the state prison system while awaiting transfer from the county jail. Mr. Baxter has made at least three serious prior suicide attempts, and the transporting officer informs the intake nurse that Mr. Baxter was on suicide precautions at the county jail following a hanging attempt a few days earlier. He also has a family history of suicide; his brother died by suicide 6 years earlier, and his mother is currently being treated for depression after a recent drug overdose. Following the initial screening process, Mr. Baxter is placed on constant observation in the mental health unit and referred to mental health staff for further assessment of his suicide risk.

Mr. Baxter is seen by the reception center psychiatrist the following morning. He denies

TABLE 22–6. Mortality review

Critically review the circumstances surrounding the incident.

Critically review jail procedures relevant to the incident.

Make a synopsis of all relevant training received by involved staff.

Review pertinent medical and mental health services/reports involving the victim.

Consider possible precipitating factors leading to the suicide.

Make recommendations, if any, for changes in policy, training, physical plant, medical or mental health services, and operational procedures.

any suicidal ideation and states, "I'm not suicidal. This is all a big mistake." The psychiatrist determines that the constant observation status is "inappropriate," and Mr. Baxter is released from suicide precautions and rehoused with the general population. He is seen by a nurse later that afternoon and appears tearful and scared. He denies any suicidal ideation and requests a cell mate. The nurse tells Mr. Baxter that she will forward his request to the shift supervisor. A few hours later, and approximately 10 hours after his release from suicide precautions, Mr. Baxter is found hanging in his prison cell.

A mortality review was subsequently conducted on George Baxter's suicide. The review found that there was uncertainty as to whether the psychiatrist had reviewed Mr. Baxter's medical file, which contained the intake medical screening form, as well as uncertainty as to whether the transporting officer's observation and the county jail records regarding Mr. Baxter's suicidal behavior were effectively communicated to reception center intake staff. Recommendations offered during the mortality review included the stipulation that inmates placed on constant observation remain on that status as clinically indicated and then be stepped down to close observation for at least another day. Inmates assigned to the mental health unit should not be discharged until their case is reviewed during the weekly treatment team meeting. In addition, a sending agency discharge summary form should be created and completed by the sending agency (e.g., county jail) and/or transporting personnel prior to the inmate's arrival at the reception center that documents any immediate concerns about the inmate.

Conclusion

> Undoubtedly, it is easier for officials to know that someone is having suicidal thoughts when that person says that he is having suicidal thoughts. However, having an inmate in custody creates a duty of care that must include enough attention to mental health concerns that inmates with obvious symptoms receive medical attention....One cannot avoid responsibility by putting one's head in the sand. (*Jutzi-Johnson v. United States* 2001)

The growth in the field of correctional mental health services has raised awareness concerning the problem of inmate suicide in correctional facilities, resulting in the development of effective suicide prevention programs becoming a standard of practice within this area of practice (Cox and Lawrence 2010; Freeman and Alaimo 2001; Goss et al. 2002; Hayes 1996; National Commission on Correctional Health Care 2008a, 2008b; *Ruiz v. Estelle* 1980).

New York experienced a significant drop in the number of jail suicides after the implementation of a statewide comprehensive prevention program (Cox and Lawrence 2010). From 1990 through 1998, the suicide rate in the Cook County (Illinois) jail system, the third largest pretrial detention system in the country, was reduced to a level of fewer than 2 suicides per 100,000 admissions (Freeman and Alaimo 2001). Texas saw a 50% decrease in the number of county jail suicides as well as almost a sixfold decrease in the rate of these suicides from 1986 through 1996, much of it attributable to increased staff training and a state requirement for jails to maintain suicide prevention policies (Hayes 1996).

One researcher reported no suicides during a 7-year time period in a large county jail after the development of suicide prevention policies based on the following principles: screening; psychological support; close observation; removal of dangerous items; clear and consistent procedures; and diagnosis, treatment, and transfer of suicidal inmates to the hospital as necessary (Felthous 1994).

In conclusion, although lacking the ability to accurately predict if and when an inmate will die by suicide, facility officials and their correctional, medical, and mental health personnel can identify, assess, and treat potentially suicidal behavior. As demonstrated by recent data showing falling rates of inmate suicide, many of these deaths are preventable. Yet because inmates can be at risk at any point during confinement, the greatest challenge for those who work in the correctional arena is to view the issue as one that requires a continuum of comprehensive suicide prevention services aimed at the collaborative identification, continued assessment, and safe management of inmates at risk for self-harm.

Key Clinical Concepts

- Inmate suicide is a serious public health problem throughout the country.
- Although there are similarities between jail and prison suicide, there are also distinct differences.
- Negative attitudes impede meaningful suicide prevention efforts.
- Communication breakdown between correctional, medical, and mental health personnel is a common factor found in the reviews of many inmate suicides.
- Suicide rates in jails and prisons are decreasing, and correctional systems that implement and maintain comprehensive suicide prevention programs have effectively reduced the incidence of inmate suicides.

References

American Correctional Association: Standards for Adult Correctional Institutions, 4th Edition. Lanham, MD, American Correctional Association, 2003

American Correctional Association: Performance-Based Standards for Adult Local Detention Facilities, 4th Edition. Lanham, MD, American Correctional Association, 2004

American Heart Association, Emergency Cardiac Care Committee and Subcommittees: Guidelines for cardiopulmonary resuscitation and emergency cardiac care. JAMA 268:2172–2183, 1992

American Psychiatric Association: Psychiatric Services in Jails and Prisons, 2nd Edition. Washington, DC, American Psychiatric Association, 2000

Appelbaum K, Dvoskin J, Geller J, et al: Report on the Psychiatric Management of John Salvi in Massachusetts Department of Corrections Facilities: 1995–1996. Worcester, University of Massachusetts Medical Center, 1997

Atlas R: Reducing the opportunity for inmate suicide: a design guide. Psychiatr Q 60:161–171, 1989

Aufderheide D: Conducting the psychological autopsy in correctional settings. J Correct Health Care 7:5–36, 2000

Beck A, Gilliard D, Greenfeld L, et al: Survey of State Prison Inmates, 1991. Bureau of Justice Statistics NCJ 136949. Washington, DC, U.S. Department of Justice, 1993, pp 1–41

Bonner R: Isolation, seclusion, and psychological vulnerability as risk factors for suicide behind bars, in Assessment and Prediction of Suicide. Edited by Maris R, Berman A, Maltsberger J, et al. New York, Guilford, 1992, pp 398–419

Bonner R: Correctional suicide prevention in the year 2000 and beyond. Suicide Life Threat Behav 30:370–376, 2000

Clark D, Horton-Deutsch S: Assessment in absentia: the value of the psychological autopsy method for studying antecedents of suicide and predicting future suicides, in Assessment and Prediction of Suicide. Edited by Maris R, Berman A, Maltsberger J, et al. New York, Guilford, 1992, pp 144–182

Cox J, Lawrence J: Suicide prevention in correctional settings, Manual of Forms and Guidelines for Correctional Mental Health. Edited by Ruiz A, Dvoskin J, Scott C, et al. Washington, DC, American Psychiatric Association, 2010, pp 121–154

Ditton PM: Mental Health and Treatment of Inmates and Probationers. Bureau of Justice Statistics Special Report NCJ 174463. Washington, DC, U.S. Department of Justice, 1999, pp 1–12

DuRand CJ, Burtka GJ, Federman EJ, et al: A quarter century of suicide in a major urban jail: implications for community psychiatry. Am J Psychiatry 152:1077–1080, 1995

Felthous A: Preventing jailhouse suicides. Bull Am Acad Psychiatry Law 22:477–488, 1994

Freeman A, Alaimo C: Prevention of suicide in a large urban jail. Psychiatr Ann 31:447–452, 2001

Frottier P, Fruehwald S, Ritter K, et al: Jailhouse blues revisited. Soc Psychiatry Psychiatr Epidemiol 37:68–73, 2002

Glaze LE: Correctional populations in the United States, 2009. Bureau of Justice Statistics Bulletin, December 2010, pp 1–8. Available at: http://bjs.ojp.usdoj.gov/content/pub/pdf/cpus09.pdf. Accessed June 24, 2011.

Goss J, Peterson K, Smith L, et al: Characteristics of suicide attempts in a large urban jail system with an established suicide prevention program. Psychiatr Serv 53:574–579, 2002

Gunter TD, Antoniak SK: Evaluating and treating substance use disorders, in Handbook of Correctional Mental Health, 2nd Edition. Edited by Scott CL. Washington, DC, American Psychiatric Publishing, 2010, pp 167–196

Hayes LM: National study of jail suicides: seven years later. Psychiatr Q 60:7–29, 1989

Hayes LM: Prison suicide: an overview and guide to prevention. Prison J 75:431–456, 1995

Hayes LM: Jail standards and suicide prevention: another look. Jail Suicide/Mental Health Update 6:9–11, 1996

Hayes LM: Suicide prevention and designing safer prison cells, in Preventing Suicide and Other Self-Harm in Prison. Edited by Dear G. New York, Palgrave Macmillan, 2006, pp 167–174

Hayes LM: National study of jail suicide: 20 years later. U.S. Department of Justice, National Institute of Corrections, 2010, pp 1–68. Available at: http://nicic.gov/Library/024308. Accessed June 24, 2011.

He XY, Felthous AR, Holzer CE, et al: Factors in prison suicide: one year of study in Texas. J Forensic Sci 46:896–901, 2001

Hughes D: Can the clinician predict suicide? Psychiatr Serv 46:449–451, 1995

Jutzi-Johnson v United States 263 F3rd 753 (7th Cir. 2001)

Kovasznay B, Miraglia R, Beer R, et al: Reducing suicides in New York State facilities. Psychiatr Q 75:61–70, 2004

Marcus P, Alcabes P: Characteristics of suicides by inmates in an urban jail. Hosp Community Psychiatry 44:256–261, 1993

Maris R: Overview of the study of suicide assessment and prediction, in Assessment and Prediction of Suicide. Edited by Maris R, Berman A, Maltsberger J, et al. New York, Guilford, 1992, pp 3–22

Meehan B: Critical incident stress debriefing within the jail environment. Jail Suicide/Mental Health Update 7:1–5, 1997

Metzner JL: Guidelines for psychiatric services in prisons. Crim Behav Ment Health 3:252–267, 1993

Metzner JL: An introduction to correctional psychiatry, part I. J Am Acad Psychiatry Law 25:375–381, 1997

Metzner JL: Class action litigation in correctional psychiatry. J Am Acad Psychiatry Law 30:19–29, 2002

Minton TD: Jail inmates at midyear 2009—statistical tables. Bureau of Justice Statistics Bulletin, June 2010, pp 1–20. Available at: http://bjs.ojp.usdoj.gov/content/pub/pdf/jim09st.pdf. Accessed June 24, 2011.

Mitchell J, Everly G: Critical Incident Stress Debriefing: An Operations Manual for the Prevention of Traumatic Stress Among Emergency Services and Disaster Workers, 2nd Edition. Ellicott City, MD, Chevron Publishing, 1996

National Commission on Correctional Health Care: Standards for Health Services in Jails. Chicago, IL, National Commission on Correctional Health Care, 2008a

National Commission on Correctional Health Care: Standards for Health Services in Prisons. Chicago, IL, National Commission on Correctional Health Care, 2008b

Noonan M: Deaths in custody: state prison deaths, 2001–2007—statistical tables. Bureau of Justice Statistics, U.S. Department of Justice, October 28, 2010a. Available at: http://bjs.ojp.usdoj.gov/index.cfm?ty=pbdetail&iid=2093. Accessed June 24, 2011.

Noonan M: Mortality in local jails, 2000–2007. Bureau of Justice Statistics Bulletin, July 2010b, pp 1–20. Available at: http://bjs.ojp.usdoj.gov/content/pub/pdf/mlj07.pdf. Accessed June 24, 2011.

Patterson P, Hughes K: Review of completed suicides in the California Department of Corrections and Rehabilitation, 1999 to 2004. Psychiatr Serv 59:676–682, 2008

Rowan JR, Hayes LM: Training Curriculum on Suicide Detection and Prevention in Jails and Lockups. Mansfield, MA, National Center on Institutions and Alternatives, 1995

Ruiz v Estelle 503 F. Supp. 1265 (S.D. Texas 1980)

Sanchez H: Inmate suicide and the psychological autopsy process. Jail Suicide/Mental Health Update 8:3–9, 1999

Severson M: Security and mental health professionals: a (too) silent partnership? Jail Suicide Update 5:1–6, 1993

Spiers EM, Pitt SE, Dvoskin JA: Psychiatric intake screening, in Clinical Practice in Correctional Medicine. Edited by Puisis M. Philadelphia, PA, Mosby Elsevier, 2006, pp 285–291

Steadman HJ, Osher FC, Robbins PC, et al: Prevalence of serious mental illness among jail inmates. Psychiatr Serv 60:761–765, 2009

Torrey EF, Kennard AD, Eslinger D, et al: More mentally ill persons are in jails and prisons than hospitals: a survey of the states. Treatment Advocacy Center, May 2010, pp 1–19. Available at: http://www.treatmentadvocacycenter.org/storage/documents/final_jails_v_hospitals_study.pdf. Accessed June 24, 2011.

U.S. Department of Homeland Security: Operations Manual ICE Performance-Based National Detention Standards. Washington, DC, U.S. Immigration and Customs Enforcement, 2008

Way BB, Sawyer DA, Barboza S, et al: Inmate suicide and time spent in special disciplinary housing in New York State prison. Psychiatr Serv 58:558–560, 2007

White TW, Schimmel DJ, Frickey R: A comprehensive analysis of suicide in federal prisons: a fifteen-year review. J Correct Health Care 9:321–343, 2002

Winter M: County jail suicides in a midwestern state: moving beyond the use of profiles. Prison J 83:130–148, 2003

Clinical Management of Suicide Risk With Military and Veteran Personnel

Mark J. Bates, Ph.D.

John C. Bradley, M.D.

Nazanin Bahraini, Ph.D.

Matthew N. Goldenberg, M.D.

Since 2001, the United States has been continuously engaged in military conflicts around the world, most notably in Afghanistan and Iraq. As a consequence of Operation Enduring Freedom (OEF), Operation Iraqi Freedom (OIF), and Operation New Dawn (OND), over 6,000 American service members have lost their lives, and more than 32,000 have been physically wounded as of June 2011 (U.S. Department of Defense 2011). Over the course of the conflicts, the so-called invisible wounds of war—physi-

This material is the result of work supported by the Veterans Integrated Service Network 19 Mental Illness Research, Education and Clinical Center. The contents do not represent the views of the U.S. Department of Defense (DoD), U.S. Department of Veterans Affairs (VA), or the United States Government. In addition, all practices, programs, and products reviewed in this report are presented for critical review and are not officially endorsed by the DoD, VA, or United States Government. This chapter is in the public domain. Citation of the source of this product is appreciated.

    Lt. Col. Mark Oordt and Maj. Robert Vanecek provided subject matter expert feedback on the description of the *Air Force Guide for Managing Suicidal Behavior.* Col. Bob Ireland of the U.S. Air Force (retired) provided valuable inputs from his experience as former chair of the DoD Suicide Prevention and Risk Reduction Committee. Dr. Craig Bryan from the University of Texas Health Science Center and Dr. David Litts from the Suicide Prevention Resource Center provided valuable input about leveraging primary care. In addition, Ms. Kathleen Sun and Dr. Jeff Rhodes ensured final review, edits, and formatting.

cal, psychological, and behavioral disturbances, including traumatic brain injury (TBI) and posttraumatic stress disorder (PTSD)—among military personnel have gained increasing attention. Because of the escalating rates in the U.S. military, the media, the public, and military officials have also focused on another type of casualty—suicide. In response, the nation has advanced efforts to understand the factors that contribute to suicide and increase resources to prevent it. This information is relevant to all caregivers working with military members and veterans.

This chapter is designed as a practical guide to help prepare and support civilian caregivers working with service members and veterans who may be at increased suicide risk. The chapter provides a discussion of relevant military culture and practices, an overview of factors that contribute to suicide among military and veteran populations, and a list of resources for preventing suicide among service members and veterans. The chapter is also intended to complement the other chapters of this book, which offers a summary of empirically based practices and standards of care for the prevention and treatment of suicide and related behaviors.

Civilian Caregivers Working With Service Members: An Increasing Phenomenon

Civilian providers are in the position to provide critical support to military members and their families for two key reasons. The first is the limited availability of clinicians in the military health system. Because clinicians are primarily colocated with military installations, shortages may still exist in rural and remote locations, despite the rise in uniformed and civilian mental health staff hired by the military departments.

A second contributing factor to this trend is the increasing utilization of U.S. reserve forces, which include each state's National Guard. Reserve and National Guard members are uniquely vulnerable to the demands of deployment operations and possess unique medical needs. Since the First Gulf War, reservists have served much like their active duty counterparts, which is a cultural shift from previously serving primarily in stateside units for one weekend a month and 15 days of annual training a year. As of 2010, nearly half of the 1.2 million National Guard and Army Reserve members have been mobilized during OEF and OIF (Bonds et al. 2010). During this period, the reserve forces have faced challenges associated with availability of personnel, preparation for deployments, and adjustments during and after deployments (Griffith 2011). When reservists return to their civilian communities and occupations, they often do not enjoy the same preestablished and geographically colocated support structure as their active duty counterparts. Furthermore, they often turn to civilian caregivers for support.

Suicide Rates Among Military Personnel

Suicide rates among military personnel are broken down between active duty and veteran populations for two important reasons. First, it is not possible to compare the rates between these populations due to the samples used to derive the rates. The active duty rates are based on the overall population of the U.S. military. In contrast, the veteran rates are based on a sample of veterans who are patients in the U.S. Department of Veterans Affairs (VA) health care system. Second, as discussed later in this chapter, there are also significant organizational and cultural differences between these populations.

Suicide Rates Among Service Members

According to the U.S. Department of Defense (DoD) Task Force on the Prevention of Suicide (TFSP) report (U.S. Department of Defense 2010), more than 1,900 service members died by suicide from 2001 to 2009. The rate of suicide across the military has risen by approximately 50% over the decade, from 10.3 deaths per 100,000 service members in 2001 and 2002 to 18.4 in 2009. Every service branch has seen increasing numbers of suicides, but the rates and increases in rates have been higher in the Army and Marines than in the Navy and Air Force. The 2009 rate in the Marines was 22.3, up from 16.7 in 2001. In 2009, some 168 Army soldiers died by suicide, for an annual rate of 21.7, more than double the rate of 9.0 in 2001; the 2009 rate was the highest rate since the Army began maintaining data in 1980. Some experts have argued that these numbers may actually underestimate the number of military suicides by as much as 20% because of misclassification of some deaths as accidental (U.S. Department of Defense 2010).

Prior to its rise over the last decade, the rate of suicide in the military was historically lower than that in the general population, especially when adjusted for the fact that the military is predominantly male (and, thus, at a higher risk for completed suicide). This lower rate has been attributed to several factors, including the exclusion from initial enlistment and the medical discharge of people with significant mental illness. It has also been thought that the lower rate may be due to certain social factors associated with military service, including higher rates of employment (by definition, 100%) among military personnel and better access to health care (including mental health treatment), as well as the inherent social support provided by the military. Over the last decade, however, as the suicide rates in the military have climbed, the overall rate of suicide among the general U.S. population has been relatively steady at approximately 12 per 100,000. After adjustment for age, gender, and ethnicity differences in the military relative to those of the general population, the civilian and overall military rates are now roughly equal, and the rates in the Army and Marines have actually exceeded matched civilian rates for the last half decade.

Suicide Rates Among Veterans

Suicide among veterans has received much attention, yet studies of suicide rates among veterans have reported inconsistent findings. Methodological issues, and in particular variability in both design and subpopulations of veterans studied, often contribute to these inconsistencies. For example, as of September 2010, there were an estimated 22.7 million veterans of the U.S. armed forces. However, the majority of studies examining suicide rates among the veteran population have focused on samples of veterans utilizing services in the Veterans Health Administration (VHA) (Desai et al. 2005; Thompson et al. 2002). Further complicating the problem is that studies using VHA samples have often been limited to high-risk patient subgroups, such as those receiving treatment for depression or other outpatient mental health services, whereas few studies have examined rates for the entire VHA patient population (McCarthy et al. 2009). Given that only 25% of veterans seek any type of care at VA facilities, studies based solely on VHA samples, especially those that focus on specific high-risk subgroups of VHA patients, may overestimate the risk of veteran suicide (U.S. Department of Veterans Affairs 2001). Moreover, such sampling issues provide a limited understanding of suicide rates and risk factors among veterans in the general population (Kaplan et al. 2007).

Although the true incidence of suicide among veterans is unknown, a number of recent studies highlight the burden of suicide in both the general veteran population and those seeking VHA care. In a prospective population-based study of suicide in male veterans, Kaplan et al. (2007) found that veterans were twice as likely to die by suicide compared with nonveterans in the general population. Another study examining 2005 data from the National Violent Death Reporting System (NVDRS) identified 1,821 suicides among former or current military personnel. This constituted 20% of all suicides in the 16 states participating in the NVDRS that year (Karch et al. 2008). This study included both active duty military personnel and veterans, because the NVDRS currently does not provide information about each group separately. In a study examining suicide mortality among all veterans seeking VHA care, McCarthy et al. (2009) found suicide risk among VHA patients was 66% higher than that observed in the general population.

Risk and Protective Factors Among Service Members

Identifying risk and protective factors that are either unique to or particularly prevalent in military populations may be an important step toward curbing the recent rise in military suicides. Although facing some significant research challenges, such efforts are able to leverage some unique sources of data about factors that potentially contribute to suicides in the military. Also, despite the research challenges, several factors have been identified that may be related to increased suicide risk. The fac-

tors that are common among suicide completers and may contribute to suicide risk include demographic characteristics (e.g., gender, race, and age); having a psychiatric diagnosis, including PTSD, or a physical injury (including TBI); substance misuse; and psychosocial stressors such as relationship problems, financial troubles, and legal problems. Although there has been speculation that multiple deployments increase risk, such an association warrants further study.

Research Challenges and Data Sources

There are a number of research challenges when studying risk and protective factors in the military population. First, the low base rate makes it difficult to find statistically significant relationships because of the limited variance that is being predicted. Second, suicide completions appear to be driven by a combination of factors rather than a single factor, which further reduces the amount of variance that any single predictor is expected to explain. Third, it is difficult to statistically determine risk factors associated with suicides in the military because of the lack of adequate control data. For example, the data may show that most young adults who die by suicide were experiencing relationship problems, but it is not possible to figure out if the rate of relationship problems is statistically higher or lower than that of their peers who do not die by suicide. Finally, all of the current research is retrospective, which limits the conclusions that can be drawn.

The DoD has been able to leverage multiple sources of data to identify potential contributing factors. Four primary sources of data about factors that potentially contribute to suicide are the DoD Suicide Event Report (DoDSER), the Health-Related Behaviors Survey (HBRS), the Mental Health Advisory Team (MHAT), and the TFSP report. The DoDSER is the primary source of data about completed suicides in the military. This standardized reporting instrument, which is completed by an authorized person after nearly every suicide in the military, provides more then 250 data points about potential contributing factors. Data can also be pulled from the HBRS, which is a confidential, anonymous standardized survey that asks active duty service members about health-related behaviors. These behaviors range from substance use (including alcohol, cigarettes, illicit drugs, and prescription drugs), suicide attempts, mental well-being, deployment issues, fitness, nutrition, and weight management to other selected national health status goals from the Department of Health and Human Services' Healthy People 2010 objectives. In addition, the HBRS randomly selects service members from the Army, Navy, Marine Corps, Air Force, and Coast Guard who represent men and women in all pay grades of the active force throughout the world.

The MHAT is another data resource that provides theater-wide assessment of deployed service member mental health and well-being, examines the delivery of behavioral health care, and provides recommendations for sustainment and improvement. Specific topics include rates of psychological problems, combat exposure, barriers to care and stigma, marital problems, resilience, and suicide. Although the first six MHAT studies focused on Army service members, the most recent, seventh MHAT study also included a sample of Marine service members.

The TFSP report provides a comprehensive review of the DoD system for preventing suicides, which includes statistics about DoD suicides and risk factors. This task force report integrates data from the DoDSER, HBRS, MHAT, and Mortality Surveillance Division, Armed Forces Medical Examiner System (AFMES). The AFMES is responsible for the critical functions of determining suicide-implied intent in deaths of DoD members and the suicide rates based on the number of suicides in a given time period divided by the population at risk (in 100,000) during the same time period.

Demographic Factors

Demographic risk factors include male gender, younger age, and divorced marital status. The TFSP reported on the relationship between gender and suicide (U.S. Department of Defense 2010). As in the general population, males in the military are more likely than women to complete suicide. From 2005 through 2009, 94% of Army suicide victims were male, compared with just 86% of the Army population as a whole. The Navy had similar statistics; from 1999 through 2009, 95% of suicide victims were male, compared with 85% of the Navy population as a whole.

In the general population, older age is associated with higher rates of suicide, and suicide rates are particularly high among those over 65. However, the military as a whole is a younger cohort, and younger service members (ages 17–24) complete suicide at higher rates than their older counterparts (Kinn et al. 2011).

Being divorced is a risk factor among the military population. In DoDSER data from 2009, just over half of military suicides were completed by married service members. The suicide rate among married persons and never-married persons was roughly the same, but divorced individuals were nearly three times more likely to die by suicide (DoDSER 2009).

Mental Health and Substance Misuse

The role of mental illness in suicide has gained much attention. Some researchers estimate that greater than 90% of suicide completers meet criteria for at least one psychiatric disorder at the time of their death (Mann 2002). In contrast, military rates of mental health disorders among people who die by suicide are typically 50% or less. The TFSP reported that fewer than half (49%) of Army suicide victims had been given a mental health diagnosis at the time of their death, including adjustment disorders (25.9%), mood disorders (21.6%), and substance use disorders (18.2%) (U.S. Department of Defense 2010). Approximately 9% of Army suicide completers had been diagnosed with PTSD at the time of their death. Between 2008 and 2009, 29% of suicide victims in the Navy had a prior psychiatric history, and just 18% had a prior history of self-injury. Forty percent of Marines who died by suicide from 1999 through 2007 had a prior psychiatric history. In the Air Force, only 26% of suicide completers were engaged in mental health treatment at the time of their death.

Substance misuse, which is a known risk factor for suicidal behavior, is tracked in the general military population as well as in military suicide completions. Alcohol misuse is thought to be extremely common among combat veterans. DoD data reveal that 35% of completed suicides involved alcohol misuse or consumption at the time of the suicide. Absolute data on the prevalence of alcohol misuse, abuse, or dependence are significant, as reported in a recent DoD survey, in which 47% of members reported binge drinking, defined as five or more drinks on the same occasion at least once a week in the past 30 days (U.S. Department of Defense 2009). This same report revealed that scores on the Alcohol Use Disorders Identification Test (AUDIT) indicated that 25% of service members were drinking at hazardous levels (AUDIT scores 8–15) and 4% were drinking at harmful levels (AUDIT scores 16–19). About 5% had symptoms that could likely lead to alcohol dependence (AUDIT score 20 or higher). The rate of drinking at or above hazardous levels (AUDIT score 8 or higher) was 47% for the Marine Corps, which was significantly higher than the 36% for the Army, 31% for the Navy and Coast Guard, and 24% for the Air Force. More than a quarter of military personnel, however, frequently or sometimes used alcohol to cope with stress. More males than females reported using alcohol (35% vs. 25%) as a coping behavior.

Psychosocial Stressors

Suicide has been associated with stressful life events; identifying and modifying psychosocial stressors may help reduce rates. Common stressors among military personnel are separation from family, relationship problems such as marital discord and divorce, multiple deployments, difficult work environments, and financial troubles. Among Navy sailors who died by suicide, almost 60% had relationship problems, 35% had legal difficulties, 31% had physical health problems, and 16% had financial troubles. Marines showed similar related stressors: relationship problems could be identified in 53% of suicides, work problems in 50%, legal or disciplinary problems in 43%, physical health problems in 33%, and financial problems in 13%. In the Air Force, 307 airmen died by suicide between 2003 and 2009. Of those, 67% had relationship problems, 39% had legal problems, and 25% had financial problems. Deployment may have been a factor for some—19% had deployed in the previous year—but certainly not a majority, because

55% of Air Force suicides occurred among airmen who had never deployed. However, most people who confront stressful life events do not die by suicide, and the rates of exposure to these stressful life events among those who did not complete suicide are not known (U.S. Department of Defense 2010).

Firearms

Access to firearms is widely considered a risk factor for completed suicide, largely because of the lethality of the guns relative to other suicidal means such as overdose. In a military population, where access to and familiarity with firearms are prevalent, understanding the relationship between gun access and suicide may be particularly important. The DoDSERs for 2008 and 2009 indicate that firearms were used in a large number of suicides and that the rates vary depending on the location (deployed versus nondeployed) and access to weapons (military issued versus nonmilitary issued). Among service members who died by suicide during their deployment to OEF/OIF, almost all (DoD total 97%, $n=38$) used a military firearm to kill themselves. In contrast, for service members who died by suicide while not deployed, the most commonly reported method was a nonmilitary issue firearm (DoD total 47%, $n=121$).

High-Risk Behaviors

In the 2008 DoD Survey of Health-Related Behaviors Among Active Duty Military Personnel (U.S. Department of Defense 2009), risk taking was assessed to objectify the associated health-related behaviors. In 2008, 46% of all services personnel were classified as high risk–takers, and 78% were classified as high sensation-seekers. High risk–takers were substantially more likely than moderate risk– or low risk–takers to use illicit drugs, including prescription drug misuse (26% vs. 17% vs. 15%) and heavy alcohol use (29% vs. 13% vs. 6%). Rates of substance use among moderate risk–takers were also significantly higher than those for low risk–takers. High risk–takers also were more likely to have seriously considered suicide in the past year (6%) than moderate risk– or low risk–takers (both 3%). Risk-taking behaviors must be assessed to determine if they adapt or pose an unnecessary risk of intentional or unintentional harm.

Acquired Capability

The Interpersonal-Psychological Theory of Suicide (IPTS) is a novel explanatory model for suicidal behavior that has gained increasing attention in recent years (Figure 23–1). The theory posits that three factors are required for one to die by suicide: 1) feelings that one does not belong with other people, 2) feelings that one is a burden on others or society, and 3) an acquired capability to overcome the fear and pain associated with suicide (Joiner 2005). Selby et al. (2010) have examined military suicide using the IPTS and have hypothesized that military service may impact all three factors. These authors also proposed that a global sense of belonging to peers may provide the most protection against suicide, whereas perceived burdensomeness may be a primary contributor to suicidal ideation, especially for those wounded in combat. Likewise, perceived burdensomeness is conceptually associated with service members who have been expelled from service or demoted or who experience survivor guilt.

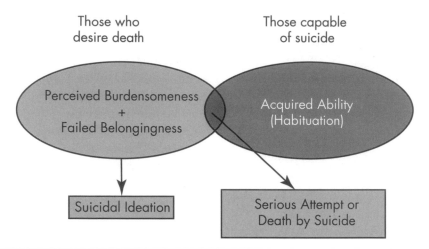

FIGURE 23–1. Interpersonal-Psychological Theory of Suicide.
Source. Adapted from Joiner 2005.

Stigma of Seeking Mental Health Care

Stigma about seeking mental health care may also contribute to suicide. Stigma has been identified as a significant threat to receiving care in the military by empirical studies (Hoge et al. 2004), operational studies (MHAT), and task force reports (e.g., TFSP report). Multiple sources of stigma have been identified. For example, because the military health system is responsible both for providing care for service members and for reporting when a service member's fitness for duty is jeopardized, service members may have a motive to limit sharing symptoms if they are concerned about possible impacts on their ability to do their job and/or stay in the military. There is also evidence that masculine values prevalent in the military can lead one to believe that in seeking help one may either be seen as weak by others or may perceive oneself as weak (Hoge et al. 2004). In addition, the collectivistic and masculine values in the military can contribute to stigma about mental health issues and help-seeking behavior.

The value of collectivism can be associated with service members' avoiding seeking help because of the impact on the unit, either taking time away from supporting the unit or possibly being pulled out of the unit.

Risk and Protective Factors Among Veterans

A number of risk factors increase the likelihood of veterans engaging in suicidal behavior. Specific factors that may elevate suicide risk include exposure to combat-related trauma, combat-related guilt, significant physical injuries, and multiple deployments. Nevertheless, it should also be noted that significant numbers of suicide deaths occur among veterans who have never been deployed. In addition, many veterans have ready access to firearms, which are used in the majority of suicide deaths. Homeless and incarcerated veterans may be at higher risk. Similar to trends found in the general population, factors such as prior suicide attempts; mental illness, including depression, PTSD, TBI, and comorbid conditions; and substance use have also been shown to elevate risk for suicide in the veteran population.

Demographic Factors

One of the most consistent findings in the literature is that male gender is associated with an increased risk of completed suicide. Given that the vast majority of veterans are males (92%; U.S. Department of Veterans Affairs 2007), the predominance of male gender increases the risk of suicide for veterans as a group compared with the general population, which is about half male. According to 2005 data from the NVDRS, nearly 97% of the veterans who died by suicide in the 16 participating states were male (Karch et al. 2008). A retrospective cohort study of 807,694 veterans receiving treatment for depression revealed that suicide rates per 100,000 person-years were more than three times higher among men than women (89.58 vs. 28.92, respectively) (Zivin et al. 2007). Other demographic risk factors for suicide among veterans include age, race, and marital status. For example, Kaplan et al. (2007) showed that compared with nonveterans who died by suicide, veteran suicide decedents were significantly more likely to be older, white, and high school graduates, and less likely to have never been married.

Mental Disorders

The presence of any psychiatric disorder has been consistently shown to increase risk for suicide among both the general population and veterans. Among veterans, completed suicide is usually associated with a mental disorder, most often depressive disorders and alcohol or other substance use disorders (Zivin et al. 2007). Ilgen et al. (2010) found that among all patients who used the VHA service in 1999, a total of 7,684 died by suicide in the following 7 years. Of those who died by suicide, nearly 47% had a psychiatric diagnosis; the most common diagnostic categories were depression (31.2%) and substance use disorders (21.3%) (Ilgen et al. 2010).

PTSD constitutes another suicide risk factor among veterans. Much debate surrounds the reasons for increased suicide risk in trauma survivors. Some studies suggest that suicide risk is higher due to the symptoms of PTSD (Amir et al. 1999; Bell and Nye 2007), yet others indicate that suicide risk is higher in those with PTSD due to comorbid psychiatric conditions, such as depression (Fontana and Rosenheck 1995). A study analyzing data from the National Comorbidity Survey, a nationally representative sample, revealed that PTSD alone was significantly associated with suicidal ideation or attempts after controlling for comorbid disorders (Sareen et al. 2005).

Combat veterans are a population shown to have an elevated risk for both PTSD (Kulka et al. 1990) and suicide (Bullman and Kang 1996). Several studies have also shown that veterans with chronic PTSD have an increased risk for both suicide attempts and completed suicide compared with both veterans without PTSD and the general population (Bullman and Kang 1994; Kramer et al. 1994). In a mixed sample of PTSD patients, high levels of intrusion significantly predicted suicide risk (Amir et al. 1999). In a sample of Vietnam combat veterans, Bell and Nye (2007) showed that reexperiencing symptoms significantly predicted severity of suicidal ideation. The authors proposed that suicidal thoughts may serve as a way to reduce or escape intolerable distress associated with intrusive symptoms. Hendin and Hass (1991) found that among veterans with combat-related PTSD, the most significant predictor of both suicide attempts and preoccupation with suicide is combat-related guilt.

Physical Injuries

Studies of suicide risk among veterans have shown a relationship between physical injuries and suicide. Among veterans who experienced combat trauma, the highest relative suicide risk is observed in those who were wounded multiple times and/or hospitalized for a wound (Bullman and Kang 1996), with the former indicating the highest risk for suicide.

Compared with the general population, patients with TBIs are at higher risk for suicidal ideation (Simpson and Tate 2002), suicide attempts (Silver et al. 2001), and suicide completions (Teasdale and Engberg 2001). Among veterans with a history of TBI, Brenner et al. (2009) identified numerous precipitating factors for suicidality, including feelings of loss due to role changes, newly experienced difficulties in cognitive functioning, and recently developed emotional and psychiatric difficulties.

Firearms

Consistent with empirical evidence linking suicide risk with the presence of firearms in the home in the United States (Kellermann et al. 1992; Miller and Hemenway 1999), possession of firearms appears to be increased in at least some subgroups of veterans, particularly combat veterans (Lambert and Fowler 1997). A study by Kaplan et al. (2007) found that veteran decedents of suicide were significantly more likely to have died using a firearm compared with nonveteran decedents of suicide. In addition, combat veterans, who are often highly trained and experienced in the use of firearms, can report feeling more secure and in control with a gun (Lambert and Fowler 1997).

Homelessness

Finding adequate, affordable housing has proven to be a burden for many veterans transitioning from active duty. Permanent housing is one of the most reported unmet needs of veterans (U.S. Interagency Council on Homelessness 2010). Approximately 10% of all people in the United States who experienced homelessness over the year identified themselves as veterans (U.S. Department of Housing and Urban Development 2010, 2011). The proportion of veterans among homeless male Americans is greater than the proportion in the general population (Rosenheck et al. 1994). Veterans constitute just under 8% of the total U.S. population, yet they account for 12% of the total homeless population (and 16% of homeless adults) on any given night.

The homeless population shares common risk factors with the general population. These risk factors include presence of psychiatric disorder (Benda 2003; Desai et al. 2003; Eynan et al. 2002), substance abuse history (Benda 2003; Desai et al. 2003; Rodell et al. 2003), and history of physical or sexual trauma (Benda 2003; Desai et al. 2003; Rodell et al. 2003). However, despite the overlap in homelessness and suicide risk factors, there is limited research and evidence about suicidal ideation and attempts among homeless adults. Benda (2003) found that longer periods of homelessness among adults are associated with suicidal ideation. A study in Los Angeles County revealed that 22% of homeless adults surveyed had attempted suicide during their lifetime, and 25% reported experiencing suicidal ideation during the past year (Gelberg et al. 1988).

Legal Problems and Incarceration

Incarceration is another outcome with adverse consequences for returning veterans.

Incarcerated veterans may be at particularly high risk for suicide (Wortzel et al. 2009). Although little is known about the suicide rates among incarcerated veterans, it is known that incarcerated veterans sit at the intersection between two populations—veterans and the imprisoned—for which elevated suicide risk has been well established (Wortzel et al. 2009). A number of similarities between the population of incarcerated veterans and those who are most likely to engage in suicidal behavior while incarcerated exist. Blaauw et al. (2005) identified several factors associated with suicide among the incarcerated: age 40 years or over, homelessness, history of psychiatric illness, history of substance abuse, and one prior incarceration and arrest or conviction for a violent offence. These characteristics, along with impulsivity and hostility (Mann et al. 1999; Renaud et al. 2008), are common among veterans who have been incarcerated (Wortzel et al. 2009).

Unemployment

Unemployment has been directly and indirectly linked to suicide risk. Stressors such as the loss of a job and financial distress can result in shame or despair, which can precipitate suicide attempts in those who are already at high risk or do not have adequate resources to cope with such adversities (Suicide Prevention Resource Center 2008). In addition, unemployment is associated with depression and substance abuse problems, both of which are independently linked to suicide risk (Suicide Prevention Resource Center 2008). Prolonged unemployment, in particular, has been shown to be a significant risk factor for both suicidal ideation and suicide attempts (Fergusson et al. 2007).

The return to civilian life for service members deployed in Iraq and Afghanistan is full of challenges, and unemployment continues to be a growing concern for this cohort. For Iraq- and Afghanistan-era veterans, many of whom are entering or reentering the job market after overseas deployments, the unemployment rate during 2010 and 2011 was consistently higher than the national average (U.S. Department of Labor 2011). It is estimated that unemployment rates among OEF/OIF veterans will continue to increase as more service members return home from overseas missions in the Middle East. Unemployment can be a significant source of distress for service members, who are likely already facing myriad challenges and psychosocial stressors as they transition to civilian life. Social isolation and exclusion from activities and routines arising from a lack of resources further contribute to the stress caused by job loss and further increase the risk of depression and subsequent suicide. For service members and veterans, the sense of burdensomeness that may arise due to difficulties providing for one's family may also increase risk for suicidal behavior, particularly when accompanied by other risk factors such as TBI and psychiatric illness.

Protective Factors

Protective factors tend to enhance resilience and may serve to counterbalance risk factors and reduce the likelihood of suicide. Protective factors include effective clinical care for mental, physical, and substance use disorders; easy access to a variety of clinical interventions and help-seeking support; restricted access to highly lethal means; strong connections to family and community support; support through ongoing medical and mental health care relationships; skills in problem solving and conflict resolution; and cultural and religious beliefs that discourage suicide and support self-preservation. Specific protective factors for veterans include camaraderie with other veterans, treatment for PTSD and depression, restricted access to guns/weapons, and increased social support. Veterans with a service-connected disability may have reduced suicide risks as a result of their greater access to VA health services and regular compensation payments that bolster and stabilize their overall income. Zivin et al. (2007) found that service connection (i.e., compensation benefits for an in-service injury) was a protective factor for suicide among veterans seeking VHA care. Desai et al. (2005) found a similar protective effect of service connection among patients who had been discharged from psychiatric inpatient units.

Military Culture

Culture has been defined by Fiske and colleagues (1998), as cited by the American Psychological Association (2003, p. 380) multicultural guidelines, as "the belief systems and value orientations that influence customs, norms, practices, and social institutions, including psychological processes (language, caretaking practices, media, educational systems) and organizations (media, educational systems)." Members of the U.S. military hail from a diverse set of geographic, ethnic, and cultural backgrounds. By enlisting or being commissioned in the military, they join an organization with its own predominant culture and subcultures. A provider's understanding and appreciation of the general military culture as well as various subcultures to which a service member ascribes may be an important component of building and maintaining an effective therapeutic relationship. The un-

derlying values in military culture can be understood by using the same dimensions that have been applied across national and organizational cultures. One such well-researched system is Hofstede's cultural value dimensions of individualism-collectivism, power distance, uncertainty avoidance, masculinity-femininity, and long- versus short-term orientation (Taras et al. 2010).

Individualism Versus Collectivism

The military favors a collectivistic orientation, which is defined as a preference for acting as part of a group instead of acting individually. Teamwork and unit cohesion are seen as critical to mission success. In addition, many features in the military are designed to reinforce conformity. These features include the standardization of appearance through the wearing of uniforms and through rules about hair length and body piercings. Standardized professional customs, courtesies, and rituals, including awards that focus on unit performance as opposed to individual awards, encourage a collectivistic mind-set.

Power Distance

The military has a high power distance, defined as an unequal distribution of power among its members. The military rank system is a primary example of power distance. A primary distinction in the rank system is between enlisted members and officers. Enlisted members can join the military without a college education, whereas officers must have at the minimum a four-year bachelor's degree. In addition, enlisted members can specialize in specific career fields. In contrast, officers are less focused on specialization and more focused on overall management and leadership responsibilities. Power distance is also exemplified by the enlisted and officer rank structures across the services. The services have the same levels (pay grades) for enlisted members and officers, but the names for the ranks associated with these pay grades can be different. Both the officer and enlisted rank scales are composed of a series of ranks or pay grades from O1 to O10 for officer ranks and from E1 to E9 for enlisted ranks. These ranks represent entry at a basic entry level and the potential to be promoted for increasing levels of responsibility and authority. Along with official organizational positions, a person's rank determines who is subordinate to whom. Although the services have different names for some of these ranks, the services share the same basic series, and the customs and courtesies afforded to senior ranks apply across services. The DoD has the following Web sites that show the pay grades, ranks, and insignias across the services:

Enlisted—www.defense.gov/about/
insignias/enlisted.aspx
Officer—www.defense.gov/about/
insignias/officers.aspx

Military organizational structures and processes also emphasize power distance. Military organizations are hierarchically organized with explicit chains of command that describe the lines of authority and responsibility, along which orders are passed. This hierarchical structure is seen as essential for effective and efficient command and control functions for commanders at all levels. The system relies on attention to the power structure and adherence to orders. The power structure describes "who outranks whom," accountability of subordinates to execute orders, accountability of leadership for the consequences of orders, rules about how feedback is transmitted in

the hierarchy, and standardized language and terminology. Examples of customs and courtesies are calling higher-ranking officers "Sir" or "Ma'am" and saluting higher-ranking officers. In addition, military organizational effectiveness is dependent on obedience to lawful orders. From entry into service, military members are taught to obey, immediately and without question, orders from people who outrank them. Likewise, those who fail to obey the lawful orders of their superiors risk serious consequences, which can range from informal to formal judicial punishments.

Uncertainty Avoidance

The military value system favors high uncertainty avoidance or a general intolerance for ambiguity. Strict adherence to rules helps manage and reduce uncertainty and risk. The low tolerance for unnecessary risk is exemplified by the careful risk management practices that are common in planning, preparing, and executing operational missions and everyday tasks. However, it is important to note that uncertainty avoidance does not necessarily mean risk avoidance as much as being "associated with preferences for clear rules and guidance" (Hofstede 2001).

Masculinity-Femininity

The distinction between masculine and feminine is based on a broad abstract conceptualization as opposed to traditional genders. Masculine cultures are characterized as more aggressive and competitive, whereas feminine cultures involve greater focus on quality of life and relationships. The military is generally characterized as a more masculine and assertive culture, as opposed to a more feminine culture focused on creating a friendly and cooperative environment. Key features of military culture associated with masculine values include the warrior ethos, task and performance focus, and acceptance of high-risk behaviors. However, there are also elements of military culture that would be classified as more feminine, such as emphases on teamwork, mutual support, and mentorship.

The tenets of the warrior ethos include different aspects of commitment to fellow service members and the unit: mission first, never accept defeat, never quit, and never leave a fallen comrade (Riccio et al. 2004). In addition, seven key attributes conceptually cut across the four tenets of the warrior ethos. These attributes are 1) perseverance, 2) ability to set priorities, 3) ability to make trade-offs, 4) ability to adapt, 5) ability to accept responsibility for others, 6) ability to accept dependence on others, and 7) motivation by a higher calling, which also relates to different cultural domains (Riccio et al. 2004). These tenets and attributes reflect values related to self-discipline and physical, moral, and spiritual strength and courage.

Performance orientation is manifest in many aspects of military activities. For example, a series of training programs start from accession and focus on developing military professional and job-specific skills. Additionally, most military activities involve a systematic plan-do-check-act type of sequence. Examples include the mission planning that is conducted before a mission to ensure clear goals and roles, as well as the after-action analysis conducted after a mission to assess success and identify learning opportunities for future missions.

Many military activities involve increased risks in both operations and training for those operations. These activities encompass conventional and asymmetrical combat, peacekeeping, search and rescue missions, and specialties such as infantry, pilots, and explosive ordnance disposal.

Furthermore, the operational tempo may be very quick, may involve high rates of information flow and ambiguity, and may rely heavily on the effectiveness of personnel and unit training, team functioning, and communication and coordination among teams and units.

Long- Versus Short-Term Orientation

Values associated with long-term orientation include persistence, thrift, and willingness to subordinate oneself for a purpose. In contrast, values related to a short-term orientation include preference for quick results and concern for fulfilling social obligations and saving face (Hofstede and Bond 1988). The military favors a long-term orientation but also integrates values from short-term orientation. This may be best reflected in how the military plans, coordinates, and conducts activities on three levels: strategic, operational, and tactical. The strategic view, which is set by the senior leaders and guides the overall activities of the military, is associated with long-term orientation. In contrast, the tactical level, which is carried out by operational units, is more short-term oriented and is concerned with swift and efficient execution of missions and tasks. In addition, most military activities involve taking time to learn from processes to update goals and tactics.

Subgroup Differences

Service members' varying values are also associated with various subgroup memberships. These subgroups include service branch and component, rank, and occupation. It is essential that a clinician consider that, as in working with anyone from a different culture, a person's level of acculturation and within-group differences may be as important as or more important than the general characteristics of the cultural group.

Services comprise the Army, Navy, Marines, and Air Force. In contrast, the components are the active duty, reserve, and National Guard forces, which can belong to different services. Each service has different identities that are associated with its primary missions, history, and traditions. The service missions are generally associated with land, sea, and air: amphibious operations (Marines), maritime operations (Navy), land operations (Army), and air operations (Air Force). However, the services also have overlapping roles in many of these areas.

As described previously, the military has two separate rank scales: officer and enlisted. The distinction between officers and enlisted members is considered important for preserving order and discipline. The services all have anti-fraternization policies that prohibit personal and business relationships between officers and enlisted ranks. The emphasis on recognizing differences in ranks and anti-fraternization leads to subcultures associated with groups sharing the same rank.

In addition, every person in the military is assigned to at least one occupational specialty or career field. These occupational specialties can encompass such diverse fields as administration, infantry, aviation, explosive ordnance disposal (bomb disposal), security forces (military police), medicine, and chaplaincy, to name a few examples. Each career field tends to develop a unique group identity and common culture.

Service Member Stages and Transitions

To more fully understand the unique culture and stressors inherent in military ser-

vice, the clinician should become familiar with a variety of standard transition phases experienced by military members, starting with the acculturation process by which a civilian becomes a member of the armed forces. The transformation that occurs is inherently and uniquely stressful. The aim of this process is to shape many of the attitudes and beliefs of the new recruit into conformity with the ideals of military service and to enhance the sense of belonging to a special subculture. This subculture is one in which the group is valued more than the individual, and the individual, in order to be valued and accepted by the group, is prepared to protect other members with his or her life in service of the mission objectives. This evolution of attitudes and beliefs reinforces a sense of trust, security, and connectedness among all members. Although the unit cohesion that results is designed to enhance survivability on the battlefield, it also has the benefit of being a significant protective factor against isolation, despair, and suicide. External stressors are necessary to form these bonds. These stressors include separation from friends, families, and loved ones; extraordinary physical demands; and real and simulated threats to safety. Adaptation to the stressors associated with basic training forms the foundation of warrior resilience and can best be thought of as a form of stress inoculation training.

Entry Into Service

The clinician should also realize the significant preselection bias associated with military recruits. Contrary to common assumptions, candidates for military service are among the more resilient and healthy members of their peer group, the lowest quartile of whom are automatically excluded from eligibility due to substance abuse, mental illness, poor health, obesity, and poor aptitude. The remainder of the eligible population is generally healthy, athletic, motivated, and prepared to accept the moral code of military service. These candidates frequently come from families with a history of military service.

Accession and Basic Training

Each military service is responsible for the recruitment, induction, and initial training of its members. The Army, Marine Corps, Navy, Air Force, and Coast Guard all have unique missions, skills, and needs. They all recruit from the same population but, because of their different missions and cultures, attract recruits with different interests. The unique missions for each service also dictate differing basic training goals. One unifying principle, however, is the need to develop service members imbued with the values of military service. This type of values-based training forms the foundation for thoughts, feelings, and behaviors for all service members and develops resilience and cohesion among service members. The skills that are developed in this environment are reinforced by a sense of purpose and belonging. The Marine Corps, for example, uses values-based training to create Marines with a strong set of core values whose sound judgment facilitates ethical decision making during highly complex situations under duress. The mental toughness developed, as guided by a moral compass, is in many ways protective against suicide.

The transformation process of basic training is deliberate and thoughtful. It begins with the recruiter, who, when working with an interested candidate, reflects the values of the particular service and educates the candidate and his or her family about the service culture, opportunities,

and initial training. This is often idealized to serve the aspirations of the potential recruit. The candidate begins the process of identifying with his or her chosen branch of service. Additional screening, including aptitude testing, background checks, and a medical examination, is performed. Upon successful screening, the recruit prepares to report to basic training. Upon arrival at the induction center, the recruit is deliberately separated from family and friends. This is usually performed under an intimidating barrage of stimuli intended to overwhelm the senses and begin to shape group cohesion. The individual identity is stripped through the relinquishment of personal property, clothing, hair, and individual behaviors. Group identity and values are forged through the issuance of uniforms, a new language, and the new communal living environment stripped of privacy. Training is performed to build the core competencies of the service; enhance the individual's mental, physical, and spiritual readiness; develop character and discipline; foster esprit de corps; and teach military culture and basic combat skills.

When negotiated successfully, developmental hurdles associated with basic training build strength and confidence. These hurdles can be obstacles for some and precipitate a suicidal crisis. Whether from homesickness or failure to achieve the goals and standards of the peer group, the loss of one's sense of purpose and place can be devastating to the individual. The recruit training anticipates this potential and is prepared to respond, first through peer support and cohesion, then through leadership, and finally through medical and psychological intervention.

One unfortunate part of military culture, reinforced in basic training, is that failure or weakness is not well tolerated. The culture fosters stoicism (Sherman 2005) and the attitude that hardship is to be expected and that the ideal warrior endures hardship without acknowledging or revealing discomfort or distress. When an individual is struggling with a developmental hurdle, individual task, or collective goal, and he or she becomes despondent or suicidal, the group often interprets this as weakness or lack of discipline or moral courage. The perception of peers and leaders regarding this crisis often lacks empathy and assumes the individual is quitting on himself or herself and his or her comrades. This assumption not infrequently leads to a belief that the person is malingering to avoid the rigors of training and is often followed with contempt, further isolating the suffering individual and increasing his or her risk for suicidal behavior. The clinician can easily fall into these assumptions as well but should be reminded that the individual in crisis is mobilizing the full extent of his or her psychological defenses and problem-solving skills. The suicidal crisis should be treated as the inability to employ a more adaptive strategy in the face of the current crisis. Clinical interventions focused on coping, problem solving, and interpersonal efficacy are the most useful to the individual, peers, and unit leaders. Rarely is a major psychiatric illness precipitated in this environment, but if present, it should be treated aggressively. When the individual is not able to recover through treatment and psychosocial support, he or she is administratively separated from the service, generally under an entry level separation or for failure to adapt to the military.

As the recruit becomes transformed into a full-fledged member of the service, numerous culture-sanctioned rites of passage are performed. These rites continue to forge identity and cohesion, enhance self-efficacy, and instill pride. This transformation is evident to anyone who witnesses a graduation ceremony at basic training: the service member is ready for specialized training.

Transitions Between Duty Stations

Relocation is an inherent part of military life, from leaving home for basic training and changing duty stations to deploying to and returning from combat. Military members must become accustomed to uprooting and reestablishing themselves in new environments. For many, this can be an exciting part of military life; for others, it is a unique stressor. On average, a service member can expect to be reassigned every 3 years. In the current operational environment, one can expect to deploy every 2–3 years for 6–12 months. The transitions, when taken together, can engender great strain for service members and their families. Recent data from the Army Suicide Prevention Task Force (U.S. Department of Defense 2010) reveal that a significant proportion of suicides occur within months of a transition. With the existing support systems of the former unit, friends, and family significantly strained, the individual becomes at risk for isolation and loss of connectedness. The new environment is naturally ill-equipped to recognize any changes from baseline for the new member, and the new member has not yet formed the social bonds that would otherwise be protective.

Deployment Cycle, Including Reintegration

The military services take great pains to prepare members for deployment to combat and to protect them from the risks associated with deployment. The DoD has learned over the past 236 years that war has both physical and mental risks; more recently, it has acknowledged risks to families and children as well. Over time, the services have employed various strategies to deal with these risks, from efforts to eliminate the most vulnerable through prescreening to the public health model in practice today. Recognizing the inherent risks to health and welfare associated with deployment to combat, the DoD has developed a robust system of population health measures to enhance wellness and protective factors (i.e., primary prevention) and also a system of screening populations at risk to identify people in need of early intervention (i.e., secondary prevention). When individuals are identified with illness, aggressive treatment is provided to restore them to health and readiness (i.e., tertiary prevention).

Many troops and families describe the return from deployment as more stressful than combat. During deployment, the rules of engagement are relatively straightforward, and the mission is clear and distractions are minimal. At home, reintegration with friends and family who have not shared the service member's experience, cannot relate to the service member's residual affective intensity, and may resent his or her deployment and return can pose certain challenges. Families become desynchronized and learn new adaptive patterns in the absence of their service member. The service member often behaves as if on vacation and may try to make up for lost time by drinking and seeking high-intensity experiences. Families often have difficulty relating to this behavior, and misunderstanding and stress result, sometimes leading to separation and divorce. Apart from the risk of death, the single greatest stressor for service members across the deployment cycle is the high potential for relationship failure. The vast majority of completed suicides while deployed or at home are related to the recent breakup of a relationship.

Service Member Health Screening

The DoD has developed a robust public health model to optimize the health of service members across the deployment life cycle. This model relies heavily on primary prevention by fostering health and wellness through physical training, ready access to health care, and health screening. The DoD performs universal screening for common illnesses across the life cycle of a service member's career as well as indicated screening for high-risk conditions at specified times.

Periodic Health Assessment

The DoD has mandated that all service members have routine biannual health screening that includes mental health issues through what is called Periodic Health Assessment. Using a two-question screen, this assessment screens for physical ailments, substance use, and depression. Figure 23–2 is an example of a question in the assessment (Post-deployment Health Re-Assessment DD Form 2900).

These questions are rated in terms of frequency, and a positive screening is followed by a more in-depth screening using the Patient Health Questionnaire–9 (PHQ-9). The PHQ-9 is a well-validated depression screen designed for primary care settings and essentially is a symptom checklist for the symptoms of a major depressive episode. It asks questions about the DSM-IV-TR symptoms associated with depressive episodes (e.g., "Over the last 2 weeks, how

14. Over the PAST MONTH, have you been bothered by the following problems?	Not at all	Few or several days	More than half the days	Nearly every day
a. Little interest or pleasure in doing things	O	O	O	O
b. Feeling down, depressed, or hopeless	O	O	O	O

FIGURE 23–2. Sample postdeployment question from the Post-Deployment Health Re-Assessment form.

often have you been bothered by [little interest or pleasure, feeling depressed, etc.?"]. Positive screening leads to follow-up with a specialist for definitive care.

Predeployment Health Assessment

Prior to deployment, time-focused screening is conducted with the Pre-Deployment Health Assessment using DD Form 2795. The purpose of this screening is twofold: to identify conditions in need of continued treatment during deployment and to identify members with conditions that would disqualify them for deployment in order to protect their health and maximize their unit's readiness. This assessment simply inquires about any mental health care within the past year and further assesses whether the behavioral health condition has been stabilized for at least 90 days prior to granting approval for deployment. One recent study reported a high degree of success in managing the majority of mental health issues on deployment through the early identification of patients and aggressive care coordination of those screened to be at risk by the unit's mental health assets in the combat theater (Warner et al. 2011).

Postdeployment Health Assessment and Reassessment

Upon return from deployment, service members are screened using the Post-Deployment Health Assessment (PDHA) (DD Form 2796) to screen for exposures to various health risks, including brain injury, psychological trauma (4-question screen), depression (2-question screen described previously), and alcohol abuse (5-question screen). This is for population surveillance as well as case finding and specialty referral. It has long been understood that redeploying troops underreport symptomatology on this screening. Hypotheses include fear that an identified health concern will delay reunion with loved ones or furlough, or simply that in the immediate aftermath of a deployment, symptoms either are not present or are not considered significant. Therefore, troops are evaluated after 3–6 months at home using the Post-Deployment Health Re-Assessment (DD Form 2900). This screening evaluates the same domains as the PDHA, with the addition of screening for domestic conflict and a specific suicide risk assessment using a two question screening instrument described previously. The most up-to-date versions of these forms and protocols can be reviewed on the Deployment Health Clinical Center's Web site (www.pdhealth.mil).

Separation and Transition to VA

Upon completion of the term of enlistment, administrative separation, or medical retirement, service members are eligible for veterans' benefits, which include health care. VA has greatly improved access to health care benefits for all service members discharged under honorable (or general) conditions within 2 years of leaving active service. There is no requirement within this time frame for establishment of a service-connected disability to receive care. This policy has greatly reduced the bureaucratic hurdles of VA enrollment and provided a bridge to continuity of care. This is especially important for the veteran suffering a suicidal crisis. It is not known what risk is imparted in the transition from active to civilian service. With no clear responsibility for tracking the outcomes for individuals in this interim status between release from active duty and official enrollment as a VA beneficiary, one can often only retrospectively include any suicide that occurred in this time frame in the suicide data collected by VA. Because local jurisdictions determine the manner of death in these cases, without any standardization or superseding organizing policy, the estimation of risk and, more importantly, the targeted intervention of any particular risks associated with this important life transition for service members can be impossible.

Entry Into VA

Eligibility for VA health care is dependent upon a number of variables, which may influence the final determination of the services for which veterans qualify. These factors include the nature of a veteran's discharge from military service (e.g., honorable, other than honorable, dishonorable), length of service, VA-adjudicated disabilities (commonly referred to as service-connected disabilities), income level, and available VA resources, among others. Generally, a veteran must be enrolled in the VA health care system to receive benefits offered in the medical benefits package. Enrollment for VA health care benefits requires completion of an application. It is VHA policy that veterans enroll once into VA's health care system and be continuously enrolled. Enrolled veterans may seek care at any VA facility without being required or requested to reestablish eligibility for VA health care enrollment purposes.

DoD Prevention and Management of Suicidal Behavior

The DoD's prevention and management strategies generally address the same issues as in the civilian population, leverage the same empirically based approaches, and emphasize coordination of resources (e.g., chain of command, primary care, and community resources). There are numerous military-specific considerations, practices, and resources that can help inform civilian providers working with military members. These areas include command consultation, reporting requirements and confidentiality, fitness for duty, increasing access and decreasing stigma, prescriptions management, weapons management, and managing high-risk behaviors. In addition, the military practice areas that overlap civilian practice can also inform civilian providers about potential resources. These areas include primary care coordination, clinical guidance, and resources for providers, service members, family members, and leaders.

Command Consultation

Command consultation has been defined as the "process of providing expert mental health advice to commanders on matters affecting the mental health and performance of military personnel, usually in the context of their military organization" (McCarroll et al. 1994). Command consultation can focus on a wide range of organization-related issues, such as risk of harm to self and others, substance abuse, family maltreatment, operational stress, disaster response, and broad community needs assessment, health promotion, and prevention. Therefore, command consultation can both directly and indirectly impact suicide risks.

There are multiple potential benefits of command consultation if the civilian provider can arrange a release from the service member to work with a person in the service member's command. First, the command can provide a range of practical support. Practical support can include arranging alternative lodging, providing continual monitoring and regular check-ins, implementing orders that restrict destructive activities, and facilitating support through medical services, community services, work activities (structure, play to strengths, emphasize value to unit), and even leisure activities (provide structure and reinforcement) to restore as much confidence and balance as possible. Second, the chain of command can also provide important collateral information about the service member's current and past functioning, resources, psychosocial stressors, and other potential challenges to effective treatment. Lastly, collaboration with the chain of command can help support leader roles and avoid splitting from this resource for the service member.

It is also important that the civilian provider know about how to engage in a command consultant role of engaging with military leadership, which is ultimately oriented toward improving the unit's capability to carry out its mission. As recognized by the DoD Task Force on the Prevention of Suicide (U.S. Department of Defense 2010, p. 80),

> Practitioners are largely unaware of military-specific considerations (e.g., the importance of command consultation and other collateral contacts) in completing a thorough risk assessment and treatment plan. Often, the default disposition is to hospitalize the patient in a local civilian psychiatric ward with little or no coordination with the service member's unit. The task force also recommended that all caregivers be trained in the governing rules applicable to appropriate and necessary information sharing among providers, outside agencies, and with service members' commands.

Each Service has a Leader's Guide for Managing Personnel in Distress that is available online and provides excellent insight into key questions and resources that military leadership wishes to address. These guides provide practical assessment tools and lists of resources and are Web-based for easy access and navigation. In addition, they cover the same wide range of topics that are addressed in other forms of command consultation. These topics include suicide risk and management, workplace violence, family maltreatment, financial problems, and legal problems. The format is a list of issues that include general information about the potential problem area, risk factors, barriers for seeking help, and ways to prevent the problem from occurring in the future. Menu options indicate how to assess a specific problem and identify appropriate resources.

Reporting Requirements and Confidentiality

Military medical providers have a unique responsibility to protect national security, which can result in a tension with standard medical confidentiality practices (American Psychological Association 2005). The medical role of military health care providers is to treat the individual patient *and* to report fitness issues that jeopardize military readiness and/or national security. Military providers typically manage this tension by being very proactive and explicit about the limits of confidentiality, starting with obtaining informed consent before initiating therapy, which can include reeducating the patient when it appears that a mandatory reporting issue could possibly be reported. Military medical providers also typically advise patients that the only military caregivers who can provide complete confidentiality are military chaplains. Also, in the event that a condition exists that a provider is mandated to report, the provider takes precautions by discussing timing and manner with the patient and ensuring that the provider reports only the minimum necessary amount of information to fulfill the reporting requirements.

The reporting requirements generally include significant threats to health or safety or a threat to a military mission. The Health Insurance Portability and Accountability Act recognizes the unique nature of the military in our society and allows that a health care provider may "disclose information regarding individuals who are members of the Armed Forces for any activities deemed necessary by appropriate military command authorities to ensure the proper execution of military mission, broadly worded" (Casciotti 2007). There are also stricter reporting requirements if the person is performing sensitive duties.

These duties may include the presidential support mission, the personnel reliability program for those involved in nuclear weapons programs, and other highly classified (top secret and above) duties. Some key implications for civilian providers include understanding their reporting requirements, discussing confidentiality practices up front with service members, and exploring if the service member is filling a sensitive job.

Fitness for Duty

The primary roles of military medical providers are to provide medical services to service members and ensure the fitness for duty of service members for their line leaders and commanders. When any medical condition is identified by a clinician that limits a service member's ability to perform his or her duties, he or she is considered not fit for duty. It is then the duty of the clinician to report these limitations to the service member's commander and establish a plan to treat the service member to restore him or her to fitness. The concept of fitness for duty applies to physical as well as psychological conditions and is governed not only by common sense, but by service medical regulations as well. Treatable conditions often require temporary limitations and accommodations by the service member's commander. Consultation with the commander to define and gain support for the treatment limitations is critical to the success of any rehabilitation plan. In the event that a condition exists that is unlikely to be resolved within a reasonable amount of time (usually up to 1 year), the service member is referred for a disability retirement evaluation known as a Medical Evaluation Board.

Suicidal behaviors interfere with military readiness and can require a conference with line leadership for two reasons. First, suicidal behavior is a mandatory reporting issue, in which the provider is required to inform the commander of the impaired state of the person in order to ensure his or her safety. Second, suicidal behavior can also trigger provisional duty restrictions (a medical profile) as well as formal evaluations of a military member's ability to stay in a specific job, deploy, and remain in the service. In addition, other incidents that precipitate a Fitness for Duty or Command-Directed Mental Health Evaluation can lead to the identification of underlying suicidality. These incidents can include a pattern of interpersonal conflicts with coworkers or supervisors, insubordination, excessive use of sick call, substance abuse, and related incidents. The general standard for determining fitness is whether the medical condition precludes the member from reasonably performing the duties of his or her office, grade, rank, or rating (DoD Instruction 1332.38; U.S. Department of Defense 1996/2006).

The medical provider typically has deep personal concern for the service member and desires to ensure military readiness and to preserve a person's career if at all possible. However, the provider's ultimate duty is to ensure the military readiness of the unit, and thus he or she must make decisions that best support the military's mission.

A Fitness for Duty Evaluation provides a systematic and comprehensive assessment of the service member's current and future ability to perform his or her duties safely and effectively. Therefore, the evaluation predominantly focuses on the service member's functional level as opposed to diagnosis. This evaluation typically integrates information from three sources: collateral contacts, psychological testing, and clinical interviews. The evaluation process generally starts with a collection of collateral information, which can include personnel records (performance reports, memos documenting performance), medical records, and internal investigation reports. However, interviews with third parties (supervisors, peers, and family members) often follow the clinical interview, the next step in the evaluation process. The interview gives the service member an opportunity to describe the problems from his or her perspective and allows the examiner to obtain a psychosocial history and conduct a current mental status examination. An important part of the interview is addressing incongruencies and identifying the value of collateral interviews and psychological testing. Psychological testing can be used as a third part of the evaluation process to assess distress and impairment, personality factors, and cognitive ability. It can add further objectivity, comprehensiveness, and defensibility to the process (Fischler 2001).

Along with evaluating if a psychological issue exists and associated impairment, the Fitness for Duty Evaluation also considers potential confounding issues such as malingering and secondary gain. A service member may be intentionally or unintentionally exaggerating or minimizing symptoms and impairment. For example, a service member may minimize symptoms out of concern for his or her career ability to get special jobs, be promoted, and stay in the service. In contrast, a service member may exaggerate symptoms in order to explain previous behaviors or to be separated from the military.

The results of a Fitness for Duty Evaluation can range from determining that behavioral issues are not related to medical issues, behavioral issues are readily treatable, or behavioral issues may be treatable and require a follow-up evaluation after sufficient time has been allowed for treatment, to determining that treatment is highly unlikely to be able to sufficiently address behavioral issues.

Command-Directed Mental Health Evaluations

Commanders and line leaders are frequently the first to notice a change in the behavior of one of their troops. When concerns arise that a condition exists that affects the health or military readiness of a service member, the commander has the ability to refer that member to the military treatment facility for a comprehensive evaluation and determination of fitness for duty. Often this occurs informally, with the member simply reporting to sick call for an evaluation, but in some cases a more formal process is required. When a behavioral health issue is suspected, service members can be encouraged to be evaluated on a voluntary basis. In this case, all of the usual privacy provisions remain in effect, and the commander will normally not receive any protected information apart from a follow-up appointment schedule unless a duty-limiting condition exists as described previously.

In the event that the commander determines the need for a behavioral health evaluation, and the service member either is reluctant to be evaluated or believes the referral to be in response to a complaint against the command, the DoD has established a provision for compulsory evaluation of the suspected behavioral health issue. DoD Directive 6490.1 and DoD Instruction 6490.4 guide the Command-Directed Mental Health Evaluation process. These documents codify and regulate the referral process in order to ensure the rights of the service member while addressing the concerns of the commander. In this process, a series of checks, balances, and protections exist to balance all interests. Upon the suspi-

cion of an impairing behavioral health issue, the commander is first required to consult with a behavioral health professional to determine whether a psychiatric emergency exists and whether a behavioral health evaluation is appropriate given the commander's concern. The service member is then informed by the commander of the reason for concern and the need for a behavioral health referral. In the case of an emergency, the service member is brought immediately for evaluation. In nonemergency situations, the service member is given at least 48 hours before the evaluation in order to consult with a chaplain, an attorney, an inspector general, a member of Congress, or any other trusted advocate. During the evaluation, the behavioral health practitioner confirms compliance with the referral process, reviews the limits of confidentiality, and proceeds with the evaluation, preparing a written report of the findings and recommendations for the service member's commander.

Increasing Access and Reducing Stigma

The military has multiple initiatives to increase access and reduce stigma-related barriers to seeking help. First, the Real Warriors Campaign is a multimedia public education campaign that features video testimonies by military personnel and their spouses about successfully dealing with psychological issues. Second, RESPECT-Mil (Re-Engineering Systems of Primary Care Treatment in the Military; Engel 2008) is a program that provides training for primary care providers on deployment and behavioral health issues. This type of primary care model has two advantages: 1) service members are regularly seen in primary care, which provides an opportunity for quick screens for potential psychological issues;

and 2) service members may be more comfortable receiving care for psychological issues in primary care than in a specialty mental health clinic. Third, the military is also embedding mental health providers in units so that the unit members can become more comfortable with these providers. Fourth, the Navy and Marine Corps have institutionalized an Operational Stress Control model that educates service members on a continuum of stress responses that can be experienced, as well as normalizes these experiences and getting necessary help. Fifth, there are a variety of services that can be accessed by phone and the Web, such as the Veterans Crisis Line operated by VA for service members and veterans, the Defense Centers of Excellence for Psychological Health and Traumatic Brain Injury (DCoE) Outreach Center, and Web sites such as afterdeployment.org, which offer anonymous self-assessments and self-help educational and skills-building modules. Information about accessing these resources is provided in the appendix to this chapter.

Prescriptions Management

The pharmacological treatment of conditions that increase risk for suicidal behavior and of suicidality itself is addressed elsewhere in this book (see Chapter 12, "Psychopharmacotherapy and Electroconvulsive Therapy") and will not be repeated here. The general principles of psychopharmacological treatment are applicable to the military and veteran population. It should be understood that with a few exceptions (lithium in bipolar depression and clozapine in schizophrenia), there exists very little evidence to support the efficacy of pharmacological intervention to target suicidality directly. This should not dissuade the aggressive bio-psycho-social treatment of the suicidal patient, but the treating clinician

should never feel reassured that treating the presenting illness alone significantly reduces the short-term or long-term suicide risk. Suicidality must be treated independently and aggressively in its own right. The most well studied and effective treatments for suicidality all have a cognitive-behavioral therapy framework. These therapies focus on correcting cognitive distortions, enhancing problem-solving skills, and building supportive relationships while avoiding risky behaviors.

When treatment includes pharmacotherapy, the clinician must weigh the risks of a particular medication with the potential benefits and alternatives to treatment as part of sound clinical management and the informed-consent process. Particular attention should be paid to the overdose potential of any prescribed medication Psychiatric medications should be carefully selected, prescribed, and dispensed to minimize the risk of overdosage during the course of treatment. The safety profiles of newer antidepressants favor serotonin reuptake inhibitors (SRIs) and serotonin-norepinephrine reuptake inhibitors (SNRIs) over tricyclic antidepressants (TCAs), but TCAs are still in use, particularly in the context of chronic pain. Antidepressant selection should take into consideration all of the medications and conditions that are present and the potential for drug interactions. Additionally, recent evidence reveals that in patients below the age of 24, the use of SRIs may transiently increase the risk of suicidal thinking and behavior and has led to a black box warning by the U.S. Food and Drug Administration (FDA) (2006). A recent review however, does not support the FDA's findings and concludes that antidepressant treatment may actually reduce the risk of suicidal behavior by 20%–40% (Leon et al. 2011). Patients must be informed of the risks and benefits of antidepressant therapy, and a safety plan must be developed and documented in the record. The risks associated with SNRIs are not as well studied, but similar caution should be exercised. Particular attention should be paid to the overdose potential of any prescribed medication.

TCAs, mood stabilizers, atypical antipsychotics, sedative-hypnotics, and narcotic analgesics are widely prescribed in the service member and veteran population, and have a high potential for adverse events—particularly when used in combination or when consumed with alcohol. Patients and families should be informed about the potential for harm as part of informed consent for treatment. It is wise to consult a pharmacologist and understand the metabolic implications when the prescription of multiple medications is necessary for effective treatment. It is also wise to consider whether self-administration of multiple medications is appropriate. The use of dispensing aids or family member support may be necessary to avoid accidental or intentional overdosing. Limitations in dispensing should be considered in suicidal, impulsive, or otherwise impaired patients to avoid ready access to lethal means by an unreliable patient. A general principle well accepted by the military services is to dispense medications weekly for the first several weeks until it can be determined that the patient is taking the medication as prescribed, demonstrating no evidence of stockpiling, responding favorably to treatment, and improving in his or her suicide risk stratification. Once the patient's compliance has been stabilized, routine prescribing practices can continue.

Weapons Management

Military providers are careful to assess and monitor access to weapons, especially given both the general access to weapons in the military and the high percentage of suicides by use of firearms in the military. The clinical implications are that very close attention should be paid to identifying if weapons are available at home or easily accessible in other locations and restricting access to firearms. The standard practice with service members who have increased suicide risk is a "lethal means counseling" approach for reduced access to firearms and other lethal means. The general forms of means restrictions in the military include removing service members from weapon-carrying duties and putting the service member's weapons in the base armory for safekeeping.

Service members, in general, are trained in the use of weapons and have a greater degree of comfort with firearms than the general population. During times of deployment, immediate access to firearms significantly increases risk of self-inflicted injury, and careful consideration must be given in the clinical assessment to restricting access to the weapon, its firing pin, or ammunition. This clinical decision must be made in the context of balancing the patient's safety with the potential for stigmatizing the soldier by removing his or her weapon and with careful consideration of the operational requirements of the situation. When access to firearms must be restricted, it should be done in consultation with the soldier's command leadership because it will require the soldier's removal from combat operations for a period of time and the leaders will need to maintain accountability of the weapon. A deployed service member without possession of a firearm is immediately conspicuous to all around him or her and may become the subject of ridicule or mistrust. In order to minimize the risk of alienating the soldier from his or her peer group, behavioral health practitioners may choose to recommend the removal of the firing pin or bolt of the weapon to maintain at least the appearance of being armed. Again, this decision is made in consultation with the soldier's command.

The clinician must remain aware that even if the soldier's personal weapon is secured, access to others' weapons is readily available. Strategies to minimize the opportunity to gain access to another weapon must be developed in collaboration with unit leaders. If access to firearms cannot be reasonably limited, the soldier must be admitted to medical care.

In the garrison environment, service members usually do not have ready access to their service weapon. Exceptions to this rule would include military police officers, armorers, and troops performing weapons training on firing ranges. Clinicians must evaluate the risks and the benefits of allowing the use of firearms for their patients, and leadership must be involved in this decision because it has a direct impact on mission readiness and service member safety.

Military members and veterans frequently own personal weapons and must be assessed for firearm ownership and access as part of any suicide risk assessment even more so than the general population. When firearms are present in the home, the clinician should determine if the firearms are locked, whether ammunition is present, and who can serve as the custodian of the firearms during the period of elevated suicide risk. Active duty unit leaders may be of assistance in securing firearms if family or trusted friends cannot do so.

Although the decision to remove access to firearms may be relatively straightforward, the clinical decision to restore access is much more complicated. There are no clear guidelines, decision tree, or risk stratification to guide the clinician in this important decision. It cannot be assumed that once firearm access is restricted the patient will not need to be continually reassessed. The clinician must take an active role in helping to determine when access can be restored rather than allowing family, friends, or unit commanders to make a uninformed decision based on the person's wishes or appearance. This decision must be informed with all available clinical information, collateral consultation, and agreement by all caregivers and leaders. This decision must be documented in the medical record as clearly as all other clinical decisions, with care taken to document the extent of the collateral consultation. It may be difficult for the clinician to fully endorse the reintroduction of lethal means to a patient with a history of suicidal behavior. This clinical decision should be "watertight" and withstand the scrutiny of risk managers, malpractice attorneys, families, and military leaders. In the event that return of firearms is not advisable, a clear plan for the sale, disposal, or permanent custody of the weapons should be a well-documented part of treatment planning.

Management of High-Risk Behaviors

An inherent need in military service is the ability to tolerate and function in high-risk and high-stress situations effectively. Service members become desensitized to many high-risk activities as part of their normal duties. Exposure to weapons and high-intensity training creates a culture in which risk is accepted and indeed welcomed. Recognizing the inherent danger of military operations, service members rigorously plan to mitigate risk but ultimately accept that danger is part of the job. Training in a high-stakes environment and participating in military operations give service members pride and unit cohesion. The adrenergic surge associated with this level of intensity increases the service member's sense of power and well-being and can become a highly desired physical state. Service members often refer to the phenomenon of becoming an "adrenaline junkie" after deployment to combat. One can hypothesize whether this occurs as a way to redirect the autonomic arousal of posttraumatic stress or whether this may represent an effort to remain sharp, as if on a razor's edge, between deployments, or whether this is simply a physiological reset and adaptation of the fear response. In any case, service members are prone to engage in many high-risk behaviors that should be assessed as part of the clinical evaluation. Activities such as speeding, racing motorcycles, drunk driving, playing "chicken," carelessly handling weapons, and engaging in extreme sports all place the individual at risk for untimely death.

Primary Care Coordination

The military health system uses multiple approaches for leveraging the role of primary care in mental health treatment and suicide prevention. The approaches include 1) training primary care managers (PCMs) to perform mental health screenings using standardized instruments like the PHQ-9 (RESPECT-Mil), 2) training PCMs to provide increased mental health treatment services (RESPECT-Mil), 3) putting behavioral health providers in primary care (Behavioral Health Optimization Program), and 4) training mental health providers to coordinate care with PCMs for patients who are at elevated suicide risk.

The fourth recommendation may be most relevant to civilian providers, especially nonphysician and nonprescribing providers, for several reasons. PCMs can provide a broader systems perspective on overall health in their role as the primary point of contact for patient care, collaborate on identifying/addressing potential physical contributions to symptoms/conditions (e.g., insomnia and pain), assess potential medication options, provide additional clinical support and monitoring, and lend credibility to the treatment plan in general. In addition, if a PCM would like additional guidance on assessment and treatment resources, the civilian provider can share information about resources from the RESPECT-Mil program (Primary Care Clinician's Manual; Oxman 2008) and Suicide Prevention Resource Center (Suicide Prevention Toolkit for Rural Primary Care; Western Interstate Commission for Higher Education and Suicide Prevention Resource Center 2009) that are described in the resource section of the appendix to this chapter.

Clinical Guidance

The *Air Force Guide for Managing Suicidal Behavior* (MSB) is a leading example of DoD clinical guidance. This description of the MSB is drawn from two seminal articles (Oordt et al. 2005, 2009). The MSB itself can be viewed and downloaded from the Air Force Suicide Prevention Program Web site in two parts:

1. The guide: http://afspp.afms.mil/idc/ groups/public/documents/afms/ ctb_016017.pdf
2. The appendices: http://afspp.afms.mil/ idc/groups/public/documents/afms/ ctb_016018.pdf

With the recognition that clinical guidelines will only be useful if they are applied consistently and effectively by clinicians, the MSB was systematically developed and implemented with careful attention to providing practical guidance and then supporting provider adaptation with an education and training program.

The Air Force developed the MSB to enhance care and increase provider confidence by integrating, standardizing, and implementing the best assessment and treatment practices that could be identified. These practices were based on a review of controlled research studies, professional guidelines, reviews, expert opinion, recognized organizational standards, lessons learned from past suicides, and feedback from leaders.

The MSB highlights five empirical findings and associated implications for managing suicidal behavior:

1. Multiple attempters are at a higher risk for future attempts than single-incident attempters and should be managed more cautiously and conservatively.
2. Treatment of clinical depression does not appear sufficient to reduce suicide risk, and it is recommended that treatment target suicidal behavior directly.
3. Short-term cognitive-behavioral interventions, including problem solving, are effective components of treatment for reducing suicidal ideation, depression, and hopelessness, and these modalities can often be used effectively in the context of outpatient care, even for higher-risk patients.
4. The period of reduction in the intensity of care after discharge from inpatient care is one of the highest-risk times for completed suicides, and simple forms of maintaining contact during periods of transition in care can be protective, so some form of ongoing care is recommended for patients who have high and chronic risk.

5. A significant number of people who die by suicide saw their primary provider within the month before their death, so the primary care provider should be included in suicide-management coordination.

The core of the clinical guide comprises 18 specific practice recommendations that are grouped into eight topic areas: 1) risk assessment, 2) decision-making framework, 3) outpatient management strategies, 4) documentation strategies, 5) coordinating with inpatient care, 6) clinic support and peer consultation, 7) ensuring continuity of care, and 8) links with the community. A key example of the topic areas is the decision-making framework that enables providers to have consistent logic for determining risk level (what provider A and provider B call "high risk" is based on the same operational criteria) and a consistent logic model for how treatment plans are aligned to these risk levels and factors. Another feature when working with military members is working closely with community resources such as unit leadership.

The MSB also provides an appendix with a set of practical tools and resources to help clinic providers and staff members implement and follow the recommendations. These resources include 1) a process-of-care flowchart, 2) a template for clinic standard operating procedures, 3) suicide assessment instruments, 4) the Suicide Status Form (SSF-II), 5) the Suicide Tracking Form (STF-I), 6) sample crisis response plan cards, 7) sample risk assessment documentation, 8) a suggested clinical-note suicide assessment overprint, 9) a sample memorandum of understanding with civilian inpatient care facilities, 10) a template client information sheet, 11) a sample "no-show" letter, and 12) an access-to-care handout.

The appendix provides both a listing of suicide assessment instruments adapted from Brown (2001) as well as modified versions of two forms, SSF and STF, from the Collaborative Approach to Managing Suicide (Jobes 2006). The SSF, which is used on the initial assessment, serves as a guide to a comprehensive and quantifiable assessment of risk factors that can be integrated into an overall risk level and attendant treatment plan. In addition, the STF is used for follow-up visits to track a core set of risk factors from the initial assessment to detect changes in risk and monitor treatment progress with suicide-specific goals.

The MSB was systemically disseminated to providers across the Air Force health system. In 2001, the dissemination strategy included a 12-hour continuing education training program that was taught to 75% of the mental health providers working across the 74 Air Force medical treatment facilities. The training included lectures, roleplays, and panel discussions, and focused not only on individual providers' clinical skills and practices, but also on establishing standardized operating procedures within the clinics. In an evaluation of this dissemination approach 6 months following the training, 44% of providers reported increased confidence in assessing suicide risk, and the majority of providers reported increased confidence in managing suicidal patients (54%), changing suicide management practices (83%), and changing clinic practices (66%).

DoD Suicide Prevention Resources

The DoD and the military services have developed a wide range of resources as part of their comprehensive and proactive prevention initiatives to address suicide risk factors. These resources target the full spectrum of prevention, including primary prevention across the military community to eliminate/mitigate risk factors and strengthen protective factors, secondary prevention for early detection and intervention, and tertiary prevention for optimal standard of care.

DoD resources are designed to meet the needs of all service members. DoD resources are also intended to respect service-specific differences and each service's role in being the primary authority for its own suicide prevention programs. The services are the primary authority on suicide prevention efforts for their service populations, and the Service Suicide Prevention office is the primary authority for overseeing service suicide prevention issues. In addition, the Services' Suicide Prevention Program Managers also work closely with one another through the DoD Suicide Prevention and Risk Reduction Committee (SPARRC) to discuss their current prevention programs and best practices.

The primary DoD suicide prevention resource is the SPARRC Web site, and the primary service-specific resources are each service's suicide prevention program's Web site. These resources, as well as additional DoD and service resources, are described in the appendix to this chapter.

VA Prevention and Management of Suicidal Behavior

Mental Health Strategic Plan

In 2004, VA developed the Mental Health Strategic Plan (MHSP). The purpose of the MHSP was to present a new approach to mental health care to focus on recovery rather than pathology and to integrate mental health care into overall health care for veteran patients. This 5-year action plan with more than 200 initiatives includes timetables and responsible offices identified for each action item. Among these action items are a number that are specifically aimed at the prevention of suicide. Specifically, those initiatives that pertain to suicide prevention follow into the following domains: Crisis Availability and Outreach, Screening and Referral, Tracking and Assessment of Veterans at Risk, Emerging Best Practice Interventions and Research, Development of an Electronic Suicide Prevention Database, and Education. MHSP initiatives pertaining to 24-hour crisis availability, outreach, referral, and development of methods for tracking veterans at risk have been implemented in multiple facilities. Initiatives focused on the development of methods for screening, assessment of veterans at risk, emerging best practice treatment interventions, education of VA health providers, and an electronic suicide prevention database have been piloted or are in the process of being piloted at selected facilities.

Mental Health Research

VA's Mental Illness Research Education, and Clinical Center in Denver, Colorado, and the Center of Excellence in Mental Health and PTSD at Canandaigua, New York, have been specifically focusing on research related to suicide prevention. The goal of these two centers is to conduct research pertaining to suicide prevention and treatment and quickly disseminate findings to the field for implementation. Ongoing studies at these centers are examining suicide risk factors for the veteran population, validating suicidal ideation screening instruments, examining the quality of mental health care and its relationship to suicide prevention, and studying the neurobiological underpinnings of suicide.

Screening

In-depth, face-to-face clinical interviews remain the best way to screen and assess for suicide risk. At present, a widely accepted and effective suicide screening tool does not exist, partly because of the complexities associated with the phenomena of suicide. However, the VHA has implemented system-wide screening by primary care providers for depression, PTSD, and substance abuse. For example, VA has implemented a policy to screen all OEF/OIF veterans for depression, PTSD, and alcohol abuse upon their initial visit to VA medical centers or clinics. Furthermore, screening for depression and alcohol abuse is required annually for all veterans, and screening for PTSD is required annually for the first 5 years after enrollment and every 5 years thereafter. Veterans who screen positive for one of these conditions are required to receive a follow-up clinical evaluation that considers both the condition(s) related to the positive screen and the risk of suicide. When this process confirms the presence of a mental disorder or suicide risk, veterans are offered mental health treatment. When there is a referral or request for mental health services, veterans must receive an initial evaluation within 24 hours. If this evaluation identifies an urgent need, treatment is to be provided immediately. Otherwise, veterans must receive a full diagnostic and treatment planning evaluation and the initiation of care within 2 weeks.

Educational Resources and Training

VA has developed a number of quick guides and educational resources to assist clinicians with different aspects of suicide risk assessment and intervention. Two primary resources are the suicide prevention coordinators and the Veterans Crisis Line, which are described below. In addition, other resources include the Suicide Risk Assessment Pocket Card and Manual, the Safety Plan Treatment Manual and Safety Plan Pocket Card, Operation SAVE gatekeeper training, the Suicide Risk Assessment Guide, the VA ACE card and brochures, the Suicide Attempt Survivor Family Resource Guide, the DoD/VA Suicide Outreach Web site, the Traumatic Brain Injury and Suicide Manual for Clinicians and Care Providers, and the Self-Directed Violence Classification System. See Table 23–1 in the appendix to this chapter for more information about these resources as well as links for additional information.

Suicide Prevention Coordinators

A central example of the VHA's ongoing and increasing efforts to enhance suicide prevention is the recent designation of suicide prevention coordinators in each medical center. These coordinators serve to facilitate implementation of suicide prevention strategies at the local level. Their primary responsibility is to support the identification of high-risk patients and to coordinate ongoing monitoring and enhancements in care. Other responsibilities include educating providers, veterans, families, and community members on risk factors and warning signs for suicide and treatment options, as well as participation in patient safety and environmental analysis to develop local suicide prevention strategies.

Veterans Crisis Line

VA has also partnered with the Lifeline Program, a grantee of the Substance Abuse and Mental Health Services Administration of the U.S. Department of Health and Human Services, to develop the Veterans Crisis Line.

Those who call 800-273-TALK are asked to press "1" if they are a veteran or are calling about a veteran. They are then connected directly to VA's hotline call center, where they speak to a VA mental health professional with real-time access to the veteran's medical records. In emergencies, the hotline contacts local emergency resources such as police or ambulance services to ensure an immediate response. In other cases, after providing support and counseling, the hotline transfers care to the suicide prevention coordinator at the nearest VA medical center for follow-up care.

DoD/VA Clinical Practice Guidelines

VA and the DoD have collaborated to develop clinical practice guidelines for the management of many health conditions (www.healthquality.va.gov). In the behavioral health arena, clinical practice guidelines have been developed for bipolar disorder in adults (2004, 2010), major depressive disorder (2008), PTSD (2004, 2010), and substance use disorders. These guidelines address suicidality only as a component of the management of the diagnostic condition, with little attention paid to the management of suicidality as a core issue. The American Psychiatric Association (APA) published, in November 2003, its guideline on the management of suicidal behaviors (psychiatryonline.org/content.aspx?bookid=28&sectionid=1673332). Although this guideline provides a thorough review of the assessment of patients with suicidal behaviors, psychiatric management and treatment with somatic and psychotherapies, and the appropriate documentation and risk management procedures, it is considered by the APA to be out of date and in need of revision. Recognizing the need for clear, evidence-based practices for the management of the most high-risk condition in our population and the need for a guideline that is compatible with the needs of the military and veteran culture, VA and the DoD have chartered a working group to draft the VA/DoD Clinical Practice Guidelines for the Management of Suicidal Behavior to fill this gap. As with all clinical practice guidelines, the process will begin with a thorough review of the applicable literature, an evaluation and scoring of the clinical evidence, a validation of a clinical pathway and an expert review, and publication is expected in 2012.

Resources for Civilian Care Providers

There is an extensive range of DoD, VA, and additional resources that can help civilian care providers who are working with military members and veterans. A list of resources is provided in the appendix to this chapter. For ease of access, the resources are organized into three categories based on the intended audience: 1) providers, 2) service members and family members, and 3) leaders. Although the resources for providers are designed to be the most accessible for care providers, the other resources can also be useful. For example, the resources for service members and family members can be a useful adjunct to work with a service member or veteran. In addition, the resources for leaders can help a civilian care provider understand how a military member's leadership and commu-

nity can be enlisted as additional support if the military member authorizes a release.

The resources are organized by source: 1) service branch, 2) DoD, 3) VA, and 4) additional sources. The emphasis on the source of resources reflects that service branches and the DoD are the primary source of information for military members, and VA is the primary source of information for veterans. Therefore, civilian care providers are advised to rely primarily on resources from DoD, services, and VA. In addition, if these general resources are not adequate, civilian care providers can also consider calling a local DoD or VA facility to request appropriate consultation resources. Locations and contact information for DoD and VA facilities can be found at the following Web sites:

1. Military installations at the DoD Military Homefront Web site: www.military-installations.dod.mil/
2. VA national facilities locator Web site: www2.va.gov/directory/guide/home.asp?isflash=1

One note of caution is that in the effort to continually improve suicide prevention programs and resources, program names, phone numbers, and Web addresses are occasionally changed. Therefore, if a phone number or Web site link does not appear to be functional, it may be wise to contact another agency to verify the resource name, phone number, or link. One simple resource for the latest information on resources is the DCoE Outreach Center.

Key Clinical Concepts

- Be mindful of the evidence for factors that contribute to suicides with service members and veterans as well as potential culture-related themes that may be influencing a person's experiences and behavior. Sensitivity to cultural themes can both help establish and maintain the therapeutic relationship and enhance the assessment and treatment process.

- Screen for mental disorders, including potential substance abuse issues, suicidality, and suicide risk factors for early detection, prevention, and intervention.

- Integrate both protective and risk factors in assessment, case conceptualization, risk level determination, and treatment planning. Also, directly treat any suicidality in addition to mental disorders.

- Coordinate a comprehensive and collaborative safety plan that includes managing access to lethal means, leveraging community resources, and coordination across the treatment team. Always consider access to weapons as part of safety planning.

- Consider leveraging military leadership and other collateral resources (military treatment facility providers, chaplains, family support, and legal resources). In addition, ensure informed consent and appropriate releases before coordinating information and support from collateral sources.

- Use the Veterans Crisis Line; general resources for service members, veterans, and family members; and provider consultation as part of safety planning.

- Be aware of the broad range of Department of Defense, Department of Veterans Affairs, and other resources, many of which are described in the appendix to this chapter.

References

American Psychological Association: Guidelines on multicultural education, training, research, practice, and organizational change for psychologists. Am Psychol 58:377-402, 2003

American Psychological Association: Report of the American Psychological Association Presidential Task Force on Psychological Ethics and National Security. Washington, DC, American Psychological Association, 2005

Amir M, Kaplan Z, Efroni R, et al: Suicide risk and coping styles in posttraumatic stress disorder patients. Psychother Psychosom 68:76–81, 1999

Bell J, Nye E: Specific symptoms predict suicidal ideation in Vietnam combat veterans with chronic post-traumatic stress disorder. Mil Med 172:1144–1147, 2007

Benda BB: Discriminators of suicide thoughts and attempts among homeless veterans who abuse substances. Suicide Life Threat Behav 33:430–442, 2003

Blaauw E, Kerkhof AJ, Hayes LM: Demographic, criminal, and psychiatric factors related to inmate suicide. Suicide Life Threat Behav 35:63–75, 2005

Bonds TM, Baiocchi D, McDonald LL: Army Deployments to OIF and OEF (DB-587-A). Santa Monica, CA, RAND Corporation, 2010

Brenner LA, Homaifar BY, Adler LE, et al: Suicidality and veterans with a history of traumatic brain injury: precipitating events, protective factors, and prevention strategies. Rehabil Psychol 54:390–397, 2009

Brown GK: A review of suicide assessment measures for intervention research with adults and older adults, 2001. Available at: http://staffweb.esc12.net/~mbooth/resources_general/mental_health/Adult_Assessment/Assessment-review-adults%5B1%5D.pdf. Accessed August 10, 2011.

Bullman TA, Kang HK: Posttraumatic stress disorder and the risk of traumatic deaths among Vietnam veterans. J Nerv Ment Dis 182:604–610, 1994

Bullman TA, Kang HK: The risk of suicide among wounded Vietnam Veterans. Am J Public Health 86:662–667, 1996

Casciotti JA: Confidentiality of mental health records in the military. Presentation at the meeting of the Department of Defense Task Force on Mental Health, Arlington, VA, 2007

Desai RA, Liu-Mares W, Dausey DJ, et al: Suicidal ideation and suicide attempts in a sample of homeless people with mental illness. J Nerv Mental Dis 191:365–371, 2003

Desai RA, Dausey D, Rosenheck RA: Mental health service delivery and suicide risk: the role of individual patient and facility factors. Am J Psychiatry 162:311–318, 2005

Engel CC, Oxman T, Yamamoto C, et al: RESPECT-Mil: feasibility of a systems-level collaborative care approach to depression and post-traumatic stress disorder in military primary care. Mil Med 173:935–940, 2008

Eynan R, Langley J, Tolomiczenko G, et al: The association between homelessness and suicidal ideation and behaviors: results of a cross-sectional survey. Suicide Life Threat Behav 32:418–427, 2002

Fergusson DM, Boden JM, Horwood LJ: Unemployment and suicidal behavior in a New Zealand birth cohort: a fixed effects regression analysis. Crisis 28:95–101, 2007

Fischler GL: Psychological fitness-for-duty examinations: practical considerations for public safety departments. Illinois Law Enforcement Executive Forum 1:77–92, 2001

Fiske AP, Kitayama S, Markus HR, et al: The cultural matrix of social psychology, in The Handbook of Social Psychology, 4th Edition, Vol 2. Edited by Gilbert DT, Fiske ST. New York, McGraw-Hill, 1998, pp 915–981

Fontana A, Rosenheck R: Attempted suicide among Vietnam veterans: a model of etiology in a community sample. Am J Psychiatry 152:102–109, 1995

Gelberg L, Linn LS, Leake BD: Mental health, alcohol and drug use, and criminal history among homeless adults. Am J Psychiatry 145:191–196, 1988

Griffith J: Decades of transition for the US reserves: changing demand on reserve identity and mental well-being. Int Rev Psychiatry 23:181–191, 2011

Hendin H, Haas AP: Suicide and guilt as manifestations of PTSD in Vietnam combat veterans. Am J Psychiatry 148:586–591, 1991

Hofstede G: Culture's Consequences: Comparing Values, Behaviors, Institutions, and Organizations Across Nations, 2nd Edition. London, Sage, 2001

Hofstede G, Bond MH: The Confucian connection: from cultural roots to economic growth. Organ Dyn 16:4–21, 1988

Hoge CW, Castro CA, Messer SC, et al: Combat duty in Iraq and Afghanistan, mental health problems, and barriers to care. N Engl J Med 351:13–22, 2004

Ilgen MA, Bohnert AS, Ignacio RV, et al: Psychiatric diagnoses and risk of suicide in veterans. Arch Gen Psychiatry 67:1152–1158, 2010

Jobes DA: Managing Suicidal Risk: A Collaborative Approach. New York, Guilford, 2006

Joiner T: Why People Die by Suicide. Cambridge, MA, Harvard University Press, 2005

Kaplan MS, Huguet N, McFarland BH, et al: Suicide among veterans: a prospective population-based study. J Epidemiol Community Health 61:619–624, 2007

Karch DL, Lubell KM, Friday J, et al; Centers for Disease Control and Prevention: surveillance for violent deaths—National Violent Death Reporting System 16 States, 2005. MMWR Surveil Summ 57:1–45, 2008

Kellermann AL, Rivara FP, Somes G, et al: Suicide in the home in relation to gun ownership. N Engl J Med 327:467–472, 1992

Kinn JT, Luxton DD, Reger MA, et al: DoD Suicide Event Report: Calendar Year 2010. Annual Report. National Center for Telehealth & Technology, Defense Centers of Excellence for Psychological Health & TBI, 2011. Available at: http://t2health.org/sites/default/files/dodser/DoDSER_2010_Annual_Report.pdf.

Kramer T, Lindy J, Green B, et al: The comorbidity of post-traumatic stress disorder and suicidality in Vietnam veterans. Suicide Life Threat Behav 24:58–67, 1994

Kulka R, Schlenger W, Fairbank J, et al: Trauma and the Vietnam War Generation: Report of Findings From the National Vietnam Veterans Readjustment Study. Philadelphia, PA, Brunner/Mazel, 1990

Lambert MT, Fowler DR: Suicide risk factors among veterans: risk management in the changing culture of the Department of Veterans Affairs. J Ment Health Adm 24:350–358, 1997

Leon AC, Solomon DA, Chunshan L, et al: Antidepressants and risks of suicide and suicide attempts: a 27-year observational study. J Clin Psychiatry 72:580–586, 2011

Mann JJ: A current perspective of suicide and attempted suicide. Ann Intern Med 136:302–311, 2002

Mann JJ, Waternaux C, Haas GL, et al: Toward a clinical model of suicidal behavior in psychiatric patients. Am J Psychiatry 156:181–189, 1999

McCarroll JE, Jaccard JJ, Radke AQ: Psychiatric consultation to command, in Military Psychiatry: Preparing in Peace for War. Edited by Jones FD, Sparacino LR, Wilcox VL, et al. Washington, DC, Borden Institute, 1994, pp 151–170

McCarthy JF, Valenstein M, Kim HM, et al: Suicide mortality among patients receiving care in the Veterans Health Administration health system. Am J Epidemiol 169:1033–1038, 2009

Miller M, Hemenway D: The relationship between firearms and suicide: a review of the literature. Aggression and Violent Behavior 4(1):59–75, 1999

Oordt MS, Jobes DA, Rudd MD, et al: Development of a clinical guide to enhance care for suicidal patients. Prof Psychol Res Pr 36:208–218, 2005

Oordt MS, Jobes DA, Fonseca VP, et al: Training mental health professionals to assess and manage suicidal behavior: can provider confidence and practice behaviors be altered? Suicide Life Threat Behav 39:21–32, 2009

Oxman TE: RESPECT-Mil Primary Care Clinician's Manual: Three-Component Model for Primary Care Management of Depression and PTSD (Military Version). August 2008. Available at: http://www.pdhealth.mil/respect-mil/downloads/PCC_Final.pdf.

Renaud J, Berlim MT, McGirr A, et al: Current psychiatric morbidity, aggression/impulsivity, and personality dimensions in child and adolescent suicide: a case-control study. J Affect Disord 105:221–228, 2008

Riccio G, Sullivan R, Klein G, et al: Warrior Ethos: Analysis of the Concept and Initial Development of Applications (U.S. Army Research Institute Research Report 1827). Vienna, VA, Wexford Group, 2004

Rodell DE, Benda BB, Rodell L: Suicidal thoughts among homeless alcohol and other drug abusers. Alcohol Treat Q 21:57–74, 2003

Rosenheck R, Frisman L, Chung A: The proportion of veterans among homeless men. Am J Public Health 84:466–469, 1994

Sareen J, Houlahan T, Cox B, et al: Anxiety Disorders Associated With Suicidal Ideation and Suicide Attempts in the National Comorbidity Survey. J Nerv Ment Dis 193:450–454, 2005

Selby EA, Anestis MD, Bender TW, et al: Overcoming the fear of lethal injury: evaluating suicidal behavior in the military through the lens of the interpersonal-psychological theory of suicide. Clin Psychol Rev 30:298–307, 2010

Sherman N: Stoic Warriors: The Ancient Philosophy Behind the Military Mind. New York, Oxford University Press, 2005

Silver JM, Kramer R, Greenwald S, et al: The association between head injuries and psychiatric disorders: findings from the New Haven NIMH Epidemiologic Catchment Area study. Brain Inj 15:935–945, 2001

Simpson G, Tate R: Suicidality after traumatic brain injury: demographic, injury, and clinical correlates. Psychol Med 32:687–697, 2002

Suicide Prevention Resource Center: Relationship Between the Economy, Unemployment and Suicide. Newton, MA, Education Development Center, 2008

Taras V, Kirkman BL, Steel P: Examining the impact of culture's consequences: a three-decade, multi-level, meta-analytic review of Hofstede's cultural value dimensions. J Appl Psychol 95:405–439, 2010

Teasdale TW, Engberg AW: Suicide after traumatic brain injury: a population study. J Neurol Neurosurg Psychiatry 71:436–440, 2001

Thompson R, Kane VR, Sayers SL, et al: An assessment of suicide in an urban VA Medical Center. Psychiatry 65:326–337, 2002

U.S. Department of Defense: DoDI 1332.38: physical disability evaluation. November 14, 1996, incorporating change 1, July 10, 2006. Available at: http://www.dtic.mil/whs/directives/corres/pdf/133238p.pdf. Accessed August 11, 2011.

U.S. Department of Defense: 2008 survey of health-related behaviors among active duty military personnel. September 2009. Available at: http://www.tricare.mil/2008HealthBehaviors.pdf. Accessed August 11, 2011.

U.S. Department of Defense: Casualty status. June 6, 2011. Available at: http://www.defense.gov/news/casualty.pdf. Accessed August 11, 2011.

U.S. Department of Defense, Task Force on the Prevention of Suicide: The Challenge and the Promise: Strengthening the Force, Preventing Suicide, and Saving Lives. Falls Church, VA, Defense Health Board, 2010

U.S. Department of Housing and Urban Development: The annual homeless assessment report to Congress, 2009. June 2010. Available at: http://www.huduser.org/publications/pdf/5thHomelessAssessmentReport.pdf. Accessed April 15, 2011.

U.S. Department of Housing and Urban Development: Veteran homelessness: a supplemental report to the 2009 annual homeless assessment report to Congress. February 2011. Available at: http://www.hudhre.info/documents/2009AHARVeteransReport.pdf. Accessed August 11, 2011.

U.S. Department of Labor, Bureau of Labor Statistics: Table A-5: employment status of the civilian population 18 years and over by veteran status, period of service, and sex, not seasonally adjusted. June 3, 2011. Available at: http://www.bls.gov/news.release/empsit.t05.htm. Accessed August 11, 2011.

U.S. Department of Veterans Affairs: 2001 National Survey of Veterans (NSV): final report. 2001. Available at: http://www.va.gov/VETDATA/docs/SurveysAndStudies/NSV_Final_Report.pdf. Accessed April 1, 2011.

U.S. Department of Veterans Affairs: Women veterans: past, present, and future. September 2007. Available at: http://www.va.gov/womenvet/docs/womenvet_history.pdf. Accessed August 11, 2011.

U.S. Food and Drug Administration: [Briefing document for Psychopharmacologic Drugs Advisory Committee.] December 13, 2006. Available at: http://www.fda.gov/ohrms/dockets/ac/cder06.html#Psychopharmacologic. Accessed August 11, 2011.

U.S. Interagency Council on Homelessness: Opening doors: homelessness among veterans. June 2010. Available at: http://www.usich.gov/resources/uploads/asset_library/FactSheetVeterans.pdf. Accessed August 11, 2011.

Warner CH, Appenzeller GN, Parker JR, et al: Effectiveness of mental health screening and coordination of in-theater care prior to deployment to Iraq: a cohort study. Am J Psychiatry 168:378–385, 2011

Western Interstate Commission for Higher Education (WICHE) and Suicide Prevention Resource Center (SPRC). Suicide prevention toolkit for rural primary care: a primer for primary care providers. 2009. Available at: http://www.sprc.org/library/PrimerModule1.pdf. Accessed August 28, 2011.

Wortzel HS, Binswanger IA, Anderson CA, et al: Suicide among incarcerated veterans. J Am Acad Psychiatry Law 37:82–91, 2009

Zivin K, Kim HM, McCarthy JF, et al: Suicide mortality among individuals receiving treatment for depression in the Veterans Affairs health system: associations with patient and treatment setting characteristics. Am J Public Health 97:2193–2198, 2007

Appendix: Service, DoD, VA, and Civilian Resources

This appendix provides a list of service branch–specific, DoD, VA, and civilian resources for service members, veterans, families, and care providers. The order is based on the recommendation that service members and families first seek primary care resources from the service branches followed by those from the DoD, while veterans are advised to consult VA resources. Since program names and contact information may change, the DCoE Outreach Center (visit www.dcoe. health.mil/24-7help.aspx, or call 866-966-1020) is a general resource that provides updated resources and other information.

TABLE 23–1. U.S. Army suicide prevention resources

Army Applied Suicide Intervention Skills Training (ASIST)	A 2-day workshop that prepares caregivers or "gatekeepers" to recognize individuals who are at risk and intervene to prevent the risk of suicidal thoughts becoming suicidal behaviors. ASIST is an Army G1-approved suicide intervention skills training. Web site: https://g1arng.army.pentagon.mil/Soldiers/ RiskReductionandSuicidePrevention/Pages/default.aspx
Army Comprehensive Soldier Fitness	A program that uses individual assessments, tailored virtual training, classroom training, and embedded resilience experts to provide resiliency skills to soldiers, family members, and Army civilians as needed. Web site: http://csf.army.mil
Army Service Leader's Guide for Managing Personnel in Distress	A Web-based guide for leaders to quickly review risk factors, assessment questions, and resources for a wide range of issues that can cause distress for service members and family members. Web site: http://www.armyg1.army.mil/hr/suicide/docs/ Leadership%20in%20Action-Strategies%20for%20Distress% 20Prevention%20and%20Management.pdf
Army Strong Bonds Program	A unit-based, chaplain-led program that assists commanders in building individual resiliency by strengthening the Army by increasing individual soldier and family readiness through relationship education and skills training. Website: http://www.strongbonds.org/skins/strongbonds/ home.aspx
Army Suicide Prevention Program	A program designed to improve readiness through the development and enhancement of the Army Suicide Prevention Program policies designed to minimize suicide behavior, thereby preserving mission effectiveness through individual readiness for soldiers, their families, and Department of the Army civilians. Website: http://www.armyg1.army.mil/hr/suicide/

TABLE 23–2. U.S. Marine Corps suicide prevention resources

Marine Corps: Assessing and Managing Suicide Risk Training for Mental Health Providers, Counselors, and Chaplains	A one-day workshop for mental health providers and chaplains that is focused on assessing and managing suicide risk. Introduces Chronological Assessment of Suicide Events, a method for recognizing suicidal ideation.
Marine Corps Behavioral Health Information Network	A Web-based clearinghouse of the latest information and tools for Marines, families, and professionals on prevention and other resources concerning behavioral health, to assist units and installation support services in their efforts to educate the military community about building resiliency, recognizing reactions, and determining the need for help. Web site: http://bhin.usmc-mccs.org
Marine Corps Deployment Cycle Training	A Marine Corps family team-building program about the normal and expected emotional responses to each phase of the deployment cycle and an opportunity for family members to have their questions answered. In the postdeployment workshop, family members learn about the combat operational stress continuum. Web site: http://www.usmc-mccs.org/suicideprevent/index.cfm
Never Leave a Marine Behind suicide prevention and awareness education series	A series that trains all ranks in fostering resiliency and in encouraging Marines to engage helping services early before problems worsen to the point of suicide risk. Content includes resiliency-building skills, warning signs of suicide, importance of intervening, how to intervene, getting help as a sign of strength, postvention best practices, and a resource directory. Web site: http://www.usmc-mcss.org/suicideprevent/ncotrng.cfm?sid=mlandmid=9
Navy & Marine Corps Public Health Center	A Web site that has a list of resources geared specifically toward the clinician. Topics include responding to a suicidal patient, working with suicidal children and youth, helping patients and families after an attempt, and risk assessment. Web site: http://www.nmcphc.med.navy.mil/healthy_living/psychological_health/suicide_prevention/suicideprev_clinicians.aspx
Unit, Personal and Family Readiness Program, Marine Corps Reserve Affairs	A multimedia intervention to educate all active duty Marines, reservists, and their families on the signs and symptoms of suicide and available resources to train providers and leaders, and to provide briefing materials, posters, brochures, and other media. Web site: http://www.usmc-mccs.org/upfrp/index.cfm?sid=fl&smid=1
Marine Corps Leader's Guide for Managing Marines in Distress	A Web-based guide for leaders to quickly review risk factors, assessment questions, and resources for a wide range of issues that can cause distress for service members and family members. Web site: http://www.usmc-mccs.org/leadersguide/downloads.cfm
Marine Corps Suicide Prevention Program	A program that is a leadership initiative to foster resilience and encourage Marines to engage helping services early, before suicide risk develops. The program seeks to eliminate suicide through surveillance, education, and training; coordination and development of research; strategic communication; and policy development. Web site: http://www.usmc-mccs.org/suicideprevent/index.cfm

TABLE 23–3. U.S. Navy suicide prevention resources

Command Program Tool: Suicide Prevention Program Checklist	Every command is required to have a suicide prevention program. This program provides tools to assist the commander in implementing a suicide program. Web site: http://www.public.navy.mil/bupers-npc/support/readiness/Documents/Checklist.doc
Navy & Marine Corps Public Health Center	A Web site that has a list of resources geared specifically toward the clinician. Topics include responding to a suicidal patient, working with suicidal children and youth, helping patients and families after an attempt, and risk assessment. Web site: http://www.nmcphc.med.navy.mil/healthy_living/psychological_health/suicide_prevention/suicideprev_clinicians.aspx
Navy Leader's Guide for Managing Sailors in Distress	A Web-based guide for leaders to quickly review risk factors, assessment questions, and resources for a wide range of issues that can cause distress for service members and family members. Web site: http://www.nmcphc.med.navy.mil/lguide/command_evaluations.aspx
Navy Suicide Prevention Leader's Guide	The purpose of the leader's guide is to help leaders at all levels to recognize distress-related behaviors, provide support to sailors within the unit, and collaborate with supporting agencies to meet individuals' needs in distress. Web site: http://www.public.navy.mil/bupers-npc/support/suicide_prevention/command/Pages/NavyLeader%27sGuide.aspx
Navy suicide prevention poster downloads	Suicide prevention posters are available for leaders to download. Web site: http://www.public.navy.mil/bupers-npc/support/suicide_prevention/command/Pages/PosterDownloads.aspx
Navy Suicide Prevention Program	A program that is intended to provide relevant and updated information on suicide prevention resources, trainings, conferences, etc. Web site: http://www.public.navy.mil/bupers-npc/support/SuicidePrevention

TABLE 23–4. U.S. Air Force suicide prevention resources

Air Force Suicide Prevention Program	A program that is a comprehensive, community-based approach for preventing suicide that focuses on decreasing risk factors for suicide and enhancing protective factors, including promoting mental health treatment for those in need. Web site: http://afspp.afms.mil
Air Force Guide for Managing Suicidal Behavior	A guide for providers on managing suicidal behavior. Web site: http://afspp.afms.mil/idc/groups/public/documents/afms/ctb_016017.pdf
Air Force Community Action Information Board/Integrated Delivery System	A program that focuses on identifying and resolving issues affecting Air Force members and their families, enhancing members' abilities to function as productive Air Force community members, and strengthening force readiness through a sense of community.
Airman's Guide for Assisting Personnel in Distress	A Web-based guide for leaders to quickly review risk factors, assessment questions, and resources for a wide range of issues that can cause distress for service members and family members. Web site: http://airforcemedicine.afms.mil/idc/groups/public/documents/kjpage/ctb_149390.pdf

TABLE 23–5. U.S. National Guard and Reserve suicide prevention resources

Directors of Psychological Health for the Guard and Reserves	State Directors of Psychological Health (DPHs) have been assigned to each of the 54 Joint Force Headquarters to serve all in the Army National Guard and Air National Guard. Each DPH is the focal point for coordinating psychological support for Guard members and their families. Web site: http://www.jointservicessupport.org/PHP/
National Guard Psychological Health Program	A program that advocates, promotes, and guides Guard members and their families by supporting psychological fitness for operational readiness. These supply behavioral health assessments and guidance on a variety of psychological health issues or concerns, clinical resources, and quality counseling services. Web site: http://www.realwarriors.net/guardreserve/treatment/NGPHP.php Web site: http://www.jointservicessupport.org/PHP/
Yellow Ribbon Reintegration Program	A program that is a supportive resource for National Guard and Reserves members and families, with information on referrals and benefits before, during, and after deployments. Web site: http://www.yellowribbon.mil Phone: 866-504-7092

TABLE 23–6. U.S. Coast Guard suicide prevention resources

Coast Guard Office of Work-Life Programs—Employee Assistance Program	A program that is designed to provide a confidential professional assessment and short-term counseling and referral services to help employees with their personal, job, or family problems. The program also provides financial, legal, and supervisory consultations. Web site: http://www.uscg.mil/worklife/employee_assistance.asp

TABLE 23–7. U.S. Department of Defense suicide prevention resources

Center for Deployment Psychology (CDP)	A center that offers a wide range of provider resources that can be viewed on the CDP home page. The CDP also offers training tailored for civilian providers. Web site: http://deploymentpsych.org Phone: 301-816-4775
Defense Centers of Excellence provider fact sheet	A handout that lists resources for health care providers treating service members, veterans, and families. Web site: http://www.dcoe.health.mil/Content/Navigation/Documents/Resources%20for%20Health%20Care%20Providers%20Treating%20Service%20Members%20Veterans%20and%20Military%20Families.pdf
InTransition program	A program that acknowledges that transitions in military service can be challenging and provides help to service members and families in any transition, be it a call to active duty, relocation, or other events. Web site: www.health.mil/inTransition Phone: 800-424-7877
Military Family Support Centers: Employment Assistance	Installation Family Centers provide counseling, education, and formation and referral to support active duty service members and their families. Specific services include employment assistance, career counseling, and skills building. Web site: http://www.defense.gov/personneltransition/military-family-support.aspx
Military OneSource	A program that is free to service members and their eligible family members and designed to help them build on their strengths, maximize their support systems, and find community resources to meet their needs. Web site: http://www.militaryonesource.com Phone: 800-342-9647
Real Warriors Campaign, Defense Centers of Excellence for Psychological Health and Traumatic Brain Injury	A campaign to promote building resilience, facilitating recovery, and supporting reintegration of returning service members, veterans, and their families. It addresses the stigma associated with seeking assistance by featuring stories of service members who have sought treatment and who are continuing to have successful military careers. Web site: http://realwarriors.net Phone: 866-966-1020
Re-Engineering Systems of Primary Care Treatment in the Military (RESPECT-Mil) from the Deployment Health Clinical Center	Primary care system and resources designed to enhance the recognition and high-quality management of posttraumatic stress disorder (PTSD) and depression to screen, assess, and treat active duty soldiers with depression and/or PTSD. The RESPECT-Mil Web site includes links to Department of Defense–Department of Veterans Affairs clinical practice guidelines and a primary care clinician's manual: http://www.pdhealth.mil/respect-mil/downloads/PCC_Final.pdf Web site: http://www.pdhealth.mil/Data/pd_contact.asp Web site: http://www.pdhealth.mil/respect-mil/index1.asp Phone: 866-559-1627

TABLE 23–7. U.S. Department of Defense suicide prevention resources *(continued)*

Service Wounded, Ill, and Injured Program	A program for families of soldiers who are assigned to warriors-in-transition battalions or units and active duty soldiers who have been injured and who are receiving inpatient or outpatient medical care for extended periods. Web site: http://www.naccrra.org Phone: (800) 424-2246
Suicide Outreach	The centerpiece of suicide intervention skills-training curriculum, which targets at-risk service members through peer- and family-led interventions. Web site: http://www.suicideoutreach.org
Understanding Military Culture When Treating PTSD	Presents important information regarding military demographics, branches, rank, status, and stressors; two programs created to help service members prevent and manage combat and operational stress; and assessment and treatment implications for clinicians. Web site: http://www.ptsd.va.gov/professional/ptsd101/course-modules/military_culture.asp
Wounded Warrior Resource Center	A center that provides immediate assistance to wounded, ill, and injured service members; their families; and caregivers with issues related to health care, facilities, or benefits. It is accessed through Military OneSource. Web site: http://www.militaryonesource.com Phone: (800) 342-9647

TABLE 23–8. U.S. Department of Veterans Affairs suicide prevention resources

PTSD Coach	An iPhone app developed by the National Center for PTSD that is designed to help individuals learn about and manage symptoms that commonly occur after trauma. It includes tools for screening and tracking symptoms as well as direct links to support and help. Web site: http://www.ptsd.va.gov/public/pages/PTSDcoach.asp
Safety plan treatment manual and pocket card	A publication that describes a brief clinical intervention that can serve as a valuable adjunct to risk assessment. This manual is intended to be used by Veterans Affairs (VA) mental health clinicians as well as other VA clinicians who evaluate, treat, or have contact with patients at risk for suicide in any VA setting. Web site: http://www.mentalhealth.va.gov/docs/ VA_SafetyPlan_quickguide.pdf Web site: http://www2.sprc.org/bpr/safety-plan-treatment-manual- reduce-suicide-risk-veteran-version
Suicide Outreach	The centerpiece of suicide intervention skills-training curriculum, which targets at-risk service members through peer- and family-led interventions. Web site: http://www.suicideoutreach.org
Suicide Risk Assessment Guide and pocket card	A publication that contains information on warning signs, factors that may increase risk, factors that may decrease risk, and tips on how to respond. Web site: http://www.mentalhealth.va.gov/docs/Suicide-Risk- Assessment-Guide.pdf
Traumatic Brain Injury (TBI) and Suicide: Information and Resources for Clinicians	An informational resource guide for clinicians and care providers working with TBI survivors. Web site: http://www.mirecc.va.gov/visn19/docs/ MANUAL_Suicide_prevention_strategies_in_TBI.pdf
VA ACE card and ACE brochure	A brochure designed to help veterans, their family members, and friends learn that they can take the necessary steps to get help through the ACE (Ask, Care, Escort) model and that summarizes the steps needed to take an active and valuable role in suicide prevention. The VA ACE Card is a pocket guide, supported by the VA ACE Brochure. Web site: http://www.mentalhealth.va.gov/docs/ VA_ACE_CARD_8_6_2009_final_version.pdf
Veterans Chat	A chat line that enables veterans, families, and friends to go online and anonymously chat with a trained Veterans Affairs (VA) counselor. If the chats are determined to be a crisis, the counselor can take immediate steps to transfer the chat to the Veterans Crisis Line, where further counseling and referral are provided. Web site: http://www.suicidepreventionlifeline.org/Veterans/ Default.aspx
Veterans Crisis Line	Those who call 800-273-TALK are asked to press "1" if they are a veteran and are connected directly to VA's hotline call center, where they speak to a VA mental health professional with real-time access to the veteran's medical records. Web site: http://www.suicidepreventionlifeline.org/Veterans/ Default.aspx Phone: 800-273-TALK

TABLE 23–9. Additional suicide prevention resources

American Association of Suicidology	A leader in the advancement of scientific and programmatic efforts in suicide prevention through research, education, and training; the development of standards and resources; and survivor support services. Web site: http://www.suicidology.org
Give an Hour	A nonprofit organization providing free mental health services to U.S. service members, providers, veterans, and families affected by the conflicts in Iraq and Afghanistan. Mental health professionals nationwide donate an hour of their time each week to provide free mental health services to military personnel and their families. Web site: http://www.giveanhour.org
Suicide Prevention Resource Center (SPRC)	A center that provides prevention support, training, and resources to assist organizations and individuals in developing suicide prevention programs, interventions, and policies, and to advance the National Strategy for Suicide Prevention. The SPRC Web site includes a Suicide Prevention Toolkit for Rural Primary Care: http://www.sprc.org/library/PrimerModule1.pdf Web site: http://www.sprc.org
Tragedy Assistance Program for Survivors	A 24/7 tragedy assistance resource for anyone who has suffered the loss of a military loved one, regardless of the relationship to the deceased or the circumstance of the death. Web site: http://www.taps.org Phone: 800-959-8277

C H A P T E R   2 4

Suicide and Gender

Liza H. Gold, M.D.

Suicide is a gendered phenomenon. Émile Durkheim, who provided the first systematic and statistical study of suicide in his 1897 work *Suicide*, observed that suicide is an "essentially male phenomenon" (Durkheim 1897/1951, p. 72). Women have consistently higher rates of two of the most widely recognized risk factors for suicide: depression and previous suicide attempts. Nevertheless, women's suicide mortality rates are remarkably low. For example, in 2007, the latest year for which statistics were available, the total number of suicide deaths per 100,000 people in the United States was 11.5. However, male suicide deaths per 100,000 were 18.3; female suicide deaths were 4.8 (American Association of Suicidology 2010a). This inverse relationship has been referred to as "the gender paradox of suicidal behavior" and has been recognized for almost 200 years (Kushner 1995).

Statistical data consistently demonstrate that deaths by suicide among males exceed those among females in every country except China (Hansen and Pritchard 2008; Nordentoft and Branner 2008). In the United States, males die by suicide at a rate three to four times that of females (see Table 24–1)

(Brockington 2001; Maris et al. 2000; Möller-Leimkühler 2003; National Institute of Mental Health 2010). In 2007, suicide was the seventh leading cause of death for males and the 15th leading cause for females (National Institute of Mental Health 2010). The highest suicide rates for women occur among white females in the range of 45–54 years (American Foundation for Suicide Prevention 2007; Hu et al. 2008). Yet even these rates are lower than the suicide rates for men of any age.

The discrepancy between men's and women's suicide mortality rates is not easily explained by what we believe we know about important aspects of suicide. For example, approximately 90% of individuals who die by suicide have a diagnosable psychiatric disorder. Affective illness (major depression, bipolar disorder, and schizoaffective disorder) is the most common diagnosis among completers, accounting for up to 60%–70% of suicide deaths (Carroll-Ghosh et al. 2003; Maris et al. 2000; Moscicki 1999; Simon 2004, 2011). Epidemiological studies have consistently demonstrated that depression is about twice as common in women as in men (Kessler et al. 1996; Regier et al. 1988). The incidence of major depres-

TABLE 24–1. Suicide rates per 100,000 population, by sex

	1998	1999	2000	2001	2002	2003	2004	2005	2006	2007
Men	18.6	17.6	17.5	17.6	17.9	17.6	17.7	17.7	17.8	18.3
Women	4.4	4.1	4.1	4.1	4.3	4.3	4.6	4.5	4.6	4.8

Source. Adapted from American Association of Suicidology 2010b.

sion ranges from 2.6% to 5.5% in men and from 6% to 11% in women. This almost 2:1 ratio has been documented across countries and ethnic groups (Dubovsky et al. 2003; Kornstein and Wojcik 2002; Kung et al. 2003; Sloan and Kornstein 2003). Nevertheless, men are more likely to die by suicide.

A history of nonfatal attempts is also an acknowledged suicide risk factor. Statistical data and clinical experience support the observation that the best clinical indicator of a future suicide attempt is a prior suicide attempt (Simon 2004, 2011). Between 7% and 12% of patients who make attempts die by suicide within 10 years. For each attempt, the risk of another attempt occurring during a 2-year follow-up period increases by 30%. Between 18% and 38% of persons who die by suicide made previous attempts (Maris et al. 2000; Moscicki 1999; Skogman et al. 2004; Zahl and Hawton 2004). One study found that individuals who had made a suicide attempt had an approximately 30-fold increase in suicide risk in the 4 years following that attempt compared with the general population (Cooper et al. 2005). In the United States, women attempt suicide at a rate three to four times that of men (American Association of Suicidology 2010a, 2010b; American Foundation for Suicide Prevention 2007; Centers for Disease Control and Prevention 2010). Nevertheless, men are more likely to die by suicide.

The gender paradox of suicide has not been adequately studied or explained. Certainly, the relationship between psychiatric illness, nonfatal suicide attempts, and eventual suicide completion is complex and involves the interaction of multiple factors. However, most theories regarding suicidal behavior have been developed on the basis of male experiences and behavior. Studies that examine suicide mortality risk factors typically are examining a low base rate phenomenon representing approximately 1.3% of all deaths (American Association of Suicidology 2010a, 2010b), occurring primarily among white males (approximately 79% of all U.S. suicides in 2006) (Centers for Disease Control and Prevention 2010). Data on mental health issues related to suicide relevant to both women and men that would most readily emerge through studies inclusive of women (as well as ethnic minorities) typically have not been available (Canetto 2001).

As a result, most of what we believe we know about suicide risk factors applies primarily to older white men. The conclusions drawn from this limited gender- and ethnicity-biased database are then often applied generically to women and non-Caucasian ethnic groups (Canetto and Lester 1995). As these authors have pointed out, "[I]t is a myth that conceptual categories developed from studying suicidal behavior in white European-American men can be generalized to women and people of other cultures" (Canetto and Lester 1995, p. 4). The gender differences in suicide mortality rates cannot be explained by differences in the male-oriented demographic risk factors these studies produce. In addition, generalization of results of male-centered research leads to the reinforcement and perpetuation of gender stereotypes in psychiatry.

The gender paradox observed in suicide behavior and mortality suggests questions that require the adoption of alternative perspectives for investigation. If we seek to understand this paradox, we must use investigative approaches that move away from the centrality of the white male experience and focus instead on the characteristics of other groups. Why are other populations less vulnerable to suicide than white males despite having many of the demographic risk factors commonly associated with suicide mortality? Which factors or behaviors protect women (and other ethnic and racial groups) from the high suicide mortality rates of white males? The answers to these questions could lead to insights that expand our understanding of suicide as well as point us toward therapeutic interventions that could decrease suicide risk.

Gender is only one of the many static demographic factors that influence suicide mortality. Multiple static and dynamic risk factors contribute to any individual's attempted or completed suicide. Although gender can be examined as a factor in and of itself, it is inextricably intertwined with other static risk factors, such as age, race, and culture (see Table 24–2). For example, whites commit 90% of all suicides in the United States (Centers for Disease Control and Prevention 2009; National Institute of Mental Health 2010), and the rates of suicide among white men are consistently at least double the rates for men in any other ethnic group for which statistics are kept. In 2007, for example, the rate of suicide among African American males was 8.4 per 100,000; among females it was 1.7 per 100,000, the lowest of any ethnic/gender subgroup. As one group of authors noted, African Amer-

ican women "are remarkably resistant to suicide compared to other demographic groups" (Garlow et al. 2005, p. 321).

Suicide rates also change relative to age across as well as within ethnic and racial groups (Garlow et al. 2005). Suicide rates for white men peak at midlife and again around age 80. Rates for white women peak in midlife and rise again after age 75, whereas rates for nonwhite men and women peak in young adult life (Garlow et al. 2005; Good and Sherrod 2001; Moscicki 1995; National Institute of Mental Health 2010; Webster Rudmin et al. 2003; Willis et al. 2003). For example, in 2007, suicide was the third leading cause of death among African American youth ages 10–19 (American Association of Suicidology 2010a). Suicide rates among Native Americans/Alaska Natives (12.1 per 100,000 in 2007), which are the highest of any racial or ethnic group other than whites, are also concentrated in lower age groups. From 1999 through 2004, individuals ages 15–24 had the highest rates among this population (Centers for Disease Control and Prevention 2011). A complete investigation of these interrelated demographic factors is beyond the scope of this discussion, but elements of these issues will inevitably arise and be noted in the course of a discussion of gender.

Case Examples

Case Example 1: Mr. Taylor

Mr. Taylor was a white, divorced, 58-year-old chief executive officer of a major corporation. He had lived alone since his divorce a number of years earlier. He had a history of escalating alcohol dependence, which had begun to impair his functioning. He sought psychiatric treatment with the encouragement and support of friends and family. He was able to discontinue alcohol use and responded well to antidepressant medication. After 2 years, he discontinued

TABLE 24–2. Suicide rates per 100,000 population, by race

Group	2003	2004	2005	2006	2007
White male	19.5	19.6	19.7	19.7	20.5
White female	4.7	5.1	5.0	5.0	5.4
Nonwhite male	9.1	9.3	9.0	9.0	9.6
Nonwhite female	2.2	2.4	2.3	2.3	2.3
Black male	8.8	9.0	8.7	8.7	8.4
Black female	1.8	1.8	1.8	1.8	1.7
Hispanic	5.0	5.3	5.1	5.1	5.4
Native American	10.4	12.9	12.4	12.4	12.1
Asian/Pacific Islander	5.5	5.6	5.2	5.2	6.1

Source. Adapted from American Association of Suicidology 2010b.

treatment because he felt he was doing well.

Soon after ending treatment, Mr. Taylor's company came under federal investigation for financial fraud. Mr. Taylor was forced out of the company, became a target of investigation, and possibly faced criminal charges. Mr. Taylor did not tell his family or friends about his work problems. He became increasingly isolative, spent his days at home, and rarely left his house. He began drinking again.

Mr. Taylor's family found out about the investigation after it made headlines in the local papers. Mr. Taylor's adult son called and spoke with his father after reading the papers. Mr. Taylor did not sound upset. He told his son not to worry and that once the whole truth came out, everything would turn out well. Later in the day, Mr. Taylor's son tried to call again, but no one answered the phone. He went to his father's house and found Mr. Taylor dead from a gunshot wound to the head, with his handgun lying next to him. The death was ruled a suicide. A blood alcohol level revealed that Mr. Taylor had been intoxicated at the time he shot himself.

Case Example 2: Ms. Smith

Ms. Smith was a white 48-year-old woman who worked in law enforcement. She had just made an appointment with a psychiatrist, Dr. Black, for a medication consultation. Ms. Smith had a history of two suicide attempts by over-the-counter medication, one at age 15 and another at age 28. The first was precipitated by problems with her physically abusive father, and the sec-

ond followed a painful divorce. Both resulted in hospitalization and successful treatment with medication. Although she stopped taking her medication some years after her first hospitalization, Ms. Smith had remained on medication since the time of her second suicide attempt. Ms. Smith reported that both of these attempts were serious and her intent had been to die.

Three years before Ms. Smith made the appointment with Dr. Black, Ms. Smith's job required that she relocate to a new state, leaving behind supportive family and friends. Since moving, she had been isolated and lonely but had remained on her medication, which she received from her internist. Despite taking her medication, Ms. Smith began experiencing more symptoms of depression and hopelessness. She had become involved in a relationship, and after 1 year she and her boyfriend began living together. However, their relationship began to deteriorate. At the same time, Ms. Smith's mother was diagnosed with terminal cancer. Because of the distance and her job responsibilities, Ms. Smith was not able to see her mother as much as she would have liked and felt increasingly guilty about this.

Ms. Smith had begun seeing a psychotherapist before contacting Dr. Black. Ms. Smith and her therapist had a good therapeutic alliance. Both Ms. Smith and her therapist were concerned that Ms. Smith's medication needed to be adjusted. The therapist referred Ms. Smith to Dr. Black. In the week prior to the scheduled consultation, Ms. Smith and her boyfriend began talking about separating. Ms. Smith developed acute suicidal ideation 3 days prior to the consultation with Dr. Black. Given her experience of surviving two previous suicide attempts by overdose, Ms. Smith wanted to make sure that if she tried to kill herself, she would succeed. She loaded her employment-issued firearm and put it to her head.

After sitting for some time with the loaded gun, Ms. Smith decided not to shoot herself. The main reason for this decision was her concern about the effect her suicide would have on her mother, although she mentally reserved the option of killing herself after her mother died. In the meantime, Ms. Smith decided to go through with the consultation to see if medication might help. Ms. Smith responded honestly to Dr. Black's questions about suicidal ideation and plans but revealed that she had not told anyone else, including her therapist, about her suicidal intent or plan.

Mr. Taylor, in the first case example, exemplifies the "typical" suicide completer: an older white male who is depressed, maybe alcoholic; lives alone or is socially isolated; has grown increasingly hopeless; has recurring work, sexual, and marital problems; has experienced a series of stressful negative life events; often sees suicide as the only permanent resolution to his persistent life problems; uses a highly lethal, irreversible method (most often a gunshot to the head); and dies after his first suicide attempt (Maris et al. 2000).

Ms. Smith, in the second case example, has a history consistent with elements of the stereotypical nonfatal suicide attempter. As a younger female, she made two suicide attempts but used less lethal methods—those having lower medical certainty of resulting in death. She was perhaps ambivalent about dying. Such attempts are often motivated by interpersonal dynamics, including changes in an important relationship. These attempts may be more impulsive and may be related to either Axis I or Axis II disorders, although those who make nonfatal suicide attempts, like those who complete suicide, tend to be depressed

and to abuse alcohol and other substances (Maris et al. 2000). The degree of Ms. Smith's current intent was indicated by her choice of a new and more lethal method based specifically on her previous experiences of failure to kill herself by overdose. Her current presentation is consistent with a high risk of suicide mortality, despite her history of lower-lethality attempts.

Demographic Risk Factors

Most of the demographic factors commonly acknowledged to increase suicide risk do not explain the differences in suicide mortality rates among groups other than white males (Canetto 1995; Canetto and Lester 1995). Demographic risk factors, such as single status, increasing age, or physical illness, are not as significant for groups other than white males or do not explain the lower or higher rates of suicide mortality in other groups. For example, the association of advanced age and suicide is almost exclusively a white-male phenomenon. The frequency of suicide among females changes relatively little across middle and late life (Maris et al. 2000), although there was a slight increase (0.7%) in the rate of suicide among white middle-aged women between the years 1999 and 2005 (Johns Hopkins Bloomberg School of Public Health 2008).

Elderly women do not have any particular advantages over elderly men in regard to the suicide risk factors most commonly mentioned in the literature. In fact, elderly women are more likely than elderly men to be exposed to conditions such as limited financial resources, loss of a spouse, living alone, and poor health that in elderly men have been thought to precipitate suicidal behavior. Yet the suicide mortality rates of elderly women are significantly lower than those of elderly men (Canetto 2001; Canetto and Lester 1995). Moreover, peak suicide rates for males in other ethnic groups, such as Native Americans and African Americans, occur at younger ages (American Association of Suicidology 2010a; Centers for Disease Control and Prevention 2011).

Other studies have confirmed that suicide among women generally is less associated with adversity and single status (Oates 2003). Notably, risk factors such as single status, lower socioeconomic status, and unemployment are at least as common among African American women as among white men (Alston and Anderson 1995). Indeed, African American women are likely to be among the most socioeconomically disadvantaged groups in the United States. Yet rates of suicide mortality for African American women are the lowest of all race-by-gender groups in the United States (American Association of Suicidology 2010a) (although their rates of violent death at the hands of others are among the highest of any subgroup; Alston and Anderson 1995).

Standard Explanations for the Gender Gap

Explanations for the gender paradox in suicide often reflect traditional gender stereotypes. Explorations of gender-related issues begin with understanding that *gender* refers to the socially constructed roles of men and women implicating different norms and cultural expectations for both sexes. These norms and expectations define characteristics typical and desirable for males and females. These characteristics are transmitted and reinforced by early socialization as well as by social institutions. Substantial disparities not supported by biological distinctions continue to exist in the construction of gender roles, myths, and stereotypes. These distinctions structure acceptable social roles as well as access to personal, social, and material resources.

Both roles and access to resources differ significantly for men and women. For this reason, gender is a significant determinant of health and illness, including psychiatric illness (Möller-Leimkühler 2003).

Early suicidologists attributed women's lower suicide mortality rates to their stereotypical female character traits, such as mental dullness and a passive nature, or to the effects of gender-based social roles. Beginning in the nineteenth century, male suicide was characterized as the result of the grave stresses inherent in men's roles and responsibilities and the consequence of adversity, such as impotence, business embarrassments, losses, and ungratified ambition. Women, in contrast, were said to die by suicide because of domestic unhappiness, loss of honor or purity (illicit love affairs), or disappointed love. Durkheim (1897/1951) theorized that women are less prone to suicide than men because of their greater emotional attachments to home and family, greater religious faith, greater patience, and less developed intellectual capacity. As outdated as such explanations may sound, they were held well into the mid-twentieth century (Canetto and Lester 1995; Kposowa and McElvain 2006; Maris et al. 2000).

Although more extreme aspects of such explanations, such as women's lower intellectual capacity, are no longer given any credence, long-standing beliefs regarding differential motives still reflect these stereotypes. The commonly held beliefs that men are more likely to kill themselves as a result of failure in some arena of achievement and that women are more likely to die as a result of romantic relationships that have gone bad still persist (McAndrew and Garrison 2007). In fact, more recent studies have generally failed to find consistent differences between factors precipitating suicide for men and women. Both men and women report mental illness, loneliness, and loss of an intimate relationship as the primary triggers for suicide (McAndrew and Garrison 2007).

Gender-based stereotypic explanations fail to provide much-needed insight into the gendered nature of suicide and create obstacles to less biased investigation. More significantly, they may lead to the underestimation of suicide risk in individuals who do not conform to gender stereotypes regarding suicide (McAndrew and Garrison 2007). Other aspects of the standard explanations for gender differences in suicide rates are reviewed in the following sections of this chapter. These other aspects also fail to provide complete explanations and may lead to similar difficulties in both research and risk assessment.

Substance Abuse or Dependence

Substance abuse is also a gendered disorder, occurring primarily in men. It has been suggested that the higher incidence of substance abuse, particularly alcohol abuse, accounts for the gender gap in suicide mortality. Alcohol abuse or dependence occurs three to four times more frequently among men than women, with the overall male-to-female ratios varying from approximately 2:1 to 5:1 (Canterbury 2002; Cotto et al. 2010; Hasin et al. 2007; Regier et al. 1990).

Could the risk of suicide associated with the use of alcohol in men outweigh the gendered risk factors of depression and suicide attempt? Alcohol abuse is the second most frequent diagnosis associated with suicide, following mood disorders (Moscicki 1999). The National Violent Death Reporting System reported that in 2006, in a total of 17 states, alcohol intoxication was present in 24% of those who died by suicide, and one-third who died by suicide were positive for alcohol at the time of death (Centers for Disease Control and Prevention 2009, 2010).

Some support for the theory of differences in rates of substance abuse as the basis of the gender gap in suicide mortality rates can be found in studies that have demonstrated a higher rate of alcoholism in males who die by suicide than in females who die by suicide (Kung et al. 2003). The Centers for Disease Control and Prevention (CDC) reports that consistent with other studies, the percentage of tested subjects with blood alcohol levels at or over the legal limit for intoxication was higher for males than for females in almost all racial/ethnic populations (Centers for Disease Control and Prevention 2009). In one such study, alcohol was detected in 28.9% of individuals who died by suicide; of these, 81.8% were male and 18.2% were female (Garlow 2002).

Gendered patterns of substance abuse in regard to comorbid illness, however, indicate that although this Axis I diagnosis and risk factor may play some role, increased rates of alcohol dependence in men do not entirely explain the gender gap. Major depression is often a primary diagnosis in women who abuse alcohol. In contrast, the majority of men who abuse alcohol demonstrate alcoholism as a primary diagnosis (Brady and Randall 1999; Canterbury 2002). Moreover, females with alcoholism have significantly more depression and anxiety disorders than do their male counterparts, and the onset of these disorders precedes the onset of substance use disorders more often in women than in men (Kessler et al. 1996; Table 24–3). In addition, one study found that differential patterns of substance abuse did not account for the lower age at suicide of African Americans, indicating that substance abuse also cannot account for other demographic differences in suicide mortality (Garlow et al. 2005).

TABLE 24–3. General patterns found in alcohol abuse/dependence relative to gender

	Men	Women
Primary diagnosis	Alcohol abuse/dependence	Major depression
Anxiety disorder present	Less often	More often
Depressive disorder present	Less often	More often
Onset of non–substance abuse disorders	More often follows onset of substance abuse	More often precedes onset of substance abuse

Male stereotypes play a role in explanations involving alcohol abuse. Although substance use disorders in general are stigmatized, substance use is more stigmatized in women than in men. This may result in the lower levels of alcohol abuse among women (Brady and Randall 1999; Maris et al. 2000). Nevertheless, when women exhibit alcohol abuse as a comorbid disorder, they exhibit higher rates of suicidal behavior and mortality (Kornstein and Wojcik 2002). In the 1993 National Mortality Followback Survey, which used natural deaths as a control group, both male and female suicide decedents were more likely to have used marijuana and alcohol (Kung et al. 2003).

Lethality of Method

The higher suicide rate among males is commonly explained at least in part by the belief that men reportedly choose relatively limited, highly lethal methods to die by suicide, particularly firearms, whereas women use a much greater variety of relatively lower-lethality methods (Kposowa and McElvain 2006; Kung et al. 2003; Maris et al. 2000). Historically, men have indeed committed the majority of firearm suicides: in 1998, the rate of suicide by such a method was more than 6.5 times the rate in women (11.4 and 1.7/100,000, respectively; Romero and Wintemute 2002).

Investigations of gender and method of suicide have concluded that the proposition that women use less lethal methods of committing suicide than men is only partially supported by data. The circumstances and explanations associated with suicide and lethality of method are more complex than a simple dichotomy between more lethal and less lethal methods (Kposowa and McElvain 2006).

More recent epidemiological data demonstrate that firearms have become the most common method of suicide for both men and women across all age groups, notwithstanding females' lower absolute rates of suicide. Women committing suicide have increasingly used firearms over past years. Each year, approximately 50% of all suicide deaths are due to firearms (Table 24–4). Of these, approximately 60% are men and 40% are women (American Association of Suicidology 2010b). In 2007, the CDC reported that of firearm suicides, 56% were male and 30% were female (National Institute of Mental Health 2010).

Analyses of methods of suicide indicate that comparable proportions of males and females use violent means to die by suicide (Judd et al. 2010) and that people use methods of suicide to which they have ready access (Elnour and Harrison 2008; Kposowa and McElvain 2006). Access to a firearm increases risk for suicide for both males and females (Hu et al. 2008; Kung et al. 2003), even in individuals with no identifiable psychopathology (Brent 2001). Women who

TABLE 24–4. Suicide methods, 2007

Method	Percentage of total suicides
Firearms	50.2
All except firearms	49.8
Suffocation/ hanging	23.6
Poisoning	18.4
Cutting/piercing	1.8
Drowning	1.0

Source. Adapted from American Association of Suicidology 2010b.

purchase handguns are at particularly high risk for suicide with a firearm. In a broad community-based study whose cohort represented all causes of death, suicide by firearm accounted for 31.2% of all deaths during the first year of gun ownership among women who purchased handguns. This rate stood in marked contrast with 0.2% of all deaths among all women in the cohort (Wintemute et al. 1999).

In a 2005 Gallup poll, 30% of the U.S. population reported owning a handgun, and another 12% reported living in a home where someone else owned a handgun. Nearly half of men (47%) reported personal ownership. Thirteen percent of women reported personal ownership, and 31% of women lived in a home with access to a firearm (Carroll 2005). The higher proportion of men committing suicide with firearms may be an artifact of higher rates of gun ownership among men rather than a reflection of men's greater preference to die by suicide using a firearm. The proportions of men versus women who use firearms to die by suicide are very similar to the gender distribution of firearm ownership and handgun ownership in the general population (Conner and Zhong 2003). Thus, lethality of method, although one possible factor,

does not itself explain the gender gap in suicide mortality.

Explanations such as those offered in regard to lethality of methods also reflect gender stereotypes. Men are said to be more familiar and comfortable with guns. The lower rates of gun ownership among women, however, may reflect social roles and norms that discourage aggression in women. In addition, social acceptability, which is related to gender stereotypes, also influences choice of suicide method (Elnour and Harrison 2008). The gender bias inherent in the investigation of lethality of method is demonstrated in the often repeated assertion that women tend to use firearms less often than men because they might cause unsightly disfigurement, implying that concerns over appearance after death may be more important to suicidal women than concerns regarding death itself (Maris et al. 2000; Stack and Wasserman 2009). This explanation reflects stereotypic beliefs regarding vanity in women and does not take into account that firearms are now a preferred method of suicide for women as well as men.

Neurobiology of Aggression, Violence, and Suicidal Ideation and Suicide Plans

In recent years, the presence of the serotonin metabolite 5-hydroxyindoleacetic acid (5-HIAA) in the cerebrospinal fluid (CSF) and its relationship to suicide, especially violent suicide, have been explored and offered as a possible explanation for various aspects of suicidal behavior, including gender differences in suicide mortality rates. A literature search of PubMed in December 2010 demonstrated more than 100 publications on these subjects in 2010 alone. One of the most consistent findings in the suicide literature, reported in both postmortem studies of suicide completers and clinical studies of suicide attempters, has been evidence of decreased brain stem levels of serotonin or 5-HIAA. More potentially lethal suicide attempts have also been associated with lower CSF 5-HIAA levels (Carroll-Ghosh et al. 2003; Mann and Arango 1999; Moscicki 1999).

Nevertheless, these findings do not as yet form the basis of a complete explanation of gender-based differences in suicide mortality rates. CSF 5-HIAA determinations, particularly those done postmortem, are an imprecise way to measure serotonin levels and activity in the living brain. Many of these studies also had small numbers of subjects. Moreover, like many types of suicide studies, most of this research on CSF concentrations of 5-HIAA has focused on male subjects (Maris et al. 2000), raising the question of whether these results can be generalized to women.

Biochemical explanations that link aggression, suicide, and gender are still incomplete. Numerous other neurotransmitters, as yet unexplored, are likely to be implicated in any complex behavior such as suicide (Carroll-Ghosh et al. 2003). In addition, other biochemical differences exist between men and women. These do not of themselves indicate a connection with greater or lesser rates of suicide mortality. Women, for example, have lower concentrations of testosterone than do men. The link between testosterone and aggression is well recognized, but there is no known direct relationship between testosterone and suicidal behavior (Maris et al. 2000).

Help-Seeking Behaviors

Women are also said to have decreased rates of suicide mortality because they are more likely than men to seek help when depressed. Multiple studies have demonstrated that emotions such as weakness, uncertainty, helplessness, anxiety, and sadness are considered common female stereotypical characteristics. A woman's identity is therefore not threatened by acknowledgment of such symptoms or the seeking of support. Women are thus believed to be more likely to seek medical or mental health services (Chrisler 2001; Kung et al. 2003; Maris et al. 2000; Möller-Leimkühler 2003).

In contrast, male stereotypes that encourage emotional isolation and suppression of distress do not promote help seeking or acknowledgment of depression. Such behaviors are considered signs of weakness and dependence and imply loss of control, autonomy, and competence. These are not consistent with perceptions of masculine identity and thus may be avoided, resulting in higher rates of suicide mortality (Good and Sherrod 2001; Maris et al. 2000; Möller-Leimkühler 2003).

Studies support the observation that women use health services more often than do men, even when visits for pregnancy and birth-related services are factored out (Chrisler 2001). One study found that a greater number of female suicide decedents were more likely than their male counterparts to have had contact with mental health services (Luoma et al. 2002). The effect of this gendered utilization of health services, however, has not been consistently demonstrated to directly correlate with suicide mortality. For example, the 1993 National Mortality Followback Survey found that both male and female suicide decedents were more likely to have used mental health services in the year prior to the suicide (Kung et al. 2003).

One recent study (Chang et al. 2009) noted that most people who die by suicide had contact with health care services and that significantly more females than males had contacted health care services prior to suicide. However, the study also found that mental disorders and major depression were largely underdiagnosed, especially in males. The Taiwanese researchers posited a cultural bias against confronting emotional or psychological problems in their Taiwanese study population.

However, in one large British study, 24% of subjects who had completed suicide had contact with mental health services in the year before death. Of these, 66% were male, a ratio of 1.93:1 (Appleby et al. 1999). Older studies found that 75% of individuals who completed suicide had had contact with a physician within 6 months prior to their death (Blumenthal 1990). Because the majority of suicide victims are men, a large proportion of the individuals who contacted physicians were also likely to be men, indicating a willingness to seek help for either a somatic or emotional problem.

Even if found to be statistically significant, gender differences in help-seeking behavior seem unlikely to fully explain lower mortality rates in women. In regard to mental health services in general, fewer than a third of people with mental disorders seek treatment, and among those who do, a significant number are misdiagnosed or suboptimally treated (Blehar and Norquist 2002; Chang et al. 2009).

Motivation and Intent

Another explanation of gender differences in the suicide mortality rate influenced by gender stereotypes focuses on beliefs regarding differences in motivation and intent in suicidal behavior. Research conducted during the 1960s served to sharpen distinctions between fatal and nonfatal suicidal behavior and portrayed the latter

as being less aimed at ending life than at changing life (McAndrew and Garrison 2007). It is now widely believed that a majority of suicidal women have little or no intent to die, resulting in low mortality rates. The nonlethal suicidal acts of women are often interpreted as maladaptive aggressive or affiliative strategies employed to solve interpersonal problems or to influence relationships rather than as a desire to end life (Stephens 1995). It is not uncommon to see suicide attempts by women described pejoratively as manipulative or passive-aggressive. Explanations that invoke character traits rather than assessment of intent both reflect and reinforce some of the most negative elements of female gender stereotypes. Help-seeking behavior is considered a female characteristic, closely equated with the negative, less mature, and less valued personality trait of dependency. Similarly, suicide attempts and gestures interpreted as manipulative or controlling behavior are closely related to both dependency and passive-aggressiveness, other negative traits that are strongly associated with women.

Gendered differences in patterns and outcomes of suicide attempts and repeated episodes of deliberate self-harm have been observed (Hawton and Harriss 2008; Skogman et al. 2004; Zahl and Hawton 2004). Nevertheless, the issue of lethal intent in women's suicidal behaviors is unresolved. Self-destructive behavior occurs on a continuum of lethality and intent. It can be difficult to determine which behaviors may be gestures without true lethal intent and which behaviors, however minimal in actual lethality, are truly intended to result in death.

Indeed, the interpretation of suicide attempts as "gestures" can result in the minimization of behavior that may have profound significance in terms of suicide assessment. Studies of suicide after a previous suicide attempt have shown conflicting results concerning the predictive value of the dangerousness of the attempt with regard to later suicide (Nordentoft and Branner 2008). These authors found that although men demonstrated higher suicidal intent, this was not associated with more frequent choice of methods with high case fatality.

In the second case example, an evaluation that focused on Ms. Smith's past attempts and use of less lethal methods to conclude that her current risk of suicide was low would have been erroneous. As Nordentoft and Branner (2008) have noted, "It is a widespread myth that choice of suicide method reflects the intention to die" (p. 209). For example, many individuals hold erroneous beliefs regarding the relative safety or lethality of commonly available over-the-counter medication or prescription medication and may be surprised to learn that 10 aspirin or 10 zolpidem tablets is not a fatal dose. Others may be devastated to find that ingestion of a bottle of acetaminopen or just a few extra lithium carbonate capsules can be fatal. Multiple authors have cautioned that the evaluation of lethality of female suicide attempters should consider the severity of the suicidal intent rather than the lethality of the method (Hawton and Harriss 2008; Simon 2004, 2011; Skogman et al. 2004).

Protective Factors in Women

The influence of gender stereotypes and gendered approaches to suicide research has obscured perspectives regarding suicide that deserve more extensive study. In the case examples, both Mr. Taylor and Ms. Smith were at high risk for suicide. A focus on risk factors such as those easily recog-

nized in the case of Mr. Taylor leads to overlooking what may be the most clinically significant question related to gender (and race, ethnicity, and culture) and suicide: Why did Mr. Taylor kill himself and Ms. Smith choose to continue living? What protects groups other than white males who demonstrate similar demographic risk factors from the high suicide mortality rates demonstrated by white males? As Kaplan and Klein (1989) observed over 20 years ago, "Perhaps the most revealing question to look at, especially in terms of future suicide prevention, is 'What keeps women alive?'" (p. 267).

The gender stereotypes noted earlier may indeed provide some protection from suicide for women, although not in the way suggested by traditional explanations based on negative female stereotypes. As noted, completed suicide is viewed as a masculine phenomenon and is considered more permissible for men. Attempted but "failed" suicide is more often identified as a feminine behavior characteristic (Canetto 2001; Canetto and Lester 1995; Kushner 1995; McAndrew and Garrison 2007). Researchers have found that both males and females who died by suicide were rated as more masculine and more potent than males and females who simply attempted suicide. Older European American men's suicides are narrated as acts of independence and courage in the face of adversity. Studies have demonstrated less empathy toward suicidal men. Nevertheless, they have also rated suicide in males as less wrong, less foolish, and less weak than suicide in females (McAndrew and Garrison 2007; Möller-Leimkühler 2003).

Because stereotypes influence behavior, women may be more inhibited from lethal suicidal behavior on the basis of cultural norms. If nonfatal suicide behavior is viewed as weaker and less masculine, males might be more likely to structure any suicidal act in such a way as to reduce the likelihood of surviving. Females, however, might feel less stigma from surviving an attempt and might therefore be likely to engage in less lethal suicidal actions (Stillion 1995). The example of the exception to the low suicide mortality rate of women may support this hypothesis. Chinese American women, who have high suicide rates, come from a culture in which suicide is considered a female behavior. China is the one country where suicide is more common among women than among men, especially in rural areas. As Canetto (2001) concluded, "The cross-cultural data suggest that it is the association of suicide with masculinity that protects most U.S. older women from suicide. Once that association is reversed, as appears to be the case in Chinese communities, women are counted among the suicidal" (pp. 192–193).

Conversely, gender stereotypes encourage men to be "tough," which means suppressing all emotions potentially associated with vulnerability. This cultural male identity often results in dysfunctional health consequences. The relative vulnerability of males to a variety of physical and emotional problems may arise from maladaptive coping strategies associated with adhering to masculine stereotypes: emotional inexpressiveness, lack of help seeking, aggressiveness, risk-taking behavior, violence, alcohol and drug abuse, and suicide. The irony inherent in the ultimate effect of such stereotypes, aimed at producing "strong men," is the evidence that "stoicism does not produce emotional strength. Indeed, rather than producing strong men, stoicism produces brittle men" (Good and Sherrod 2001, p. 205).

Other explorations of the factors that decrease suicide mortality in women look to psychological theory, which has proposed alternative models of healthy female psychological development and mental health (Gilligan 1993; Jordan 1997; Jordan et al. 1991; Miller 1987). This model, based on the centrality of relationships, posits a continuous path of relational development that moves beyond a traditional psychodynamic focus on individual psychological development. Interdependency, reciprocity, and mutual empathy are seen as characteristics of healthy relationships. Although members of both sexes can and do engage in such an exchange, powerful cultural norms tend to reinforce relational development in girls to a greater extent than in boys (Kaplan and Klein 1989). The significance of relatedness to others and the importance of social supports appear to serve women as protection against suicidal urges.

Relational theorists propose that both women and men experience increased psychological difficulties when opportunities to enter into and sustain healthy relationships are unavailable (Kaplan and Klein 1989). This is supported by recent studies that demonstrate that both men and women who die by suicide reported loneliness and rejection in an intimate relationship as primary triggers for suicide (see McAndrew and Garrison 2007). More traditional psychodynamic frameworks interpret women's need for and maladaptive attempts to maintain relationships in negative terms such as *dependency, passivity,* or *manipulativeness.* From the perspective of relational theory, suicidal action becomes a mode by which a woman makes a desperate plea for mutual engagement: "When a woman's relational priorities and needs are so blocked or distorted that she perceives no further possibilities for growth within relationships, her vulnerability to suicide will be greater" (Kaplan and Klein 1989, p. 259).

Women may also be protected from suicide by an adherence to ethics based on the centrality of relationships and principles of interdependence, mutuality of caretaking, and responsibility for the well-being of others. These ethics differ from the predominantly male ethic of justice, which centers on principles of right and wrong (Gilligan 1993). This proposed female "ethic of care" defines a moral responsibility to avoid hurting others. This may prevent women from taking actions such as suicide that would cause pain to others, particularly to dependent children (Canetto 2001; Kushner 1995). For a woman, the decision to kill herself and to therefore abandon her relationships with or hurt others "stands in direct opposition to the values most central to her core identity as a relational being" (Kaplan and Klein 1989, p. 260).

The importance of relationships and relatedness to others (including childbearing and child care) may provide a core framework for understanding suicidal behavior in women (Maris et al. 2000). Epidemiological data indicate that having a child in the home under age 18 reduced the risk of suicide in women but not in men (Kung et al. 2003; Maris et al. 2000; Young et al. 1994). Clinical observations indicate that the psychological experience of a seriously suicidal woman often includes feeling torn by an anguished struggle between the need to alleviate her own unbearable pain and her sense of responsibility to avoid hurting those who would be affected by her death (Kaplan and Klein 1989).

The clinical implications of these protective factors are profound. In a case example presented earlier in this chapter, Ms. Smith ultimately chose not to kill herself because of the effect her death would have on her mother. Should Ms. Smith's mother die, and Ms. Smith's level of depression and access to a firearm remain unchanged, her risk for suicide would increase considerably. It is possible that had Mr. Taylor (in the other case example presented earlier) been more engaged with his adult children, the risk of his committing suicide in response to his problems would have been decreased.

Women also demonstrate more adaptational and flexible coping styles than do men. Many women demonstrate a willingness to try to resolve problems in a variety of ways and in ways that include connecting with others. Studies of suicide prevention center utilization confirm the significantly greater tendency for women to seek and benefit from contact with these helping facilities, although as noted, this factor cannot entirely explain the gender gap in mortality rates. Nevertheless, gender differences in suicidal behavior may reflect a tendency for males to respond with a more rigid position to stress, conflict, and frustration. Females may have a greater tendency to adopt problem-solving strategies that include seeking help, thus maximizing their chances for attachment and assistance (Canetto and Lester 1995; Maris et al. 2000). In contrast, men "tend to move more readily to a position of giving up and ending a perceived intolerable state of being" (Maris et al. 2000, p. 157), increasing their risk of suicide.

The relational model may also explain the differential effects of more traditionally recognized suicide risk factors. For example, marriage is commonly cited as a protective factor against suicide (Maris et al. 2000; Slaby 1998). Nevertheless, it appears that marriage protects men from suicide more than it does women (Kposowa 2000). The relational model provides insight into how the social and psychological benefits provided by marriage differ for men and women. Males are less socially integrated and report fewer sources of support. Often the only source of support is their spouse, who may also mediate their relationships with children, other family members, and friends. When men lose their spouses, their social relationships are more disrupted. Women, on the other hand, seem to form greater supportive networks, such as meaningful friendships, regardless of their marital status. Accordingly, even when a marriage ends in divorce or death, women can fall back on resources of social bonds and support often unavailable to men (Kposowa 2000; Möller-Leimkühler 2003).

More research needs to be done to find the factors that protect women and other groups from the high rates of suicide associated with older white men and some younger ethnic groups. This perspective requires a reversal of the pattern of allowing gender stereotypes to define problems as well as approaches to answering these problems. The suicide "gender paradox" offers an opportunity to develop interventions that can reduce the risk of suicide in those groups that lack the protective factors more commonly found in women.

Gendered Issues in Suicide

Exploration of the role of gender in suicide has included a number of speculative investigations, some of which implicitly reinforce gender stereotypes. Some researchers have proposed the existence of a "male depressive syndrome," a subtype of depression clinically limited to men, in which suicide is more common (Walinder and Rutz 2001). The validity of this concept has limited support. Other explorations of gender have included investigations of whether male and female suicide completers jump from different heights (apparently not; Lester 2003) and whether suicide notes written by men and women differ (maybe; Maris et al. 2000).

Certain gendered issues related to suicide have been explored with research that demonstrates some clinical significance or epidemiological validity. These gender-related issues are worth reviewing both in and of themselves and for their ability to elucidate gender-related protective factors as well as suicide risk factors.

Childhood Sexual Abuse

A history of childhood sexual abuse is another recognized suicide risk factor. Childhood sexual abuse is associated with a higher rate of adult psychopathology in general, including adult suicide behaviors (Maris et al. 2000; Martin et al. 2004; Simon 2004, 2011). This factor is also more commonly associated with women than with men, because childhood sexual abuse is more common among women (Finkelhor 1994; Molnar et al. 2001; Roy and Janal 2006). Research studies consistently confirm the strong association between childhood sexual abuse and suicide attempts, with attributable risk consistent with the more prevalent exposure to sexual abuse among women (Bebbington et al. 2009; Roy and Janal 2006).

Strikingly, although more common among girls, the experience of childhood sexual abuse carries more consequences for boys in regard to alcohol and drug use, aggressive behavior, truancy, and suicidal ideation and plans. Community-based studies have found the risk of suicide death in abused boys to be markedly elevated not only when compared with nonabused boys but also when compared with abused girls (Martin et al. 2004; Molnar et al. 2001). The possibility that gender-related protective factors might mitigate the risk of suicide completion in sexually abused girls, particularly when compared with the highly elevated risk of suicide attempts (Roy and Janal 2006), remains to be investigated.

Women Physicians and Suicide

Studies examining rates of suicide in women physicians consistently report substantially higher rates of suicide for this professional group: four times higher than the national female rate. Research into the association of specific occupations and suicide has been marked by methodological problems and inconsistencies (Frank and Dingle 1999; Stack 2000). Research on the incidence of suicide among physicians is marked by considerable debate over the extent to which physicians generally are at risk for suicide or whether the high rates noted reflect the demographics associated with white males, who make up the majority of this profession (Stack 2000).

One study comparing suicide to other causes of mortality in physicians found that physicians in general are at substantially lower risk of dying compared with the general population for all causes of death except suicide (Torre et al. 2005). A meta-analysis reviewing the research in this area noted that both male and female physicians show elevated suicide ratios when compared with the general population. Although the male physicians' rate was modestly elevated, at 1.41, the female physicians' rate was highly elevated, at 2.27. However, the issue of the bias of the studies regarding female physicians and suicide was also noted, especially in regard to creating an appearance of elevated rates that may in fact not be accurate (Schernhammer and Colditz 2004).

A number of groups of professionals are noted to have elevated suicide rates. These include physicians, nurses, pharmacists, veterinarians, chemists, lawyers, and psychologists (Stack 2000). High suicide rates have been found among female chemists, psychologists, and university professors, as well as physicians (Yang and Lester 1995).

Researchers have also observed the preponderance of professions that have access to lethal methods of suicide in these groups. Thus, studies that have found elevated risk of suicide in female members of these professions may indeed reflect the elevated risk in these occupations due to such access (Brockington 2001; Frank and Dingle 1999; Stack 2000). This finding implies that whatever protective factors may be associated with gender can be outweighed by access to lethal means of suicide.

The prevalence of suicide among women physicians in the United States and the presence of associated factors such as psychiatric disorders and suicidal behavior have actually received little systematic investigation. Available studies are methodologically flawed in a variety of ways, including the problems associated with small sample sizes (Frank and Dingle 1999; Schernhammer and Colditz 2004; Yang and Lester 1995). Depression, drug abuse, and alcoholism are often associated with suicides of physicians. Women physicians in particular have been shown to have a higher frequency of alcoholism and a higher incidence of depression than women in the general population (Schernhammer and Colditz 2004).

Nevertheless, although the suicide completion rate of female physicians seems to be higher than that of other women and higher than the rate of male physicians, their suicide attempt rate may be lower. One study (Frank and Dingle 1999) found that 1.5% of women physicians reported having attempted suicide, and 19.5% reported a history of depression. Those with a history of depression were substantially more likely to have attempted suicide than were those without a history of depression (7% and 0.2%, respectively). The rate of 1.5% for suicide attempts is low even compared with the rate of attempts (about 4%) reported generally among U.S. women. Women physicians may therefore have lower rates of suicidal intent and/or higher rates of completion than women in the general population (Frank and Dingle 1999).

Various hypotheses have been advanced to explain physician suicide generally and the higher rates in women physicians in particular. Affective disorders and substance abuse are the most common psychiatric diagnoses noted, and as in other gender subgroups, the risk associated with these disorders appears to outweigh any protective factors. The possibility of higher rates of completion relative to occupational access to lethal methods and increased incidence of drug and alcohol abuse may decrease some of the association of gender-related issues. Other explanations take social and cultural perspectives. Many believe that the practice of medicine poses additional stresses for women, including prejudice and discrimination, the lack of women role models, role conflict, and inadequate family and institutional support (Bowman and Allen 1985; Frank and Dingle 1999; Stack 2000; Yang and Lester 1995).

Gender stereotypes both suggest and support such explanations. However, gendered beliefs also have their own effect on assumptions underlying research and thus may be a source of distortion in both results and interpretation of data. Most of the research on women, employment, and suicide mortality has focused on those occupations with the highest prestige, such as women physicians, whereas research on men has considered the full range of occupational types (Yang and Lester 1995). This may be an artifact of the practice, persistent since the nineteenth century, of barring or limiting women from professional types of employment.

In fact, evidence on suicide mortality generally does not support the assumption that working outside the home, regardless of type of occupation, leads to more psychopathology and suicide in women. At the aggregate level, participation in the labor force is associated with a lowered risk of death from suicide for women, even though some groups of professional women do appear to have an increased risk of death from suicide. In addition, suicidal behavior in women demonstrates the same pattern in response to employment as that found in men: for both, unemployment, as well as certain professional careers, seems to increase the risk of suicide (Yang and Lester 1995).

Cosmetic Breast Implants and Suicide

Several studies have reported that women with cosmetic breast implants have a two to three times higher rate of death from suicide than similar-age women in the general population (Lipworth and McLaughlin 2010; McLaughlin et al. 2003). The amount of attention this suicide-related issue has garnered, given other less investigated gender-related suicide issues, is remarkable. Nevertheless, the largest investigation of this subject has found no difference in the rates of suicide among women who received breast implants and among women who underwent other forms of cosmetic surgery (Sarwer et al. 2007).

The Sarwer et al. (2007) study suggests that cosmetic breast implants as a risk factor for suicide in women are only one aspect of a possible increase in psychopathology associated with achieving a socially defined "ideal" body image. Women in particular are strongly influenced by this social norm. The conclusion that the focus on breasts implants and suicide is gender biased is hard to avoid, given, for example, the widespread recognition of high morbidity and mortality rates of predominantly female psychiatric disorders associated with the socially defined "ideal" female body, such as anorexia nervosa.

Personality Disorders

Patients with personality disorders are at seven times greater risk for suicide than the general population. Of all patients who die by suicide, 30%–40% have personality disorders (Simon 2004, 2011). Cluster B diagnoses, and especially borderline personality disorder (BPD), are associated with suicidal acts. Studies have found rates of suicide in BPD to range from 4% to 9.5% (Jacobs et al. 1999). BPD is in fact the only personality disorder in which recurrent suicidal threats, gestures, or behavior or self-mutilatory behaviors are one of the formal diagnostic criteria. The comorbidity of Axis I disorders makes suicidal acts more likely (Maris et al. 2000; Simon 2004, 2011).

BPD is also a diagnosis primarily associated with women. The rate of BPD in the general population is 2%–3%, but the ratio of women to men who meet the criteria for BPD is 2:1 or even higher (Phillips et al. 2003). The influence of gender stereotypes in the construction of this diagnosis has been extensively discussed and is the subject of ongoing debate (Hensley and Nurnberg 2002). The association of female stereotypical characteristics with criteria for this diagnosis of psychopathology, including suicide gestures and attempts, has been well documented.

Also consistent with female gender stereotypes, the incidence of suicide attempts outnumbers that of suicide completions. Actual suicide attempts (as opposed to suicide threats or gestures) occur in 60%–70% of borderline patients, and this group usually makes multiple attempts, with an average of three. In contrast, the rate of suicide in clinical samples of BPD is about 9%—

about 400 times the rate of suicide in the general population and more than 800 times the rate in young females. Still, when contrasted with the 60%–70% of borderline patients who make multiple suicide attempts, the 9% figure actually reflects the high frequency with which borderline patients make suicide attempts that do not result in death (Gunderson and Ridolfi 2001). Because depression is a common comorbid diagnosis, and given the number of suicide attempts, higher rates would be expected. These findings again raise questions about protective factors associated with women.

Antisocial personality disorder is another gendered Cluster B diagnosis, one found more frequently in men than in women. About 3% of men and 1% of women meet criteria for this diagnosis (Phillips et al. 2003). It is associated primarily with externally directed violence but is also associated with a suicide rate of 5% (Perry 1999). Although some research has been done in recent years in regard to the association of antisocial personality and suicide (Douglas et al. 2008; Verona et al. 2001), the extent of such research is limited. The 5% rate of completed suicides cited may include persons with concurrent Axis I depressive disorders, substance use disorders, or personality disorders that themselves increase the risk of suicide (Jacobs et al. 1999; Perry 1999; Weiss and Hufford 1999).

Suicide During Pregnancy and the Postpartum Period

Despite high rates of psychiatric morbidity, including elevated levels of depression during childbearing years as well as the postpartum period (Marzuk et al. 1997; Nonacs and Cohen 2003; Sloan and Kornstein 2003), studies have found a low risk of fatal self-harm in childbearing women. Pregnancy and recent motherhood appear to protect against suicidal behavior, consistent with research indicating that having a child in the home under age 18 decreases the risk of suicide. The suicide rates for women during pregnancy and up to 2 years postpartum are fractions of those expected after adjustment for age (Appleby 1996; Oates 2003; Samandari et al. 2011). In one Canadian study (Turner et al. 2002), only 0.02%–0.2% of maternal deaths resulted from suicide in the period between 20 weeks of gestation and 42 days postpartum. In the period of 43 days to 225 days postpartum, 0.5%–1.0% of deaths were due to suicide. The researchers concluded, "Although postpartum depression clearly affects many women, it apparently does not result in an increased incidence of suicide" (Turner et al. 2002, p. 35).

Notably, the risk of suicide associated with severe psychiatric illness, particularly psychosis, appears to outweigh the protection conferred by pregnancy and childbirth. Although postnatal women in general may have a low rate of suicide, those who develop severe postpartum illness are at high risk, particularly during the first year after childbirth (Appleby et al. 1998). In one study in which suicide was the leading cause of all maternal deaths either during pregnancy or up to 1 year postdelivery, 85% of the women had psychiatric problems that had been brought to clinical attention and were receiving treatment. At least 68% were psychotic or had severe depressive illness (Oates 2003). In another study, deaths by suicide that did occur were among women suffering from psychosis (Appleby 1996). One group of researchers found that the overall risk of suicide in women admitted to psychiatric hospitals in the year following childbirth increased 70-fold. This figure is consistent with the elevated suicide rates found within the first year of discharge of individuals who were hospitalized for psy-

chosis (Appleby et al. 1998) and in particular in the first week after discharge (Qin and Nordentoft 2005).

Murder-Suicide

Gendered patterns are also prominent in the rare but tragic incidence of murder-suicide. This event occurs much less frequently than either simple suicide or homicide. Homicide-suicide rates seem to be relatively stable in the United States, with an incidence of 0.2–0.3 per 100,000 persons (Eliason 2009; Liem et al. 2011). The majority of homicide-suicides are intimate-partner related (42%–69%), followed by filicide-suicide (18%–47%) (Logan et al. 2008). Homicide-suicides with victims younger than 15 are primarily committed by parents (see Eliason 2009).

The most frequent subtype of murder-suicide, killing the spouse at the same time as committing suicide, is mainly a white male behavior pattern. Consistently, across multiple studies, those who commit murder-suicide tend to be men, are in or have been in an intimate relationship with the victims, and use a firearm, and victims tend to be women (Eliason 2009; Liem et al. 2011; Logan et al. 2008; Warren-Gordon et al. 2010). In an analysis based on data from the National Violent Death Reporting System, one study found that between 2003 and 2005, most incidents of murder-suicide were committed with a firearm (88.2%) and perpetrated by males (91.4%), a majority of whom were white (77.0%). Over 70% of all victims are female (Felthous et al. 2001; Logan et al. 2008; Malphurs and Cohen 2002).

In contrast, the gender differential in spousal murder is less pronounced: women committed almost half of the spousal homicides, yet they very rarely committed murder-suicide (Eliason 2009). A recent study found that among older adults, men commit 42% of spousal murders, and women commit 25% (Bourget et al. 2010). However, women who kill their husbands are much less likely to die by suicide afterward. In an older study across age groups (Nock and Marzuk 1999), 19%–26% of male spouse murderers died by suicide, compared with only 0%–3% of females. In the Bourget et al. (2010) study, older men who killed their spouses were much more likely to kill themselves (51%) than were women (25%). A history of domestic violence is a major risk factor for female and male victims of any age (Bourget et al. 2010).

Filicide-suicide, the second most common type of murder-suicide, also demonstrates gendered patterns. In contrast to homicide-suicide associated with intimate partners, over half (51.5%) of filicide-suicide perpetrators are female (Logan et al. 2008; Malphurs and Cohen 2002). Among men, victims of murder-suicide were children in only 4% of cases. In the reported literature, a large proportion of filicides are filicide-suicides, with 16%–29% of mothers and 40%–60% of fathers committing suicide after murdering their own children over 1 year of age (Hatters Friedman et al. 2005). This percentage falls to 2.3% of mothers and 10.5% of fathers when one considers only infanticide-suicides (Malphurs and Cohen 2002).

A mother tends to kill only her children and herself. In contrast, a father who kills his children is more likely to kill his entire family, including his spouse (Malphurs and Cohen 2002; Nock and Marzuk 1999). In one study, the authors found that 65% of fathers attempted to kill their wives as well as their children, whereas no mothers attempted to kill their husbands. In all, 55% of fathers, but none of the mothers, attempted familicide (Hatters Friedman et al. 2005).

In addition, mothers with severe postpartum depression and psychotic disorders commit a significant percentage of reported infanticides. One study found that among mothers who commit infanticide, 62% die by suicide (Attia et al. 1999; Brockington 1996). In one of the studies of suicide during pregnancy and the postpartum period reviewed in the previous section, 5% of the women who died by suicide also committed infanticide (Appleby 1996). One group of authors concluded that infant homicide followed by a suicide is "largely preventable by preempting postpartum depression" (Bell and McBride 2010).

These women are generally motivated from the wish to spare the children from some external impending harm or from enduring the pain of being motherless after the mother commits suicide (Brockington 1996; Hatters Friedman et al. 2005). In one study, 90% of women who committed filicide-suicide did so out of altruistic motives, real or delusional. However, there was evidence of depression in 70% of mothers and of psychosis in 30% of mothers (Hatters Friedman et al. 2005). These findings provide a chilling reminder that even a powerful protective factor can give way to fatal consequences in the context of severe psychiatric disorder, the most significant risk factor for suicide.

Conclusion

Suicide is a complex behavior, and many factors besides gender play a role in determining the precipitants and outcome of any individual's suicide attempt, whether ultimately fatal or not. Sociodemographic, psychiatric, biological, familial, and situational risk factors are not mutually exclusive. They can and do co-occur, and it is their comorbidity that may carry the greatest risk for suicide (Simon 2011). In any discussion of gender, we should bear in mind that there is no generic female, just as there is no generic male. Factors such as race, religion, and culture will result in as many differences among women and men as there may be similarities. Moreover, some of the protective factors associated with women will apply to some men and will also not apply to some women.

Nevertheless, protective factors specific to women (and certain ethnic and age groups) require further elucidation. One of the challenges for suicide research is to explain the gender paradox of suicide without falling into the subtle errors gender bias can cause. Such an approach recognizes the importance of preventing suicide by elucidating both risk factors and protective factors. Investigations from this perspective can provide opportunities to further our understanding of suicidal behavior. Insights developed through such research may well result in therapeutic interventions that could be utilized to reduce the suicide rates of high-risk populations as well as those of individuals in low-risk populations who may develop risk factors that increase their suicide potential.

Key Clinical Concepts

- Women demonstrate more depressive illness and suicide attempts than do men. Despite the association of these two major risk factors with suicide completion, women have lower suicide mortality rates.
- Risk factors for older white males, the group with the highest rates of suicide, cannot be generalized as risk factors for women and nonwhite ethnic or racial groups.
- Protective factors related to gender decrease the risk of suicide mortality in women. These include the role of relationships in women's psychological development and mental health and women's sense of responsibility to others based on an ethic of caring and avoiding harm to others.
- More research is needed that examines the risk factors and protective factors in suicide in women and nonwhite male groups.
- Further elucidation of these and other as yet unknown gender-related protective factors can be utilized to assist high-risk populations and individuals by suggesting therapeutic interventions that may reduce their risk of suicide.

References

Alston MH, Anderson SE: Suicidal behavior in African-American women, in Women and Suicidal Behavior. Edited by Canetto SS, Lester D. New York, Springer, 1995, pp 133–143

American Association of Suicidology: Suicide Statistics Archive 1996–2007. 2010a. Available at: http://mypage.iusb.edu/~jmcintos/datayrarchives.htm. Accessed June 23, 2011.

American Association of Suicidology: U.S.A. Suicide: 2007 official final data. 2010b. Available at: http://www.suicidology. org/web/guest/stats-and-tools/statistics. Accessed June 23, 2011.

American Foundation for Suicide Prevention: Facts and figures by gender. 2007. Available at: http://www.afsp.org/index.cfm? fuseaction=home.viewPage&page_id =04ECB949-C3D9-5FFA-DA9C65C381 BAAEC0. Accessed June 23, 2011.

Appleby L: Suicidal behavior in childbearing women. Int Rev Psychiatry 8:107–115, 1996

Appleby L, Mortensen PB, Faragher EB: Suicide and other causes of mortality after post-partum psychiatric admission. Br J Psychiatry 173:209–211, 1998

Appleby L, Shaw J, Amos T, et al: Suicide within 12 month of contact with mental health services: national clinical survey. BMJ 318:1235–1239, 1999

Attia E, Downey J, Oberman M: Postpartum psychoses, in Postpartum Mood Disorders. Edited by Miller LJ. Washington, DC, American Psychiatric Press, 1999, pp 99–117

Bebbington PE, Cooper C, Minot S, et al: Suicide attempts, gender, and sexual abuse: data from the 2000 British Psychiatric Morbidity Survey. Am J Psychiatry 166:1135–1140, 2009

Bell CC, McBride DF: Commentary: homicide-suicide in older adults—cultural and contextual perspectives. J Am Acad Psychiatry Law 38:312–317, 2010

Blehar MC, Norquist G: Mental health policy and women, in Women's Mental Health: A Comprehensive Textbook. Edited by Kornstein SG, Clayton AH. New York, Guilford, 2002, pp 613–627

Blumenthal SJ: An overview and synopsis of risk factors, assessment, and treatment of suicidal patients over the life cycle, in Suicide Over the Life Cycle: Risk Factors, Assessment and Treatment of Suicidal Patients. Edited by Blumenthal SJ , Kupfer DJ. Washington, DC, American Psychiatric Press, 1990, pp 685–733

Bourget D, Gagné P, Whitehurst L: Domestic homicide and homicide-suicide: the older offender. J Am Acad Psychiatry Law 38:305–311, 2010

Bowman MA, Allen DI: Stress and Women Physicians. New York, Springer-Verlag, 1985

Brady KT, Randall CL: Gender differences in substance use disorders. Psychiatr Clin North Am 22:241–252, 1999

Brent DA: Firearms and suicide. Ann N Y Acad Sci 932:225–240, 2001

Brockington IF: Motherhood and Mental Health. Oxford, UK, Oxford University Press, 1996

Brockington IF: Suicide in women. Int Clin Psychopharmacol 16(suppl):S7–S19, 2001

Canetto SS: Elderly women and suicidal behavior, in Women and Suicidal Behavior. Edited by Canetto SS, Lester DL. New York, Springer, 1995, pp 215–233

Canetto SS: Older adult women: issues, resources, and challenges, in Handbook of the Psychology of Women and Gender. Edited by Unger RK. New York, Wiley, 2001, pp 183–197

Canetto SS, Lester D: Women and suicidal behavior: issues and dilemmas, in Women and Suicidal Behavior. Edited by Canetto SS, Lester D. New York, Springer, 1995, pp 3–7

Canterbury RJ: Alcohol and other substance use, in Women's Mental Health: A Comprehensive Textbook. Edited by Kornstein SG, Clayton AH. New York, Guilford, 2002, pp 222–243

Carroll J: Gun ownership and use in America. Gallup, November 22, 2005. Available at: http://www.gallup.com/poll/20098/ gun-ownership-use-america.aspx?version=print. Accessed June 23, 2011.

Carroll-Ghosh T, Victor BS, Bourgeois JA: Suicide, in The American Psychiatric Publishing Textbook of Clinical Psychiatry, 4th Edition. Edited by Hales RE, Yudofsky SC. Washington, DC, American Psychiatric Publishing, 2003, pp 1457–1483

Centers for Disease Control and Prevention: Alcohol and suicide among racial/ethnic populations—17 states, 2005–2006. June 19, 2009. Available at: http://www.cdc. gov/mmwr/preview/mmwrhtml/ mm5823a1.htm. Accessed June 23, 2011.

Centers for Disease Control and Prevention: Suicide facts at a glance. 2010. Available at: http://www.cdc.gov/violenceprevention/ pdf/Suicide_DataSheet-a.pdf. Accessed June 23, 2011.

Centers for Disease Control and Prevention, National Center for Injury Prevention and Control: Injury Prevention & Control: Data & Statistics (WISQARS). February 24, 2011. Available at: http://www.cdc. gov/injury/wisqars/index.html. Accessed December 23, 2010.

Chang CM, Liao SC, Chiang HC, et al: Gender differences in healthcare service utilisation 1 year before suicide: national record linkage study. Br J Psychiatry 195:459–460, 2009

Chrisler JC: Gendered bodies and physical health, in Handbook of the Psychology of Women and Gender. Edited by Unger RK. New York, Wiley, 2001, pp 201–214

Conner KR, Zhong YY: State firearm laws and rates of suicide in men and women. Am J Prev Med 25:320–324, 2003

Cooper J, Kapur N, Webb R, et al: Suicide after deliberate self-harm: a 4-year cohort study. Am J Psychiatry 162:297–303, 2005

Cotto JH, Davis E, Dowling GJ, et al: Gender effects on drug use, abuse, and dependence: a special analysis of results from the National Survey on Drug Use and Health. Gend Med 7:402–413, 2010

Douglas KS, Lilienfeld SO, Skeem JL, et al: Relation of antisocial and psychopathic traits to suicide-related behavior among offenders. Law Hum Behav 32:511–525, 2008

Dubovsky SL, Davies R, Dubovsky AN: Mood disorders, in The American Psychiatric Publishing Textbook of Clinical Psychiatry, 4th Edition. Edited by Hales RE, Yudofsky SC. Washington, DC, American Psychiatric Publishing, 2003, pp 439–542

Durkheim E: Suicide: A Study in Sociology (1897). Translated by Spaulding JA, Simpson G. New York, Free Press, 1951

Eliason S: Murder-suicide: a review of the recent literature. J Am Acad Psychiatry Law 37:371–376, 2009

Elnour AA, Harrison J: Lethality of suicide methods. Inj Prev 14:39–45, 2008

Felthous AR, Hempel AG, Heredia A, et al: Combined homicide-suicide in Galveston County. J Forensic Sci 46:586–592, 2001

Finkelhor D: The international epidemiology of child sexual abuse. Child Abuse Negl 19:409–417, 1994

Frank E, Dingle AD: Self-reported depression and suicide attempts among U.S. women physicians. Am J Psychiatry 156:1887–1894, 1999

Garlow SJ: Age, gender and ethnicity differences in patterns of cocaine and ethanol use preceding suicide. Am J Psychiatry 159:615–619, 2002

Garlow SJ, Purselle D, Heninger M: Ethnic differences in patterns of suicide across the life cycle. Am J Psychiatry 162:319–323, 2005

Gilligan C: In a Different Voice: Psychological Theory and Women's Development, 2nd Edition. Cambridge, MA, Harvard University Press, 1993

Good GE, Sherrod NB: The psychology of men and masculinity: research status and future directions, in Handbook of the Psychology of Women and Gender. Edited by Unger RK. New York, Wiley, 2001, pp 201–214

Gunderson JG, Ridolfi ME: Borderline personality disorder: suicidality and self-mutilation. Ann N Y Acad Sci 932:61–73, 2001

Hansen L, Pritchard C: Consistency in suicide rates in twenty-two developed countries by gender over time 1874–78, 1974–76, and 1998–2000. Arch Suicide Res 12:251–262, 2008

Hasin DS, Stinson FS, Ogburn E, et al: Prevalence, correlates, disability, and comorbidity of DSM-IV alcohol abuse and dependence in the United States: results from the National Epidemiological Survey on Alcohol and Related Conditions. Arch Gen Psychiatry 64:830–842, 2007

Hatters Friedman S, Hrouda DR, Holden CE, et al: Filicide-suicide: common factors in parents who kill their children and themselves. J Am Acad Psychiatry Law 33:496–504, 2005

Hawton K, Harriss L: How often does deliberate self-harm occur relative to each suicide? A study of variations by gender and age. Suicide Life Threat Behav 38:650–660, 2008

Hensley PL, Nurnberg HG: Personality disorders, in Women's Mental Health: A Comprehensive Textbook. Edited by Kornstein SG, Clayton AH. New York, Guilford, 2002, pp 323–343

Hu G, Wilcox HC, Wissow L, et al: Mid-life suicide: an increasing problem in U.S. whites, 1999–2005. Am J Prev Med 35:589–593, 2008

Jacobs DG, Brewer M, Klein-Benheim M: Suicide assessment: an overview and recommended protocol, in The Harvard Medical School Guide to Suicide Assessment and Intervention. Edited by Jacobs DG. San Francisco, CA, Jossey-Bass, 1999, pp 3–39

Johns Hopkins Bloomberg School of Public Health: U.S. suicide rate increases. October 21, 2008. Available at: www.jhsph.edu/publichealthnews/press_releases/2008/baker_suicide.html. Accessed June 23, 2011.

Jordan JV (ed): Women's Growth in Diversity: More Writings From the Stone Center. New York, Guilford, 1997

Jordan JV, Kaplan AG, Miller JB, et al (eds): Women's Growth in Connection: Writings From the Stone Center. New York, Guilford, 1991

Judd F, Jackson H, Komiti A, et al: The profile of suicide: changing or changeable? Soc Psychiatry Psychiatr Epidemiol October 30, 2010 [Epub ahead of print]

Kaplan AG, Klein RB: Women and suicide, in Suicide: Understanding and Responding: Harvard Medical School Perspectives. Edited by Jacobs D, Brown HN. Madison, CT, International Universities Press, 1989, pp 257–282

Kessler RC, Nelson CB, McGonagle KA, et al: The epidemiology of co-occurring addictive and mental disorders: implications for prevention and service utilization. Am J Orthopsychiatry 66:17–31, 1996

Kornstein SG, Wojcik BA: Depression, in Women's Mental Health: A Comprehensive Textbook. Edited by Kornstein SG, Clayton AH. New York, Guilford, 2002, pp 147–165

Kposowa AJ: Marital status and suicide in the National Longitudinal Mortality Study. J Epidemiol Community Health 54:254–261, 2000

Kposowa AJ, McElvain JP: Gender, place, and method of suicide. Soc Psychiatry Psychiatr Epidemiol 41:435–443, 2006

Kung HC, Pearson JL, Liu X: Risk factors for male and female suicide decedents ages 15–64 in the United States: results from the 1993 National Mortality Followback Survey. Soc Psychiatry Psychiatr Epidemiol 38:419–426, 2003

Kushner HI: Women and suicidal behavior: epidemiology, gender, and lethality in historical perspective, in Women and Suicidal Behavior. Edited by Canetto SS, Lester D. New York, Springer, 1995, pp 11–34

Lester D: Do male and female suicides jump from different heights? Percept Mot Skills 96:798, 2003

Liem M, Barber C, Markwalder N, et al: Homicide-suicide and other violent deaths: an international comparison. Forensic Sci Int 207:70–76, 2011

Lipworth L, McLaughlin JK: Excess suicide risk and other external causes of death among women with cosmetic breast implants: a neglected research priority. Curr Psychiatry Rep 12:324–328, 2010

Logan J, Hill HA, Black ML, et al: Characteristics of perpetrators in homicide-followed-by-suicide incidents: National Violent Death Reporting System—17 US States, 2003–2005. Am J Epidemiol 168:1056–1064, 2008

Luoma JB, Martin CE, Pearson JL: Contact with mental health and primary care prior to suicide: a review of the evidence. Am J Psychiatry 159:909–916, 2002

Malphurs JE, Cohen D: A newspaper surveillance study of homicide-suicide in the United States. Am J Forensic Med Pathol 23:142–148, 2002

Mann JJ, Arango V: The neurobiology of suicidal behavior, in The Harvard Medical School Guide to Suicide Assessment and Intervention. Edited by Jacobs DG. San Francisco, CA, Jossey-Bass, 1999, pp 98–114

Maris RW, Berman AL, Silverman MM: Comprehensive Textbook of Suicidology. New York, Guilford, 2000

Martin G, Bergen HA, Richardson AS, et al: Sexual abuse and suicidality: gender differences in a large community sample of adolescents. Child Abuse Negl 28:491–503, 2004

Marzuk PM, Tardiff K, Leon AC, et al: Lower risk of suicide during pregnancy. Am J Psychiatry 154:122–123, 1997

McAndrew FT, Garrison AJ: Beliefs about gender differences in methods and causes of suicide. Arch Suicide Res 11:271–279, 2007

McLaughlin JK, Lipworth L, Tarone RE: Suicide among women with cosmetic breast implants: a review of epidemiologic evidence. J Long Term Eff Med Implants 13:445–450, 2003

Miller JB: Toward a New Psychology of Women, 2nd Edition. Boston, MA, Beacon Press, 1987

Möller-Leimkühler AM: The gender gap in suicide and premature death, or why are men so vulnerable? Eur Arch Psychiatry Clin Neurosci 253:1–8, 2003

Molnar BE, Berkman LF, Buka SL: Psychopathology, childhood sexual abuse and other childhood adversities: relative links to subsequent suicidal behavior in the US. Psychol Med 31:965–977, 2001

Moscicki EK: Epidemiology of suicide. Int Psychogeriatr 7:137–148, 1995

Moscicki EK: Epidemiology of suicide, in The Harvard Medical School Guide to Suicide Assessment and Intervention. Edited by Jacobs DG. San Francisco, CA, Jossey-Bass, 1999, pp 40–51

National Institute of Mental Health: Suicide in the U.S.: Statistics and Prevention. September 27, 2010. Available at: http://www.nimh.nih.gov/health/publications/suicide-in-the-us-statistics-and-prevention/index.shtml. Accessed June 28, 2011.

Nock MK, Marzuk PM: Murder-suicide: phenomenology and clinical implications, in The Harvard Medical School Guide to Suicide Assessment and Intervention. Edited by Jacobs DG. San Francisco, CA, Jossey-Bass, 1999, pp 188–209

Nonacs R, Cohen LS: Assessment and treatment of depression during pregnancy: an update. Psychiatr Clin North Am 26:547–562, 2003

Nordentoft M, Branner J: Gender differences in suicidal intent and method among suicide attempters. Crisis 29:209–212, 2008

Oates M: Suicide: the leading cause of maternal death. Br J Psychiatry 183:279–281, 2003

Perry JC: Personality disorders, suicide and self-destructive behavior, in The Harvard Medical School Guide to Suicide Assessment and Intervention. Edited by Jacobs DG. San Francisco, CA, Jossey-Bass, 1999, pp 157–169

Phillips KA, Yen S, Gunderson JG: Personality disorders, in The American Psychiatric Publishing Textbook of Clinical Psychiatry, 4th Edition. Edited by Hales RE, Yudofsky SC. Washington, DC, American Psychiatric Publishing, 2003, pp 803–832

Qin P, Nordentoft M: Suicide risk in relation to psychiatric hospitalization: evidence based on longitudinal registers. Arch Gen Psychiatry 62:427–432, 2005

Regier DA, Boyd JH, Burke JD Jr, et al: One-month prevalence of mental disorders in the United States: based on five Epidemiologic Catchment Area sites. Arch Gen Psychiatry 45:977–986, 1988

Regier DA, Farmer ME, Rae DS, et al: Comorbidity of mental disorders with alcohol and other drug abuse: results from the Epidemiologic Catchment Area (ECA) study. JAMA 264:2511–2518, 1990

Romero MP, Wintemute GJ: The epidemiology of firearm suicide in the United States. J Urban Health 79:39–48, 2002

Roy A, Janal M: Gender in suicide attempt rates and childhood sexual abuse rates: is there an interaction? Suicide Life Threat Behav 36:329–335, 2006

Samandari G, Martin SL, Kupper LL, et al: Are pregnant and postpartum women at increased risk for violent death? Suicide and homicide findings from North Carolina. Matern Child Health J 15:660–669, 2011

Sarwer DB, Brown GK, Evans DL: Cosmetic breast augmentation and suicide. Am J Psychiatry 164:1006–1013, 2007

Schernhammer ES, Colditz GA: Suicide rates among physicians: a quantitative and gender assessment. Am J Psychiatry 161:2295–2301, 2004

Simon RI: Assessing and Managing Suicide Risk: Guidelines for Clinically Based Risk Management. Washington, DC, American Psychiatric Publishing, 2004

Simon RI: Preventing Patient Suicide: Clinical Assessment and Management. Washington, DC, American Psychiatric Publishing, 2011

Skogman K, Alsén M, Ojehagen A: Sex differences in risk factors for suicide after attempted suicide: a follow-up study of 1052 suicide attempters. Soc Psychiatry Psychiatr Epidemiol 39:113–120, 2004

Slaby AE: Outpatient management of suicidal patients, in Risk Management With Suicidal Patients. Edited by Bongar B, Berman AL, Maris RW, et al. New York, Guilford, 1998, pp 34–64

Sloan DME, Kornstein SG: Gender differences in depression and response to antidepressant treatment. Psychiatr Clin North Am 26:581–594, 2003

Stack S: Work and the economy, in Comprehensive Textbook of Suicidology. Edited by Maris RW, Berman AL, Silverman MM. New York, Guilford, 2000, pp 193–221

Stack S, Wasserman I: Gender and suicide risk: the role of wound site. Suicide Life Threat Behav 39:13–20, 2009

Stephens BJ: The pseudosuicidal female: a cautionary tale, in Women and Suicidal Behavior. Edited by Canetto SS, Lester D. New York, Springer, 1995, pp 85–108

Stillion JM: Through a glass darkly: women and attitudes toward suicidal behavior, in Women and Suicidal Behavior. Edited by Canetto SS, Lester D. New York, Springer, 1995, pp 71–84

Torre DM, Wang NY, Meoni LA, et al: Suicide compared to other causes of mortality in physicians. Suicide Life Threat Behav 35:146–153, 2005

Turner LA, Kramer MS, Liu S, et al: Cause-specific mortality during and after pregnancy and the definition of maternal death. Chronic Dis Can 23:31–36, 2002

Verona E, Patrick CJ, Jointer TE: Psychopathy, antisocial personality, and suicide risk. J Abnorm Psychol 110:462–470, 2001

Walinder J, Rutz W: Male depression and suicide. Int Clin Psychopharmacol 16(suppl):S21–S24, 2001

Warren-Gordon K, Byers BD, Brodt SJ, et al: Murder followed by suicide: a newspaper surveillance study using the New York Times Index. J Forensic Sci 55:1592–1597, 2010

Webster Rudmin F, Ferrada-Noli M, Skolbekken JA: Questions of culture, age and gender in the epidemiology of suicide. Scand J Psychol 44:373–381, 2003

Weiss RD, Hufford MR: Substance abuse and suicide, in The Harvard Medical School Guide to Suicide Assessment and Intervention. Edited by Jacobs DG. San Francisco, CA, Jossey-Bass, 1999, pp 300–310

Willis LA, Coombs DW, Drentea P, et al: Uncovering the mystery: factors of African American suicide. Suicide Life Threat Behav 33:412–429, 2003

Wintemute GJ, Parham CA, Beaumont JJ, et al: Mortality among recent purchasers of handguns. N Engl J Med 341:1583–1589, 1999

Yang B, Lester D: Suicidal behavior and employment, in Women and Suicidal Behavior. Edited by Canetto SS, Lester D. New York, Springer, 1995, pp 97–108

Young MA, Fogg LF, Scheftner WA, et al: Interactions of risk factors in predicting suicide. Am J Psychiatry 151:434–435, 1994

Zahl DL, Hawton K: Repetition of deliberate self-harm and subsequent suicide risk: long-term follow-up study of 11,583 patients. Br J Psychiatry 185:70–75, 2004

PART VI

Special Topics

C H A P T E R   2 5

Neurobiology of Suicidal Behavior

J. John Mann, M.D.

Dianne Currier, Ph.D., M.P.H.

Suicide and nonfatal suicide attempts are complex, multidetermined behaviors that occur generally in the context of a diathesis or predisposition. This diathesis is characterized by traits in multiple domains, including clinical, cognitive, behavioral, and biologic aspects (see Mann and Currier 2008 for an overview). Research over the past 30 years has revealed much about neurobiological dysfunction associated with suicidal behavior and underlying other traits that characterize the diathesis, including impulsive aggression, deficits in executive function, negative or rigid cognitive processes, and recurrent mood disorders. These neurobiological deficits and the associated clinical, behavioral, and cognitive traits are likely to originate from combinations of genes and early life experiences during critical formative developmental periods. In this chapter we describe neurobiological abnormalities observed in suicide and suicide attempts, relate those findings to traits characterizing the diathesis for suicide, and present recent evidence from genetic stud-

ies suggesting possible origins for those abnormalities. Research into the biological underpinnings of suicidal behavior is ongoing, and in the final section of this chapter we outline newer fields of investigation.

Evidence of Abnormal Function in Major Neurotransmitter Systems in Suicidal Behavior

The serotonergic and noradrenergic neurotransmitter systems have been the most intensively investigated, with an accumulating body of evidence that abnormalities in both systems are involved in suicidal behavior.

Serotonergic System

Evidence from multiple sources has confirmed that altered serotonergic function is a biological trait and is related to suicidal behavior. In a pioneering study, Åsberg et al. (1976) observed a greater likelihood of lower cerebrospinal fluid (CSF) 5-hydroxyindoleacetic acid (5-HIAA) levels, indicative of less serotonin (5-HT) release, in depressed individuals who had either attempted suicide by violent means or later died by suicide. Since that time, the function of the serotonergic system in suicide and attempted suicide has been examined in many paradigms, and although not all studies agree, there is substantial consensus that individuals who die by suicide or who make serious nonfatal suicide attempts exhibit a deficiency in 5-HT neurotransmission in parts of the brain involved in decision making and mood regulation.

Evidence of serotonergic system impairment or hypofunction comes from CSF studies in living patients and from postmortem brain tissue studies of individuals who have died by suicide. 5-HIAA is the major metabolite of 5-HT, and the level of CSF 5-HIAA is indicative of 5-HT activity in parts of the brain, including the prefrontal cortex. Meta-analysis of prospective studies of CSF 5-HIAA in mood disorders found that CSF 5-HIAA levels below the mean increased the chance of death by suicide by approximately 4.6-fold compared with those higher than the mean over follow-up periods ranging from 1 to 14 years (Mann et al. 2006). Lower concentration of CSF 5-HIAA has also been found in suicide attempters compared with nonattempters in studies of patients with other psychiatric disorders such as schizophrenia, bipolar disorder, and personality disorders. These results are consistent with findings of low levels of 5-HT and/or 5-HIAA in the brain stems of suicide completers of a similar magnitude across diagnostic categories (Mann et al. 2001). Because these findings are associated with suicide and suicide attempts and transcend diagnostic or syndromal boundaries, they indicate an association with the diathesis for suicidal behavior more so than with a specific psychiatric illness.

Postmortem studies of the brains of suicides have suggested a model of hypofunction and homeostatic response. Evidence of serotonergic hypofunction in suicide includes lower serotonin transporter (SERT) binding localized to the ventromedial prefrontal cortex and anterior cingulate, brain areas involved in willed action or decision making (Arango et al. 1995; Mann et al. 2000); and deficient serotonergic transmission, evidenced by low 5-HIAA in CSF and brain and low 5-HT and/or 5-HIAA in the brain stem. Less SERT binding on the 5-HT nerve terminal could be a compensatory acceleration of internalization of the transporter in response to lower intrasynaptic levels of 5-HT, due to fewer nerve terminals or due to less gene expression as a result of gene variants or epigenetic mechanisms. Moreover, morphometric analysis of 5-HT neurons in the brain stem shows greater neuronal density in depressed suicides compared with nonsuicides, suggesting it is dysfunctional cells rather than fewer neurons that underlie observed reduction in 5-HT activity. A recent study (Underwood et al. 2011) looking at both neuron density and SERT binding found lower neuron density and lower SERT binding index in the prefrontal cortex regions in depressed suicides. SERT binding and 5-HT$_{1A}$ binding were negatively correlated, suggesting a postsynaptic receptor upregulation that is independent of differences in neuron density.

Further evidence of impaired serotonergic function is provided by neuroendocrine challenge studies in surviving suicide attempters using fenfluramine. Fenfluramine is a 5-HT-releasing agent and a reuptake inhibitor and may also directly stimulate postsynaptic 5-HT receptors. The release of 5-HT following the administration of fenfluramine results in an increase in serum prolactin levels, which thus provides an indirect index of central serotonergic responsivity. Depressed patients with a history of suicide attempts have a more blunted prolactin response to fenfluramine challenge compared with depressed patients with no history of attempting suicide, and there is evidence that the effect is more pronounced in those who make more serious or medically damaging attempts (Kamali et al. 2001). The latter is consistent with findings that individuals who use violent methods to die by suicide or who make nonfatal attempts of higher lethality have lower CSF levels of 5-HIAA (Cooper et al. 1992; Mann and Malone 1997; Sher et al. 2006). Brain imaging studies also report localized differences in serotonergic function in individuals who make more serious nonfatal suicide attempts. In a study using positron emission tomography (PET), depressed high-lethality suicide attempters had lower fluorodeoxyglucose (^{18}F) regional cerebral glucose metabolic rates (rCMRGlu) in response to fenfluramine administration in anterior cingulate and superior frontal gyri, compared with depressed low-lethality suicide attempters (Oquendo et al. 2003). The lethality of the most serious lifetime suicide attempt was negatively correlated with rCMRGlu in the anterior cingulate and right superior frontal and right medial frontal gyri, consistent with prefrontal cortex hypofunction seen in depressed high-lethality suicide attempters (Oquendo et al. 2003).

Other studies have found evidence of enhanced serotonergic function, which is postulated to reflect a homeostatic response to lower levels of 5-HT and/or 5-HIAA in the brain stem of suicide completers and lower CSF 5-HIAA levels in serious suicide attempters (for review, see Mann et al. 2001). Upregulation of serotonergic postsynaptic receptors, including 5-HT$_{1A}$ and 5-HT$_{2A}$,

and a decrease in the number of 5-HT reuptake sites (Mann et al. 2001) are likely examples of such compensatory responses. In individuals who died by suicide, irrespective of depression diagnosis, 5-HT$_{2A}$ receptors were found to be upregulated in the dorsal prefrontal cortex but not the rostral prefrontal cortex. In depressed individuals who died by suicide, elevated 5-HT$_{2A}$ binding has also been observed in the amygdala (Hrdina et al. 1993). Thus, the picture emerging from postmortem studies of greater 5-HT$_{2A}$ receptor binding in the frontal cortex of depressed suicides, fewer brain stem 5-HT$_{1A}$ autoreceptors, and fewer SERTs in the cortex, in conjunction with findings of greater tryptophan hydroxylase (TPH) immunoreactivity in 5-HT nuclei in the brain stem (Boldrini et al. 2005), points to homeostatic response to deficient serotonergic transmission as evidenced by low levels of 5-HIAA in CSF and brain, low levels of 5-HT and 5-HIAA in the brain stem, and blunted prolactin response to fenfluramine challenge.

Findings that serotonergic system deficits are observed in suicidal behavior across psychiatric disorders indicate that this biological abnormality characterizes suicidal behavior itself rather than any specific psychiatric disorder. This understanding of serotonergic dysfunction as a trait belonging to the diathesis for, or predisposition to, suicidal behavior provided the basis for the next wave of studies, which went on to explore the pathways and mechanisms through which serotonergic deficits relate to suicidal behavior directly as well as via intermediate phenotypes such as cognitive deficits and aggression.

The complexity of suicidal behavior, as well as evidence that it is heritable, means an endophenotype approach is well suited to developing an understanding of the pathogenic pathways that include molecular, behavioral, cognitive, and environmental-level factors. In terms of the serotonergic system, a number of behavioral and cognitive correlates of suicidal behavior are potentially related to serotonergic dysfunction. Impulsive-aggressive traits are proposed to be part of the diathesis for suicidal behavior (Mann et al. 1999). Increased aggression has been observed in those who die by suicide and in those who make more highly lethal suicide attempts, whereas impulsivity has been more strongly related to the probability of nonfatal suicide attempts (Oquendo et al. 2004). Studies examining several indices of serotonergic function have found evidence that reduced activity of the serotonergic system is implicated in impulsive violence and aggression, including low CSF levels of 5-HIAA in individuals with personality and other psychiatric disorders who have a lifetime history of aggressive behavior (Brown and Goodwin 1986; Stanley et al. 2000); a blunted prolactin response to fenfluramine challenge in patients with personality disorders that in the absence of a mood disorder correlates with aggressive trait severity (Coccaro et al. 1989; New et al. 2004); and a correlation between platelet 5-HT$_{2A}$ binding and aggressive behavior in patients with personality and other psychiatric disorders (Coccaro et al. 1997; McBride et al. 1994). Finally, a postmortem study of suicides observed a positive correlation between level of lifetime aggression and 5-HT$_{2A}$ binding in several regions of the prefrontal cortex (Oquendo et al. 2006).

Brain imaging studies using PET studies comparing aggressive impulsive individuals with control subjects have observed a deficient response to serotonergic challenge in the orbitofrontal cortex, medial frontal, and cingulate regions in impulsive-aggressive individuals compared with control subjects (New et al. 2002; Siever et al. 1999) and

lower SERT binding in the anterior cingulate cortex (Frankle et al. 2005). Others have found lower uptake of the tryptophan analogue [^{11}C]methyltryptophan in orbital prefrontal cortex that correlates inversely with suicidal intent (Leyton et al. 2006). The prefrontal cortex is an important region involved in the inhibitory control of behavior, including impulsive and aggressive behavior (de Almeida et al. 2006). If, then, the diathesis for suicidal behavior is characterized by aggressive/impulsive traits related to serotonergic dysfunction, an individual with the diathesis might engage in those behaviors, resulting in self-harm when he or she is confronted by stressful situations or powerful emotions. This tendency might be thought of as a diminution in natural inhibitory circuits or as a volatile cognitive decision style related to impulsiveness. Another potential endophenotype related to cognitive function is suggested by the finding that 5-HT$_{2A}$ binding negatively correlated with levels of hopelessness, a correlate of suicide and suicide attempt, although based on suicide studies in the brain and platelet studies in attempters, one would have predicted a positive correlation (van Heeringen et al. 2003). Hopelessness has been shown in clinical studies to be associated with both suicide and nonfatal suicide attempt (Beck et al. 1975; Oquendo et al. 2004).

Noradrenergic System

The noradrenergic system has been less intensively investigated than the serotonergic system. Nonetheless, as a major stress response system it is an obvious target for research into the neurobiology of suicidal behavior. Again, postmortem studies provide evidence of abnormalities in suicide. In postmortem studies in depressed suicides a number of findings indicate noradrenergic dysfunction, including higher β-adrenergic binding in the frontal cortex of suicide victims, fewer noradrenergic neurons in the locus coeruleus, less α_1-receptor binding in layers IV and V of the prefrontal cortex, α_2-receptor binding in the locus coeruleus, and greater tyrosine hydroxylase immunoreactivity in the locus coeruleus (Mann 2003). Taken together, these changes suggest a pattern of cortical noradrenergic overactivity that may result from excessive norepinephrine release in response to stress that then leads to depletion due to the smaller population of norepinephrine neurons found in individuals who died by suicide.

In living patients, 3-methoxy-4-hydroxyphenylglycol (MHPG) is a metabolite of norepinephrine that, in the CSF, has been studied as an indicator of brain noradrenergic activity. Although evidence has been largely negative in cross-sectional studies of CSF MHPG and past suicide attempt in studies of patients of varied psychiatric diagnoses (reviewed in Lester 1995), two studies reported significantly lower CSF levels of MHPG in suicide attempters compared with nonattempters in major depression (Agren and Niklasson 1986) and offenders (Linnoila et al. 1989). Likewise, results have been generally negative in cross-sectional studies of the relationship between violence and/or lethality of suicide attempts and CSF MHPG levels in various diagnostic groups (Mann 2003). The stress-responsive nature of the noradrenergic system may underlie the negative findings, reflecting the inadequacy of cross-sectional and retrospective study designs in assessing associations between state-dependent biological alterations and past behaviors. Prospective study may be better able to observe state-dependent biological alterations occurring in closer time proximity to the behavior of interest. There have been few pro-

spective studies of CSF MHPG and suicidal behavior. A prospective study of depressed patients found that 20% of patients with low CSF MHPG attempt suicide in follow-up compared with 5% of high-MHPG patients (Galfalvy et al. 2009). Moreover, lower CSF levels of MHPG were associated with higher lethality suicide attempts. In another study, hospitalized suicide attempters who made a further suicide attempt or died by suicide in the year following their index attempt were more likely to have CSF MHPG levels above the median (Träskman et al. 1981). That result, however, was not tested statistically. Follow-up studies using records to track deaths 1–12 years after the index hospital admission for a suicide attempt found no differences in baseline CSF MHPG between those who did or did not die by suicide during follow-up (Engstrom et al. 1999; Nordström et al. 1994; Sunnqvist et al. 2008), and other studies reported no difference in CSF MHPG levels between patients who did and did not attempt suicide during an 11-year follow-up of schizophrenia (Cooper et al. 1992) or in a 2-year follow-up of bipolar disorder (Sher et al. 2006).

Hypothalamic-Pituitary-Adrenal Axis and Suicidal Behavior

The stress-diathesis model of suicidal behavior posits that suicidal behavior occurs in the context of the combination of a set of biological and behavioral traits making up the diathesis for, or predisposition to, suicidal behavior and experiencing current or acute stressful circumstances. Thus, altered functioning of stress response systems is likely a key element of the diathesis. Besides the rapid short-term noradrenergic system stress response, the hypothalamic-pituitary-adrenal (HPA) axis is the other major stress response system and provides a short- and longer-term stress response. When encountering environmental stress, the HPA axis is activated by the release of corticotropin-releasing hormone (CRH) from the hypothalamus, which acts on the CRH_1 receptor in the pituitary to stimulate the release of adrenocorticotropic hormone (ACTH), which in turn is responsible for peripheral release of cortisol from the adrenal cortex (Goldstein and Kopin 2007). CRH also acts directly as a neurotransmitter on several central brain regions, including the brain stem and amygdala, which we shall see later are potentially involved in suicidal behavior.

One test of HPA axis function evaluates cortisol feedback inhibition of this system using dexamethasone. A meta-analysis found a more than fourfold risk of dying by suicide in depressed individuals who were cortisol nonsuppressors compared with suppressors on the dexamethasone suppression test (DST challenge) (Mann et al. 2006). This feedback defect may be related to reported childhood abuse in suicide completers that resulted in greater DNA methylation, and lower expression, of the glucocorticoid receptor gene (McGowan et al. 2009), which was also reported to occur in mouse models of maternal deprivation in infancy along with the consequent lower gene expression (Plotsky and Meaney 1993). This receptor mediates feedback inhibition of the higher levels of cortisol seen in stress responses. Other markers of HPA axis hyperactivity associated with suicide death include higher levels of plasma and urinary cortisol and larger pituitary and adrenal gland volumes (Mann 2003). Lower CRH receptor binding has been observed in the frontal cortex in suicides (Nemeroff 1988) and higher CSF CRH in major depression (Arató et al. 1989), suggesting that a state of excessive CRH-release downregulating CRH receptors may be present in depressed individuals who

die by suicide (Nemeroff et al. 1988). With respect to nonfatal suicidal behavior, although DST nonsuppression is not clearly related to future nonfatal suicide attempt, some report an association with serious or violent attempts (for review, see Mann and Currier 2007). However, when other indices of HPA axis function are considered, lower CSF levels of CRH (Brunner et al. 2001; but no difference in plasma CRH or plasma cortisol levels), higher urinary levels of cortisol in violent attempters (van Heeringen et al. 2000), and higher serum levels of cortisol after 5-hydroxytryptophan challenge (Meltzer et al. 1984) were associated with nonfatal suicide attempt.

The HPA axis and serotonergic system have a bidirectional relationship (Meijer and de Kloet 1998). CRH neurons project to the 5-HT raphe nuclei, and serotonergic projections from the raphe nuclei extend to brain regions that contain CRH and are involved in stress response (Owens and Nemeroff 1991). Through these pathways, the hyperactivity of the HPA axis observed in suicidal patients potentially mediates or moderates some of the 5-HT abnormalities seen in these patients (López et al. 1997). CRH_1 and CRH_2 receptors act on the dorsal raphe nucleus controlling the release of 5-HT to the forebrain, and modulation of 5-HT receptors by corticosteroids in response to stress may have important implications for the pathophysiology of suicide (López et al. 1997; Stoff and Mann 1997). Further studies are required to clarify these relationships with respect to suicidal behavior.

There is also a bidirectional relationship between the HPA axis and the noradrenergic system. Both the HPA axis and locus coeruleus, the major source of norepinephrine neurons in the brain, are activated by stress. Locus coeruleus neurons influence the neuroendocrine stress response system through their broad innervation of the paraventricular nucleus projection pathways (Dunn et al. 2004). CRH projections from the central amygdala to CRH_1 in the locus coeruleus alter noradrenergic locus coeruleus neuron firing, affecting hippocampus and amygdala function. The reciprocal interactions connect cerebral norepinephrine and CRH systems and may generate a feed-forward loop. Thus, severe anxiety in response to stress may be related to norepinephrine overactivity and hyperactivity of the HPA axis and thereby contribute to suicide risk (Brown et al. 1988). CRH_1 also interacts with dopamine receptors in the amygdala and is involved in controlling glutamate transmission to the medial prefrontal cortex. The medial prefrontal cortex is an important part of the circuitry for emotion regulation and decision making, both of which can be dysregulated in suicide attempters. Finally, there is a debate about whether noradrenergic antidepressants are as effective in reducing the risk of suicidal behavior compared with selective serotonin reuptake inhibitors (SSRIs) (Grunebaum et al. 2012).

Other Biological Systems

Beyond the serotonergic and stress response systems, other biological systems have been examined with respect to suicidal behavior. There is evidence that suicide death is more common in groups with very low cholesterol levels or after cholesterol lowering by diet (reviewed in Golomb 1998). Studies of nonhuman primates on a low-fat diet found lower serotonergic activity and increased aggressive behaviors (Muldoon et al. 1993), suggesting that the observed relationship between cholesterol and suicide may be mediated by serotonergic function. Long-chain polyunsaturated fatty acids, particularly omega-3, may also be a mediating factor in the relationship between low cholesterol

and increased risk for depression and suicide (Brunner et al. 2002). In a 2-year follow-up study (Sublette et al. 2006), depressed patients with a lower docosahexaenoic acid (DHA) percentage of total plasma polyunsaturated fatty acids and a higher omega-6/omega-3 ratio were at greater risk for suicide attempt in follow-up, and lower eicosapentaenoic acid has been found in red blood cells of suicide attempters compared with control subjects (Huan et al. 2004). A recent study of male soldiers in the U.S. Army reported that risk of suicide death was 14% higher per standard deviation of lower DHA percentage, and risk of suicide death was 62% higher with low serum DHA status (Lewis et al. 2011).

Signal transduction pathways have been investigated because they may underlie some of the observed functional alterations in receptors. A number of signaling systems have been studied postmortem in the brains of individuals who died by suicide. Components of the phosphoinositide and adenylyl cyclase signaling systems, including protein kinase C, protein kinase A, cAMP-response element-binding protein, and brain-derived neurotrophic factor (BDNF), have been implicated in the pathophysiology of youth suicide (see Pandey and Dwivedi 2010 for more details).

Neurogenesis is reported to be inhibited in mice under stress and increased in mice administered weeks of antidepressants. This effect may occur in patients as suggested recently by the finding that greater neurogenesis was present in the dentate gyrus in depressed individuals with a history of recent antidepressant treatment who died by suicide compared with untreated depressed and nonpsychiatric control subjects (Boldrini et al. 2009). Whether childhood adversity is related to less neurogenesis in adulthood in the dentate gyrus remains to be determined.

Stress, Genes, and the Neurobiology of Suicidal Behavior

It is generally accepted that both early-life environment and genes, and the interaction between the two, are involved in the abnormal development and subsequent dysfunction in later life of neurobiological systems implicated in suicidal behavior.

Early-Life Environment

Reported early-life adversity, including sexual or physical abuse, neglect, parental loss, and severe family discord, has been associated with suicidal behavior (Brodsky and Stanley 2008; Fergusson et al. 1996). Reported sexual and physical abuse are independently associated with repeated suicide attempts after adjustment for other childhood adversities (Ystgaard et al. 2004). Exposure to early-life adversity and trauma may potentially have effects on neurodevelopment that affect neurobiological function in multiple systems later in life, and thus the observed neurobiological dysfunctions in suicidal behavior may originate, in part, in early-life adversity, explaining the association between the two. Epigenetic mechanisms, such as DNA methylation, may mediate part of the effect of environment on the developing brain.

Studies of adult rodents who experienced early-life stress of maternal separation show alteration in multiple markers of serotonergic function, including increased 5-HT and 5-HIAA levels in the dorsal raphe nucleus and elevated 5-HIAA levels in the nucleus accumbens; decreased 5-HT cell firing in the raphe nuclei in response to increased doses of the SSRI citalopram, suggestive of alterations in 5-HT transporter and/or 5-HT_{1A} autoreceptors; decreased 5-HT_{2C} messenger RNA editing, reduced 5-HT level in the dorsal hippocampus, and lower 5-HT in the medial prefrontal cortex in males; and decreased sensitivity of α_1-adrenergic receptors mediating excitation of 5-HT neurons in the dorsal raphe nucleus and of 5-HT_{1A} receptors regulating 5-HT release in the frontal cortex (for review, see Mann 2003).

In adult rhesus macaques, lower levels of CSF 5-HIAA (Higley et al. 1992) and lower SERT binding on PET scanning (Ichise et al. 2006) were observed in a subgroup of macaques who experienced maternal deprivation in infancy and were carriers of the lower-expressing SERT gene 5′-upstream regulatory region (5-HTTLPR) alleles.

In humans, PET scanning has found lower transporter binding in depressed adults who report childhood abuse (Miller et al. 2009). In studies of children and adolescents, depressed children who have experienced abuse have increased prolactin but normal cortisol responses to L-5-hydroxytryptophan, compared with nonabused depressed children and control subjects (Kaufman et al. 1998). Furthermore, increased prolactin response to fenfluramine challenge was seen in boys in juvenile detention who had experienced adverse rearing environments (Pine et al. 1997). These alterations in childhood appear to persist into adulthood. Adult women with borderline personality disorder who report a history of severe childhood abuse have a blunted prolactin response to the serotonergic agonist m-chlorophenylpiperazine (Rinne et al. 2000).

Alterations in stress-response function have also been reported in animal and human studies of the effects of early-life environment on both the noradrenergic system and the HPA axis. In animal studies, rhesus monkeys separated from their mothers in infancy had elevated CSF norepinephrine in adulthood (Kraemer et al. 1989), and adult rats exposed to early-life stress had altered noradrenergic response to stress, showing evidence of overactivity in adulthood and subsequent depletion (Liu et al. 2000). There have been few studies of early-life stress and norepinephrine activity in humans. One study, however, found that suicide attempters who reported sexual abuse during childhood and adolescence had significantly higher levels of CSF MHPG and urinary norepinephrine/epinephrine compared with those with no history of abuse (Sunnqvist et al. 2008). Noradrenergic response to stress in adulthood also appears related to childhood adversity, with greater response being observed in adults reporting an abusive experience in childhood (Heim and Nemeroff 2001).

Early-life stress also leads to lasting alterations in HPA axis stress response, perhaps through pathways involving lasting alteration of CRH expression in limbic regions involved in the regulation of the HPA axis (Brunson et al. 2001). In animal models, early-life adversity altered glucocorticoid receptor gene expression in hippocampus and frontal cortex, two brain regions implicated in the negative-feedback regulation of CRH (Liu et al. 2000; Meaney et al. 1996), and resulted in excessive corticosterone and ACTH release under stress in adulthood. Thus, stress in early life might diminish glucocorticoid gene expression within the brain through DNA methylation, leading to enduring modifications in HPA axis function, which in turn later in life result in abnormal responses to further stressful stimuli (Avishai-Eliner et al. 2001; Plotsky and Meaney 1993).

In humans, early adversity or abuse has also been associated with abnormal HPA axis function in adulthood. Mineralocorticoid receptor gene overexpression has been reported in maternally deprived mice in adulthood, which mediates the feedback loop for lower concentrations of corticosterone in the resting state (Plotsky and Meaney 1993). In a study of women with varied psychiatric diagnoses, a history of childhood abuse was associated with hypersuppression of salivary cortisol concentrations in response to dexamethasone (Stein et al. 1997). This indicates a supersensitivity of the corticosteroid feedback inhibitory mechanisms. This is found in posttraumatic stress disorder and contrasts with the opposite effect in major depression. In other markers of HPA axis function, women with a history of childhood abuse had lower basal plasma cortisol concentrations (Heim et al. 2001), and abused women with or without current depression had markedly increased plasma ACTH and increased cortisol responses in response to laboratory stress compared with control subjects and depressed women without early-life stress (Heim et al. 2000). That picture is consistent with mineralocorticoid receptor overexpresssion and glucocorticoid receptor underexpression.

Genes and Suicidal Behavior

Twin, adoption, and family studies all provide evidence that genes play a role in suicidal behavior independently of psychiatric disorder (Brent and Mann 2005; Brent and Melhem 2008). The contribution of additive genetic factors is estimated to be between 30% and 50% for a broad phenotype of suicidal behavior (ideation, plans, and/or attempts) (Voracek and Loibl 2007). Monozygotic twins have a higher concordance rate for suicide compared with dizygotic twins (24.1% vs. 2.8%) (Voracek and Loibl 2007), and adoption studies find higher suicide rates in biological parents of adoptees who died by suicide (Schulsinger et al. 1979; Wender et al. 1986) compared with biological parents of adoptees who did not die by suicide. With respect to nonfatal suicide attempt, family studies show that offspring of depressed suicide attempters are more likely to become suicide attempters themselves compared with offspring of depressed parents who have not attempted suicide (Brent and Melhem 2008).

Given the observed neurobiological dysfunctions in suicidal behavior, the early investigation of genes potentially involved in suicidal behavior has largely focused on the serotonergic system and HPA axis. More recently, given the understanding that inheritance is likely polygenic, functional genomic methodologies, such as microarray technologies for profiling expression of thousands of genes simultaneously (for an overview, see Sequeira and Turecki 2006) and genome-wide arrays for hundreds of thousands of single nucleotide polymorphisms (SNPs), are becoming more prevalent. Despite the evolving approaches, early candidate gene studies offered preliminary indications of the role of genes in both the association of behavioral phenotypes with suicidal behavior and potential structural and functional neurobiological pathways underlying those phenotypes.

The lower-expressing S (or L_G) alleles of the relatively functional polymorphism of 5-HTTLPR in SLC6A4 have shown the most consistent evidence of association with suicidal behavior or major depression (for review, see Tsai et al. 2011), although there is no consensus on the effect of genotype on structural or functional characteristics of the serotonergic system either in postmortem studies of 5-HTTLPR genotype and SERT density in individuals who died by suicide (Arango et al. 2002; Du et al. 1999) or in vivo (Bah et al. 2008; Parsey et al. 2006). There is some concurrence that the lower-expressing SS genotype is related to increased amygdala activity in healthy individuals matching angry or fearful faces, negative words, or aversive pictures (reviewed in Brown and Hariri 2006). Given that the amygdala, the seat of emotional memory, is densely innervated by serotonergic neurons and has abundant 5-HT receptors, this association is not surprising. Other genes related to the serotonergic system investigated include TPH1 (tryptophan hydroxylase, the rate-limiting enzyme in the synthesis of 5-HT outside the brain after birth but also in the brain in utero), which has been associated with suicidal behavior (Bellivier et al. 2004) and aggression (Rujescu et al. 2002); and TPH2, which has been associated with suicide (Zill et al. 2004) and suicide attempt (Ke et al. 2006; Lopez et al. 2007), major depression (Haghighi et al. 2008), and hopelessness (Lazary et al. 2012). Monoamine oxidase A gene (MAOA) variants have been associated with aggression, especially in males reporting childhood adversity (Brunner et al. 1993; Cases et al. 1995), and MAOA–upstream variable number of tandem repeats (uVNTR) lower-expressing polymorphisms are associated with greater impulsivity in males (Huang et al. 2004).

Serotonergic-related genes have been shown to be involved in decision making. One study of suicide attempts found that genetic polymorphisms in 5-HTTLPR (of SLC6A4), TPH1, and MAOA modulate the learning process necessary for making advantageous choices in the Iowa Gambling Task (Jollant et al. 2010). For all of these genes, however, there have been studies that have failed to find these associations, and no clear association with the 5-HT$_{2A}$ receptor gene has been shown in patients with mood disorder who attempted suicide (Anguelova et al. 2003). Brain imaging studies have reported associations between the low-expressing alleles of the MAOA–

upstream VNTR (uVNTR) and increased risk of violent behavior and alterations in the corticolimbic circuitry involved in affect regulation, emotional memory, and impulsivity (Meyer-Lindenberg et al. 2006); an effect of *MAOA* genotype on performance during response tasks indicative of impulsivity (Passamonti et al. 2006); and an association between *TPH2* genotype and altered amygdala response (Furmark et al. 2008) and altered functioning in prefrontal and parietal brain regions (Reuter et al. 2008).

Genes relating to other biological systems implicated in suicidal behavior, primarily stress response systems, have been less studied, and there have been few consistent findings in the noradrenergic system or HPA axis–related genes (for review, see Currier and Mann 2008). However, there is an increasing interest in genetic studies of these systems, particularly the HPA axis, where CRH-related genes are seen as promising candidates. In a recent study (Tyrka et al. 2009), the CRH subtype 1 receptor (CRH$_1$) gene was reported to be associated with cortisol response to dexamethasone challenge. In studies of suicidal behavior, there was an association of CRH$_1$ genotype and suicidality in depressed males exposed to low levels of life stressors (Wasserman et al. 2008), CRH$_1$ and CRH binding protein (CRHBP) were associated with suicide attempt and severity of suicidal behavior in schizophrenia patients (De Luca et al. 2010), and a haplotype variation of the CRH subtype 2 receptor (CRH$_2$) gene was associated with suicidal behavior in bipolar disorder (De Luca et al. 2007). Other candidate genes investigated for association with suicidal behavior include those related to neurotrophic factors such as BDNF, polyamine genes such as arginase II, *S*-adenosylmethionine decarboxylase 1, and antizymes 1 and 2 (*OAZ1* and *OAZ2*).

Interaction of Genes and Early-Life Environment

The role of early-life environment is now recognized as an important consideration for genetic studies, particularly the interactive effects of environment and genes on neurodevelopment that have lasting effects into adulthood. Animal studies have demonstrated that early-life adversity interacts with genotype to produce biological and behavioral alterations that endure into adulthood (Barr et al. 2004; Bennett et al. 2002). Multiple studies in humans of early-life environment–5-HTTLPR interaction and vulnerability for psychiatric disorder report an effect (for review, see Uher and McGuffin 2008), although not all do. With respect to studies of gene–early-life environment interactions in suicidal behavior, reported childhood maltreatment in those with the lower-expressing 5-HTTLPR S allele increased risk for suicide attempt (Caspi et al. 2003), and 5-HTTLPR reported childhood adversity–genotype interactions increased risk for suicidal behavior in mixed-diagnosis inpatients (Gibb et al. 2006) and among abstinent African-American substance-dependent patients (Roy et al. 2007). A recent meta-analysis has called into question the finding of a gene-environment interaction for this variant (Risch et al. 2009). For males only, early-life adversity in combination with a lower-expressing variant of *MAOA* was found to contribute to the development of antisocial behavior and increased impulsivity, both of which may contribute to suicidal behavior (Caspi et al. 2002; Huang et al. 2004).

Similar findings of interaction effects are being reported in more recent studies of genes related to the HPA axis. One study (Roy et al. 2011) reported that CRHBP SNPs interacted with history of childhood trauma in suicide attempters. Other studies have not examined suicidal behavior directly but instead reported on behavioral/clinical outcomes and functional biological alterations that are relevant, or even part of the diathesis, for suicidal behavior. For example, one study (Bradley et al. 2008) found an interaction effect between CRH_1 haplotype and early-life stress on the severity of depression, whereas another found that CRH_1 SNPs showed significant gene-environment interactions with childhood abuse on development of elevated HPA reactivity in adults (Tyrka et al. 2009). A related finding is that childhood adversity interacted with the FKBP5 gene to increase risk for suicide attempt in an African-American sample (Roy et al. 2011). FKBP5 is a protein known to lower glucocorticoid sensitivity, and elevated levels of it might result in impairment of the HPA axis negative-feedback loop. Decreased expression and greater DNA methylation of the glucocorticoid receptor have been detected in the hippocampus of suicide victims with reported childhood trauma (McGowan et al. 2009), and *FKBP5* SNPs have been associated with suicide attempt in bipolar patients (Willour et al. 2009), making it a promising candidate gene for future studies.

Genome-wide arrays are now available with more than 2,000,000 SNP probes, and the next step should be to move from candidate genes from genome-wide association studies (GWASs) to deep sequencing or functional analysis. Matching GWAS findings with brain expression data may shed more light on functionality of new candidate genes, but such sample sizes will always be limited.

Epigenetics

Another avenue for investigation of the role of genes in the etiology of neurobiological alterations related to suicidal behavior is epigenetics. *Epigenetics* involves the modulation of gene expression through biochemical modification of function of the primary DNA sequence and can result in different patterns of expression for a selective effect as for different copies of the same gene in a given cell nucleus. *Methylation* is an epigenetic modification that affects gene expression and involves methyl groups attaching to DNA and blocking transcriptional factors from gaining access to the gene and thus effectively altering or generally suppressing or reducing expression of the gene. The same thing can happen when histone tails are acetylated and chromatin becomes more or less tightly packed, affecting access of transcription factors to regulatory sites on genes. Thus, the same allele on different chromosomes may show different expression levels due to epigenetic effects. Methylation is compatible with a model of gene–early-life experience interaction whereby the familial transmission of suicidal behavior is not simply a case of direct intergenerational transmission of a vulnerability gene but may also occur in the context of early-life environment effects on epigenetic mechanisms that in turn have developmental effects on neurobiological function.

Adverse experiences such as physical or sexual abuse, which have been shown to be transmitted intergenerationally (Brodsky and Stanley 2008), may alter gene expression and behavior through methylation of key genes. Thus, gene function may be similarly affected across generations by familial transmission of adversity or behavior and mimic a structural gene difference that is transmitted genetically. For example, rodent maternal deprivation affects HPA axis gene expression (Liu et al. 1997), and DNA methylation of the glucocorticoid and mineralocorticoid genes is one potential mechanism for this alteration. In rats, adult offspring born to low-maternal-care mothers had elevated levels of DNA methylation in the glucocorticoid receptor promoter region 1_7 in hippocampal tissues compared with adult offspring of high-maternal-care mothers, consistent with decreased levels of glucocorticoid receptor expression found in low-maternal-care offspring (Weaver et al. 2004). Microarray technologies permit whole-genome DNA methylation profiling in human tissues, including the brain, and can provide data on total and allele-specific methylation. Such studies may reveal suicide-related alterations in DNA methylation.

Emerging Targets and Methodologies

New areas of inquiry, as well as new methodological approaches, offer the means to expand current understanding of suicidal behavior and begin to untangle the complex network of neurobiological abnormalities, traits, and environmental effects that underlie suicide and nonfatal suicidal behavior.

Genetic studies are at the forefront of new approaches to elucidate the neurobiological etiology of suicidal behavior as well as being hypothesis-generating in terms of identifying potential new candidate neurobiological systems and/or pathways that may be involved in suicidal behavior. One novel approach, adopted in a recent pilot study (Galfalvy et al. 2011), was used to examine correlations between candidate genes and gene expression in the prefrontal cortex of suicide completers, with a focus on identifying correlations that were independent of mood disorder diagnosis. Genes identified in that study as related to suicidal behavior had not been previously identified in candidate gene studies of suicide; however, they do overlap with the broad domains of biological ontology identified in earlier expression studies in suicide, including central nervous system development, homophilic cell adhesion, regulation of cell proliferation, and transmission of nerve impulse (Galfalvy et al. 2011; Sequeira et al. 2007; Thalmeier et al. 2008). Of interest, *CD44*, a gene connected with the immune system, has been identified in three studies of suicides (Sequeira and Turecki 2007; Thalmeier et al. 2008; Galfalvy et al. 2011), and Galfalvy et al. (2011) additionally found that its expression in both Brodmann areas 9 and 24 was significantly low. Immune system dysregulation is reported in major depression (Mendlovic et al. 1997, 1999), but little is known about whether it plays a role in suicide, suggesting a new target for research. Moreover, a hypothesis of depression has been proposed (Maes 2009) in which neurodegeneration and reduced neurogenesis are thought to be caused by inflammation, cell-mediated immune activation, and their long-term sequelae. Disordered neuroimmune function may be present in suicide and its pathogenesis related to genes identified in the previous studies.

Another area of emerging interest is a possible link between suicide and allergic reactions that may alter the function of the orbital prefrontal cortex (Postolache et al. 2007, 2010). Interleukin-2 is a cytokine immune signaling molecule, and higher CSF interleukin-2 receptor concentration is reported in suicide attempters (Nässberger and Träskman-Bendz 1993; Rothenhäusler et al. 2006). Other potential targets for investigation are likely to be revealed by GWASs of SNPs, DNA methylation and gene expression in the brains of suicide completers, and white blood cells from nonfatal suicide attempters.

Key Clinical Concepts

- Neurobiological systems are implicated in suicide and nonfatal suicide attempt independently of abnormal brain findings related to major psychiatric disorders such as major depression.

- The abnormal brain findings related to suicidal behavior are thought to be part of the diathesis for or predisposition to suicidal behavior.

- Abnormalities in the serotonin system have been linked to recurrent depression and aggression, the probability of risky decision making, and suicidal intent. Abnormalities in stress response systems such as the noradrenergic system and the HPA axis are related to mood instability and to cognitions that favor more lethal suicidal behavior.

- Studying the environmental and genetic factors that underlie the development of the neurobiological anomalies observed in suicidal behavior in adulthood has identified much about intermediate biologic phenotypes.

- Understanding the causal relationships of neurobiological deficits, genes, and environment to the behavioral, clinical, and cognitive factors that compose the diathesis for suicidal behavior requires further investigation using both human studies and valid animal models.

References

Agren H, Niklasson F: Suicidal potential in depression: focus on CSF monoamine and purine metabolites. Psychopharmacol Bull 22:656–660, 1986

Anguelova M, Benkelfat C, Turecki G, et al: A systematic review of association studies investigating genes coding for serotonin receptors and the serotonin transporter, II: suicidal behavior. Mol Psychiatry 8:646–653, 2003

Arango V, Underwood MD, Gubbi AV, et al: Localized alterations in pre- and postsynaptic serotonin binding sites in the ventrolateral prefrontal cortex of suicide victims. Brain Res 688:121–133, 1995

Arango V, Underwood MD, Mann JJ: Serotonin brain circuits involved in major depression and suicide. Progr Brain Res 136:443–453, 2002

Arató M, Bánki CM, Bissette G, et al: Elevated CSF CRF in suicide victims. Biol Psychiatry 25:355–359, 1989

Åsberg M, Träskman L, Thorén P: 5-HIAA in the cerebrospinal fluid: a biochemical suicide predictor? Arch Gen Psychiatry 33:1193–1197, 1976

Avishai-Eliner S, Eghbal-Ahmadi M, Tabachnik E, et al: Down-regulation of hypothalamic corticotropin-releasing hormone messenger ribonucleic acid (mRNA) precedes early life experience–induced changes in hippocampal glucocorticoid receptor mRNA. Endocrinology 142:89–97, 2001

Bah J, Lindstrom M, Westberg L, et al: Serotonin transporter gene polymorphisms: effect on serotonin transporter availability in the brain of suicide attempters. Psychiatry Res 162:221–229, 2008

Barr CS, Newman TK, Shannon C, et al: Rearing condition and rh5-HTTLPR interact to influence limbic-hypothalamic-pituitary-adrenal axis response to stress in infant macaques. Biol Psychiatry 55:733–738, 2004

Beck AT, Kovacs M, Weissman A: Hopelessness and suicidal behavior: an overview. JAMA 234:1146–1149, 1975

Bellivier F, Chaste P, Malafosse A: Association between the TPH gene A218C polymorphism and suicidal behavior: a meta-analysis. Am J Med Genet B Neuropsychiatr Genet 124B:87–91, 2004

Bennett AJ, Lesch KP, Heils A, et al: Early experience and serotonin transporter gene variation interact to influence primate CNS function. Mol Psychiatry 7:118–122, 2002

Boldrini M, Underwood MD, Mann JJ, et al: More tryptophan hydroxylase in the brainstem dorsal raphe nucleus in depressed suicides. Brain Res 1041:19–28, 2005

Boldrini M, Underwood MD, Hen R, et al: Antidepressants increase neural progenitor cells in the human hippocampus. Neuropsychopharmacology 34:2376–2389, 2009

Bradley RG, Binder EB, Epstein MP, et al: Influence of child abuse on adult depression: moderation by the corticotropin-releasing hormone receptor gene. Arch Gen Psychiatry 65:190–200, 2008

Brent DA, Mann JJ: Family genetic studies, suicide, and suicidal behavior. Am J Med Genet C Semin Med Genet 133:13–24, 2005

Brent DA, Melhem N: Familial transmission of suicidal behavior. Psychiatr Clin North Am 31:157–177, 2008

Brodsky BS, Stanley B: Adverse childhood experiences and suicidal behavior. Psychiatr Clin North Am 31:223–235, 2008

Brown GL, Goodwin FK: Cerebrospinal fluid correlates of suicide attempts and aggression. Ann N Y Acad Sci 487:175–188, 1986

Brown RP, Stoll PM, Stokes PE, et al: Adrenocortical hyperactivity in depression: effects of agitation, delusions, melancholia, and other illness variables. Psychiatry Res 23:167–178, 1988

Brown SM, Hariri AR: Neuroimaging studies of serotonin gene polymorphisms: exploring the interplay of genes, brain, and behavior. Cogn Affect Behav Neurosci 6:44–52, 2006

Brunner HG, Nelen M, Breakefield XO, et al: Abnormal behavior associated with a point mutation in the structural gene for monoamine oxidase A. Science 262:578–580, 1993

Brunner J, Stalla GK, Stalla J, et al: Decreased corticotropin-releasing hormone (CRH) concentrations in the cerebrospinal fluid of eucortisolemic suicide attempters. J Psychiatr Res 35:1–9, 2001

Brunner J, Parhofer KG, Schwandt P, et al: Cholesterol, essential fatty acids, and suicide. Pharmacopsychiatry 35:1–5, 2002

Brunson KL, Avishai-Eliner S, Hatalski CG, et al: Neurobiology of the stress response early in life: evolution of a concept and the role of corticotropin releasing hormone. Mol Psychiatry 6:647–656, 2001

Cases O, Seif I, Grimsby J, et al: Aggressive behavior and altered amounts of brain serotonin and norepinephrine in mice lacking MAOA. Science 268:1763–1766, 1995

Caspi A, McClay J, Moffitt TE, et al: Role of genotype in the cycle of violence in maltreated children. Science 297:851–854, 2002

Caspi A, Sugden K, Moffitt TE, et al: Influence of life stress on depression: moderation by a polymorphism in the 5-HTT gene. Science 301:386–389, 2003

Coccaro EF, Siever LJ, Klar HM, et al: Serotonergic studies in patients with affective and personality disorders: correlates with suicidal and impulsive aggressive behavior. Arch Gen Psychiatry 46:587–599, 1989

Coccaro EF, Kavoussi RJ, Sheline YI, et al: Impulsive aggression in personality disorder correlates with platelet 5-HT2A receptor binding. Neuropsychopharmacology 16:211–216, 1997

Cooper SJ, Kelly CB, King DJ: 5-Hydroxyindoleacetic acid in cerebrospinal fluid and prediction of suicidal behaviour in schizophrenia. Lancet 340:940–941, 1992

Currier D, Mann JJ: Stress, genes and the biology of suicidal behavior. Psychiatr Clin North Am 31:247–269, 2008

de Almeida RM, Rosa MM, Santos DM, et al: 5-HT(1B) receptors, ventral orbitofrontal cortex, and aggressive behavior in mice. Psychopharmacology (Berl) 185:441–450, 2006

De Luca V, Tharmalingam S, Kennedy JL: Association study between the corticotropin-releasing hormone receptor 2 gene and suicidality in bipolar disorder. Eur Psychiatry 22:282–287, 2007

De Luca V, Tharmalingam S, Zai C, et al: Association of HPA axis genes with suicidal behaviour in schizophrenia. J Psychopharmacol 24:677–682, 2010

Du L, Faludi G, Palkovits M, et al: Frequency of long allele in serotonin transporter gene is increased in depressed suicide victims. Biol Psychiatry 46:196–201, 1999

Dunn AJ, Swiergiel AH, Palamarchouk V: Brain circuits involved in corticotropin-releasing factor–norepinephrine interactions during stress. Ann N Y Acad Sci 1018:25–34, 2004

Engstrom G, Alling C, Blennow K, et al: Reduced cerebrospinal HVA concentrations and HVA/5-HIAA ratios in suicide attempters: monoamine metabolites in 120 suicide attempters and 47 controls. Eur Neuropsychopharmacol 9:399–405, 1999

Fergusson DM, Horwood LJ, Lynskey MT: Childhood sexual abuse and psychiatric disorder in young adulthood, II: psychiatric outcomes of childhood sexual abuse. J Am Acad Child Adolesc Psychiatry 35:1365–1374, 1996

Frankle WG, Lombardo I, New AS, et al: Brain serotonin transporter distribution in subjects with impulsive aggressivity: a positron emission study with [11C]McN 5652. Am J Psychiatry 162:915–923, 2005

Furmark T, Appel L, Henningsson S, et al: A link between serotonin-related gene polymorphisms, amygdala activity, and placebo-induced relief from social anxiety. J Neurosci 28:13066–13074, 2008

Galfalvy H, Currier D, Oquendo MA, et al: Lower CSF MHPG predicts short-term risk for suicide attempt. Int J Neuropsychopharmacol 12:1327–1335, 2009

Galfalvy H, Zalsman G, Huang YY, et al: A pilot genome wide association with gene expression array study of suicide with and without major depression. World J Biol Psychiatry November 7, 2011 [Epub ahead of print]

Gibb BE, McGeary JE, Beevers CG, et al: Serotonin transporter (5-HTTLPR) genotype, childhood abuse, and suicide attempts in adult psychiatric inpatients. Suicide Life Threat Behav 36:687–693, 2006

Goldstein DS, Kopin IJ: Evolution of concepts of stress. Stress 10:109–120, 2007

Golomb BA: Cholesterol and violence: is there a connection? Ann Intern Med 128:478–487, 1998

Grunebaum MF, Ellis SP, Duan M, et al: Pilot randomized clinical trial of an SSRI vs. bupropion: effects on suicidal behavior, ideation, and mood in major depression. Neuropsychopharmacology 37:697–706, 2012

Haghighi F, Bach-Mizrachi H, Huang YY, et al: Genetic architecture of the human tryptophan hydroxylase 2 gene: existence of neural isoforms and relevance for major depression. Mol Psychiatry 13:813–820, 2008

Heim C, Nemeroff CB: The role of childhood trauma in the neurobiology of mood and anxiety disorders: preclinical and clinical studies. Biol Psychiatry 49:1023–1039, 2001

Heim C, Newport DJ, Heit S, et al: Pituitary-adrenal and autonomic responses to stress in women after sexual and physical abuse in childhood. JAMA 284:592–597, 2000

Heim C, Newport DJ, Bonsall R, et al: Altered pituitary-adrenal axis responses to provocative challenge tests in adult survivors of childhood abuse. Am J Psychiatry 158:575–581, 2001

Higley JD, Suomi SJ, Linnoila M: A longitudinal assessment of CSF monoamine metabolite and plasma cortisol concentrations in young rhesus monkeys. Biol Psychiatry 32:127–145, 1992

Hrdina PD, Demeter E, Vu TB, et al: 5-HT uptake sites and 5-HT2 receptors in brain of antidepressant-free suicide victims/depressives: increase in 5- HT2 sites in cortex and amygdala. Brain Res 614:37–44, 1993

Huan M, Hamazaki K, Sun Y, et al: Suicide attempt and n-3 fatty acid levels in red blood cells: a case control study in China. Biol Psychiatry 56:490–496, 2004

Huang YY, Cate SP, Battistuzzi C, et al: An association between a functional polymorphism in the monoamine oxidase A gene promoter, impulsive traits and early abuse experiences. Neuropsychopharmacology 29:1498–1505, 2004

Ichise M, Vines DC, Gura T, et al: Effects of early life stress on ^{11}CDASB positron emission tomography imaging of serotonin transporters in adolescent peer- and mother-reared rhesus monkeys. J Neurosci 26:4638–4643, 2006

Jollant F, Lawrence NS, Olie E, et al: Decreased activation of lateral orbitofrontal cortex during risky choices under uncertainty is associated with disadvantageous decision-making and suicidal behavior. Neuroimage 51:1275–1281, 2010

Kamali M, Oquendo MA, Mann JJ: Understanding the neurobiology of suicidal behavior. Depress Anxiety 14:164–176, 2001

Kaufman J, Birmaher B, Perel J: Serotonergic functioning in depressed abused children: clinical and familial correlates. Biol Psychiatry 44:973–981, 1998

Ke L, Qi ZY, Ping Y, et al: Effect of SNP at position 40237 in exon 7 of the TPH2 gene on susceptibility to suicide. Brain Res 1122:24–26, 2006

Kraemer GW, Ebert MH, Schmidt DE, et al: A longitudinal study of the effect of different social rearing conditions on cerebrospinal fluid norepinephrine and biogenic amine metabolites in rhesus monkeys. Neuropsychopharmacology 2:175–189, 1989

Lazary J, Viczena V, Dome P, et al: Hopelessness, a potential endophenotype for suicidal behavior, is influenced by TPH2 gene variants. Prog Neuropsychopharmacol Biol Psychiatry 36:155–160, 2012

Lester D: The concentration of neurotransmitter metabolites in the cerebrospinal fluid of suicidal individuals: a meta-analysis. Pharmacopsychiatry 28:77–79, 1995

Lewis MD, Hibbeln JR, Johnson JE, et al: Suicide deaths of active-duty US military and omega-3 fatty-acid status: a case-control comparison. J Clin Psychiatry 72:1585–1590, 2011

Leyton M, Paquette V, Gravel P, et al: alpha-[11C]Methyl-L-tryptophan trapping in the orbital and ventral medial prefrontal cortex of suicide attempters. Eur Neuropsychopharmacol 16:220–223, 2006

Linnoila M, De Jong J, Virkkunen M, et al: Family history of alcoholism in violent offenders and impulsive fire setters. Arch Gen Psychiatry 46:613–616, 1989

Liu D, Diorio J, Caldji C, et al: Maternal care, hippocampal glucocorticoid receptors, and hypothalamic-pituitary-adrenal responses to stress. Science 277:1659–1662, 1997

Liu D, Caldji C, Sharma S, et al: Influence of neonatal rearing conditions on stress-induced adrenocorticotropin responses and norepinephrine release in the hypothalamic paraventricular nucleus. J Neuroendocrinol 12:5–12, 2000

López JF, Vázquez DM, Chalmers DT, et al: Regulation of 5-HT receptors and the hypothalamic-pituitary-adrenal axis: implications for the neurobiology of suicide. Ann N Y Acad Sci 836:106–134, 1997

Lopez VA, Detera-Wadleigh S, Cardona I, et al: Nested association between genetic variation in tryptophan hydroxylase II, bipolar affective disorder, and suicide attempts. Biol Psychiatry 61:181–186, 2007

Maes M: Inflammatory and oxidative and nitrosative stress pathways underpinning chronic fatigue, somatization and psychosomatic symptoms. Curr Opin Psychiatry 22:75–83, 2009

Mann JJ: Neurobiology of suicidal behaviour. Nat Rev Neurosci 4:819–828, 2003

Mann JJ, Currier D: A review of prospective studies of biologic predictors of suicidal behavior in mood disorders. Arch Suicide Res 11:3–16, 2007

Mann JJ, Currier D: Suicide and attempted suicide, in The Medical Basis of Psychiatry. Edited by Fatemi SH, Clayton PJ. Philadelphia, PA, Humana Press, 2008, pp 561–576

Mann JJ, Malone KM: Cerebrospinal fluid amines and higher-lethality suicide attempts in depressed inpatients. Biol Psychiatry 41:162–171, 1997

Mann JJ, Waternaux C, Haas GL, et al: Toward a clinical model of suicidal behavior in psychiatric patients. Am J Psychiatry 156:181–189, 1999

Mann JJ, Huang YY, Underwood MD, et al: A serotonin transporter gene promoter polymorphism (5-HTTLPR) and prefrontal cortical binding in major depression and suicide. Arch Gen Psychiatry 57:729–738, 2000

Mann JJ, Brent DA, Arango V: Neurobiology and genetics of suicide and attempted suicide: a focus on the serotonergic system. Neuropsychopharmacology 24:467–477, 2001

Mann JJ, Currier D, Stanley B, et al: Can biological tests assist prediction of suicide in mood disorders? Int J Neuropsychopharmacol 9:465–474, 2006

McBride PA, Brown RP, DeMeo M, et al: The relationship of platelet 5-HT2 receptor indices to major depressive disorder, personality traits, and suicidal behavior. Biol Psychiatry 35:295–308, 1994

McGowan PO, Sasaki A, D'Alessio AC, et al: Epigenetic regulation of the glucocorticoid receptor in human brain associates with childhood abuse. Nat Neurosci 12:342–348, 2009

Meaney MJ, Diorio J, Francis D, et al: Early environmental regulation of forebrain glucocorticoid receptor gene expression: implications for adrenocortical responses to stress. Dev Neurosci 18:49–72, 1996

Meijer OC, de Kloet ER: Corticosterone and serotonergic neurotransmission in the hippocampus: functional implications of central corticosteroid receptor diversity. Crit Rev Neurobiol 12:1–20, 1998

Meltzer HY, Perline R, Tricou BJ, et al: Effect of 5-hydroxytryptophan on serum cortisol levels in major affective disorders, II: relation to suicide, psychosis, and depressive symptoms. Arch Gen Psychiatry 41:379–387, 1984

Mendlovic S, Doron A, Eilat E: Short note: can depressive patients exploit the immune system for suicide? Med Hypotheses 49:445–446, 1997

Mendlovic S, Mozes E, Eilat E, et al: Immune activation in non-treated suicidal major depression. Immunol Lett 67:105–108, 1999

Meyer-Lindenberg A, Buckholtz JW, Kolachana B, et al: Neural mechanisms of genetic risk for impulsivity and violence in humans. Proc Natl Acad Sci U S A 103:6269–6274, 2006

Miller JM, Kinnally EL, Ogden RT, et al: Reported childhood abuse is associated with low serotonin transporter binding in vivo in major depressive disorder. Synapse 63:565–573, 2009

Muldoon MF, Rossouw JE, Manuck SB, et al: Low or lowered cholesterol and risk of death from suicide and trauma. Metabolism 42 (suppl 1):45–56, 1993

Nässberger L, Träskman-Bendz L: Increased soluble interleukin-2 receptor concentrations in suicide attempters. Acta Psychiatr Scand 88:48–52, 1993

Nemeroff CB: The neurobiology of aging and the neurobiology of depression: is there a relationship? Neurobiol Aging 9:120–122, 1988

Nemeroff CB, Owens MJ, Bissette G, et al: Reduced corticotropin releasing factor binding sites in the frontal cortex of suicide victims. Arch Gen Psychiatry 45:577–579, 1988

New AS, Hazlett EA, Buchsbaum MS, et al: Blunted prefrontal cortical 18fluorodeoxyglucose positron emission tomography response to meta-chlorophenylpiperazine in impulsive aggression. Arch Gen Psychiatry 59:621–629, 2002

New AS, Trestman RF, Mitropoulou V, et al: Low prolactin response to fenfluramine in impulsive aggression. J Psychiatr Res 38:223–230, 2004

Nordström P, Samuelsson M, Åsberg M, et al: CSF 5-HIAA predicts suicide risk after attempted suicide. Suicide Life Threat Behav 24:1–9, 1994

Oquendo MA, Placidi GP, Malone KM, et al: Positron emission tomography of regional brain metabolic responses to a serotonergic challenge and lethality of suicide attempts in major depression. Arch Gen Psychiatry 60:14–22, 2003

Oquendo MA, Galfalvy H, Russo S, et al: Prospective study of clinical predictors of suicidal acts after a major depressive episode in patients with major depressive disorder or bipolar disorder. Am J Psychiatry 161:1433–1441, 2004

Oquendo MA, Russo SA, Underwood MD, et al: Higher postmortem prefrontal 5-HT2A receptor binding correlates with lifetime aggression in suicide. Biol Psychiatry 59:235–243, 2006

Owens MJ, Nemeroff CB: Physiology and pharmacology of corticotropin-releasing factor. Pharmacol Rev 43:425–473, 1991

Pandey GN, Dwivedi Y: What can post-mortem studies tell us about the pathoetiology of suicide? Future Neurol 5:701–720, 2010

Parsey RV, Hastings RS, Oquendo MA, et al: Effect of a triallelic functional polymorphism of the serotonin-transporter-linked promoter region on expression of serotonin transporter in the human brain. Am J Psychiatry 163:48–51, 2006

Passamonti L, Fera F, Magariello A, et al: Monoamine oxidase-a genetic variations influence brain activity associated with inhibitory control: new insight into the neural correlates of impulsivity. Biol Psychiatry 59:334–340, 2006

Pine DS, Coplan JD, Wasserman GA, et al: Neuroendocrine response to fenfluramine challenge in boys: associations with aggressive behavior and adverse rearing. Arch Gen Psychiatry 54:839–846, 1997

Plotsky PM, Meaney MJ: Early, postnatal experience alters hypothalamic corticotropin-releasing factor (CRF) mRNA, median eminence CRF content and stress-induced release in adult rats. Brain Res Mol Brain Res 18:195–200, 1993

Postolache TT, Lapidus M, Sander ER, et al: Changes in allergy symptoms and depression scores are positively correlated in patients with recurrent mood disorders exposed to seasonal peaks in aeroallergens. ScientificWorldJournal 7:1968–1977, 2007

Postolache TT, Mortensen PB, Tonelli H, et al: Seasonal spring peaks of suicide in victims with and without prior history of hospitalization for mood disorders. J Affect Disord 121:88–93, 2010

Reuter M, Esslinger C, Montag C, et al: A functional variant of the tryptophan hydroxylase 2 gene impacts working memory: a genetic imaging study. Biol Psychol 79:111–117, 2008

Rinne T, Westenberg HG, den Boer JA, et al: Serotonergic blunting to meta-chlorophenyl-piperazine (m-CPP) highly correlates with sustained childhood abuse in impulsive and autoaggressive female borderline patients. Biol Psychiatry 47:548–556, 2000

Risch N, Herrell R, Lehner T, et al: Interaction between the serotonin transporter gene (5-HTTLPR), stressful life events, and risk of depression: a meta-analysis. JAMA 301:2462–2471, 2009

Rothenhäusler HB, Stepan A, Kapfhammer HP: Soluble interleukin 2 receptor levels, temperament and character in formerly depressed suicide attempters compared with normal controls. Suicide Life Threat Behav 36:455–466, 2006

Roy A, Hu XZ, Janal MN, et al: Interaction between childhood trauma and serotonin transporter gene variation in suicide. Neuropsychopharmacology 32:2046–2052, 2007

Roy A, Hodgkinson CA, Deluca V, et al: Two HPA axis genes, CRHBP and FKBP5, interact with childhood trauma to increase the risk for suicidal behavior. J Psychiatr Res October 4, 2011 [Epub ahead of print]

Rujescu D, Giegling I, Bondy B, et al: Association of anger-related traits with SNPs in the TPH gene. Mol Psychiatry 7:1023–1029, 2002

Schulsinger F, Kety SS, Rosenthal D, et al: A family study of suicide, in Origin, Prevention, and Treatment of Affective Disorders. Edited by Schou M, Strömgren E. New York, Academic Press, 1979, pp 277–287

Sequeira A, Turecki G: Genome wide gene expression studies in mood disorders. OMICS 10:444–454, 2006

Sequeira A, Klempan T, Canetti L, et al: Patterns of gene expression in the limbic system of suicides with and without major depression. Mol Psychiatry 12:640–655, 2007

Sher L, Carballo JJ, Grunebaum MF, et al: A prospective study of the association of cerebrospinal fluid monoamine metabolite levels with lethality of suicide attempts in patients with bipolar disorder. Bipolar Disord 8:543–550, 2006

Siever LJ, Buchsbaum MS, New AS, et al: d,1-Fenfluramine response in impulsive personality disorder assessed with [18 F]fluorodeoxyglucose positron emission tomography. Neuropsychopharmacology 20:413–423, 1999

Stanley B, Molcho A, Stanley M, et al: Association of aggressive behavior with altered serotonergic function in patients who are not suicidal. Am J Psychiatry 157:609–614, 2000

Stein MB, Yehuda R, Koverola C, et al: Enhanced dexamethasone suppression of plasma cortisol in adult women traumatized by childhood sexual abuse. Biol Psychiatry 42:680–686, 1997

Stoff DM, Mann JJ: Suicide research: overview and introduction. Ann N Y Acad Sci 836:1–11, 1997

Sublette ME, Hibbeln JR, Galfalvy H, et al: Omega-3 polyunsaturated essential fatty acid status as a predictor of future suicide risk. Am J Psychiatry 163:1100–1102, 2006

Sunnqvist C, Westrin A, Träskman-Bendz L, et al: Suicide attempters: biological stressmarkers and adverse life events. Eur Arch Psychiatry Clin Neurosci 258:456–462, 2008

Thalmeier A, Dickmann M, Giegling I, et al: Gene expression profiling of post-mortem orbitofrontal cortex in violent suicide victims. Int J Neuropsychopharmacol 11:217–228, 2008

Träskman L, Åsberg M, Bertilsson L, et al: Monoamine metabolites in CSF and suicidal behavior. Arch Gen Psychiatry 38:631–636, 1981

Tsai SJ, Hong CJ, Liou YJ: Recent molecular genetic studies and methodological issues in suicide research. Prog Neuropsychopharmacol Biol Psychiatry 35:809–817, 2011

Tyrka AR, Price LH, Gelernter J, et al: Interaction of childhood maltreatment with the corticotropin-releasing hormone receptor gene: effects on hypothalamic-pituitary-adrenal axis reactivity. Biol Psychiatry 66:681–685, 2009

Uher R, McGuffin P: The moderation by the serotonin transporter gene of environmental adversity in the aetiology of mental illness: review and methodological analysis. Mol Psychiatry 13:131–146, 2008

Underwood MD, Kassir SA, Bakalian MJ, et al: Neuron density and serotonin receptor binding in prefrontal cortex in suicide. Int J Neuropsychopharmacol 9:1–13, 2011

van Heeringen K, Audenaert K, Van de Wiele L, et al: Cortisol in violent suicidal behaviour: association with personality and monoaminergic activity. J Affect Disord 60:181–189, 2000

van Heeringen C, Audenaert K, Van Laere K, et al: Prefrontal 5-HT2a receptor binding index, hopelessness and personality characteristics in attempted suicide. J Affect Disord 74:149–158, 2003

Voracek M, Loibl LM: Genetics of suicide: a systematic review of twin studies. Wien Klin Wochenschr 119:463–475, 2007

Wasserman D, Sokolowski M, Rozanov V, et al: The CRHR1 gene: a marker for suicidality in depressed males exposed to low stress. Genes Brain Behav 7:14–19, 2008

Weaver IC, Cervoni N, Champagne FA, et al: Epigenetic programming by maternal behavior. Nat Neurosci 7:847–854, 2004

Wender PH, Kety SS, Rosenthal D, et al: Psychiatric disorders in the biological and adoptive families of adopted individuals with affective disorders. Arch Gen Psychiatry 43:923–929, 1986

Willour VL, Chen H, Toolan J, et al: Family based association of FKBP5 in bipolar disorder. Mol Psychiatry 14:261–268, 2009

Ystgaard M, Hestetun I, Loeb M, et al: Is there a specific relationship between childhood sexual and physical abuse and repeated suicidal behavior? Child Abuse Negl 28:863–875, 2004

Zill P, Buttner A, Eisenmenger W, et al: Single nucleotide polymorphism and haplotype analysis of a novel tryptophan hydroxylase isoform (TPH2) gene in suicide victims. Biol Psychiatry 56:581–586, 2004

C H A P T E R   2 6

Combined Murder-Suicide

Carl P. Malmquist, M.D., M.S.

Understanding murder followed by suicide has all the complexities of understanding each entity by itself as well as the added interaction between them. A theoretical issue is whether murder-suicide should be given emphasis more as a form of murder or of suicide, or whether it is a generic entity of its own. A mixture of motives and background factors has led to diverse attempts at classification, both by clinicians and by social scientists or epidemiologists. If the person attempting suicide survives, he or she is usually prosecuted legally for some degree of murder. A common typology is to divide murder-suicide into four categories (Roberts 2003):

1. Domestic violence connected to a murder-suicide
2. Elderly murder-suicide
3. Infanticidal murder-suicide
4. Murder-suicide related to mental illnesses

The difficulty with such a grouping is that psychiatric disorders are not a discrete group. In many cases, they overlap with the other categories. Diverse psychiatric diagnoses can appear in the backgrounds of in-dividuals in all of the other categories when data are available to study. Difficulties in classification thus appear to reflect problems encompassing the possibility of personal psychopathology as well as an adverse social environment that contributes to such a final outcome of a murder-suicide. A classification of murder-suicide based on victims is presented in Table 26–1, and motivational and diagnostic backgrounds of the perpetrators are discussed later in this chapter.

Difficulties in Assessing Murder-Suicide

A major, and obvious, limitation in assessment is that in most cases the perpetrator is dead. Hence the only opportunity to evaluate such individuals directly is through those who survive a suicide effort. Some researchers have attempted to study those who commit a homicide with a subsequent attempted suicide (a parasuicide) in an effort to determine whether the combined acts more resemble a homicide or suicide or a unique phenomenon (Liem et al. 2011). In most cases, the behavior leading up to the final outcome needs to be reconstructed by

TABLE 26–1. Classification of murder-suicide by victim

I.   Domestic violence
    A. Spouse
    B. Partner
       1. Male
       2. Female

II. Perpetrated by the elderly
    A. Spouse
    B. Offspring
    C. Companion

III. Minors
    A. Feticide
    B. Neonaticide
    C. Infanticide (up to 1 year)
    D. Pedicide (older than 1 year)

IV. Mass murder-suicides
    A. Familicide
    B. Workplace murders
    C. School shootings
    D. Acts of revenge

outside information and from those in contact with the person, along with any past medical or counseling records and notes left.

Another complication is that a standardized definition of murder-suicide does not exist. A question arises as to whether an attempted homicide followed by a suicide or a homicide followed by an incomplete suicide would qualify as murder-suicide. The time issue is also debatable, such as how much time can have elapsed after the homicide to qualify for a murder-suicide. Some see the acts as one unitary event, occurring perhaps within minutes of each other, whereas others use a day, a week, or some other basis to connect the acts (Marzuk et al. 1992). Reports may use a selected group, such as a small sample, or focus on homicide-suicide in one city, region, or state, and thus their findings may not be generaliz-

able. Sometimes studies ignore the various types of homicide-suicide in drawing conclusions. Data from different countries also have the obvious limitations in making comparisons.

An individual who has killed an intimate partner may first go into a state of hibernation and hiding and die by suicide some time later when he or she is about to be apprehended. The emotional and legal significance of killing one's lover may emerge only gradually. It may lead to a suicidal act while awaiting trial some time later or even after a trial when incarcerated. A mother who has murdered her infant while in a psychotic depression may be treated for the depression while incarcerated. When her clinical psychotic state goes into remission, she reflects not only on her future situation of spending many years in prison but also on her guilt, which may lead to suicide. The phenomenon of mass killings—whether these are acts of familicide, school killings, or cult killings followed by suicides—presents yet other difficulties. Explanations for these events often involve different clinical and social features than in the murder-suicide of a couple in an intimate relationship.

Epidemiological Perspectives

The following is a survey of articles and reports on murder-suicide. Some reports are from an earlier period, and some are from different countries and cultures. No standard methodology was used in these different reports. National data for homicide-suicide in the United States are not available. The hope was expressed in a newspaper surveillance approach that the Centers for Disease Control and Prevention (CDC) would have such data in the future through its National Violent Death Reporting System (Warren-Gordon et al. 2010).

An early study in 1928 of 39 murder-suicides was followed by a dearth of studies (Cavan 1928). In the interval, there were individual case reports, and murder-suicide continued to be covered by the media. In a study of murder-suicide in England and Wales, West (1966) found that 1 in 3 murders was followed by a suicide, but only 1 in 100 suicides was coupled with a previous murder. Interestingly, he did not find an increased incidence of "insanity" in comparison with more common types of homicide. A 1980 study of murder-suicide in the United States found a rate of 6.22 per 100,000 (Palmer and Humphrey 1980). A review by Coid (1983) of 17 studies involving 10 countries, including the United States, from 1900 to 1979 focused on "abnormal homicides" (in which a verdict of not guilty by reason of insanity or diminished responsibility or its equivalent in the country of origin was found) and murder followed by suicide. The murder-suicide rates were quite similar and consistent in different countries, with an average of 0.20–0.30 per 100,000, despite considerable differences in the overall rates of homicide. It was found that the higher the rate of homicide in a given population, the lower the percentage of offenders who were seen as mentally abnormal or who died by suicide.

However, it should be noted that similarity in rates does not indicate the percentage of murder-suicides among all homicides in a given country. The latter varies widely. Thus, the percentage of murder-suicide combinations in the United States was 4%, whereas in Denmark it was 42%. The variation is due to the principle that the higher the overall rate of homicide in a given country, such as the United States, the lower the proportion of murder-suicides.

A study from England and Wales examined 52 cases of homicide-suicide from 1975 through 1992. The rates varied from 0.05 in Scotland in comparison with 0.55 in Miami, Florida (Milroy 1995). However, this variation may not be that surprising given the number of elderly couples in the Miami region, where a partner may be terminally ill and facing continued suffering and isolation. The most common precipitating factor for a murder-suicide was the dissolution of a relationship, with the subsequent emergence of mental symptoms of depression or murderous jealousy. Alcohol abuse factored in 29% of the cases.

A Florida study compared two regions over 6 years regarding the incidence of murder-suicide for those younger than 55 years and those age 55 years or older (Cohen et al. 1998). The annual incidence rates ranged from 0.3 to 0.7 per 100,000 persons younger than 55 years, and from 0.4 to 0.9 for those age 55 years or older, with higher rates found in the older group every year but two.

The odds of an increased rate of suicide or homicide were studied for 16,245 homicides in the files of the Chicago Police Department for the years 1965 through 1990, during which time 267 murder-suicides occurred (Stack 1997). After sociodemographic variables were controlled for, murder of an ex-spouse or a lover increased the risk for suicide the most—by 12.68 times. Killing a child increased the risk by 12.28 times, killing a current spouse by 8.00 times, killing a girlfriend or boyfriend by 6.11 times, and killing a friend by 1.88 times. The conclusion of the study was that the principal source of frustration in murder-suicide cases is a chaotic intimate relationship marked by jealousy and ambivalence. Nock and Marzuk (1999) concluded that in the United States, 1.5% of all suicides and 5.0% of all homicides occur in the context of a murder-suicide.

A 5-year study of 16 cases of murder-suicide occurring within a week of the homicide was carried out in New Hampshire (Campanelli and Gilson 2002). New Hampshire is a state with a low homicide rate, and hence the combination accounted for 14.7% of all the homicides in the state. The findings were typical: 94% of the perpetrators were males, and firearms were used in most cases.

More recent studies from the United States have broadened the groups studied. A study in west-central Florida compared older men who died by suicide with those who committed homicide and then died by suicide (Malphurs et al. 2001). Depression was prominent in both groups, but the former had more physical illnesses, and 50% of the latter were in caregiving roles compared with 17% of the former. The same data suggest that homicide-suicide rates may be increasing in Florida and in other states with aging populations because of the older population (Cohen et al. 1998). Data from the Hemlock Society indicate that most mercy killings are by an older man who kills his sick wife and then dies by suicide (Canetto and Hollenshead 2000–2001).

A California study examined the murders of all intimate partners in 1 year to determine whether differences were seen when a suicide followed (Lund and Smorodinsky 2001). Forty percent died by suicide, and the differences noted were that those who completed suicide were all males, were older, almost always used a gun, and were less likely to be black men. Almost all of the older homicide perpetrators took their own lives, whereas fewer than half of those younger than 40 years did so, which suggests different bases for carrying out a homicide.

Various studies from different countries have continued to appear. Spousal murder-suicide was studied in Quebec, Canada, over 8 years (1991–1998). Among 388 cases of death by intrafamilial violence in the Que-

bec coroner's office, 145 were conjugal homicides, and in 58 of these cases, the homicidal spouses killed themselves (Bourget et al. 2000). The perpetrators were mainly men who were separated from their spouses and who used a firearm. Most were seen as clinically depressed. A Swiss study of "double suicide" and homicide-suicide found that the precipitating factors were similar to those in suicides (Haenel and Elsässer 2000). Stressors such as physical illness, isolation, and social losses were correlated with depression, borderline disturbances, and narcissistic neuroses.

An epidemiological study used death certificates for all those who died by homicide-suicide (in which the suicide followed the homicide within 3 days) in England and Wales (Barraclough and Harris 2002). In 144 incidents, 327 people died; 88% involved members of the same family, 75% of the victims were females, and 85% of the suspects were males. Car exhaust and firearms accounted for 40% of the victims' and 50% of the suspects' deaths. The conclusion was that in England and Wales, homicide-suicide is mostly a "family affair."

The findings of a study in Fiji analyzing murder-suicide over a 10-year period (Adinkrah 2003) were consistent with those in studies of Western developed countries, with the exception that perpetrators were equally divided between men and women, and no firearms were used. Another study, focusing on Hong Kong, was the first systematic research of murder-suicide in a Chinese society (Chan et al. 2004). According to records from the police and coroner's court over a 10-year period, most cases involved spouses and lovers and were motivated by separation or the end of a marital relationship. Depression was the most common mental disorder, and economic factors were seen as having high relevance. In contrast to Western societies, firearms were used infrequently; the most frequent modes of killing were strangulation or suffocation (carried out in 26% of cases) and stabbing or chopping (14%). In Finland, the ratio of homicide-suicide to homicide declined from 15% to 6% from the 1960s to 2000 (Kivivuori and Lehti 2003). The rates of intimate partner murders and parent-child killings have declined but have consistently remained highest among those in the middle classes.

Over a 90-year period (1900–1990) in four cities—two in Canada (Toronto and Vancouver) and two in the United States (Buffalo and Seattle)—there were 451 homicide-suicide cases, with 88% of the offenders being male (Gartner and McCarthy 2009). However, the distribution differed from other types of homicides, with female intimate partners being the victim in 72% of the cases. In contrast, most of the victims of women offenders were children. In this study, the trend in homicide-suicide rates seemed independent of the trend in total homicide rates, and to some degree the homicide-suicide trend was associated more with the trend for *suicides* than homicides. This finding raises unresolved issues, with some studies showing a relatively fixed rate of homicide-suicide (Eliason 2009), and others finding a variation of rates up to 100-fold (Large et al. 2009). The latter study analyzed 64 samples from 49 publications and found that the United States had a significant association between homicide-suicide rates and other types of *homicides* in contrast to 17 other countries and Greenland, which did not. Another 15-year study examined infant homicide rates using World Health Organization and CDC data and found that these rates were significantly and independently associated with both total homicide and total suicide rates (Large et al. 2010).

A comparison of the homicide-suicide rates in the Netherlands, Switzerland, and the United States was made with the suicide occurring within 24 hours after the homicide (Liem et al. 2011). Certain subtypes of homicide are frequently followed by suicide, such as when men kill an intimate partner with a firearm and, in over half of the incidents, subsequently die by suicide. In all three countries the homicide-suicide acts were more likely than other homicides to involve multiple victims and more likely than homicide only or suicide only to take place at home. The homicide-suicide rates in Switzerland and the United States were substantially higher than in the Netherlands, with the difference attributed to the availability of firearms in the home. Switzerland has a militia system that requires every male citizen to serve in the military, with the weapons kept at home.

The National Violent Death Reporting System is a surveillance system in which 17 states were enrolled by 2008. From 2003 through 2005, there were 408 homicide-suicide incidents identified (Logan et al. 2008). Eighty-eight percent of the incidents were committed with a firearm, 91% by males, 98% by those older than 19 years, and 77% by white individuals. However, 51.5% of filicide-suicides were by females. When a comparison was made between males in the homicide-suicide group and a suicide alone group, 55% of the former group had intimate partner conflicts, compared with 26% of the latter. Of the 208 male homicide-suicide perpetrators with intimate partner conflicts, 191 were believed to have been retaliating for a breakup or divorce request. Over 85% of the homicide-suicide perpetrators were not suspected of having a depressed mood or having a current mental health problem, whereas only 67% of the filicide-suicide perpetrators were so classified. Further, the majority did not have prior reports of alcohol or substance abuse problems, but 1 in 5 perpetrators was suspected of being intoxicated at the time of the incident.

It is not news that high schools and colleges experience violence, but the onset of shootings that involve suicides following homicides has begun to attain high publicity. The CDC studied school-associated violence with a population-based surveillance from media databases, state and local agencies, and police and school officials for the years 1994–1999 (Anderson et al. 2001). The 220 events resulted in 253 deaths, with 11 of the cases being homicide-suicides. During the period of the study, the homicide rates for students killed in multiple-victim events increased; 172 cases were by students, and in 120 of them, a note, threat, or other action indicating potential violence prior to the offense was found. Subsequently, many high-profile school shootings with suicides in high school and colleges have occurred, from Columbine in 1999 onward (Malmquist 2006). This has led to many discussions and conferences regarding such tragedies (Newman and Fox 2009).

A recurrent question in murder-suicide acts involves the role of alcohol or other drugs. Alcohol or drug use can play a role in bringing about the final act through the resulting poor judgment, impulsivity in deciding to act, and preexisting depressive and paranoid elements that may be present under the surface. Most studies have not included data on this variable. One study of murder-suicide did find that 10% of perpetrators and 7% of victims had been using street drugs (Cooper and Eaves 1996). The acute effects of drugs need to be distinguished from perpetrators with chronic substance abuse problems. The New Hampshire study showed 30% of perpetrators positive for alcohol and 16% having chronic alcohol problems (Campanelli and Gilson 2002). Another study that focused on jealousy and paranoia found 21% legally in-

toxicated and 27% using alcohol (Palermo et al. 1997).

Clinical Factors

Descriptive and motivational factors may vary depending on the type of murder-suicide. Many overlapping factors of perpetrators are commonly found, such as being clinically depressed, paranoid to some degree, jealous, or ambivalent; having poor control of aggression; wanting revenge; being influenced by alcohol or drugs; and feeling a sense of hopelessness in their lives. Hopelessness may arise in diverse contexts, such as in a relationship per se involving unfaithfulness, or when there is despair in a terminally ill spouse or a sensed betrayal by a superior at work. Consistent with homicide data, most perpetrators are men (about 90%), with the exception of filicidal mothers who murder and then die by suicide. In reviewing several studies, Felthous and Hempel (1995) found that about 80% of the victims in murder-suicide were female.

Depression in connection with murder-suicide is viewed hypothetically as having more in common with suicidal acts than with homicidal acts. The loss of hope in a relationship or disillusionment with someone is seen as a key element. It is like a reaction to the loss of a major element in a person's life—be it a spouse, lover, job, health, or goal one is pursuing. The situation is like a deficit in the ability to grieve a major loss or to manage disappointment but raises a key question: why does the actor not just die by suicide instead of commiting the murder first? Diverse dynamics are possible, such as not wanting the other to survive and enjoy a life, the desire to punish or seek vengeance, or the fantasy that they will both be happy and later reunited in some new sphere of existence. If an element of blame or faultfinding with others, or some component of society, is seen as responsible for the person's misery, a type of mass killing may occur, such as in a violent outburst in public settings where persons unknown to the perpetrator are killed. Elements of humiliation and helplessness without any way seen to alleviate the situation may play a large role in some cases. Shootings in public places and school shootings are examples in which the perpetrator expects to be shot or to die by suicide. Mass killings are usually seen as a form of suicide but with the added element of needing first to destroy others.

Specific Types of Murder-Suicide

Disappointments in Relationships

Spouse or lover murder-suicide represents the major category in terms of frequency, accounting for an estimated 50%–75% of all murder-suicides. When a murder results, it represents the point of no return in a love relationship that has gone awry. Some of these individuals may have psychotic delusions leading to the final act, but most are rather experiencing deep jealousy and resentment that their once hopeful and happy relationship is not capable of continuing. The idea is the Othello syndrome: instead of allowing for the possibility that the other should live and have a happy future, the decision is, rather, "If I can't live and be happy, neither will you."

Narcissistic entitlement is seen when the person believes that his or her own unhappiness entitles him or her to take another's life. The killing may occur in an explosive and impulsive manner when the spouse or lover leaves or is about to do so. The perpetrator is then convinced that all

hope for the relationship is gone. Yet why are men more likely than women to kill in this situation? The explanation often given is that for the woman, murder in a spousal or lover relationship is connected to an abusive situation. Hence, perpetrating a murder alone suffices. However, in one subtype, the children or the ex-spouse's or ex-lover's new partner may be killed as well.

Case Example 1

A middle-aged man discovers that his wife has developed a sexually intimate relationship with another woman. He first denies that this is possible, but when denial is no longer possible, he begins brooding and becomes deeply depressed. When he asks his wife about it, she first denies it, but after her return from a vacation with her female friend, she informs him that she wants to leave him to live with her friend and confirms that they are in love. For a few months, his wife and he continue to live together while arrangements are made for her to move out. On returning home from a holiday family gathering in a rural setting, he stops the car and tells his wife he has to get out to urinate. On returning to the car, he opens the trunk, takes out his shotgun, and shoots his wife. He then attempts suicide with the shotgun but cannot place it accurately, and he survives the shooting. Five years later he is still hospitalized after being committed with a diagnosis of psychotic depression.

The emotional state in these individuals before the killing is that of being deeply shamed. It is as though they have been not only exposed but also destroyed. Hence, their life is over, and the life of the person or people who have done this to them should also be over. There seems to be a need to complete—or end—the story.

This explanation is relevant to several of the mass murder-suicides that have occurred. An example is that at Jonestown, Guyana, where the Reverend James Jones's psychotic thinking blurred his own self-concept into the extended family of 913 other people at the settlement he ran (Chidester 1988). Jones had had sexual relationships and fathered children with several women in "the family." To kill himself involved first convincing others in the cult to die by suicide with him so that his act would feel complete; those who did not comply were murdered.

Dependent personalities may show a variation of this type of despair (Malmquist 2006). The joint murder-suicide act in these situations is not only to destroy the person who has been the source of deep disappointment to him or her but also, it is hoped, to be reunited with that person. The dependency killings occur in the background of an overidealized relationship that has ended but without a realization of how distorted the relation was. A variation is seen in which military personnel about to be deployed overseas to a combat zone murder their spouse or lover and then die by suicide. A mixture of motives may be present, from separation and depression, and the act represents an escape from the military and an angry accusation against the military or politicians that have placed them in that situation. In some cases there may be a suicide pact.

Thernstrom (1997) described the following murder-suicide by a student with a dependent personality:

> Two female Harvard University students became roommates in an unplanned way. They were both immigrant students from different cultures, but their personalities were even more different. One was popular and outgoing, whereas the other was reticent and self-loathing. The brooding girl was proud and idealized who she had acquired as a roommate, but the other girl progressively ignored her in developing her own life. When the popular girl informed her roommate that she would not be rooming with her the next year, her roommate began pleading and

attempted to cajole her not to leave her but to no avail. During final examination week, changes were noted in the brooding girl, who began to dress in a more provocative manner and seemed happy for a change. The culmination came when she stabbed her roommate 45 times one morning and then hung herself. At the beginning of the school year, she had written in her diary, "If I ever grow desperate enough to seek power and a fearful respect through killing, she would be the first one I would blow off. ...You know what annoys me the most that situations would never reverse for me to be the strong and her to be the weak. She'll live on tucked in the warmth and support of her family while I cry alone in the cold....The bad way out I see is suicide and the good way out killing, savoring their fear and [then] suicide. But you know what annoys me the most, I do nothing."

Illness and Declining Health

A second main type of homicide-suicide emerges when one or both persons in a committed relationship develop a serious illness or realize their health is rapidly declining and both may be depressed. They will be left in a state of dependency because they will not be able to care for themselves. The perpetrator, whose partner is dying of an incurable disease or is becoming helpless, may commit a mercy killing. However, the decision to murder also may be based on a practical factor; that is, their financial assets are dwindling, and living some extra time with pain and disability is not a benefit comparable to leaving something to loved ones. The person also may realize that his or her resources will not permit him or her to receive the quality care he or she has been receiving. A Quebec study using coroner files of 27 homicide cases of those over 65 years found 19 cases with a homicide-suicide dynamic (Bourget et al. 2010). There were 13 suicides, with 5 failed attempts. Nearly half of the offenders had a preexisting medical condition, but 80% of the victims did.

Case Example 2

A middle-aged man's wife has developed multiple sclerosis. Over a period of years, she has had remissions and exacerbations, but she is now in a state of needing to be fed by him, and she is confined to a wheelchair. She has lost bowel and bladder control. She has always made clear to him that she never wants to end up in a nursing home, but continuing to care for her at home has become impossible. Thoughts of helping her die come and go, and after a few months, he concludes that he owes his wife a dignified ending rather than her having to remain in the state she is in. While she is in her wheelchair, he kisses her good-bye and, crying, strangles her with his belt while standing behind her. He then makes three unsuccessful attempts to hang himself, which leave rope burns on his neck. Finally, he drives to an isolated country road with a gun and sits in a ditch for hours while putting the gun to his head, but he is not able to pull the trigger. He returns home and keeps his wife's body in a freezer in the garage for several weeks until relatives of his wife report that they are not able to contact anyone about her, which leads to an investigation. He is prosecuted and pleads guilty to second-degree murder, receiving a mitigated sentence.

Suicide Pacts

Suicide pacts are sometimes called *double suicides* and are seen as joint ventures. In contrast to the Romeo and Juliet scenario, it is customarily older couples with increased dependency needs who carry out the acts. These may be difficult to distinguish from a murder-suicide if outside confirmatory material is lacking. When both parties totally independently agree that for diverse reasons, one is becoming too ill to be cared for and that they will both die by suicide, it would be viewed as a pact. However, if the party initiating the pact idea is more dominant or persuasive in the relationship, the

issue can become blurred between a pact and a murder-suicide. The suicide pact of noted author Arthur Koestler *(Darkness at Noon)* and his third wife is an example (Maris et al. 2000). Koestler was 77 years old and had Parkinson disease and leukemia, whereas she, 55 years old, was his caregiver but in good health. They both overdosed on barbiturates, and in her death note, she wrote, "I cannot face life without Arthur."

Familicides

Familicides are another variation of a homicide-suicide group. The goal of the perpetrator is to eliminate all members of the family who are present. In these cases, it is not a matter of seeking out someone, such as a sibling, who has left home. The victims are rather those family members who are at the scene, which suggests a degree of impulsivity. The motives may vary. In some cases, the person who is the prime source of financial support is no longer able to continue in that role. The perpetrator believes that the family needs to be relieved of an ensuing burden. Killing all the family members relieves them from a troubled future, so the perpetrator kills them and then commits suicide.

In other cases, there may be a marital life with unresolved conflicts that continue. In the state of ongoing disturbances and depression, the father, or occasionally the mother, decides that destroying the entire family and then committing suicide is the best solution for all of them in such an unhappy situation (Malmquist 1980). A variation is a depressed or psychotic adolescent who takes such action.

Infanticides and Pedicides

Killings of a child younger than 1 year and of a child age 1–17 years are actually separate types of killings but are often grouped under acts of "filicide." Infanticide involves the complexities of postpartum conditions that arise in the puerperal period. These can vary from mild depressive states ("the blues") to severe psychotic states with delusional content. Postpartum depressions may take on an altruistic theme to save the child from a miserable existence on earth, and lead to the murder of the child and suicide by the mother. If the disorder is schizophrenia, the mother may have grandiose delusions and exaltations, sometimes of a religious nature, that result in a homicide-suicide of the child and mother because of the idea that they will be in Heaven together. The sad case of Andrea Yates, who drowned her five children while in a postpartum psychotic state, is an example of the homicidal behavior that can occur, although no suicide occurred in this case (O'Malley 2004).

Women in the postnatal period ordinarily have a low suicide rate, but those with a postpartum illness, such as a psychotic depression or schizophrenia, in which a murder-suicide may occur, are in a high-risk group (Appleby et al. 1998). A host of diverse factors are usually involved and lead to the murder of a child and subsequent suicide. Precipitants can include psychosocial problems, isolation, immaturity, lack of an adequate social support system, earlier physical or sexual trauma, and a pervasive sense of hopelessness (Spinelli 2003). These situations may also arise when a mother gives birth to a child with multiple disabilities.

Political Killings

Political killings may be perpetrated by members of cults or terrorist organizations and are a type of murder-suicide in which the victims are usually strangers, such as occurred in the September 11, 2001, attack on the World Trade Center in the United States.

In most cases, the perpetrators are committed to dying, either in the course of the acts or by a direct suicide. These disgruntled individuals may externalize their inner states of discontent into a mass act of violence, or they may view themselves as carrying out some praiseworthy act to achieve political martyrdom, and within their group they may be viewed as heroes. Such altruistic suicides may reflect a fusion of personal identity with a group, in the context of a sense of moral agency that develops to sacrifice their own lives on behalf of the group (Swann et al. 2010).

Murders in the Workplace

Murders in the workplace are often connected to a disappointed and depressed employee or ex-employee who comes into his or her place of present or past employment, shoots others, and then commits suicide. Simon (2008) has suggested several variations of workplace violence besides disgruntled employees:

- Angry spouses or relatives may stalk employees at work.
- Violence may occur during criminal acts, such as robberies at a place of employment.
- People who work in dangerous occupations such as law enforcement may experience violence.
- Victims of acts of terrorism may be simply employees on-site, such as at the 2001 destruction of the World Trade Center or the 2011 shootings in Arizona in which Congresswoman Gabrielle Giffords was shot and other people attending her talk outside a supermarket were killed or wounded.

Fortunately, many of these acts of violence in the workplace do not result in a murder-suicide. Similar acts have been noted in academic centers (besides high schools), post offices, health care facilities, and courthouses or lawyers' offices. Displaced marital anger can lead to the shooting death of the spouse or former companion and whoever may be in the way. In one case, the shooting of a separated spouse occurred in workplace and was followed by the spouse's suicidal jump from the window in the office building.

The killings are often part of a personal agenda arising from the combination of the perpetrator's own specific social situation and psychopathology. Sometimes the goal is to kill a specific person and then others indiscriminately before committing suicide. Mullen (2004) refers to these types of killings as *autogenic (self-generated) massacres.* The perpetrators are seen as social isolates, often bullied in their childhoods, and they have not established themselves adequately in a work role. They often have paranoid and narcissistic traits. When they believe they have been rejected or encounter a disappointment, such as failing to obtain a promotion or not receiving an expected appointment or assignment, they decide to get their revenge and end it all (Copeland 1985). Some of the victims may be those who have failed them, but the act is often indiscriminate, and whoever is present gets killed. The final act by the perpetrator is a suicide by shooting him- or herself or a shoot-out with police in which the goal is to be killed ("suicide by cop"). It is estimated that police kill nearly 400 civilians a year in situations in which the officers are used as an instrument of suicide (Dahl 2011). Although the FBI keeps information on police officers killed in the line of duty (about 50 a year), information on people killed by police is not kept.

There are many overlaps between this type of mass murder-suicide by adults and school shootings by adolescents. The clinical question always lurks as to the degree of depression mixed with a personality disorder in a psychologically wounded person. As a clinician I am impressed by the number of persons who harbor such thoughts but keep them on a fantasy level or abort an act, sometimes by a fortunate clinical intervention.

Conclusion

Many questions remain beyond this brief discussion that need to be addressed involving the assessment of people who are suicidal but who also may be homicidal. The diversity of types of murder-suicide is the key; clinicians must assess the degree of hurt and rejection, the pattern of externalizing, the person's thoughts as mainly obsessional brooding or delusional, disturbances in attachments that lead the person to believe that he or she cannot go on in the absence of a particular person or attachment, past suicide attempts, stalking, and past homicidal levels of violence. Cult or terrorist acts are the most difficult in which to intervene because they are closely kept secrets and are not likely to be divulged by associates.

Key Clinical Concepts

- Murder-suicide occurs in various contexts: situations of domestic violence with mass shootings, familicides, planned deaths of the elderly or those with a terminal illness, infanticidal acts, and mass killings as a response to personal disappointment or disillusionment.

■ The subtype of a man killing an intimate partner with a firearm and then committing suicide is the most prevalent pattern of murder-suicide.

■ In all contexts, one must discern the degree of psychopathology, the situation, and possible diagnoses. Some of these individuals are psychotic, but many are not. The difficulty is when so many of the perpetrators die by suicide.

■ The central theme of all murder-suicides, despite their diversity, is often the overvaluation of a relationship or goal.

■ The question of whether homicide-suicides are more closely related to acts of homicide or suicide continues to be debated. Epidemiological and clinical studies have gone in both directions. Perhaps the lack of specificity for the type of homicide-suicide in studies contributes to the ambiguity.

■ Homicidal acts often follow the end or threatened end of a relationship (in a marital, romantic, or personal context), the terminal illness of a loved one, or the narcissistic blow of a rejection or disappointment and the need to retaliate. They may also involve the killing of an infant to shorten his or her supposed suffering on earth.

■ The relevant theme running through many of these diverse situations is a disorder in the realm of attachments that has never been resolved. The vulnerability is reflected in difficulties in handling stress regulation and the lack of mental capacity to assess the consequences of causing innocent deaths. Because these persons are not able to perceive a remedy for their more immediate disorganized and insecure state, their solution is to end it all. The narcissistic blow and emerging depression are not seen as repairable. Although patients with borderline personality disorder seem especially prone to this "solution," allowance must be made for some of these acts to be part of a delusional psychotic state. At the other extreme are mass killings carried out as part of a cult or terrorist group whose members view their acts as a service for the right cause and worthy to die for.

References

Adinkrah M: Homicide-suicide in Fiji: offense patterns, situational factors, and sociocultural contexts. Suicide Life Threat Behav 33:65–73, 2003

Anderson M, Kaufman J, Simon TR, et al: School associated violent deaths in the United States, 1994–1999. JAMA 286:2695–2702, 2001

Appleby L, Mortenson PB, Faragher EB: Suicide and other causes of mortality after post-partum psychiatric admission. Br J Psychiatry 173:209–211, 1998

Barraclough B, Harris EC: Suicide preceded by murder: the epidemiology of homicide-suicide in England and Wales, 1988–1992. Psychol Med 32:577–584, 2002

Bourget D, Gagné P, Maomai U: Spousal homicide and suicide in Quebec. J Am Acad Psychiatry Law 28:179–183, 2000

Bourget D, Gagné P, Whitehurst L: Domestic homicide and homicide-suicide: the older offender. J Am Acad Psychiatry Law 38:305–311, 2010

Campanelli C, Gilson T: Murder-suicide in New Hampshire, 1995–2000. Am J Forensic Med Pathol 23:248–251, 2002

Canetto SS, Hollenshead JD: Older women and mercy killing. Omega (Westport) 42:83–89, 2000–2001

Cavan R: Suicide. Chicago, IL, University of Chicago Press, 1928

Chan CY, Beh SL, Broadhurst RG: Homicide-suicide in Hong Kong, 1989–1998. Forensic Sci Int 140:261–267, 2004

Chidester D: Salvation and Suicide: An Interpretation of Jim Jones, the Peoples Temple, and Jonestown. Bloomington, Indiana University Press, 1988

Cohen D, Llorente M, Eisdorfer C: Homicide-suicide in older persons. Am J Psychiatry 155:390–396, 1998

Coid J: The epidemiology of abnormal homicide and murder followed by suicide. Psychol Med 13:855–860, 1983

Cooper M, Eaves D: Suicide following homicide in the family. Violence Vict 11:99–112, 1996

Copeland AR: Dyadic death—revisited. J Forensic Sci 25:181–188, 1985

Dahl J: How to stop suicide by cop. Miller-McCune 4:67–73, 2011

Eliason S: Murder-suicide: a review of the recent literature. J Am Acad Psychiatry Law 37:371–376, 2009

Felthous AR, Hempel A: Combined homicide-suicides: a review. J Forensic Sci 40:846–857, 1995

Gartner R, McCarthy B: Twentieth-century trends in homicide followed by suicide in four North American cities, in Histories of Suicide. Edited by Weaver J, Wright D. Toronto, University of Toronto Press, 2009, pp 281–303

Haenel T, Elsässer PN: Double suicide and homicide-suicide in Switzerland. Crisis 21:122–125, 2000

Kivivuori I, Lehti M: Homicide followed by suicide in Finland: trend and social locus. Journal of Scandinavian Studies in Criminology and Crime Prevention 4:223–236, 2003

Large M, Smith G, Nielssen O: The relationship between the rate of homicide by those with schizophrenia and the overall homicide rate: a systematic review and meta-analysis. Schizophr Res 112:123–129, 2009

Large M, Nielssen O, Lackersteen S, et al: The associations between infant homicide, homicide, and suicide rates; an analysis of World Health Organization and Centers for Disease Control statistics. Suicide Life Threat Behav 40:87–97, 2010

Liem M, Barber C, Markwalder N, et al: Homicide-suicide and other violent deaths: an international comparison. Forensic Sci Int 207:70–76, 2011

Logan J, Hill HA, Black ML, et al: Characteristics of perpetrators in homicide-followed-by-suicide incidents: National Violent Death Reporting System—17 US states, 2003–2005. Am J Epidemiol 168:1056–1064, 2008

Lund LE, Smorodinsky S: Violent death among intimate partners: a comparison of homicide and homicide followed by suicide in California. Suicide Life Threat Behav 31:451–459, 2001

Malmquist CP: Psychiatric aspects of familicide. Bull Am Acad Psychiatry Law 8:298–304, 1980

Malmquist CP: Homicide: A Psychiatric Perspective, 2nd Edition. Washington, DC, American Psychiatric Publishing, 2006

Malphurs JE, Eisdorfer C, Cohen D: A comparison of antecedents of homicide-suicide and suicide in older married men. Am J Geriatr Psychiatry 9:49–57, 2001

Maris RW, Berman AL, Silverman MM (eds): Comprehensive Textbook of Suicidology. New York, Guilford, 2000

Marzuk PM, Tardiff K, Hirsch CS: The epidemiology of murder-suicide. JAMA 267:3179–3183, 1992

Milroy CM: Reasons for homicide and suicide in episodes of dyadic death in Yorkshire and Humberside. Med Sci Law 35:213–217, 1995

Mullen PE: The autogenic (self-generated) massacre. Behav Sci Law 22:311–323, 2004

Newman K, Fox C: Repeat tragedy: rampage shootings in American high school and college settings, 2002–2008. Am Behav Sci 52:1309–1326, 2009

Nock MK, Marzuk PM: Murder-suicide: phenomenology and clinical implications, in The Harvard Medical School Guide to Suicide Assessment and Intervention. Edited by Jacobs DG. San Francisco, CA, Jossey-Bass, 1999, pp 188–209

O'Malley S: "Are You There Alone?" The Unspeakable Crime of Andrea Yates. New York, Simon & Schuster, 2004

Palermo GB, Smith MD, Jentzen JM, et al: Murder-suicide of the jealous paranoia type: a multicenter statistical pilot study. Am J Forensic Med Pathol 18:374–383, 1997

Palmer S, Humphrey J: Criminal homicide followed by offender's suicide. Suicide Life Threat Behav 10:106–118, 1980

Roberts AT: Murder-suicide, in Encyclopedia of Murder and Violent Crime. Edited by Hickey E. Thousand Oaks, CA, Sage, 2003, pp 324–326

Simon RI: Bad Men Do What Good Men Dream: A Forensic Psychiatrist Illuminates the Darker Side of Human Behavior. Washington, DC, American Psychiatric Publishing, 2008

Spinelli MG (ed): Infanticide: Psychosocial and Legal Perspectives on Mothers Who Kill. Washington, DC, American Psychiatric Publishing, 2003

Stack S: Homicide followed by suicide: an analysis of Chicago data. Criminology 35:435–453, 1997

Swann WB, Gomez A, Dovidio JF, et al: Dying and killing for one's group: identity fusion moderates responses to intergroup versions of the trolley problem. Psychol Sci 21:1176–1183, 2010

Thernstrom M: Halfway Heaven: Diary of a Harvard Murder. New York, Doubleday, 1997

Warren-Gordon K, Byers BD, Brodt SJ, et al: Murder followed by suicide: a newspaper surveillance study using the New York Times Index. J Forensic Sci 55:1592–1597, 2010

West DJ: Murder Followed by Suicide. Cambridge, MA, Harvard University Press, 1966

C H A P T E R   2 7

Suicide and the Internet

Patricia R. Recupero, J.D., M.D.

Within the past two decades, Internet use has become ubiquitous among individuals from nearly all walks of life and throughout most developed and developing countries in the world. Today, the Internet is relevant to nearly every aspect of our daily lives: how we communicate, how we work, how we shop, how we deal with health and illness, and even how we deal with death and dying.

As Tam et al. (2007) note, the Internet can be a "double-edged tool" when it comes to suicide. On the one hand, the Internet can be a source of tremendous support to individuals who are lonely or struggling with feelings of hopelessness and depression. On the other hand, reports of "cybersuicide" (i.e., suicide attempts and completed suicides facilitated by the Internet) (Alao et al. 2006) have raised concerns about how suicide information on the Internet, or even the sociological implications of the Internet in general, may affect vulnerable persons. On the Internet one may find chat rooms (BBC News 2008) and Web sites (Baker and

Fortune 2008) devoted exclusively to the topic of suicide. Whether these forums are beneficial or harmful is the subject of a great deal of controversy.

Preliminary data are inconclusive but raise some interesting questions. In a cross-national study using data from the World Health Organization and the United Nations Web sites, Shah (2010) found a positive statistical correlation between the prevalence of Internet users and general population suicide rates among both males and females. This relationship was found independently among males in multiple regression analysis, and in females the independent relationship approached statistical significance. Yang et al. (2011) analyzed a side-by-side comparison of Internet search trends and mortality data for suicide deaths over several years for a large urban area and found that search terms related to suicide risk factors (such as "divorce" and "major depression") either coincided with or temporally preceded related deaths by suicide for the region. However, McCarthy (2010) reports that Internet searches for "suicide" are lowest during summer months, when reported rates of suicide are higher.

From the psychiatrist's perspective, the Internet is relevant to many aspects of suicide risk assessment and management. Tam et al. (2007) summarized the main concerns about the Internet and its role in suicide:

> [T]he emergence of suicide pacts on the web has brought more attention to the web as a means by which ideas of suicide methods, ranging from access to means, can be actively exchanged and encouraged. The ease with which online orders of prescription drugs or other poisons bypass government regulations and custom controls also bridges the gaps of locality and accessibility, which previously formed a natural divide in selecting the means of suicide....the internet plays a much more influential role in bringing down the threshold for suicide. It provides not just the information, but also access to the means, as well as dynamic interactions among those who are like-minded. (p. 454)

There have been some attempts to restrict access to pro- and how-to suicide Web sites through regulation, primarily in Australia (Pirkis et al. 2009) and Europe, but the legal, ethical, and practical issues raised by such efforts are complicated and numerous (Mishara and Weisstub 2007).

Three Ways the Internet May Be Changing Suicide

Because it is impossible within the confines of a single textbook chapter to detail all of the ways in which the Internet may be relevant to psychiatrists treating patients at risk

for suicide, this discussion focuses on three key trends that can provide a framework for further study and reflection: 1) problematic behaviors, 2) information access, and 3) social networking.

Problematic Behaviors

In the early years of the Internet, problems that had been common in "techie" and computer gaming communities (such as "flaming" on Listservs and discussion forums) began to spread throughout the rest of the Internet. Many of these problematic behaviors related to the anonymity enjoyed by most early Internet users. Peter Steiner's cartoon in the *New Yorker* showing two dogs at a computer terminal, the one saying to the other, "On the internet, nobody knows you're a dog," became a popular adage for illustrating the sociological aspects of the Internet. Anonymity and depersonalization have contributed to the rise of "cyberbullying," harassment, suicide voyeurism, and addictive-like behaviors.

Internet Harassment and Cyberbullying

In more recent years, concern has arisen over the prevalence of harassment, bullying, and deliberately hurtful behaviors on the Internet, particularly among adolescents and young adults. Media coverage of suicides of youth who were bullied or harassed online prior to their deaths[1] has prompted controversy over how best to deal with problems like cyberbullying (Cloud 2010). Some of these suicides have been termed "bullycides." Although an analysis of the differences between cyberbullying and

---

[1] A partial listing of some of the youth who have died by suicide after being subjected to cyberbullying or Internet harassment includes Ryan Patrick Halligan (www.ryanpatrickhalligan.org), Jeff Johnston, William Lucas, Tyler Clementi, Asher Brown, Seth Walsh, Jesse Logan, and Megan Meier.

other forms of Internet harassment is beyond the scope of this chapter, it is important for psychiatrists to understand these phenomena and the effects they may have on patients and patients' relative risk for suicide.

Internet harassment has been linked to symptoms of depression (Ybarra 2004), and numerous studies have demonstrated a correlation between bullying behaviors and suicidal ideation among youth (Klomek et al. 2011). Because of links between cyberbullying victimization or perpetration and psychosocial and psychosomatic dysfunction, researchers recommend including questions about cyberbullying in the psychiatric evaluation and assessment of adolescents (Sourander et al. 2010). Young adolescent victims *and* perpetrators of cyberbullying behaviors are almost twice as likely as their peers to report having attempted suicide (Hinduja and Patchin 2010). More frequent involvement in bullying has been linked to increased levels of depression and suicidality among adolescents (Klomek et al. 2007). The customary mental status examination for adolescents has always included inquiries about friends and school. Today, the mental status examination might also include specific questions about friends and conflict related to Internet use (Recupero 2010b).

Adults may also be involved in Internet harassment or cyberbullying behaviors, either as victims or as perpetrators. The Korean actress Choi Jin-sil was the subject of a vicious campaign of rumors and insults through the Internet; when she died by suicide, the insults toward her on the Internet were cited as a primary reason for the suicide (Sang-Hun 2008). In the widely publicized "MySpace suicide" case, Megan Meier, a young girl, was taunted online by an adult female neighbor who had posed online as a boy Megan's age in order to gain her trust; when Megan hanged herself, it was discovered that the "boy" had insulted her and told her that the world would be a better place without her (Ruedy 2008). Similarly, a man in the United Kingdom died by suicide by hanging (and broadcast his suicide by Web cam) after participating in an Internet chat room in which members exchanged insults (BBC News 2007). Depressed persons may seek reinforcement of their negative cognitions in Internet venues. Low self-esteem and loneliness are two factors that have been linked with a heightened suicide risk, and being the recipient (or perhaps even the instigator) of a campaign of insults and harassment on the Web may further increase these risk factors among vulnerable individuals.

One critical way in which Internet harassment or bullying may affect an individual's suicide risk is in the ease and speed with which someone can be publicly humiliated before a large, even worldwide, audience. Impending or recent humiliation has been identified as a risk factor for "shame suicides" (see Chapter 1, "Suicide Risk Assessment: Gateway to Treatment Management," this volume), and this appears to have been a factor in several suicides that have been linked to humiliation through the Internet. In the fall of 2010, 18-year-old college student Tyler Clementi plunged to his death by jumping off a bridge after his roommate filmed a romantic encounter between Clementi and a male partner and streamed the video live on the Internet. Although the video had not gone "viral" at the time that he died by suicide, Clementi had expressed distress about the surreptitious surveillance and broadcasting when he first discovered it (Foderaro and Hu 2010). Presumably, he had a legitimate concern that the video *would* go viral and that he would be exposed and humiliated. As Schwartz (2010) notes,

Public humiliation and sexual orientation can be an especially deadly blend. In recent weeks, several students have died by suicide after instances that have been described as cyberbullying over sexual orientation, including Seth Walsh, a 13-year-old in Tehachapi, Calif., who hanged himself from a tree in his backyard last month and died after more than a week on life support. (p. 1)

Another 18-year-old student, Jesse Logan, killed herself when her ex-boyfriend sent nude photographs of her to her classmates; Logan had sent the photos to the boyfriend in a practice known as "sexting" (Celizic 2009).

Baiting and Suicide Voyeurism

Related to Internet-based harassment is the problem of baiting and suicide voyeurism. Baiting behaviors (although not necessarily for suicide) are common on Internet forums, and individuals who deliberately taunt and provoke others to negative emotional reactions in order to disrupt these forums are termed "trolls" (Polder-Verkiel 2010). Internet baiting and voyeurism are exemplified by the case of Brandon Vedas, a teen who was egged on by chat partners to take a fatal overdose of various prescription medicines while on his Web cam (BBC News 2003b). The prescriptions were obtained legally from a doctor and a psychiatric nurse, and Brandon had been treated for depression, but the chat transcript suggests that he did not intend to die by the overdose (Kennedy 2003). Although voyeuristic behaviors toward others' misfortunes and suffering are not new (e.g., the phenomenon of "rubbernecking" as traffic passes an accident), the Internet enables these behaviors to escalate and spread rapidly. For example, in Los Angeles, a police chase of a man that was followed by several television news helicopters

also attracted the attention of laypersons in the area, who, using mobile phones, began posting live updates from their cell phones to the popular social networking site Twitter. The chase "ended when, surrounded by police cars, cameras, and people busily live-tweeting from their phones, the man shot himself" (Kiume 2009).

Although Brandon Vedas's overdose was not intentionally fatal, there have been several media accounts of individuals who broadcast their suicides over the Internet through a Web cam after indicating their intention to do so (BBC News 2007). In late 2008, 19-year-old Abraham Biggs posted on a Web-based bodybuilding forum his intention to kill himself by taking a lethal overdose of prescription drugs and provided a link to a live Web cam streaming site where his suicide would be broadcast to the public. The live video had numerous viewers, but the authorities were not notified until after the young man became unconscious, and they did not arrive in time to rescue him. The Biggs case has prompted comparisons to the bystander effect noted in the 1964 Kitty Genovese murder, when neighbors apparently observed an assault and did not alert police in time to save the victim (Polder-Verkiel 2010). Biggs reportedly suffered from bipolar disorder, was in treatment for depression, and had threatened suicide on the Internet forum in the past (Stelter 2008). In offline scenarios, it is common for even family members and friends of a suicidal person to ignore suicide hints (such as "I'm writing a will") and not to mobilize to get the person into treatment; the tendency to underestimate the severity of the problem or to feel that one is not responsible for helping may be dramatically greater among anonymous Internet chat partners who are strangers to one another "IRL" ("in real life").

Problematic Internet Use

Problematic Internet use (PIU), the excessive use or otherwise problematic misuse of the Internet and related technologies, can affect suicide risk in several ways. PIU is correlated with depression and suicidal ideation (Kim et al. 2006), and depression symptoms are prevalent among heavy users of social media such as Facebook (giving rise to the term "Facebook depression" [O'Keeffe et al. 2011]). Messias et al. (2011) found that "teens who reported 5 hours or more of video games/Internet daily use in the 2009 [and 2007] YRBS [Youth Risk Behavior Survey] had a significantly higher risk for sadness,…suicidal ideation,…and suicide planning" (p. 1). PIU has been implicated in extreme emotional states, even contributing to violent behavior in some instances (BBC News 2005). Block (2007) presents a compelling argument for the role that PIU (or, more specifically, immersion in online gaming combined with related psychosocial risk factors) played in the Columbine school shootings.

Other Problematic Behaviors

Numerous other problematic behaviors linked to Internet use may be relevant in a suicide risk assessment or affect an individual's risk for suicide. For example, researchers have called attention to the potential of the Internet to normalize and reinforce self-destructive behaviors, such as deliberate self-harm, which is common among persons with borderline personality disorder. On the popular video sharing site YouTube, videos containing graphic images of self-injurious behaviors have many viewers, and comments posted in response are frequently positive and reinforcing of the behavior (Lewis et al. 2011). Robert Simon, summarizing work by Stone et al. (1987), notes that

"although self-mutilation is considered to be parasuicidal behavior (without lethal intent), the risk of suicide is doubled when self-mutilation is present" (see Chapter 1, "Suicide Risk Assessment," this volume).

Additionally, videos of potentially fatal self-injurious behaviors, such as helium inhalation to the point of unconsciousness, have been posted and shared on YouTube by adolescents (Ogden 2010). Many of these videos may have been inspired by shows such as *Jackass,* in which dangerous pranks are performed for humor. Also to be found on these Web sites are videos of adolescents getting drunk and having physical fights, deliberately sickening themselves in "ipecac challenges," and assaulting other youth in a practice known as "happy slapping." Whereas it remains to be seen how these types of problematic behaviors relate to suicide risk, it would seem that they reflect many of the risk factors for suicide among adolescents and young adults, such as impulsivity and aggression (American Academy of Child and Adolescent Psychiatry 2001). The Internet may be involved in cases of accidental death; for example, death by autoerotic asphyxiation may be associated with the use of Internet pornography (Vennemann and Pollak 2006).

Interaction online between troubled persons can lead to problematic behaviors and mutual reinforcement of maladaptive and dysfunctional coping strategies. For example, in addition to sharing tips on suicide methods, people in Internet discussion groups also "trade tips on how to fake symptoms to con a doctor into prescribing pain relievers, tranquilizers, stimulants, and sedatives" (Kennedy 2003, p. 1). Web sites and communities that promote anorexia and bulimia as a "lifestyle choice" are known as "pro-ana" or "pro-mia" groups, in which persons with eating disorders exchange "thinspiration" advice on how to hide the behavior from others and offer criticism of the medical profession (Borzekowski et al. 2010). Problematic behavior on the Internet may precipitate the development of a crisis or increase situational risk factors (Recupero 2008). For example, pathological gambling at Internet casinos might lead to severe financial hardship. PIU, such as excessive online gaming, could adversely affect school or work performance, leading to academic problems or unemployment. Excessive use of Internet pornography, cybersex, or the development of an "online affair" (or even offline infidelity facilitated through Internet dating sites) could lead to divorce or the breakup of a serious relationship.

Psychopathology may manifest itself in an individual's behavior on the Internet. Richard et al. (2000) described a case example of a suicidal man with multiple sclerosis whose correspondence with clinicians and with other members of a discussion board for physician-assisted suicide suggested that he might have been suffering from a manic phase of bipolar disorder. The authors commented,

> Over a period of weeks, his apparent self-presentation shifted from a lone and anguished seeker to a leader and prophet, urging others toward suicide with overt excitement and glee. This phase highlighted not only the probable worsening mania but also the clinical quandaries inherent in the Internet as a connection between dangerously distressed people who might rely solely on nonprofessional sources of input. (p. 222)

The Internet may change the way in which a patient deals with the symptoms of mental illness. As in the previous example, a patient with bipolar disorder, for example, may find an "audience" online that responds positively and affirmatively to problematic behaviors that might cause concern in a face-to-face scenario. Similarly, a person suffering from major depressive disorder may use the Internet to engage in isolative or avoidant behaviors, withdrawing from normal activities and real-life social supports in favor of "virtual" connections. Conversely, patients with mental illness may also use the Internet adaptively to reduce or manage symptoms, such as participating in an online support group before attending one in person or seeking out healthier friendships through the Web when one's real-life relationships are unsupportive or dysfunctional.

Information Access

The Internet has enabled both a literal and a virtual international search for suicide support and methodology as well as international access to unusual suicide methods alleged to be both painless and foolproof. The ease and speed of information access through the Web is one of the critical factors for considering the Internet's impact on suicide.

"Googling" Suicide

Suicide information is easily and immediately accessible through Internet search engines. In a survey of Web sites that appeared through popular Internet search engines for the terms "suicide," "how to commit suicide," "suicide methods," and "how to kill yourself," the majority of the hits returned were antisuicide and suicide-neutral sites (Recupero et al. 2008). However, explicitly prosuicide Web sites and detailed instructions for unusual and highly lethal suicide methods were also among the top results of the searches (Recupero et al. 2008). A similar study found that the top three most frequently occurring results in similar queries were prosuicide Web sites and that the top four hits provided information evaluating various methods of suicide, including "detailed information about speed, certainty, and the likely amount of pain associated with a method" (Biddle et al. 2008, p. 800). The existence of prosuicide and how-to suicide sites on the Internet has generated much concern and controversy. However, greater awareness of potentially harmful Internet sources has spurred an increase in suicide prevention and crisis intervention efforts online. Now, when someone "Googles" suicide, a pop-up box with the phone number of a crisis hotline is likely to appear on the screen (Boyce 2010).

Prosuicide Ideology

Most of the prosuicide resources located through Internet search engines are generated by a relatively small number of groups (including content added by members of these groups). The Euthanasia Research & Guidance Organization (ERGO), formerly known as the Hemlock Society, has a Web site (www.finalexit.org) and links to a large amount of literature and resources on the "right to die," physician-assisted suicide, and "death with dignity" advocacy "for the rights of the terminal or hopelessly physically ill, competent adult."

Other groups, such as the Church of Euthanasia (COE) and the Voluntary Human Extinction Movement, have raised more concern because they openly advocate suicide regardless of a person's medical status or psychiatric illness. Prosuicide groups and Web sites such as these have a significant presence on the Web (Sawer 2008). Some prefer to refer to themselves as "pro-choice" suicide sites (Sinderbrand 2003). The alt.suicide.holiday (a.s.h.) discussion group is a related forum that will be discussed in more detail in the following section. Material from a.s.h. appears frequently among results of

search engine queries for suicide information. These groups and their role in completed and attempted suicide have been discussed in more detail elsewhere (see, e.g., Recupero et al. 2008).

How-To Suicide Instructions

One of the critical ways that the Internet is changing suicide is through the rapid spread of information about particular suicide methods. Much of the information about specific suicide methods is linked to the a.s.h. discussion group's "methods file," but as more stories have appeared in news media, blogs, and other discussion forums online, the spread of such information has had a snowball effect. The spread of new trends in suicide methods is not a new phenomenon or unique to the Internet. For example, the publication of the book *Final Exit* (which included a recommendation for suffocation by plastic bag as a suicide method) in 1991 preceded a 30.8% increase in the rate of suicide by plastic bags in the United States (Ogden 2010). The speed with which information spreads through Internet channels and the wide reach of its distribution are unprecedented.

Internet-derived instructions for committing suicide have been reported in suicide attempts requiring emergency treatment as early as 1998 (Nordt et al. 1998) (i.e., nearly as long as the Internet has been available to the public in the United States). Suicide "fads" communicated through news media and the Internet have been particularly troubling in East Asia, where charcoal burning has become an increasingly common method for suicide, often in connection with suicide pacts formed on the Internet (Lee et al. 2005). The rise in charcoal-burning suicides began around 2003 following news coverage of the suicide of a Japanese teenager who used the method (Hagihara et al. 2010), charcoal burning has become the most common method used in suicide pacts in Japan (Yip and Lee 2007). Data indicate that the publication of information regarding this method around the turn of the twenty-first century actually increased suicide rates (e.g., in Hong Kong) rather than merely changing the distribution of suicide methods among total suicides (Yip and Lee 2007).

In 2008, a "suicide craze" involving homemade hydrogen sulfide gas, in which the method and past successful attempts were described, spread rapidly in Japan through news and Internet message boards (Truscott 2008). In a brief period, over only several months, more than 208 suicidal people took their lives by that method, and in several cases the poisonings were serious enough to kill family members and others who attempted to rescue the victims. As researchers warned, "This fad has rapidly spread by Internet communication, and can happen anywhere in the world" (Morii et al. 2010). The chemicals required for producing a large amount of the gas in lethal concentration levels are freely available for purchase on the Internet.

Gas asphyxiation suicides are rare, but anecdotal evidence suggests that they may be on the rise, in part because of the spread of step-by-step, how-to information about this method on the Internet. Several case reports in toxicology journals have noted that printouts of pages from the Internet detailing the method were found alongside the deceased. Asphyxiation by inhalation of helium gas is advocated by the COE and ERGO and has been used in several completed suicides (Gallagher et al. 2003; Ogden 2010; Sinderbrand 2003). Literature from the right-to-die and death-with-dignity movement has contributed to wider awareness of these methods:

The first edition of *Final Exit* dismissed gas methods for suicide. But, in 2000 detailed information about the lethality of helium asphyxiation was published in *Supplement to Final Exit* and a separate video/Digital Video Disc (DVD). By 2002 the third edition of the book had a full chapter on helium asphyxia titled, "A Speedier Way: Inert Gases." (Ogden 2010, p. 156)

Other methods that have been linked to instructions downloaded from the Internet include plastic-bag inhalation of diethyl ether (Athanaselis et al. 2002), nicotine poisoning through extraction of nicotine from tobacco (Corkery et al. 2010; Schneider et al. 2010), ingestion of castor oil beans (Alao et al. 1999), and excess consumption of water (Alao et al. 1999). In one case report, a man was found to have killed himself by inhalation of hydrogen cyanide through a complicated, multistep method; his body was found in a car with a camping stove, chemicals, and information from the Internet about potassium ferrocyanide and potassium cyanide (Musshoff et al. 2011).

Use of the Internet to Acquire Lethal Means

One of the most critical risk factors for suicide is the availability of lethal means, especially firearms, to the suicidal person. The Internet also increases suicidal persons' access to other lethal means of suicide, such as drugs that can be used in suicide attempts or that have the potential for abuse and accidental fatality (Boyer et al. 2007; Logan et al. 2009). Unusual methods of poisoning have also broken down geographic boundaries that would formerly have made specific toxins inaccessible to persons from distant areas. In one case, a suicidal young man in New York required emergency treatment after he ingested seeds of the plant *Abrus precatorius*, which he had purchased online from Asia after reading about the seeds as a recommended suicide method on the Internet (Jang et al. 2010). Wang et al. (2007) report two cases of potentially fatal poisonings by arsenic trioxide and mercuric chloride; in both cases, the chemicals were purchased on the Internet (the arsenic through an online auction site, and both for under $40). Poisons are available for purchase at low cost on Internet sites such as eBay (Cantrell 2005), and the range of potential lethal means is vastly increased by the ease with which a suicidal person can purchase a preferred method online.

The Internet also provides access to specific information about how to acquire lethal means by masquerading as a gardener, welder, jeweler, or some other professional (Sawer 2008). In one case, a teenage girl purchased cyanide with advice from other members of the a.s.h. discussion group:

> To get the materials, [she] used a trick recommended by other group members. Posing as a jeweler, she ordered the cyanide online, ostensibly to polish metal. She also requested several other chemicals to make her order look genuine. [Her] order, billed to "Winston Jewelers," didn't raise a red flag at the Massachusetts chemical manufacturer, which in turn sold her the poison. (Scheeres 2003, p. 1)

Individuals on prosuicide forums have instructed others on methods to evade detection, listed locations where supplies for a suicide attempt may be purchased, and provided mechanical drawings illustrating how to create a lethal apparatus.

Suicide Contagion and the "Werther Effect"

The Internet may increase suicide risk by facilitating the rapid spread of sensational-

istic or romanticized media coverage of suicides as well as by giving suicidal persons a larger audience. Researchers have suggested that the Internet may contribute to a "Werther effect" (Becker and Schmidt 2004; Mehlum 2000), a phenomenon whereby copycat suicides or suicide clusters follow a widely publicized suicide, particularly when the deceased individual was a celebrity or shared characteristics with which vulnerable others identify, often among youth (Mesoudi 2009). ("Werther effect" alludes to a series of copycat suicides following the publication of Johann Wolfgang von Goethe's novel *The Sorrows of Young Werther,* in which the young hero kills himself while suffering from hopeless, unrequited love.) This phenomenon may have been a factor in the cluster of suicides by sexual minority youth within a very short time frame, which received a great deal of news coverage. To reduce the risk of suicide contagion, preventive education "should refrain from overemphasizing the link between cyberbullying and suicide (e.g., showing videos of youth who have killed themselves after being bullied). While well-intentioned, these efforts may inadvertently present rewards for the suicide act" (Klomek et al. 2011).

When a suicide occurs, the Internet has almost instantaneous news coverage and viral videos related to the event that are accessible through Internet search engines. In many cases, suicide notes are posted and archived online or forwarded among readers in an e-mail chain. For example, when a man shot himself at Harvard Yard, his mother revealed that he had posted a 1,905-page, heavily footnoted "suicide note" online, which he had e-mailed to some of his family and friends and which is still publicly and freely accessible on the Web at the time of this writing (Abel 2010; Newcomer and Srivatsa 2010). The book is in large part an attempt at a scholarly defense of the man's decision to kill himself, complete with a section called "Open Your Mind to Death" (Heisman 2010). Web pages for news media coverage of the man's suicide referenced and provided links to the suicide note; this level of coverage of the suicide would have been burdensome and rare in the days prior to the Internet.

The risk for suicide contagion and suicide clusters may be particularly acute among adolescents and young adults. After the suicide of an entertainment celebrity or a heavily covered suicide in the news, it may be helpful for psychiatrists to be familiar with the Internet coverage of the event and its potential influence on patients who may be at risk for suicide.

Beneficial Education on the Internet for Suicide Prevention

Although the Internet's potential to increase suicide risk is alarming, it is critical for psychiatrists to appreciate the Internet's beneficial effect on suicide risk factors for many individuals. Public awareness of suicide and the recognition of suicide warning signs and risk factors have spread rapidly through Internet channels. A concerned acquaintance or family member of a vulnerable person can learn a great deal about how to help the person by conducting research online or using the Internet to connect with supportive resources. An e-mail received by volunteers at the suicide prevention charity Befrienders International read as follows:

> Thank you for saving my brother. He want to suicide himself because father say he have no pride for family. I don't know what to do, so I look your website. Then I sit very quiet and listen him. He is alive now because of you. Thank you, thank you, thank you. (Bale 2001, p. 11)

The Internet contains plentiful information about common suicide warning signs, including many listed as important risk factors by the American Psychiatric Association (e.g., giving away prized possessions, isolation or withdrawal, risk-taking or reckless behavior) (Mandrusiak et al. 2006).

Not every suicidal person will use the Internet merely to access harmful or prosuicide information. In a study of Internet search trends and suicide rates, McCarthy (2010) reports that "there is an inverse correlation between Internet searches and suicides in the general population," suggesting that "the internet is used by many to seek help or otherwise reduce suicide risk" (p. 278). Eichenberg (2008) found that the majority of members of a prominent suicide forum used the forum for constructive (e.g., seeking support and understanding) rather than harmful (e.g., forming suicide pacts or researching suicide methods) purposes. The psychiatrist may find the Internet a valuable resource for helping the patient to modify dynamic suicide risk factors such as poor psychosocial support. For example, a Web search may help the patient to find local support groups, Web discussion forums, and even self-help resources like education about developing strong and healthy coping strategies.

Social Networking

Social networking has become a critical function of the Internet in recent years. Once considered primarily the virtual playground of teens and young adults, social networking sites such as MySpace and Facebook are increasingly popular among older demographic groups. On these interactive sites, users stay in touch with friends, family, and colleagues through posting "status updates," photos, videos, notes, hyperlinks to content elsewhere on the Web, and so forth. Social networking also takes place through support groups and discussion forums on nearly every topic imaginable, including suicide and self-harm.

Suicide and Self-Harm Communities

Suicide forums, even those with a prosuicide bias, may be helpful to suicidal persons who value the opportunity to communicate openly and anonymously with others who understand them and who struggle with similar problems (Harris et al. 2009). For someone in the midst of a crisis, suicide prevention sites may be less helpful, particularly when their tone is patronizing or proselytizing (Harris et al. 2009). Supportive communication among peers in an interactive online discussion board often contains helpful advice and empathic understanding; many participants offer suggestions based on their own past experiences and struggles (Miller and Gergen 1998). General suicide discussion groups may be communities in which the suicidal person feels "at home," and they may help to give the person a sense of belonging. As Baker and Fortune (2008) explain:

> A community member is someone who belongs to a group, is socially integrated, and socially valid. This represents another positive identity for people who use self-harm and suicide websites. Outsiders may lack important knowledge shared by the community and may be unhelpful or even threatening. (p. 120)

Miller and Gergen (1998) found that self-disclosure—that is, "the revealing of personal problems in such a way that help is invited"), which was frequently "highly intimate in character and...charged with emotional energy" (p. 195)—was one of the most frequent forms of communication among participants in an online suicide discussion board. For many people, achieving a sense of belonging and community through these forums may help to reduce suicide risk factors like loneliness and isolation.

However, there are other risks associated with the use of these forums. There may be subtle pressure from one's peers in the group to construct an identity of being "authentically" suicidal; participants in these groups often struggle with the need to be taken seriously by fellow members and to have their suicidal feelings validated by others (Horne and Wiggins 2009). Thus, there may be an incentive to ignore or suppress nonsuicidal feelings, because these characteristics could lead to alienation from other members of the group. Furthermore, when a patient's condition improves and he or she begins to feel less suicidal, embracing an identity as a person who is *not* suicidal or does *not* self-harm may mean that one no longer feels a sense of belonging to the community, and leaving may result in a loss of psychosocial support and affirmation:

> A 13-year-old can go on the internet and instantly find community and get hitched to this behavior. When they don't want to self-injure anymore, it means they have to leave a community. (Janis Whitlock, quoted in Brody 2008, p. 1)

Adolescents involved with the a.s.h. group have described the group as a "scene," with discussions involving knowledge sharing and feedback similar to what might be found on a music genre discussion board, except that the discussions in suicide forums tend to have death, depression, and suicide as the primary topics and shared interests among the members (Aderet 2009).

Internet Suicide Pacts

Suicide pacts are typically formed between close acquaintances, often a married couple (American Psychiatric Association 2003). However, tools for social networking on the Internet (such as suicide groups or other discussion forums) can bring together suicidal individuals who share suicidal intent but who are otherwise strangers (Rajagopal 2004). "Net suicide" pacts are well known in Japan (Ozawa-de Silva 2008), where in 2007 there were over 60 deaths that year linked to pacts formed online (Naito 2007). In Japanese culture, an individual's identity is closely tied to his or her role as a member of a group, and the desire to be part of a group likely contributed to the popularity of Internet group suicides in Japan (Ozawa-de Silva 2010). Internet suicide pacts have occurred throughout the world, including several countries in Europe (Mishara and Weisstub 2007; Naito 2007). Individuals who form such pacts often travel considerable distances to meet each other. In 2000, a young Norwegian man and a 17-year-old Austrian girl who had formed a pact through an Internet suicide discussion group jumped to their death from a scenic cliff in Norway (Mehlum 2000).

Social networking can also lead to the formation of potentially harmful relationships between depressed individuals and others who are eager to exploit their vulnerability. William Francis Melchert-Dinkel, a former nurse from Minnesota, was found guilty of two felony counts of advising and encouraging suicides for his role in the suicides of two individuals (a man from the United Kingdom and a woman from Canada) with whom he had corresponded on the Internet (Winter 2011). Melchert-Dinkel acknowledged entering into suicide pacts with five people through the a.s.h. suicide forum; he discussed with suicidal individuals the pros and cons of various suicide methods through e-mail and instant messaging or chat room correspondence and cited his experience as an emergency nurse in support of his knowledge about the desirability or effectiveness of different methods (*State of Minnesota v. William Francis Melchert-Dinkel* 2011). The 2008 film *Downloading Nancy* dramatized the true story of a suicidal, masochistic woman who met a man through the Internet who murdered her at her request. The woman upon whom the story was based, Sharon Lopatka, had been involved with pornographic Web sites on the Internet and prior to her death had indicated in Internet postings that she fantasized about being tortured until the point of death (Bell 2011). The case has been described as "consensual homicide," and Lopatka's story is not unique (BBC News 20003a). These true stories illustrate the harmful potential of social networking for people at risk for suicide.

Disclosure of Suicidal Ideation on the Internet

Patients at risk for suicide are often reluctant to volunteer information about their suicidal ideation to others. The seeming anonymity one may feel in computer-mediated communication may make the disclosure of suicidal thoughts or feelings less intimidating (Janson et al. 2001). In a comparison of statements made to volunteers at a crisis center through a telephone hotline, on an asynchronous message board, and on a personal chat online, Gilat and Shahar (2007) discovered that explicit threats of suicide were more frequently voiced in the asynchronous message board than in the other forums. One of the protective aspects of Internet social networking is that when a depressed person voices a suicide threat online, his or her chat partners or online acquaintances may be able to get help for the person. Janson et al. (2001) discuss two suicide threats that were disclosed in Internet chat rooms (in one, a man on his Web cam pointed a gun at his head) and reported to police by other chatters; in both cases, the suicidal persons were taken for emergency medical treatment. Baume et al. (1997) describe posts on interactive forums like the a.s.h. newsgroup as "the open declaration of suicide notes" (p. 75). Psychiatrists with child and adolescent patients might consider encouraging parents to monitor what their children post online, particularly when suicide risk factors are elevated.

The Internet and Mental Health Professionals

The Internet and the Clinician-Patient Relationship

The Internet can have a dramatic impact on the clinician-patient relationship. Patients today use the Internet to research their health difficulties (e.g., "cyberchondria") or to network with other patients (e.g., through health-related sites like PatientsLikeMe), and they may expect to take on a more active role in their care planning and treatment decision making. Patients frequently do not tell their doctors what they learned online (Hart et al. 2004), and although often the information they seek is helpful (e.g., educational resources about living with depression), occasionally they may encounter information that can be detrimental to the therapeutic alliance (e.g., prosuicide forums). On the Internet there are numerous Web sites and groups that are highly critical of psychiatry and mental health treatment, and there is also a great deal of inaccurate information about treatments like electroconvulsive therapy and psychotropic medications. Because lack of a strong therapeutic alliance is a significant risk factor for suicide

(see Chapter 1, "Suicide Risk Assessment," this volume), a patient's reliance on antipsychiatry Web sites, for example, could be a significant risk factor to consider when performing a suicide risk assessment.

Traditionally, the clinician-patient relationship is conceptualized as a supportive alliance between a patient seeking treatment and a clinician who uses professional knowledge and skills to exercise a fiduciary duty. In the age of the Internet, however, relationships between many medical professionals and consumers seeking health care do not always conform to the standard model. For example, a consumer may visit an Internet pharmacy Web site in the hopes of acquiring a prescription without having to visit a doctor in person. When psychiatrists issue such prescriptions on the basis of an unknown consumer's responses to a questionnaire (and in the absence of a physical examination of the patient), significant ethical concerns are raised. For example, a psychiatrist from Colorado was charged with the unlicensed practice of medicine when he issued a prescription for an antidepressant to a college student in California on the basis of an Internet pharmacy questionnaire; the student subsequently killed himself (Neimark 2009).

Psychiatrists may also receive requests to perform evaluations on disabled persons who are seeking authorization for physician-assisted suicide. As Simon and Shuman (2007) note, "Such a role represents a radical departure from the physician's code of ethics, which prohibits an ethical doctor's participation in any intervention that hastens death" (p. 159). Richard et al. (2000) discuss a case example of a disabled man who contacted a physician via the Internet regarding his "rational" desire to die by suicide; through correspondence with the man, it became evident that he likely suffered from a treatable mental illness. The authors offer helpful suggestions for physicians who are contacted by patients about physician-assisted suicide, noting the ethical implications of responding or deciding not to respond to such inquiries.

Patient Evaluation and Assessment

Implications of the Internet for Face-to-Face Evaluations

When the mental status examination is being conducted, it can be helpful to ask patients about their use of the Internet; suggested questions to ask during the evaluation and examples of how the Internet relates to the assessment are available (Recupero 2010b). For a patient at risk for suicide, the psychiatrist may inquire directly as to whether the patient has sought information online about suicide and what the patient found. It is also helpful for the psychiatrist to be familiar with the terminology and slang that may be common in Internet suicide discussion forums. As Simon notes, "To perform an adequate suicide risk assessment, the clinician must be able to understand idiomatic phrases and slang expressions" (p. 23).

If a patient discloses that he or she uses suicide forums or similar Web sites or groups, the psychiatrist may want to learn more about which site(s) the patient visits and their culture. For example, in the a.s.h. group, suicide is often referred to as "transition" or "catching the bus"; patients may use these terms without realizing that the clinician is not familiar with them. Eichenberg (2008) provides a helpful and detailed typology of users of suicide discussion boards on the Internet, which may be especially useful to the psychiatrist in trying to better understand a patient.

Collateral Information and Research

The Internet can be valuable as a tool to aid in conducting research and obtaining collateral information about a patient. Although the ethical implications of "Googling" a patient are controversial, it is worth noting the potential benefits of Internet research for conducting a suicide risk assessment. Neimark et al. (2006) describe a case example in which a Google search of a patient in emergency treatment services produced a newspaper article about a prior suicide attempt that the patient had not disclosed to the treatment team. Particularly when working with a patient who is evasive or uncommunicative, a Web search may turn up important risk factors as well as relevant protective factors to consider in the assessment. Because the psychiatrist may not have time to conduct extensive Internet research on an individual patient, it may be helpful to warn the patient's family or significant others to report any recent troubling communications from Facebook or any other social media.

Forensic Evaluations

Although this chapter is focused primarily on the provision of psychiatric treatment to patients at risk for suicide, the Internet can also be relevant to forensic evaluations (Recupero 2010a). A psychiatrist may be asked to consult in a case alleging intentional or negligent infliction of emotional distress (e.g., to conduct an evaluation of a victim or perpetrator in a cyberbullying case), violation of privacy (e.g., to determine whether a violation of privacy by the Internet proximately caused the victim psychic harm), or malpractice (e.g., to determine if a psychiatrist issued a prescription to a patient through an Internet pharmacy but never examined the patient in person), and in various other types of cases. Information and transcripts of communications stored on the Internet can be especially pertinent for psychological autopsies.

Risk Assessments

An individual's behavior online may prompt a referral for psychiatric assessment. For example, a patient may be referred when others notice hints about suicidal thoughts or plans in an acquaintance's activities online, such as blog entries containing expressions of a desire to die. Similarly, worsening psychiatric symptoms may manifest themselves as unusual behavior online, such as excessive or bizarre status updates, the posting of inappropriate material on a social networking site such as Facebook, or uploading troubling content (such as photographs of the user posing with a gun). In such circumstances, a risk assessment may be necessary to determine whether the individual poses a threat to him- or herself or others. Furthermore, a person's Internet use is often relevant to psychiatric risk assessments in general, even if the Internet use was not a reason for the appointment or referral (Recupero 2010b).

Cultural and demographic factors that are relevant to an individual's risk for suicide may also affect the relevance of the person's Internet use to the psychiatric risk assessment. It is important to consider the cultural context for the person's use of the Internet and how it may relate to suicide risk factors. For example, as Naito (2007) reports, "historically, suicide has been regarded as a crime in western societies whereas in Japanese history there was a period when suicide was considered as an honourable way of escaping failure when one was confronted by inevitable defeat" (p. 587) or in self-imposed punishment for the humiliation associated with failure. Cultural attitudes toward suicide in Japan likely played a role in the "Net suicide" phenomenon and the popularity of

group suicide pacts formed through the Internet, but many of the same phenomena occur in other cultures.

It is important to note that the Internet can also break down geographical boundaries that may have previously kept specific cultural beliefs or attitudes confined to a specific region or demographic group. A depressed person in the United States, for example, may learn about another culture's more permissive attitude toward suicide. Conversely, Western ideas about mental health treatment and suicide prevention may influence the ways in which other regions address psychosocial problems. These trends spread rapidly, and it is important for the psychiatrist to stay up to date on evidence-based practice for suicide risk assessments.

Although it is impossible to detail all of the demographic factors at play in an Internet user's suicide risk, there are important considerations for the risk assessment, depending on the patient's general age group and developmental stage. Some unique factors might be seen when working with youth, adult, and elderly populations.

Youth. Suicide is the third most common cause of death among people 15–24 years old (Frierson 2007), and today most adolescents and young adults are described as members of the "wired" generation. A young person's Internet use could be relevant to nearly every aspect of the psychiatric evaluation, and his or her risk for suicide is no exception. When evaluating a child, adolescent, or young adult patient for suicide risk, it is important for the psychiatrist to stay informed of recent literature regarding Internet use among others in this demographic group. Although Internet searches for "suicide" were inversely correlated with rates of completed suicide for the general population, "internet searches are positively correlated with self-injury and suicide among youth, suggesting this group uses the internet to facilitate self-injury" (McCarthy 2010, p. 279).

As O'Keefe et al. (2011) note, "A large part of this generation's social and emotional development is occurring while on the Internet and on cell phones" (p. 800). Although it is not yet clear what long-term impact this may have on human development, this fact underscores the vital importance of the Internet and information technology for children and young adults when compared with their parents' and grandparents' generations. Many young people turn to the Internet for support and guidance when they are in crisis. Becker et al. (2004) present a case report of an adolescent girl who used suicide forums initially for support but later to obtain information and access to suicide methods:

> Predisposed by recurring sub-depressive mood, feelings of inferiority and dependent personality traits, disappointed by conversations with friends in real life whom she considered (because of differing opinions) to be nonsupportive, she looked for like-minded chat partners on the Web. (p. 113)

With respect to adolescents' susceptibility to potentially harmful prosuicide messages that they may encounter online, Becker et al. (2004) note that "youths with dependent, insecure, frightened and evasive traits may especially be at risk, as well as those who cannot express their worries, fears and sadness to a parent and thus look for guidance on the Internet" (p. 114).

Adults. During middle age, the risk for suicide lessens, and the role of the Internet in an adult's life may have a different relationship to his or her unique suicide risk factors. If the psychiatrist determines that the patient uses the Internet, it may be helpful to take an "Internet history" to help identify patients whose Internet use may have implications for their suicide risk and treatment recommendations (Cooney and Morris 2009). Rajagopal (2004) recommends specifically asking "whether a depressed patient uses the internet to obtain information about suicide" (p. 1299). A clinical profile including shyness and PIU (Internet "addiction") related to depression, low self-esteem, and lower life satisfaction may carry a greater risk of susceptibility to the negative aspects of suicide forums (Grimland and Apter 2009). Prior (2004) suggests that individuals who attempt suicide using methods learned on the Internet may be more likely to have "rigid, concrete, or maladaptive coping strategies" (p. 1501). If a patient discloses a suicide plan that involves an unusual, complicated, or unfamiliar method of suicide (such as asphyxiation by inert gas), the psychiatrist should consider the possibility that the patient has been researching suicide methods online. Asking the patient what gave him or her the idea to use that particular method may elicit further information about the seriousness of the suicidal intent and the relevant risk factors at play.

The elderly. When evaluating and treating elderly patients, the psychiatrist should avoid the common assumption that older adults are unfamiliar with information technology like the Internet. Although it may be true that many older adults do not use the Internet, today Internet adoption is so widespread that the stereotype of the senior citizen as a technophobe is often an outdated misconception. At the time of this writing, the oldest known American blogger is 109 years old, another began blogging at the age of 107, and a number of older adults enjoy a significant following on sites like Twitter and YouTube.[2] In a cross-national study, Shah (2010) found an independent association between the spread of Internet adoption and an increase in rates of suicide among the elderly, suggesting that even older individuals may be seeking suicide information on the Internet, although data are currently insufficient to support a causal relationship. It is important to consider recent media coverage of suicides when evaluating suicide risk; as Frei et al. (2003) have noted, publicized accounts of assisted suicide may trigger a "Werther effect" of similar suicide attempts, even among the elderly, particularly when the deceased had similar life characteristics.

When conducting a risk assessment, the psychiatrist may find it helpful to identify problematic or protective functions of the patient's Internet use. Eichenberg (2008) provides a helpful table of "potential risks and benefits of suicide forums" on the Internet, contrasting "endangering effects" and "suicide-preventative effects," along with references for further reading on these factors.

Prevention and Intervention

The Internet plays an important role in suicide prevention today (Mandrusiak et al. 2006). Professional organizations (e.g., American Psychiatric Association), crisis intervention agencies (e.g., American Foundation for Suicide Prevention), and government agencies (e.g., National Institute of Mental Health) have numerous suicide prevention resources online that are easily accessible to the public. The Samaritans (www.samaritans.org.uk/) maintain 24-hour crisis support, including confidential e-mail exchanges for individuals who are feeling suicidal. The Internet has also become an important forum for outreach to vulnerable populations and individuals at heightened risk for suicide. For example, in response to several highly publicized suicides by lesbian, gay, bisexual, or transgender (LGBT) youth in a short time frame, older members of the LGBT community developed the It Gets Better Project (www.itgetsbetter.org), which aims to spread messages of hope to adolescent victims of homophobic bullying.

Psychiatrists and other clinicians can download and provide informational resources, such as pamphlets, to parents whose children may be accessing suicide information on the Web (Coombes 2008). Referrals to online support groups may be useful, and Internet resources (e.g., "15 Ways to Support a Loved One With Serious Mental Illness" [Tartakovsky 2011]) can facilitate the provision of supportive psychoeducation that performs a risk management function. The Centers for Disease Control and Prevention Web site (www.cdc.gov/ViolencePrevention/suicide/index.html) has numerous helpful resources and links for psychiatrists, patients, educators, families, and other members of the public.

The Internet may also play a useful role in the provision of mental health screening and treatment. Web-based depression screening is available through many informational and health care Web sites and search engines (see, e.g., www.mental-healthscreening.org/). In one study of Web-based screening followed by interactive online communication between at-risk students and a counselor who encouraged them to seek treatment, the students who chatted with the counselor were three times

---

[2]See, for example, Wikipedia: "Old Age." Available at: http://en.wikipedia.org/wiki/Old_age). Accessed July 22, 2011.

more likely subsequently to see a clinician for a face-to-face evaluation (Haas et al. 2008). Researchers have begun conducting randomized controlled trials of Internet-based intervention, self-help, and treatment to help reduce suicidal thoughts (van Spijker et al. 2010) and other suicide risk factors. Numerous support groups are available on the Web (Gilat and Shahar 2009), and there are guidelines to assist clinicians who use the Internet to counsel suicidal persons (Lester 2008–2009).

The Internet in the Aftermath of a Suicide

The Internet is credited with helping to facilitate the bereavement process for individuals who have lost a close acquaintance through suicide by hosting interactive online memorial pages and social networking channels for communication with others about the death (Chapple and Ziebland 2011). After a patient has completed suicide, the psychiatrist may refer grieving family members and other survivors to specific resources on the Web for support (see Chapter 34, "Aftermath of Suicide: The Clinician's Role," this volume). Rather than providing merely a pro forma referral to "check out the Internet for support groups," the psychiatrist can provide the family with links to specific reputable Web sites. It bears noting that a suicide can have an impact not only on the person's family and friends in real life but also on his or her chat and Web friends; Hsiung (2007) has provided some useful guidance for clinicians about facilitating the bereavement process for someone who has lost an Internet acquaintance to suicide.

Conclusion

The assessment and treatment of persons at risk for suicide has always been a compli-

cated process for the clinician. In the old paradigm, people could use the library or read the newspaper and learn harmful or beneficial information, but times have changed. There is now a wealth of information, and one does not need to leave the house in order to conduct in-depth research or to communicate with others on very specific topics, including suicide. The Internet has several features that distinguish its role in suicide risk assessment from the role of information outlets in the past. Unlike newspapers or books, the Internet enables the formation of interactive communities of suicidal persons, and the magnitude of information access online is unprecedented. Three key ways in which the Internet may be changing suicide are in the development of problematic behaviors (such as cyberbullying or suicide baiting), the vast expansion of information access (e.g., prosuicide ideology), and the facilitation of social networking (including suicide pacts or suicide support groups). It seems likely that public knowledge of highly lethal and formerly unusual suicide methods (such as gas asphyxiation by helium inhalation) will continue to increase in response to news media and Internet dissemination of information on these methods (Grassberger and Krauskopf 2007). These factors may complicate the clinician's evaluation of a patient's potential suicide risk.

The Internet has already begun to change behaviors with regard to suicide, but we are only at the very beginning stages of understanding the implications of these changes and how they will impact the assessment and management of suicidal patients in the future. Much of the available research and knowledge to date is based on specific case studies and is anecdotal. Furthermore, many trends (such as the spread of charcoal-burning suicides) appear to be culture specific. It is nearly impossible to predict how the Internet will develop within the next decade, but it seems reasonable to expect that suicide assessment and management will not get *easier* for the clinician but rather more complicated because of rapidly changing risk and protective factors. The prudent clinician will try to take the Internet into consideration when working with a patient at risk for suicide. The existing standards for the assessment and treatment of suicidal patients can help to guide judgments about the relevance of the Internet in the clinical scenario.

As with the treatment of patients prior to the spread of the Internet, clinicians can mitigate risk by applying traditional suicide risk management strategies. For example, it may be helpful to involve third parties in the risk management strategy; just as the psychiatrist might direct family members to remove firearms and lethal medications from the home, it may be helpful to ask families to install Internet content filters or to monitor a child's Internet activity and to report any unusual circumstances to the clinician (e.g., if a teen receives an unusual package in the mail). Finally, it is advisable for clinicians to learn more about the Internet and its potential effect on suicide by reading the academic literature and following relevant news stories to understand emerging trends and factors relating to suicide risk.

Key Clinical Concepts

- The Internet is changing suicide in three major ways: 1) through problematic behaviors, such as cyberbullying or suicide voyeurism; 2) through information access, by increasing access to prosuicide ideology and unusual suicide methods; and 3) through social networking, which connects suicidal and vulnerable persons to one another and to others in new ways.

- Internet harassment and cyberbullying may increase the risk of suicide in both perpetrators and victims. Although these behaviors occur online, they often have significant real-life consequences for those involved.

- Depressed and suicidal persons may be encouraged by others online to go through with a suicidal act; online acquaintances may even provide the person with specific instructions on how to obtain lethal means, how to evade detection, and which methods are most likely to result in death.

- Suicide reporting by the media can contribute to suicide contagion, or a "Werther effect"; online, news stories about suicides often contain sensationalistic or romanticized portraits of the deceased and links to suicide notes. It may be helpful to follow such events in the news and be aware of the impact they may have on persons at risk for suicide.

- Suicide communities can help suicidal persons to feel a sense of connection with others and may thereby *reduce* a person's suicide risk; conversely, it is also possible that they may result in baiting toward suicide or that an improvement in depression symptoms would necessitate alienation from the group, thereby increasing risk.

- The Internet is relevant to many aspects of patient evaluation and assessment. If a patient uses the Internet, inquiring about how he or she uses it can help to identify risk and protective factors for suicide.

- The Internet is a powerful tool for suicide prevention and intervention. Clinicians can direct patients and their families or significant others to reliable, beneficial psychoeducation online, such as specific support groups or informational pages from recognized professional organizations and government agencies.

- In the aftermath of a suicide, the Internet may be useful in helping survivors through the grief process, such as by enabling online memorial pages and social networking with others who have lost a loved one to suicide.

References

Abel D: What he left behind: a 1,905-page suicide note. The Boston Globe, September 27, 2010. Available at: http://www.boston.com/news/local/massachusetts/articles/2010/09/27/book_details_motives_for_suicide_at_harvard/?page=1. Accessed June 24, 2011.

Aderet A: Alert: the dark side of chats—internet without boundaries. Isr J Psychiatry Relat Sci 46:162–166, 2009

Alao AO, Yolles JC, Armenta W: Cybersuicide: the internet and suicide. Am J Psychiatry 156:1836–1837, 1999

Alao AO, Soderberg M, Pohl EL, et al: Cybersuicide: review of the role of the internet on suicide. Cyberpsychol Behav 9:489–493, 2006

American Academy of Child and Adolescent Psychiatry: Practice parameter for the assessment and treatment of children and adolescents with suicidal behavior. J Am Acad Child Adolesc Psychiatry 40(suppl):24S–51S, 2001

American Psychiatric Association, Work Group on Suicidal Behaviors: Practice Guideline for the Assessment and Treatment of Patients With Suicidal Behaviors, November 2003. Available at: http://www.psychiatry-online.com/pracGuide/pracGuideTopic_14.aspx. Accessed June 24, 2011.

Athanaselis S, Stefanidou M, Karakoukis N, et al: Asphyxial death by ether inhalation and plastic-bag suffocation instructed by the press and the Internet. J Med Internet Res 4:E18, 2002

Baker D, Fortune S: Understanding self-harm and suicide websites: a qualitative interview study of young adult website users. Crisis 29:118–122, 2008

Bale C: Befriending in cyberspace: challenges and opportunities. Crisis 22:10–11, 2001

Baume P, Cantor CH, Rolfe A: Cybersuicide: the role of interactive suicide notes on the internet. Crisis 18:73–79, 1997

BBC News: German cannibal tells of fantasy. BBC News, December 3, 2003a. Available at: http://news.bbc.co.uk/2/hi/europe/3286721.stm. Accessed June 24, 2011.

BBC News: Net grief for online 'suicide.' BBC News, Technology, February 4, 2003b. Available at: http://news.bbc.co.uk/1/hi/technology/2724819.stm. Accessed June 24, 2011.

BBC News: Chinese gamer sentenced to life. BBC News, April 8, 2005. Available at: http://news.bbc.co.uk/2/hi/technology/4072704.stm. Accessed June 24, 2011.

BBC News: Inquest held after webcam death. BBC News, March 30, 2007. Available at: http://news.bbc.co.uk/go/pr/fr/-/2/hi/uk_news/england/shropshire/6509523.stm. Accessed June 24, 2011.

BBC News: Call to ban 'suicide chatrooms.' BBC News, January 18, 2008. Available at: http://newsvote.bbc.co.uk/mpapps/pagetools/print/news.bbc.co.uk/2/hi/uk_news/7194134.stm. Accessed June 24, 2011.

Becker K, Schmidt MH: Internet chat rooms and suicide. J Am Acad Child Adolesc Psychiatry 43:246–247, 2004

Becker K, Mayer M, Nagenborg M, et al: Parasuicide online: can suicide websites trigger suicidal behaviour in predisposed adolescents? Nord J Psychiatry 58:111–114, 2004

Bell R: Internet assisted suicide: the story of Sharon Lopatka. truTV.com, 2011. Available at: http://www.trutv.com/library/crime/notorious_murders/classics/sharon_lopatka/1.html. Accessed June 24, 2011.

Biddle L, Donovan J, Hawton K, et al: Suicide and the internet. BMJ 336:800–802, 2008

Block JJ: Lessons from Columbine: virtual and real rage. Am J Forensic Psychiatry 28:5–34, 2007

Borzekowski DLG, Schenk S, Wilson JL, et al: e-Ana and e-Mia: a content analysis of pro-eating disorder web sites. Am J Public Health 100:1526–1534, 2010

Boyce N: Pilots of the future: suicide prevention and the internet. Lancet 376:1889–1890, 2010

Boyer EW, Lapen PT, Macalino G, et al: Dissemination of psychoactive substance information by innovative drug users. Cyberpsychol Behav 10:1–6, 2007

Brody JE: The growing wave of teenage self-injury. The New York Times, May 6, 2008. Available at: http://www.nytimes.com/2008/05/06/health/06brod.html. Accessed June 24, 2011.

Cantrell FL: Look what I found! Poison hunting on eBay. Clin Toxicol (Phila) 24:375–379, 2005

Celizic M: Her teen committed suicide over 'sexting.' MSNBC.com, March 6, 2009. Available at: http://www.msnbc.msn.com/id/29546030. Accessed June 24, 2011.

Chapple A, Ziebland S: How the internet is changing the experience of bereavement by suicide: a qualitative study in the UK. Health (London) 15:173–187, 2011

Cloud J: Bullied to death? Time 176:60–63, 2010

Coombes R: Safety nets. BMJ 336:803, 2008

Cooney GM, Morris J: Time to start taking an internet history? (letter) Br J Psychiatry 194:185, 2009

Corkery JM, Button J, Vento AE, et al: Two UK suicides using nicotine extracted from tobacco employing instructions available on the internet. Forensic Sci Int 199:E9–E13, 2010

Eichenberg C: Internet message boards for suicidal people: a typology of users. Cyberpsychol Behav 11:107–113, 2008

Foderaro LW, Hu W: Before a suicide, hints in online musings. The New York Times, September 30, 2010. Available at: http://www.nytimes.com/2010/10/01/nyregion/01suicide.html. Accessed June 24, 2011.

Frei A, Schenker T, Finzen A, et al: The Werther effect and assisted suicide. Suicide Life Threat Behav 33:192–200, 2003

Frierson RL: The suicidal patient: risk assessment, management, and documentation. Psychiatric Times, April 15, 2007. Available at: http://www.psychiatrictimes.com/display/article/10168/53981. Accessed June 24, 2011.

Gallagher KE, Smith DM, Mellen PF: Suicidal asphyxiation by using pure helium gas: case report, review, and discussion of the influence of the internet. Am J Forensic Med Pathol 24:361–363, 2003

Gilat I, Shahar G: Emotional first aid for a suicide crisis: comparison between Telephonic hotline and internet. Psychiatry 70:12–18, 2007

Gilat I, Shahar G: Suicide prevention by online support groups: an action theory–based model of emotional first aid. Arch Suicide Res 13:52–63, 2009

Grassberger M, Krauskopf A: Suicidal asphyxiation with helium: report of three cases. Wien Klin Wochenschr 119:323–325, 2007

Grimland M, Apter A: Commentary: street lights on the dark side of the net. Isr J Psychiatry Relat Sci 46:172–181, 2009

Haas A, Koestner B, Rosenberg J, et al: An interactive web-based method of outreach to college students at risk for suicide. J Am Coll Health 57:15–22, 2008

Hagihara A, Miyazaki S, Tarumi K: Internet use and suicide among younger age groups between 1989 and 2008 in Japan. Acta Psychiatr Scand 121:485–486, 2010

Harris KM, McLean JP, Sheffield J: Examining suicide-risk individuals who go online for suicide-related purposes. Arch Suicide Res 13:264–276, 2009

Hart A, Henwood F, Wyatt S: The role of the Internet in patient-practitioner relationships: findings from a qualitative research study. J Med Internet Res 6:e36, 2004

Heisman M: Suicide note. 2010. Available at: http://www.suicidenote.info/ebook/suicide_note.pdf. Accessed June 25, 2011.

Hinduja S, Patchin JW: Bullying, cyberbullying, and suicide. Arch Suicide Res 14:206–221, 2010

Horne J, Wiggins S: Doing being 'on the edge': managing the dilemma of being authentically suicidal in an online forum. Sociol Health Illn 31:170–184, 2009

Hsiung RC: A suicide in an online mental health support group: reactions of the group members, administrative responses, and recommendations. Cyberpsychol Behav 10:495–500, 2007

Jang DH, Hoffman RS, Nelson LS: Attempted suicide, by mail order: Abrus precatorius. J Med Toxicol 6:427–430, 2010

Janson MP, Alessandrini ES, Strunjas SS, et al: Internet-observed suicide attempts (letter). J Clin Psychiatry 62:478, 2001

Kennedy H: He takes fatal OD as internet pals watch: chatroom vultures egged him to pop more Rx pills. Daily News, Washington Bureau, February 2, 2003. Available at: http://www.nydailynews.com/archives/news/2003/02/02/2003-02-02_he_takes_fatal_od_as_interne.html. Accessed June 25, 2011.

Kim K, Ryu E, Chon MY, et al: Internet addiction in Korean adolescents and its relation to depression and suicidal ideation: a questionnaire survey. Int J Nurs Stud 43:185–192, 2006

Kiume S: Suicide hashtag livetweeting. World of Psychiatry blog, February 11, 2009. Available at: http://www.psychcentral.com/blog/archives/2009/02/11/suicide-hashtag-livetweeting/. Accessed June 25, 2011.

Klomek AB, Marrocco F, Kleinman M, et al: Bullying, depression, and suicidality in adolescents. J Am Acad Child Adolesc Psychiatry 46:40–49, 2007

Klomek AB, Sourander A, Gould MS: Bullying and suicide: detection and intervention. Psychiatric Times 28:1–6, February 10, 2011. Available at: http://www.psychiatrictimes.com/display/article/10168/1795797. Accessed June 25, 2011.

Lee DT, Chan KP, Yip PS: Charcoal burning is also popular for suicide pacts made on the internet (letter). BMJ 330:602, 2005

Lester D: The use of the internet for counseling the suicidal individual: possibilities and drawbacks. Omega (Westport) 58:233–250, 2008–2009

Lewis SP, Heath NL, St Denis JM, et al: The scope of nonsuicidal self-injury on YouTube. Pediatrics 127:E552–E557, 2011

Logan BK, Goldfogel G, Hamilton R, et al: Five deaths resulting from abuse of dextromethorphan sold over the internet. J Anal Toxicol 33:99–103, 2009

Mandrusiak M, Rudd MD, Joiner TE, et al: Warning signs for suicide on the internet: a descriptive study. Suicide Life Threat Behav 36:263–271, 2006

McCarthy MJ: Internet monitoring of suicide risk in the population. J Affect Disord 122:277–279, 2010

Mehlum L: The internet, suicide, and suicide prevention. Crisis 21:186–188, 2000

Mesoudi A: The cultural dynamics of copycat suicide. PLoS One 4:e7252, 2009

Messias E, Castro J, Saini A, et al: Sadness, suicide, and their association with video game and internet overuse among teens: results from the Youth Risk Behavior Survey 2007 and 2009. Suicide Life Threat Behav 41:305–315, 2011

Miller JK, Gergen KJ: Life on the line: the therapeutic potentials of computer-mediated conversation. J Marital Fam Ther 24:189–202, 1998

Mishara BL, Weisstub DN: Ethical, legal, and practical issues in the control and regulation of suicide promotion and assistance over the Internet. Suicide Life Threat Behav 37:58–65, 2007

Morii D, Miyagatani Y, Nakamae N, et al: Japanese experience of hydrogen sulfide: the suicide craze in 2008. J Occup Med Toxicol 5:28, 2010

Musshoff F, Kirschbaum KM, Madea B: An uncommon case of a suicide with inhalation of hydrogen cyanide. Forensic Sci Int 204:E4–E7, 2011

Naito A: Internet suicide in Japan: implications for child and adolescent mental health. Clin Child Psychol Psychiatry 12:583–597, 2007

Neimark G: Boundary violation. J Am Acad Psychiatry Law 37:95–97, 2009

Neimark G, Hurford MO, DiGiacomo J: The internet as collateral informant. Am J Psychiatry 163:1842, 2006

Newcomer EP, Srivatsa NN: Suicide note found online. The Harvard Crimson, September 22, 2010. Available at: http://www.thecrimson.com/article/2010/9/22/heisman-harvard-mother-death/. Accessed June 27, 2011.

Nordt SP, Kelly K, Williams SR, et al: "Black Plague" on the internet. J Emerg Med 16:223–225, 1998

Ogden RD: Observation of two suicides by helium inhalation in a prefilled environment. Am J Forensic Med Pathol 31:156–161, 2010

O'Keeffe GS, Clarke-Pearson K; Council on Communications and Media: The impact of social media on children, adolescents, and families. Pediatrics 127:800–804, 2011

Ozawa-de Silva C: Too lonely to die alone: internet suicide pacts and existential suffering in Japan. Cult Med Psychiatry 32:516–551, 2008

Ozawa-de Silva C: Shared death: self, sociality, and internet group suicide in Japan. Transcult Psychiatry 47:392–418, 2010

Pirkis J, Neal L, Dare A, et al: Legal bans on pro-suicide web sites: an early retrospective from Australia. Suicide Life Threat Behav 39:190–193, 2009

Polder-Verkiel SE: Online responsibility: bad samaritanism and the influence of internet mediation. Sci Eng Ethics, December 16, 2010 [Epub ahead of print]

Prior TI: Suicide methods from the internet. Am J Psychiatry 161:1500–1501, 2004

Rajagopal S: Suicide pacts and the internet: complete strangers may make cyberspace pacts. BMJ 329:1298–1299, 2004

Recupero PR: Forensic evaluation of problematic internet use. J Am Acad Psychiatry Law 36:505–514, 2008

Recupero PR: Forensic psychiatry and the internet, in Textbook of Forensic Psychiatry, 2nd Edition. Edited by Simon RI, Gold LH. Washington, DC, American Psychiatric Publishing, 2010a, pp 587–615

Recupero PR: The mental status examination in the age of the internet. J Am Acad Psychiatry Law 38:15–26, 2010b

Recupero PR, Harms SE, Noble JM: Googling suicide: surfing for suicide information on the internet. J Clin Psychiatry 69:878–888, 2008

Richard J, Werth JL Jr, Rogers JR: Rational and assisted suicidal communication on the internet: a case example and discussion of ethical and practice issues. Ethics Behav 10:215–238, 2000

Ruedy MC: Repercussions of a MySpace teen suicide: should anti-cyberbullying laws be created? North Carolina Journal of Law and Technology 9:323–346, 2008

Sang-Hun C: Korean star's suicide reignites debate on web regulation. The New York Times, October 13, 2008. Available at: http://www.nytimes.com/2008/10/13/technology/internet/13suicide.html. Accessed June 27, 2011.

Sawer P: Predators tell children how to kill themselves. The Telegraph, February 17, 2008. Available at: http://www.telegraph.co.uk/news/uknews/1578945/Predators-tell-children-how-to-kill-themselves.html. Accessed June 27, 2011.

Scheeres J: A virtual path to suicide: depressed student killed herself with help from online discussion group. San Francisco Chronicle, June 8, 2003. Available at: http://www.sfgate.com/cgi-bin/article.cgi?f=/c/a/2003/06/08/MN114902.DTL&ao=all. Accessed June 27, 2011.

Schneider S, Diederich N, Appenzeller B, et al: Internet suicide guidelines: report of a life-threatening poisoning using tobacco extract. J Emerg Med 38:610–613, 2010

Schwartz J: Bullying, suicide, punishment. The New York Times, Week in Review, October 2, 2010. Available at: http://www.nytimes.com/2010/10/03/weekinreview/03schwartz.html. Accessed June 27, 2011.

Shah A: The relationship between general population suicide rates and the internet: a cross-national study. Suicide Life Threat Behav 40:146–150, 2010

Simon RI, Shuman DW: The suicidal patient, in Clinical Manual of Psychiatry and the Law. Washington, DC, American Psychiatric Publishing, 2007, pp 131–163

Sinderbrand R: Point, click and die: "prochoice" suicide sites come under legal scrutiny. Newsweek, June 30, 2003, p 28

Sourander A, Klomek AB, Ikonen M, et al: Psychosocial risk factors associated with cyberbullying among adolescents: a population-based study. Arch Gen Psychiatry 67:720–728, 2010

State of Minnesota v William Francis Melchert-Dinkel, No. 66-CR-10-1193 (Minn. Dist. Ct., 3d Judicial Dist., 2011)

Stelter B: Web suicide viewed live and reaction spur a debate. The New York Times, November 25, 2008. Available at: http://www.nytimes.com/2008/11/25/us/25suicides.html. Accessed June 27, 2011.

Stone MH, Stone DK, Hurt SW: Natural history of borderline patients treated by intensive hospitalization. Psychiatr Clin North Am 10:185–206, 1987

Tam J, Tang WS, Fernando DJ: The internet and suicide: a double-edged tool. Eur J Intern Med 18:453–455, 2007

Tartakovsky M: 15 ways to support a loved one with serious mental illness. PsychCentral, April 11, 2011. Available at: http://psychcentral.com/lib/2011/15-ways-to-support-a-loved-one-with-serious-mental-illness/. Accessed June 27, 2011.

Truscott A: Suicide fad threatens neighbours, rescuers. CMAJ 179:312–313, 2008

van Spijker BA, van Straten A, Kerkhof AJ: The effectiveness of a web-based self-help intervention to reduce suicidal thoughts: a randomized controlled trial. Trials 11:25, 2010

Vennemann B, Pollak S: Death by hanging while watching violent pornographic videos on the Internet—suicide or accidental autoerotic death? Int J Legal Med 120:110–114, 2006

Wang EE, Mahajan N, Wills B, et al: Successful treatment of potentially fatal heavy metal poisonings. J Emerg Med 32:289–294, 2007

Winter M: Former Minn. nurse guilty of using chats to encourage 2 suicides. USA Today, March 15, 2011. Available at: http://content.usatoday.com/communities/ondeadline/post/2011/03/former-minn-nurse-guilty-of-using-chats-to-encourage-2-suicides/1?csp=34. Accessed June 27, 2011.

Yang AC, Tsai SJ, Huang NE, et al: Association of internet search trends with suicide death in Taipei City, Taiwan, 2004–2009. J Affect Disord 132:179–184, 2011

Ybarra ML: Linkages between depressive symptomatology and internet harassment among young regular internet users. Cyberpsychol Behav 7:247–257, 2004

Yip PS, Lee DT: Charcoal-burning suicides and strategies for prevention. Crisis 28 (suppl 1):21–27, 2007

C H A P T E R   2 8

Patient Suicide and Litigation

Charles L. Scott, M.D.

Phillip J. Resnick, M.D.

In 2007, suicide was the 11th leading cause of death in the United States, accounting for 34,598 deaths (Xu et al. 2010). Studies indicate that during the course of his or her career, a psychiatrist has a 50% chance of losing a patient to suicide (Chemtob et al. 1988). A review of psychiatric claims in all 50 states from 1998 through 2009 found that suicide and attempted suicide were the most frequently identifiable cause of loss (Professional Risk Management Services 2011). Despite the inherent increased risk of suicide in a psychiatric population, only 22.2% of psychiatrists report that they have ever had a medical malpractice claim filed against them for any reason (Kane 2010).

In this chapter, we examine psychiatrists' roles in two areas of litigation. In the first section, we provide an overview of malpractice litigation when the psychiatrist is a defendant in a lawsuit. In the second section, we review retrospective psychiatric evaluations conducted to determine whether a person's death was due to a suicide or resulted from other causes. In both situations, it is important that the psychiatrist be familiar with the legal principles that are rele-

vant in approaching the referral issue. In the following case example, the psychiatrist received a formal legal complaint against him alleging psychiatric malpractice.

Case Example 1

Mr. A is a 44-year-old married man being treated in an outpatient psychiatric clinic for major depression and narcissistic personality disorder. Mr. A has a past history of suicide attempts that include an attempted hanging while intoxicated when he was 33 years old. During the first week of his hospitalization after that attempt, Mr. A denied having suicidal feelings and was taken off suicide precautions. Within 20 minutes of his change in status level, Mr. A attempted to hang himself with torn sheets. After 3 weeks of inpatient care, Mr. A was discharged, and he has been followed as an outpatient on a weekly basis.

At his last outpatient psychiatric appointment, Mr. A tells his psychiatrist that his wife informed him that morning that she is in love with a coworker. He is despondent and tearful. Mr. A denies any specific suicide plan but also refuses to answer questions related to current homicidal or suicidal thoughts. The psychiatrist learns that Mr. A received a driving under the influence citation the prior week, and he smells alcohol on Mr. A's breath during the interview. Mr. A refuses inpatient psychiatric admission, and the psychiatrist schedules a routine follow-up appointment for 4 weeks later. The following morning, the psychiatrist learns that Mr. A went home, shot and killed his wife, and then shot himself. The psychiatrist subsequently receives a formal legal complaint against him alleging psychiatric malpractice.

Suicide and Malpractice Litigation

Legal Concepts

Knowledge of general legal concepts assists the clinician both in providing mental health treatment and in understanding medical-legal disputes that may arise when a patient dies. Tort law governs the legal resolution of complaints regarding medical treatment. A *tort* is a civil wrong. Tort law seeks to financially compensate individuals who have been injured or who have suffered losses because of the conduct of others. In cases involving suicide, the plaintiff is generally a surviving spouse or family member who seeks financial compensation for the loss of his or her loved one. Torts are typically divided into three categories: 1) strict liability, 2) intentional torts, and 3) negligence (Table 28–1).

Strict liability imposes liability on defendants without requiring any proof of lack of due care, and this standard is not used in malpractice litigation involving suicide. The most common example of strict liability is harm caused to an individual resulting from a product proven to be unreasonably dangerous and defective (Schubert 1996). *Intentional torts* involve actions in which an individual either intends harm or knows that harm may result from his or her behavior (Schubert 1996). Examples of intentional torts that involve mental health care include assault (an attempt to inflict bodily injury), battery (touching without

TABLE 28–1. Types of torts

Strict liability	Liability imposed without proof of lack of due care
Intentional tort	Individual intends harm or knows harm will result from his or her actions
Negligence	Individual's behavior unintentionally causes an unreasonable risk of harm to another

consent), false imprisonment, and violation of a person's civil rights.

Negligence occurs when a clinician's behavior unintentionally causes an unreasonable risk of harm to another. This type of tort is typically used in a lawsuit against a clinician involving a suicide. Medical malpractice is based on the theory of negligence. The four elements required to establish medical negligence are commonly known as the four *D*'s. These include a *dereliction* of *duty* that *directly* results in *damages*. A duty is most commonly established for a clinician when the patient seeks treatment and treatment is provided. The provision of services does not require the patient's presence and can even extend to assessment and treatment provided over the telephone. Dereliction of duty is usually the most difficult component of negligence for the plaintiff to establish. Dereliction of duty is divided into acts of commission (providing substandard care) and acts of omission (failure to provide required care).

The standard of care does not have to be perfect care but care provided by a reasonable practitioner. This standard requires that the provider exercise, in both diagnosis and treatment, "that reasonable degree of care which a reasonably prudent person or professional should exercise in same or similar circumstances" (Black 1979). In contrast to the standard of care, the *quality of care* represents the adequacy of total care delivered. The quality of care may be influenced by the patient's own health care decisions as well as available resources and may be below, equal to, or above the standard of care as previously defined (Simon 2006). Two aspects of causation generally cited as establishing negligence in suicide cases include the foreseeability of the suicide and the clinician's role in directly causing the harm.

Damages are the amount of money the plaintiff is awarded in a lawsuit. Various types of damages may be awarded. *Special damages* are those actually caused by the injury and include payment for lost wages and medical bills. *General damages* are more subjective in nature and provide financial compensation for the plaintiff's pain and suffering, mental anguish, loss of future income, and loss of companionship. A third category of damages, referred to as *exemplary* or *punitive damages,* may be awarded when the defendant has been determined to have acted in a malicious or grossly reckless manner. Because punitive damages generally involve harm that is intentionally caused, they are rarely awarded in suicide malpractice cases. Table 28–2 summarizes the four key components necessary to successfully establish a claim of medical negligence.

TABLE 28–2. Four *D*'s of negligence

Duty	Established when a professional treatment relationship exists between a clinician and a patient
Dereliction	Deviations from minimally acceptable standards of care
Directly causing	Relation between dereliction of duty and harm caused
Damages	Amount of money awarded the plaintiff to compensate for harm caused

Treatment Settings and Malpractice Litigation

The possibility of a patient committing suicide represents one of the greatest emotional and legal concerns of clinicians. This concern is realistic in view of the fact that 10%–15% of patients with major psychiatric disorders will die by suicide (Brent et al. 1988a). Lawsuits involving suicide usually involve one of three scenarios: 1) an inpatient suicide in which the facility and its practitioners provide inadequate care or supervision, 2) a recently discharged inpatient who commits suicide, or 3) an outpatient who commits suicide (VandeCreek and Knapp 1983).

Suicidality is the most common reason for inpatient psychiatric hospitalization (Friedman 1989). When a patient is admitted to the hospital because of thoughts of self-harm, the clinician is on notice that the patient is at an increased risk for suicidal behavior. Nearly one-third of inpatient suicides result in a lawsuit (Litman 1982). Malpractice actions often name the hospital in addition to the treating clinicians. For example, when hospital staff members are aware of the patient's suicidal tendencies, then the hospital assumes the duty to take reasonable steps to prevent the patient from inflicting self-harm (Robertson 1988). Common allegations for psychiatric malpractice following inpatient and outpatient suicides are outlined in Table 28–3 and Table 28–4, respectively.

Stages of Malpractice Litigation

A malpractice case usually begins because there is a bad outcome coupled with the survivors' bad feelings toward the clinician (Appelbaum and Gutheil 1991). Malpractice litigation goes through several steps before the case actually reaches trial. Laws

TABLE 28–3. Common allegations of negligence following inpatient suicides

The treater(s) failed to

Diagnose or foresee the suicide

Control, supervise, or restrain

Evaluate suicidal intent adequately

Provide appropriate pharmacotherapy

Provide adequate monitoring

Gather an adequate history

Remove potentially harmful items such as belts or shoelaces

Provide a safe, secure environment

Source. Robertson 1988.

TABLE 28–4. Common allegations of negligence following outpatient suicides

The treater(s) failed to

Evaluate properly the need for psychopharmacological intervention or provide suitable pharmacotherapy

Implement hospitalization

Maintain an appropriate clinician-patient relationship

Obtain supervision and consultation

Evaluate for suicide risk at intake and at management transitions

Secure records of prior treatment or perform adequate history taking

Conduct a mental status examination

Diagnose a patient's symptoms appropriately

Establish a formal treatment plan

Safeguard the outpatient environment

Document clinical judgments, rationales, and observations adequately

Source. Packman et al. 2004.

governing the rules of civil procedure vary from state to state but typically have the following components. The party believed to be injured first seeks legal advice to determine if there is a basis for a malpractice claim. The attorney may provide a summary of the facts to a potential expert to determine merit before selecting a psychiatrist to review the records. At this early stage, a plaintiff's attorney often sends the medical records to a mental health expert to review the merits of the case.

A review by a mental health professional is important to determine whether potential negligence has occurred. Experts working with plaintiff's counsel may be asked to identify deviations from the standard of care. Defense attorneys may seek help in defending any alleged deviations in care and in identifying critical areas to review as part of their deposition preparation. The reviewing experts on either side may be asked whether they believe the hospital staff fell below the standard of care in addition to the care provided by the defendant physician.

Some states require that 50%–75% of the expert's time be spent in practice and teaching for the expert to be allowed to testify

on standard of care in malpractice cases. Furthermore, experts should clarify with attorneys involved in cases outside their home state if they are required to have a license in that state before giving expert testimony (Simon and Shuman 1999). Psychiatrists should also refer out those cases they are not qualified to do, such as a case involving complex psychopharmacology.

If the plaintiff's attorney decides to pursue the case, he or she then drafts a document known as the *complaint*. The complaint outlines specific claims of negligence, the form of relief sought (generally monetary), and the specific names of sued defendants. The complaint may be overly inclusive in both allegations of negligence and the number of parties sued. For an inpatient suicide, there are likely to be multiple defendants. During the process of litigation, certain parties may eventually be dropped when there is insufficient evidence to support a cause of action against them.

Once the parties being sued are served with the complaint, they must provide a formal response, known as the *answer,* within a specified time. In the answer to the complaint, the responding party outlines his or her defense to each claim asserted and either admits or denies the claims as outlined in the plaintiff's complaint. In certain situations, the response to the complaint involves a *demurrer,* or a motion to dismiss for failure to state a cause of action. A demurrer is a written response to the complaint that requests dismissal based on the point that even if the facts as outlined in the complaint were true, there is no legal basis for the lawsuit. A judge holds a hearing to determine the validity of the demurrer and decides if the case should be dismissed.

If a demurrer is not granted, litigation moves to the next stage, known as *discovery.* The discovery phase involves an exchange of information so that each side has knowledge of the facts and anticipated testimony and is not surprised should the case proceed to trial. Information may be exchanged through a series of written documents known as *interrogatories.* Interrogatories are a set of written questions posed by one party to the other that requires a written response (also termed *answer to interrogatories)* under oath within a specified time frame. Interrogatory questions commonly request detailed specifics about the suicide, care providers, and treatment provided. The discovery process can involve demands for production of documents such as nursing policies regarding suicide precautions or a mental health examination of a plaintiff alleging emotional damages.

During the discovery stage of litigation, *depositions* of parties and potential witnesses are usually requested. Discovery depositions in suicide malpractice cases usually involve three phases: 1) depositions of the parties, the treating health care professionals, and fact witnesses; 2) depositions of the various standard of care experts, 3) depositions of the causation experts and damage experts. During a deposition, the testimony of a fact or expert witness is taken under oath before a court reporter, and a written transcript of this proceeding can be used to assist in trial preparation or to impeach the testimony of a witness during trial.

After the discovery phase has concluded, either party may file a *motion for summary judgment.* A motion for summary judgment asserts that there is no need for a trial because there is no dispute as to any material fact issues in the case, and the law clearly favors judgment for the moving party. If the court grants summary judgment for the requesting party, the case ends at this point.

If the case is not dismissed, an *arbitration* or *settlement conference* may be arranged to determine whether the parties can agree to a settlement and avoid the time and expense of a trial. Various factors that influence whether a case settles include an assessment of the defendant physician's demeanor as caring versus arrogant, the ability of the experts, the strength of the attorneys, the attitude of the particular judge, and the nature of the local jury pool. If the legal parties are unable to settle the case, litigation then proceeds to *trial,* at which the evidence is presented to the *trier of fact.* The trier of fact is either a judge (bench trial) or a jury and is responsible for determining the outcome of the litigation, known as the *judgment.* The types of damages resulting from the judgment are discussed earlier in this section.

Litigation and Retrospective Analysis of Suicidal Intent

The psychiatrist's evaluation of suicidal intent plays a pivotal role in various types of litigation surrounding an individual's death. Whereas the actual cause of death may be clear (e.g., gunshot wound to the head or crush injury from a car accident), the mode of death requires an examination of the person's intent to die. When assessing the mode of death, the examiner addresses if the death was from natural causes, an accident, a suicide, or a homicide (Ebert 1987). In 5%–20% of death cases reviewed by medical examiners (coroners), the mode of death is unclear (Schneidman 1981). Common situations in which the cause of death is clear but the *mode* of death is not include autoerotic asphyxia, a fatal car crash, and death resulting from Russian roulette. Any one of these scenarios could result from suicidal intentions or from a tragic accident. When the circumstances surrounding a death are unclear, litigation may follow to answer such unresolved questions, especially if there are financial consequences. Multiple areas of potential litigation may follow a death from unclear reasons, and some of these are noted in Table 28–5 (Simon 1990).

Robins et al. (1959) conducted the first retrospective psychological study of suicides through their detailed analysis of 134 consecutive suicides that occurred during a 1-year period. This retrospective investigation of a victim's mental state was further developed by the Suicide Prevention Center in Los Angeles, California, during the 1950s to assist coroners' accuracy in the determination of death (Beskow et al. 1990; Curphey 1961; Jobes et al. 1986).

The term *psychological autopsy* was coined by Schneidman (1981) to describe the method by which an evaluator conducts a retro-

TABLE 28–5. Areas of potential litigation following death from unclear reasons

Life, health, or disability benefits from insurance policies that allow financial recovery for accidents but not suicides

Homeowners' policies that exclude coverage for intentionally violent acts

Legal actions related to workers' compensation benefits

Malpractice actions alleging suicide

Product liability claims

Motor vehicle insurance claims

Contested wills

Awarding of military benefits to surviving family members

Criminal prosecution when homicide by a third party rather than suicide of the decedent is alleged

Determination of whether death from police intervention was "suicide by cop"

Source.   Simon 1990.

spective review in equivocal deaths to determine whether the death involved suicidal *intent*. Three important legal components of intent are

> 1) that it is a state of mind, 2) about consequences of an act [or omission] and not about the act itself, and 3) it extends not only to having in mind a purpose [or desire] to bring about given consequences but also to having in mind a belief [or knowledge] that given consequences are substantially certain to result from the act. (Keeton et al. 1984, p. 34)

More simply stated, suicidal intent involves a person's understanding that an action he or she takes will result in his or her own death.

Whereas suicidal intent involves an appreciation of the permanent consequences of the suicidal act, *motive* refers to the reasons that the person wants to die. Such reasons may include a desire to have insurance money cover a family debt in the face of overwhelming financial stress or the hope that suicide will provide an escape from personal problems or emotional pain. In a review of large psychological autopsy studies from around the world, Foster (2011) found that nearly all persons who died by suicide had experienced at least one adverse life event within 1 year of death, with interpersonal conflict posing the greatest risk for suicide. Retrospective reviews of suicidal intent and motive are potentially helpful in a variety of civil and criminal matters and are discussed in the following sections (Simon 2002).

Psychological Autopsies in Litigation

Life Insurance Claims

Many life insurance policies differentiate the extent of death benefits based on whether the death was due to natural or accidental causes rather than suicide, as in the following case example.

Case Example 2

Mrs. and Mr. B are enjoying their routine Sunday morning coffee and newspaper. Mr. B leaves the room to take his shower while Mrs. B begins tackling the weekly crossword puzzle. After 5 minutes, Mrs. B hears a loud shot from their bedroom and rushes to the room, where she discovers her husband lying dead on the floor. His .45-caliber revolver is in his right hand, and he has a fatal gunshot wound to his head. Mr. B never communicated to her any suicidal thoughts, and she reports that he was not depressed. Mr. B and Mrs. B each took out a life insurance policy 18 months ago that included an exclusion clause for any suicide occurring within the first 2 years of the policy. The insurance company refuses to pay benefits to Mrs. B, stating that her husband's death was a suicide, and she is therefore not entitled to the life insurance benefits. Mrs. B's attorney contacts a psychiatrist, asking his assistance in conducting a psychological autopsy

to offer an opinion about whether the decedent died by suicide.

When conducting an assessment of a deceased person's suicidal intent, the evaluator should see the relevant insurance policy language. In particular, the psychiatrist should examine if the policy governed by the relevant jurisdictional statute and case law distinguishes "sane" from "insane" suicides. In some jurisdictions, a person who commits suicide but is assessed as "insane" is judged not to have intentionally committed the suicide; therefore, the beneficiaries have a right to the policy proceeds. One definition of an *insane suicide* was described more than 100 years ago in the U.S. Supreme Court case *Mutual Life Insurance Company v. Terry* (1873, p. 242). In this 1873 case, the Court wrote:

> If the death is caused by the voluntary act of the assured, he knowing and intending that his death shall be the result of his act, but when his reasoning faculties are so far impaired that he is not able to understand the moral character, the general nature, consequences and effect of the act he is about to commit, or when he is impelled thereto by an insane impulse, which he has not the power to resist, such death is not within the contemplation of the parties to the contract and the insurer is liable.

The following case example illustrates a situation in which life insurance benefits may be granted if insane suicides are not specifically excluded from policy coverage.

Case Example 3

Mr. C, a psychotic man, shoots himself in the head with a revolver in the delusional belief that he is immortal and cannot be killed. Although Mr. C may have understood that he was pulling the trigger of a loaded weapon, if his delusional beliefs prevented him from understanding that he would die as a result of this gunshot wound, his death could be determined an insane suicide.

Some insurance companies have revised their policies to specifically exclude the recovery of benefits by suicide, whether sane or insane. In *Bigelow v. Berkshire Life Insurance Company* (1876), the Supreme Court upheld the exclusion of insane suicides from coverage under a particular life insurance policy, thereby preventing the distribution of life insurance benefits following a suicide, regardless of the mental state of the deceased.

Workers' Compensation Claims

Workers' compensation awards monetary benefits when mental harms are determined to have been caused by a work-related injury. When an employee commits suicide following a work-related injury, can a family member seek workers' compensation survivor benefits? In this situation, a psychological autopsy may be useful in determining the relationship, if any, between a work-related injury and a suspected suicide. In the 1984 Montana case *Campbell v. Young Motor Co.*, the court allowed Dr. Walters, a psychologist who conducted a psychological autopsy, to testify whether a back injury Raymond Campbell sustained working as a car body repairman was a proximate cause of his suicide 5 years after the injury occurred. The trial court found that there was a causal connection between the injury and the suicide and commented as follows:

> Where can this Court find the bright line that distinguishes the act, the act premeditated by intellect, from the act that is the result of the diseased mind? This Court must, and can only, discover this line by examining the pre-accident and post-accident conduct of the decedent, conduct which steps forward and speaks on his behalf, and the expert tes-

timony of the psychologist who performed the psychological autopsy. (*Campbell v. Young Motor Co.* 1984)

In the subsequent 1992 Kansas case of *Rodriguez v. Henkle Drilling and Supply Company*, a deceased man's wife sued for benefits, alleging that injuries her husband sustained while working on irrigation wells resulted in constant pain, decreased self-esteem, and depression that resulted in his suicide 2 years later. The employer presented findings from two psychological autopsies that indicated that the deceased had difficulties with alcohol and drug use, prior suicidal threats, and marital problems. The experts conducting the psychological autopsy testified that work-related injuries were not a significant cause of the man's suicide. The trial court found that although a worker's suicide does not automatically preclude compensation, the claimant failed to prove that her husband's work injuries resulted in his suicide (*Rodriguez v. Henkle Drilling and Supply Company* 1992). In both of these workers' compensation cases, the findings from the psychological autopsies were allowed into evidence to assist the court's understanding of the relationship between a work-related injury and the employee's later suicide.

Inheritance Litigation

A psychological autopsy may be helpful in determining if an individual was sane or insane regarding his or her estate's legal right to a potential inheritance following the individual's commission of a homicide-suicide. In general, a perpetrator who takes a person's life cannot inherit or profit from his or her crime. For example, if a son shoots his father because his father was about to alter his will to exclude his son, the son could not profit from his father's death. Does this principle apply if a person commits a homicide and then takes his or her own life? Would the homicide victim's assets be included in the deceased perpetrator's estate if this perpetrator was included in the victim's will? In some states, the answer to this question requires a determination of whether the killer would have met the state's legal test of criminal insanity at the time of the homicide. For example, in New York, if the court finds that the deceased perpetrator would have met the criminal test for insanity, then the killer's estate may profit from the victim's estate (Goldstein 1986).

Criminal Cases

The psychological autopsy may also provide useful information in the evaluation of defendants involved in the criminal justice system. Most commonly, a psychological autopsy may be requested from a defendant charged with homicide to support his or her defense that the death with which he or she is charged was actually a result of the victim's suicide. In the case of *United States v. St. Jean* (1995), a husband charged with the premeditated murder of his wife argued that his wife's death was as likely a result of a suicide as a homicide and therefore reasonable doubt existed as to his guilt. To rebut this assertion, the prosecutor called an expert who had conducted a psychological autopsy of the victim and was prepared to testify that none of the factors normally associated with suicide was present. The defense challenged the admissibility of the psychological autopsy results, alleging that they were unreliable and that the evaluator was not an expert in suicidology. The court allowed the expert's testimony, and the results of the psychological autopsy were deemed admissible on appeal (Biffl 1996; *United States v. St. Jean* 1995).

Results from psychological autopsies may also be allowed in cases involving criminal child abuse. *Jackson v. State* (1989) is a frequently cited case in which a psychological autopsy examined the alleged relationship between a mother's alleged abusive behavior and her daughter's subsequent suicide. In this case, a mother altered her 17-year-old daughter's birth certificate so that she could work as a nude dancer in a nightclub. The teenager subsequently shot herself, and a psychiatrist was prepared to testify that the mother's behavior was a substantial factor in the daughter's suicide. Although the defense argued that psychological autopsies are not reliable and therefore not admissible, the court reasoned that the jury could determine the reliability of this testimony and allowed the psychological autopsy results into evidence. Dr. Douglas Jacobs, a psychiatrist specializing in suicidology, testified that the abusive relationship with the mother was a substantial contributing cause to the teenager's suicide. The mother was found guilty of child abuse and this verdict was challenged. A Florida appellate court held that the state had presented sufficient evidence to establish that psychological autopsies examining suicides had gained acceptance in the field of psychiatry and that the trial judge did not err in allowing the psychiatrist's testimony (*Jackson v. State* 1989).

In a subsequent Ohio case, a father was alleged to have repeatedly sexually abused his daughter. After she died by suicide, he was charged with nine counts of sexual battery and involuntary manslaughter. A psychological autopsy was conducted to determine if there was a connection between the father's alleged sexual abuse and his daughter's suicide. The father filed a motion to exclude the results of the psychological autopsy. Although the court ultimately determined that the father could not be charged with involuntary manslaughter for his daughter's suicide, it commented that the results of the psychological autopsy could be relevant to the charges of sexual abuse. The court also emphasized that the possible relationship of the father's sexual abuse to his daughter's suicide could be considered as evidence during his sentencing phase (*State v. Huber* 1992).

Components of the Psychological Autopsy

Schneidman (1981) recommended that forensic evaluators review 14 areas when conducting the psychological autopsy (Jacobs and Klein-Benheim 1995). Table 28–6 outlines important areas to review when conducting a psychological autopsy.

TABLE 28–6. Areas to review for psychological autopsy

Basic identifying information (e.g., age, gender, marital status, occupation)

Specific details of the death

Outline of the victim's history, to include previous suicide attempts

Family psychiatric history (i.e., suicides and mood disorders)

Victim's personality and lifestyle characteristics

Victim's historical pattern of reaction to stress and emotional lability

Recent stressors or anticipated conflicts

Relation of alcohol and drugs to the victim's lifestyle and death

Quality of the victim's interpersonal relationships

Changes in the victim's routine, schedule, and habits before death

Information relating to the "lifeside" of the victim (i.e., successes and plans)

Rating of lethality

Reaction of informants to the victim's death

Assessment of suicidal intent

Source. Jacobs and Klein-Benheim 1995; Schneidman 1981.

To accomplish such an analysis, the evaluator examines two sources of information when conducting the psychological autopsy (Isometsä 2001). The first source involves extensive interviews of family members, friends, and other individuals close to the victim. Such interviews are considered the more important source of information (Hawton et al. 1998). The second source is a thorough review of collateral records. Collateral documents that should be considered for review include the victim's psychiatric records, medical records, suicide notes, personal journals, computer hard drive, employment records, academic records (when indicated), and relevant legal documents such as the person's will or new insurance policies; police reports; witness statements; accident reports; and autopsy reports.

Although often admitted into evidence in a courtroom proceeding, psychological autopsies have been criticized for lacking basic psychometric test qualities such as reliability and validity. To address these concerns, the Centers for Disease Control and Prevention developed Empirical Criteria for Determination of Suicide (ECDS). This instrument has 16 items that review a person's mental state at the time of his or her death and has been shown to be 92% accurate in differentiating between a suicide and an accident. The 16 items included on this instrument are listed in Table 28–7 (Jobes et al. 1986; Simon 1998).

The ECDS serves to supplement the evaluator's clinical judgment and may provide useful data to submit to support opinions reached in the psychological autopsy (Simon 1998).

Conducting the Psychological Autopsy

Surviving family members, friends, and colleagues may be reluctant to speak with an

TABLE 28–7. Suicide and mental state checklist

1. Pathological evidence (autopsy) indicates self-inflicted death.
2. Toxicological evidence indicates self-inflicted harm.
3. Statements by witnesses indicate self-inflicted death.
4. Investigatory evidence (e.g., police reports, photographs from scene) indicates self-inflicted death.
5. Psychological evidence (observed behavior, lifestyle, personality) indicates self-inflicted death.
6. States of the deceased indicate self-inflicted death.
7. Evidence indicates that decedent recognized high potential lethality of means of death.
8. Decedent had suicidal thoughts.
9. Decedent had recent and sudden change in affect (emotions).
10. Decedent experienced serious depression or mental disorder.
11. Decedent made an expression of farewell, indicated desire to die, or acknowledged impending death.
12. Decedent made an expression of hopelessness.
13. Decedent experienced stressful events or significant losses (actual or threatened).
14. Decedent experienced general instability in immediate family.
15. Decedent had recent interpersonal conflicts.
16. Decedent had history of generally poor physical health.

Source. Jobes et al. 1991; Simon 1998.

examiner following the victim's death. Because the evaluator may have only one opportunity to interview a key informant, it is helpful to carefully review in advance the collateral documents when formulating interview questions. The evaluator should be sensitive to a variety of feelings that the person interviewed may experience. Such feel-

ings range from extreme grief accompanied by guilt, sadness, or anger to suspicion and mistrust about the examiner's role. In some circumstances, if the examiner determines that death resulted from an intentional suicide, the individual being interviewed may suffer a financial loss and therefore may have substantial reluctance to participate in the postmortem analysis. Such individuals may also have significant motivation to misrepresent information. In litigation, important sources of information may be required by law to respond in a deposition.

Although some family members may be reluctant to discuss suicidal communications, a sudden death from suicide may be genuinely surprising to most family members. Research indicates that only one-third to one-half of all victims examined in a psychological autopsy had communicated explicit statements of suicidality to their family members or health care professionals during the months before their death (Barraclough et al. 1974; Isometsä et al. 1994; Robins et al. 1959). Likewise, a clinician may not know that his or her patient was contemplating taking his or her own life. In a Finnish review of 100 suicides of persons who had met with a health care professional on the day of their suicide, only 21% had communicated their suicidal intent to their clinician (Isometsä 2001; Isometsä et al. 1995).

When is the best time to conduct the interviews? Postmortem researchers of suicide have conducted interviews of informants ranging from a few weeks to 6 months after the victim's death. Brent et al. (1988b) found that when interviews were performed between 2 and 6 months after the suicide, no significant relationship was found between the timing of the interview and the reporting of important diagnostic history and familial variables. However, studies have also found that survivors are more satisfied when interviews are conducted less than 10 weeks following the suicide rather than later (Runeson and Beskow 1991).

Various approaches have been proposed for contacting informants to arrange the interview. Researchers have found that contacting informants by letter followed by a telephone call 1 week later resulted in a high acceptance rate, with 77% of the approached families agreeing to be interviewed (Brent et al. 1988b). In contrast, other researchers have achieved a low rejection rate by first contacting the survivors by telephone before sending a letter. By speaking directly with the informant during the initial contact, the evaluator is able to assess the reaction of the survivor (Beskow et al. 1990). When a letter is used to contact a close survivor, improved outcomes may be achieved through attempts to personalize the letter by referring to the deceased as "your son," "your wife," or "your partner," or using another appropriate phrase (Cooper 1999). Procedures that require the informant to complete a personality inventory of the deceased in advance of the interview have generated negative reactions from interviewees and are not recommended (Beskow 1979).

The evaluator must use caution in setting up the interview on potentially sensitive dates such as the victim's birthday or the anniversary of his or her death. The examiner needs to be flexible and sensitive to the emotional needs of the interviewee. In a pilot study of factors that increase the acceptability of the interview, Cooper (1999) determined that asking questions surrounding the death during an early stage of the inter-view was recommended to alleviate anxiety as soon as possible. In addition, the use of the phrase "sudden death" instead of "suicide" was generally preferred, especially in those cases in which the informant did not believe the death was a result of suicide.

The evaluator needs to anticipate the potential grief, guilt, or distress that an informant may experience during the interview. A refusal to participate during the first contact should be respected. The examiner may invite the individual to contact him or her when and if he or she is ready to do so. Several authors have described a therapeutic aspect of the psychological autopsy for those interviewed. Aspects of the interview process that were deemed helpful include allowing the interviewee to find meaning in the suicide, to contribute to the understanding of the person's death, to obtain psychological support and a connection with others, to accept the loss, and to better understand his or her own functioning (Henry and Greenfield 2009). Only a minority of those questioned about a suicide report finding the experience more distressing than expected (Wong et al. 2010). Although the investigator may discuss the factual circumstances of the death, information that has been concealed from relatives or close friends should generally not be revealed (Beskow et al. 1990). In summary, the psychological autopsy is a delicate examination that balances the need to obtain sufficient relevant information with the requirement to treat both the survivors and the deceased with dignity and respect.

Key Clinical Concepts

- The most common malpractice claims against psychiatrists are those that involve a patient's suicide.
- To successfully establish malpractice, the plaintiff must prove that there was a dereliction of duty that directly resulted in damages.

- Psychological autopsies have been accepted into evidence in legal proceedings and can play a critical role in the outcome of both civil and criminal litigation.

- The psychological autopsy involves a combination of in-depth interviews with surviving family members and friends and an extensive review of collateral records.

References

Appelbaum PS, Gutheil TG: Malpractice and other forms of liability, in Clinical Handbook of Psychiatry and the Law, 2nd Edition. Edited by Appelbaum PS, Gutheil TG. Baltimore, MD, Williams & Wilkins, 1991, pp 136–213

Barraclough BM, Bunch J, Nelson B, et al: A hundred cases of suicide: clinical aspects. Br J Psychiatry 125:355–373, 1974

Beskow J: Suicide and mental disorder in Swedish men. Acta Psychiatr Scand Suppl 277:1–138, 1979

Beskow J, Runeson B, Asgard U: Psychological autopsies: methods and ethics. Suicide Life Threat Behav 20:307–323, 1990

Biffl E: Psychological autopsies: do they belong in the courtroom? Am J Crim Law 24:123–145, 1996

Bigelow v Berkshire Life Insurance Company 93 US 284 (1876)

Black HC: Black's Law Dictionary. St Paul, MN, West Publishing Company, 1979

Brent DA, Kupfer DJ, Bromet EJ, et al: The assessment and treatment of patients at risk for suicide, in American Psychiatric Press Review of Psychiatry. Edited by Frances AJ, Hales RE. Washington, DC, American Psychiatric Press, 1988a, pp 353–385

Brent D, Perper J, Kolko D, et al: Psychological autopsy: methodological considerations for the study of adolescent suicide. J Am Acad Child Adolesc Psychiatry 27:362–366, 1988b

Campbell v Young Motor Co., 684 P2d 1101 (Mont. 1984)

Chemtob CM, Hamada RS, Bauer G, et al: Patients' suicides: frequency and impact on psychiatrists. Am J Psychiatry 145:224–228, 1988

Cooper J: Ethical issues and their practical application in a psychological autopsy study of suicide. J Clin Nurs 89:467–475, 1999

Curphey TJ: The role of the social scientist in the medicolegal certification of death from suicide, in The Cry for Help. Edited by Farberow NL, Schneidman ES. New York, McGraw-Hill, 1961

Ebert BW: Guide to conducting a psychological autopsy. Prof Psychol Res Pr 18:52–53, 1987

Foster T: Adverse life events proximal to adult suicide: a synthesis of findings from psychological autopsy studies. Arch Suicide Res 15:1–15, 2011

Friedman RS: Hospital treatment of the suicidal patient, in Suicide: Understanding and Responding: Harvard Medical School Perspectives. Edited by Jacobs DG, Brown HN. Madison, CT, International Universities Press, 1989

Goldstein R: When it pays to be insane: three unusual legacies of insanity. Bull Am Acad Psychiatry Law 14:253–262, 1986

Hawton K, Appleby L, Platt S, et al: The psychological autopsy approach to studying suicide: a review of methodological issues. J Affect Disord 50:269–276, 1998

Henry M, Greenfield B: Therapeutic effects of psychological autopsies. Crisis 30:20–24, 2009

Isometsä ET: Psychological autopsy studies—a review. Eur Psychiatry 16:379–385, 2001

Isometsä ET, Henriksson MM, Sro HM, et al: Suicide in major depression. Am J Psychiatry 151:530–536, 1994

Isometsä ET, Heikkinen ME, Marttunen MJ, et al: The last appointment before suicide: is suicidal intent communicated? Am J Psychiatry 152:919–922, 1995

Jackson v State, 553 So. 2d 719, 720 (Fla. Dist. Ct. App. 1989)

Jacobs D, Klein-Benheim M: The psychological autopsy: a useful tool for determining proximate causation in suicide cases. Bull Am Acad Psychiatry Law 23:165–182, 1995

Jobes DA, Berman AL, Josselson AR: The impact of psychological autopsies on medical examiners' determination of manner of death. J Forensic Sci 31:177–189, 1986

Jobes DA, Casey JO, Berman AL, et al: Clinical criteria for the determination of suicide manner of death. J Forensic Sci 36:244–256, 1991

Kane CK: Policy research perspectives: medical liability claim frequency: a 2007–2008 snapshot of physicians. American Medical Association. 2010. Available at: http://www.ama-assn.org/resources/doc/health-policy/prp-201001-claim-freq.pdf. Accessed September 10, 2011.

Keeton W, Dobbs D, Keeton R, et al: Prosser and Keeton on Torts, 5th Edition. St. Paul, MN, West Publishing Company, 1984, pp 33–66

Litman RE: Hospitals and suicides: lawsuits and standards. Suicide Life Threat Behav 12:212–220, 1982

Mutual Life Insurance Company v Terry, 15 Wall 21 LEd 236, 242 (1873)

Packman WL, Pennuto TO, Bongar B, et al: Legal issues of professional negligence in suicide cases. Behav Sci Law 22:697–713, 2004

Professional Risk Management Services: Psychiatric claims by cause of loss: all states: 1998–2009. 2011. Available at: http://www.psychprogram.com/claims/COL2010.pdf. Accessed September 12, 2011.

Robertson JD: Psychiatric Malpractice: Liability of Mental Health Professionals. New York, Wiley Law Publications, 1988

Robins E, Gassner S, Kayes J, et al: The communication of suicidal intent: a study of 134 consecutive cases of successful (completed) suicide. Am J Psychiatry 115:724–733, 1959

Rodriguez v Henkle Drilling and Supply Company, 828 P2d 1335 (Kan. Ct. App. 1992)

Runeson B, Beskow K: Reactions of survivors of suicide victims to interviews. Acta Psychiatr Scand 83:169–173, 1991

Schneidman ES: The psychological autopsy. Suicide Life Threat Behav 11:325–340, 1981

Schubert FA: Grilliot's Introduction to Law and the Legal System, 6th Edition. Boston, MA, Houghton Mifflin, 1996, pp 537–541

Simon RI: You only die once—but did you intend it? Psychiatric assessment of suicide intent in insurance litigation. Tort Insur Law J 25:650–662, 1990

Simon RI: Murder masquerading as suicide: postmortem assessment of suicide risk factors at the time of death. J Forensic Sci 43:1119–1123, 1998

Simon RI: Retrospective assessment of mental states in criminal and civil litigation: a clinical review, in Retrospective Assessment of Mental States in Litigation. Edited by Simon RI, Shuman DW. Washington, DC, American Psychiatric Publishing, 2002, pp 1–20

Simon RI: Commentary: medical errors, sentinel events, and malpractice. J Am Acad Psychiatry Law 34:99–100, 2006

Simon RI, Shuman DW: Conducting forensic examinations on the road: are you practicing your profession without a license? J Am Acad Psychiatry Law 27:75–82, 1999

State v Huber, 597 NE2d 570 (Ohio C.P. 1992)

United States v St. Jean, WL 106960, at 1 (A.F. Ct. Crim. App. 1995)

VandeCreek L, Knapp S: Malpractice risks with suicidal patients. Psychotherapy: Theory, Research, and Practice 10:274–280, 1983

Wong PW, Chan WS, Beh PS, et al: Research participation experiences of informants of suicide and control cases. Crisis 31:238–246, 2010

Xu J, Kochanek KD, Murphy SL, et al: Deaths: final data for 2007. Natl Vital Stat Rep 58:1–136, 2010

C H A P T E R   2 9

Therapeutic Risk Management of the Suicidal Patient

Robert I. Simon, M.D.

The law has come to play a pervasive role in the practice of psychiatry (Simon and Shuman 2007a). The contours of the doctor-patient relationship are no longer defined solely by the psychiatrist and the patient. Courts, legislatures, and administrative agencies also shape the practice of psychiatry. Knowledge of the legal regulation of psychiatry that informs clinical practice is no longer optional for psychiatrists. The requirements of the law must be integrated with best practices to achieve optimal therapeutic benefits. Effective management of the risks inherent in the practice of psychiatry that are enhanced by the risks that external regulation generates is a reality of psychiatric practice (Simon and Shuman 2009).

Therapeutic risk management assures that in addition to clinical competence, there is an optimal therapeutic accord to be found in each case that demands a working knowledge of the law regulating the practice of psychiatry (Simon and Shuman 2007b). Successful resolution of clinical-legal dilemmas requires an understanding of the legal process that helps clinicians to provide good patient care and to avoid unnecessary and counterproductive defensive practices (Simon and Shuman 2009). Most clinicians are not lawyers or forensic psychiatrists, but an understanding of how the law and psychiatry interact in frequently occurring clinical situations is essential. In most instances, because the law derives its requirements from professional practice, good clinical care and good laws are often complementary (Wexler and Winick 1991, 1996).

Therapeutic risk management affirms the clinician's role in the treatment of the suicidal patient (Table 29–1). It informs appropriate clinical management of legal concerns that frequently arise regarding suicidal patients in crisis. For example, clinical-legal matters often involve confidentiality, informed consent, freedom of movement (least-restrictive alternative), involuntary treatment (medication, hospitalization), and electroconvulsive therapy.

Defensive psychiatry can be divided into preemptive and avoidant practices (Simon 1985). Preemptive defensive practices use

TABLE 29–1. Therapeutic risk management of suicidal patients: objectives

Apply legally informed solutions to clinical-legal dilemmas

Manage psychiatric-legal issues clinically, to the extent possible

Support good clinical care

Prevent patient injury or harm

Avoid harmful defensive practices

Avoid a malpractice suit or provide a legal defense, if sued

Source. Adapted from Simon and Shuman 2007b.

procedures and treatments designed to prevent or limit liability; for example, unnecessarily hospitalizing a patient at risk for suicide who could be treated safely as an outpatient (Brown and Rayne 1989). Avoidant defensive practices forgo necessary procedures or treatments for fear of lawsuits, even though the patient would likely benefit from these interventions. An example would be failing to involuntarily hospitalize a treatment-refusing, acute, high-risk suicidal patient.

When defensive practices direct rather than support clinical decision making, the outcome can be harmful to patient care, to the doctor-patient relationship, and to the professional integrity of the practitioner. For example, psychiatric residents often display a paralytic fear of lawyers and lawsuits that impairs their clinical decision-making. Paradoxically, inappropriate defensive practices, often the result of clinical-legal misunderstandings, can invite a lawsuit. The goal of therapeutic risk management is to address clinical-legal dilemmas effectively while maintaining the integrity of the patient's treatment.

Good clinical care is not always synonymous with therapeutic risk management. Although good clinical care is necessary, it

may not be sufficient in reducing malpractice risk. Good clinical care can deteriorate into inappropriate defensive practices when clinicians are confronted by difficult clinical-legal dilemmas. Therapeutic risk management upholds and maintains good clinical care. For example, an exception to informed consent allows the psychiatrist to treat the high-risk suicidal patient in an emergency. The emergency exception is embodied in case law in some states and in statutory laws in others, with the definition of what constitutes an emergency varying from state to state. Under the common law as well as statutory codifications, informed consent has not been required in an emergency in which the clinician is unable to obtain the patient's competent consent.

The legal standard of care does not require the psychiatrist to adhere to best practices or even to provide good clinical care to the patient. The laws articulating the standard of care, in both the legislative and judicial voices, vary among the states from customary practice to the practice of the reasonable, prudent practitioner (Simon and Shuman 2007a). Although the provision of good clinical care and a working understanding of clinical-legal management cannot construct an impenetrable carrier against a malpractice suit, they provide an important strategic option.

Risk management is a reality of psychiatric practice, especially in the assessment and management of patients at risk for suicide. Risk management guidelines often recommend *ideal* or *best* practices, whereas the actual standard of care required of a psychiatrist is the skill and care "ordinarily provided," or reasonable, prudent care. These standards can be confused by expert witnesses who testify in malpractice cases (Simon 2005). Moreover, suicide cases are challenging, multifaceted, and nuanced, making it difficult to provide precise assessment and management guidelines. Obtaining a consultation and keeping adequate documentation are sound therapeutic risk management measures.

Clinically based risk management is patient centered. It supports the treatment process and the therapeutic alliance (see Table 29–1). At a minimum, it follows the fundamental ethical principle in medicine of "first do no harm." A working knowledge of the legal regulation of psychiatry enables the psychiatrist to manage clinical-legal issues more effectively. Clinically based risk management provides the psychiatrist with a significant measure of practice comfort that permits continued maintenance of the treatment role with patients at risk for suicide.

Good clinical care provides the best risk management. For example, performing systematic suicide risk assessments that inform treatment and management interventions is good clinical care and, secondarily, sound clinically based risk management. Documentation of the risk assessments supports good patient care and substantiates clinical judgment (American Psychiatric Association 2002). In malpractice litigation, what is not recorded by a physician may be considered not to have been performed (Simon 2001). Good care of patients at suicidal risk requires the clinician's full commitment to the patient's evaluation, treatment, and management. This clinical imperative also holds true in collaborative treatment relationships with other mental health professionals.

Risk management practices that are not clinically tempered and patient centered interfere with the patient's treatment and undermine the therapeutic alliance. They are undertaken to avoid malpractice liability or to provide a legal defense against a malpractice claim. For example, an undue reliance on suicide prevention contracts

("no-harm contracts") may be the result of the clinician's attempt to reduce the anxiety associated with treating suicidal patients (Miller et al. 1998). Some erroneously believe that the suicide prevention contract legally binds the patient to refrain from self-harm. Suicide prevention contracts may falsely reassure the clinician, often preempting adequate suicide risk assessment and increasing the patient's risk for suicide.

Consulting with a colleague is good clinical practice when the clinician is confronted with complex diagnostic, treatment, and management issues. As a clinically based risk management technique, consultation supports and guides good clinical care by providing a "biopsy" of the standard of care. The clinician's uncertainty, even anxiety, must be contained within reasonable limits to treat the patient's condition effectively. The clinician should "never worry alone" (T.G. Gutheil, personal communication, December 2002). In certain cases, consulting with a risk manager or an attorney can be helpful. Clinical risk management helps the psychiatrist avoid defensive practices that are harmful to both the patient and the clinician. The clinician must focus on providing good care while carrying sufficient malpractice insurance.

Suicide and Malpractice Litigation

A clinical axiom states that there are three kinds of psychiatrists: 1) those who have had a patient die by suicide, 2) those who will have a patient die by suicide, and 3) those who will have more than one patient die by suicide. Patient suicide is an unavoidable occupational hazard of psychiatric practice that is accompanied by increased malpractice liability exposure. When a patient commits suicide, a lawsuit may follow (Figure 29–1). Although the potential for malpractice suits remains high for psychiatrists who treat suicidal and violent patients, the plaintiff's success rate in malpractice actions is only 2 or 3 out of every 10 litigated claims.

Generally, malpractice claims against psychiatrists for a patient's suicide are brought under the following theories of negligence:

- Failure to diagnose the patient's condition properly
- Failure to assess suicide risk adequately
- Failure to implement an appropriate treatment plan (use reasonable treatment interventions and safety precautions)

Ordinarily, only the patient with whom the psychiatrist has established a doctor-patient relationship can file a malpractice claim. No duty is owed to family members. Wrongful-death statutes, however, allow survivors to recover money damages for a death caused by another person's wrongful act. The right to sue for wrongful death belongs to individuals who experience financial or other loss because of the patient's death.

Families may bring malpractice suits under the Federal Tort Claims Act (1946) if the individual who died was employed by the U.S. government and the government is accused of wrongdoing. This federal statute permits the government to be sued like any citizen in similar circumstances. It is an exception to the doctrine of sovereign immunity.

Courts evaluate the psychiatrist's assessment and management of the patient who attempted or completed suicide to determine the *reasonableness* of the suicide risk assessment process and whether the patient's suicide attempt or suicide was foreseeable (Simon 2001). *Foreseeability* is a legal term of art rather than a scientific construct. It is a commonsense, probabilistic concept. There is, however, an imperfect fit between legal and medical terminology. Foreseeability is legally defined as the reasonable anticipation that harm or injury is likely to result from certain acts or omissions (Black 1999). The law does not require defendants to "foresee events which are merely possible but only those that are reasonably foreseeable" (*Hairston v. Alexander Tank and Equip. Co.* 1984). Foreseeability should not be confused with the predictability of suicide, for which no professional standard exists (Pokorny 1983). Imminence of suicide is an illusion of short-term prediction. It is not synonymous with foreseeability (Simon 2006). Moreover, foreseeability is not the same as preventability. In hindsight, a suicide may have been preventable but not foreseeable at the time of the assessment.

The assessment of suicide risk is determinable and, therefore, foreseeable. Reasonable clinical basis exists for assessing the patient's suicide risk, but the prediction of suicide is not possible. Contemporaneous documentation of systematic suicide risk assessments provides the court with guidance. When adequate suicide risk assessments are not performed or documented, the court is less able to evaluate the clinical complexities and ambiguities that exist in the assessment, treatment, and management of patients at risk for suicide. The failure to perform an adequate suicide risk assessment is frequently alleged along with other claims of negligence. It is rarely the only complaint.

Basic Elements of Malpractice

Psychiatric malpractice is medical malpractice. Malpractice lawsuits are civil actions that allege negligence, not intentional wrongdoing. A malpractice claim has four

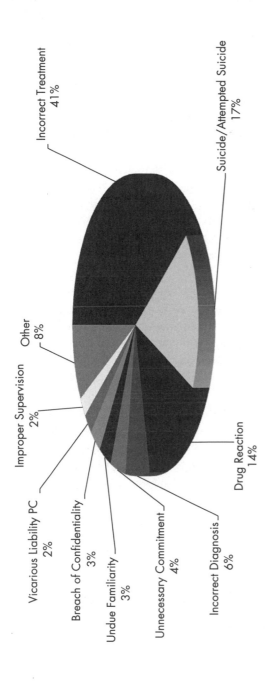

FIGURE 29–1. Most common malpractice claims against psychiatrists, by cause of loss: United States, 2000–2009.

Note. "Other" includes libel/slander, fen-phen, third party (e.g., parents), forensic, other/not specific, administrative, lack of informed consent, Tarasoff, none, abandonment, boundary violation, and premises liability.

The "cause of loss" represents the main allegation in the claim of the lawsuit. In almost all lawsuits, multiple allegations of negligence are asserted. These data are collected based on the chief allegation or complaint. Thus, the category of "incorrect treatment" may be alleged in a lawsuit based on a patient suicide, but the main or chief allegation/complaint is stated as "incorrect treatment." Suicide/attempted suicide is the most frequently identifiable cause of loss. The "drug reaction" category used here encompasses all types of drug/medication misadventures, including errors in prescribing, adverse reactions to medications, mismanagement of a patient's medication regimen, and other unanticipated outcomes related to medication use.

Source. The Psychiatrists' Program, the APA-Endorsed Psychiatrists' Liability Insurance Program, 2009.

basic elements, sometimes referred to as the four *D*'s (see Table 29–2).

Duty of Care

A legal duty of care derives from the existence of a doctor-patient relationship. Usually, a psychiatrist-patient relationship is created knowingly and voluntarily by both parties. No duty of care is owed to a patient unless a psychiatrist-patient relationship exists. However, a psychiatrist–patient relationship may be established unwittingly. Unless working in an emergency department or a similar setting where psychiatrists are legally obligated to treat all individuals who seek help, the psychiatrist owes no duty of care to a prospective patient.

A court will determine whether a psychiatrist-patient relationship existed if a malpractice suit is brought. Several actions may be construed as creating a doctor-patient relationship (Table 29–3). Online consultations may create a doctor-patient relationship with a duty of care. Individuals at risk for suicide should not have their conditions assessed or managed online. Face-to-face psychiatrist-patient interaction is necessary. Psychiatrists also may be vicariously liable for the negligence of others under their supervision or employ.

Deviation From Standard of Care

The standard of care, like the duty of care, is a legal concept. States define by statute the standard of care required of physicians. The precise definition of the standard of care varies from state to state. The specific statutory language is applied to the facts of a malpractice case to determine whether the physician's treatment of the patient was negligent. For example, in *Stepakoff v. Kantar* (1985), the standard of care applied by the court in a suicide case was the "duty to exercise that degree of skill and care ordinarily

TABLE 29–2. Basic elements (four *D*'s) of a malpractice claim

DUTY of care (a doctor-patient relationship must exist)

DEVIATION from the standard of care

DAMAGE to the patient

DIRECT damage caused by the deviation from the standard of care

Source. Adapted from Simon and Shuman 2007a.

employed in similar circumstances by other psychiatrists." The court defined the duty of care as that of the "average psychiatrist." Thus, an adequate suicide risk assessment should meet the standard of care in malpractice litigation. "Best practices" would exceed the "care ordinarily employed" by the "average psychiatrist" (Simon 2005).

The standard of care is determined by expert testimony, practice guidelines, the psychiatric literature, hospital policies and procedures, and other authoritative sources. Managed care protocols and utilization review procedures are entrepreneurial based and are not necessarily clinically authoritative. Guidelines and policies are general concepts that must be applied to highly specific fact patterns of complex cases in litigation. The standard of care is not a fixed legal concept.

Official practice guidelines evolve and change according to new developments in practice and science, necessitating frequent updating. Studies show that no more than 90% of practice guidelines are valid after 3.6 years (Shekelle et al. 2001). At 5.8 years, half of such guidelines are outdated. Sponsoring organizations, such as the American Psychiatric Association (2003), in its "Practice Guideline for the Assessment and Treatment of Patients With Suicidal Behaviors," issue disclaimers that practice guidelines do not represent the standard of care.

TABLE 29–3. Some actions by therapists that may create a doctor-patient relationship

Providing online consultations

Giving advice to prospective patients, friends, and neighbors

Making psychological interpretations

Writing a prescription or providing sample medications

Supervising treatment by a nonmedical therapist

Having a lengthy telephone conversation with a prospective patient

Treating an unexamined patient by mail

Giving a patient an appointment

Telling walk-in patients that they will be seen

Covering for a psychiatrist or other mental health professional

Providing treatment during an evaluation

Source. Adapted from Simon and Shuman 2007a.

The standard of care must be distinguished from the quality of care (Simon 1997). *Quality of care* refers to the adequacy of total care that the patient receives from the psychiatrist and other health care professionals and providers, including third-party payers. The quality of care is also influenced by the patient's health care decisions and the allocation and availability of psychiatric services. The quality of care that is provided by the psychiatrist may be below, be equal to, or even exceed the acceptable standard of psychiatric care.

Generally, a psychiatrist who exercises the "skill and care ordinarily employed" by the "average psychiatrist" will not be held liable for any resulting injury (*Stepakoff v. Kantar* 1985). Mistakes alone are not a basis for liability if the standard of care is not breached. If the court finds that the psychiatrist did not deviate from the standard of care, then no basis for a malpractice claim exists. In psychiatry, the standard of care is broadly defined. For example, a depressed suicidal patient can receive a wider range of treatment than that provided by other specialists for patients with life-threatening illnesses (Hillard 2004).

Although a lawsuit may follow a patient's suicide, the suicide by itself does not establish that the psychiatrist was negligent. In *Siebert v. Fink* (2001), the court held that a clinician is not automatically liable when a patient commits suicide, provided that careful examination and assessment took place that directed the decision-making process. Experts for both the plaintiff (estate of deceased patient) and the defendant psychiatrist provide testimony regarding the standard of care.

The "skill and care ordinarily employed" standard is undergoing change. Tort law generally allows physicians to set their own standard of care; for example, the practice of the "average physician" is the measure applied to negligence claims. Defendants in ordinary tort claims are expected to use reasonable care under the same or similar circumstances. Physicians, however, have needed only to conform their provision of care to the customs of their peers (Peters 2000).

An increasing number of states are rejecting the "medical custom" standard in favor of the "reasonable, prudent physician" standard (Peters 2000). This standard goes beyond a statistical "head count." For example, even if 99 out of 100 psychiatrists do not perform and document adequate suicide risk assessments, such omission constitutes negligent practice that is potentially harmful to patients. Courts have held that negligence cannot be excused simply because others practice the same kind of negligence (Simon 2002). Thus, actual practice must bear a relation to a reasonable, prudent standard of care.

Damage to the Patient

Even if a deviation in the standard of care occurs, legal liability cannot be assessed when the patient is not harmed. The courts rely on the testimony of expert witnesses to determine the presence or absence of harm to the plaintiff. The determination of emotional injury can be difficult because psychiatric disorders or conditions often preexist. Also, the emotional injury claimed may be the result of the natural progression of the patient's psychiatric disorder rather than the harm caused by the psychiatrist's alleged negligence.

Malpractice suits require plaintiffs to prove their allegations by a preponderance of the evidence. *Preponderance of the evidence* is defined as the weight of evidence (51% vs. 49%) for the plaintiff to prevail. The law, however, does not assign a percentage to the standard of proof.

Because malpractice cases are determined by a preponderance of the evidence, the outcome of these suits is often difficult to predict. Defendants who perceive themselves to be vulnerable to substantial monetary awards may choose to settle for a given amount rather than risk open-ended liability.

Direct Damage Caused by Deviation From Standard of Care

If a psychiatrist deviates from the standard of care in the diagnosis and treatment of a patient, no malpractice liability can be found unless the harm to the patient is the direct result of the deviation from the standard of care.

In *Paddock v. Chacko* (1988/1989), a Florida appeals court concluded that the psychiatrist was not liable for the self-inflicted injuries of a patient he had seen only once. The patient had placed herself in her parents' care and custody. The parents disregarded the psychiatrist's recommendation that their daughter be hospitalized. The parents' unwillingness to heed the psychiatrist's recommendation represented a "superseding" factor that intervened between the patient's injuries and the psychiatrist's care.

Therapeutic Risk Management Strategies

- Fully commit to the overall care and treatment of the patient at risk for suicide.
- Carefully document suicide risk assessments. Such documentation shows the provision of good clinical care and provides a sound legal defense in malpractice litigation. Defensible cases are settled or lost as the result of inadequate, altered, or absent documentation.
- Do not unwittingly create a doctor-patient relationship.
- Avoid online assessment and management of patients at risk for suicide. Face-to-face evaluation is clinically necessary.
- Never worry alone. Consider obtaining consultation when confronted by complex, difficult problems in treatment and management of patients at risk for suicide.
- Gain a working knowledge of the legal regulations of psychiatry, which will enable you to manage clinical-legal issues without harming the patient's treatment.
- Use therapeutic risk management that supports both the treatment process and the psychiatrist-patient alliance. At a minimum, risk management should not interfere with patient treatment or introduce destructive defensive practices.

Suicide Risk Assessment

The national suicide rate in the general population for the year 2007 was 11.3 per 100,000 (National Institute of Mental Health

2010). The suicide rate or absolute risk of suicide for individuals with bipolar disorder is estimated to be 193 per 100,000, a relative risk 18 times greater than in the general population (Baldessarini et al. 2003). Thus, 99,807 patients with bipolar disorder do not die by suicide in a given year. On a statistical basis alone, the vast majority of bipolar patients do not die by suicide. Suicide is a low base rate event for all psychiatric disorders. The clinical challenge is to identify and treat those patients who are at significant risk for suicide at any given time (Jacobs et al. 1999). An adequate risk assessment systematically evaluates both risk and protective factors. Perfect assessments of suicide risk are not possible; exhaustive assessments are not necessary. Suicide risk assessment based on current research enables the clinician to make evidence-based treatment and safety management decisions.

Therapeutic Risk Management Strategies for Suicide Assessment

- Effective treatment and safety management of the suicidal patient require a full commitment of time and effort from the clinician (Simon 2011).
- Systematic suicide risk assessment informs the treatment and safety management of patients at risk for suicide. It is a core competency requirement (Scheiber et al. 2003) and is only secondarily, although importantly, a risk management technique.
- Suicide risk assessment is an evolving process, not an event. Psychiatric inpatients should have suicide risk assessments conducted at admission and discharge and at other important clinical decision points during their treatment. A

similar risk assessment process also applies to outpatient treatment.
- The uncertainty that clouds the treatment and safety management of the suicidal patient can be lessened by the process of systematic suicide risk assessment.
- Suicide prevention contracts do not supplant conducting systematic suicide risk assessments.
- Contemporaneous documentation of suicide risk assessments is essential to good clinical care and represents standard psychiatric practice.
- Systematic suicide risk assessment performed at the time of discharge informs the patient's readiness for discharge and postdischarge planning.
- For inpatients at risk for suicide, obtain information of clinical importance from family members or others who know the patient regarding prior or current suicide threats, ideation, plan, or attempts. Whenever possible, the patient's permission should be obtained. Just listening does not violate the patient's confidentiality.
- During the treatment of outpatients at significant risk for suicide, it may become necessary to contact family members or others to facilitate hospitalization, mobilize support, and provide information of clinical importance to the clinician. Whenever possible, the patient's permission should be obtained before contacting family members or others.
- Suicide risk assessment is the responsibility of the psychiatrist. Do not delegate it to others.
- Clinicians have a professional, ethical, and legal duty to provide adequate care to their patients, regardless of managed care protocols and other restrictions. Managed care limitations on patient care should not be allowed to heighten a patient's risk for suicide.

- Personal factors that may potentially interfere with the care of the suicidal patient must be considered. The clinician must make a realistic self-appraisal regarding the number of suicidal patients he or she can competently treat or treat at all.

Suicide Prevention Contracts

The suicide prevention contract has achieved wide acceptance, although no studies find that it is effective in preventing suicide (Stanford et al. 1994). Instead, these contracts often interfere with adequate suicide risk assessment. The suicide prevention contract goes by a variety of names, such as the "no-harm contract," the "no-suicide contract," and the "contract for safety." It is used by psychiatrists and other mental health professionals in outpatient and inpatient settings and in hospital emergency departments. Suicide prevention contracts are now an integral part of nursing assessments (Egan 1997).

With the advent of the managed care era, mental health professionals have come to rely on suicide prevention contracts to manage a patient's risk for suicide (Simon 1999). In both outpatient and inpatient settings, most patients are treated briefly. The length of stay for patients in acute-care psychiatric units and hospitals is, on average, 5 days or less. The most frequent admissions are severely mentally ill patients who are at substantial risk for suicide. The admission requirements usually exceed substantive criteria for involuntary hospitalization.

The therapeutic alliance often fails to develop in managed care settings because of limitations on treatment sessions and an increased reliance on medications. Empathic interaction, pivotal to the development of a therapeutic alliance, is difficult to maintain in managed care settings where a large volume of mentally ill patients are rapidly treated, stabilized, and discharged. Yet these settings are precisely where such contracts are heavily used.

Suicide prevention measures that are not based on a therapeutic alliance are often unreliable. The therapeutic alliance is a dynamic, changeable interaction between the clinician and the patient that is influenced by the course of the patient's illness and by situational and other factors. The therapeutic alliance that supports a patient's safety during one session may dissipate before a next scheduled session because of an acute exacerbation of the illness or other factors. The status of the therapeutic alliance should be assessed regularly and documented. The absence or presence of a therapeutic alliance can be a key suicide risk or preventive factor. Also, health care decision-making capacity, the foundation of the patient's ability to cooperate with a suicide prevention contract or plan, often varies with the patient's clinical course.

Therapeutic Risk Management Strategies for Suicide Prevention Contracts

- If used, the suicide prevention contract should be adjunct to the comprehensive psychiatric evaluation, to ongoing suicide risk assessment, and to safety management planning.
- Suicide prevention contracts cannot take the place of systematic suicide risk assessment. The contract establishes that the patient is a suicide risk but does not establish that suicide risk has been assessed.
- Safety management is an evolving process. A suicide prevention contract is usually an event. If a suicide prevention contract is used, reevaluate it regularly

with the patient, and document rationale for continued use.

- The suicide prevention contract is not viable risk management. Using a suicide prevention contract puts the clinician on notice that systematic risk assessment is necessary.
- A suicide prevention contract is a clinical, not a legal, contract. It is a mutual understanding reached between the clinician and the patient regarding collaboration to prevent suicide. The trustworthiness of the arrangement is contingent on many variables.
- Suicide prevention contracts have little or no utility in emergency settings.
- Mental health professionals need to be aware of the limitations and misuse of suicide prevention contracts.

Outpatients

Most patients at low to moderate risk for suicide, and even some patients at high suicide risk, are treated in outpatient settings. Many patients who were formerly treated as inpatients are now treated as outpatients, some after only a brief hospital stay. Heretofore, lawsuits against therapists for outpatient suicides have been relatively infrequent. Courts have reasoned that when an outpatient attempts or commits suicide, the therapist may not necessarily have breached a duty to protect the patient from self-harm because of the difficulty in controlling the patient (*Bellah v. Greenson* 1978; *Speer v. United States* 1981/1982). In *Kockelman v. Segals* (1998), however, a patient treated for depression as an outpatient died by suicide by taking an overdose of medications. The psychiatrist's attorney moved to dismiss the case on the basis of a California law that did not impose a duty on a psychiatrist to prevent an outpatient from committing sui-

cide. The appellate court held that a psychiatrist owes a duty of care to a patient who commits suicide, whether the patient is an outpatient or an inpatient.

Insurance benefits for the treatment of outpatients are limited by third-party payers. Severely ill inpatients are discharged to outpatient treatment after a brief hospitalization, some at significant risk for suicide. Therapists ("providers") approved by managed care organizations receive patient referrals to provide outpatient psychotherapy. Patients who are at moderate to high risk for suicide require time-intensive psychotherapy. However, only a few sessions may be authorized. When the therapist simply abandons the patient after insurance coverage ends, the liability risk is high if the patient attempts or commits suicide.

Summary discharge of patients when insurance benefits end is an invitation for lawsuits alleging negligent treatment and abandonment of the suicidal patient (Simon and Gutheil 2003). The therapist's professional responsibility to the patient exists independently of managed care organization payments for treatment (Simon 1998b). The therapist's duty of care to the patient is not defined or limited by managed care arrangements.

Currently, outpatient psychiatrists are just as likely as inpatient psychiatrists to be sued for malpractice for alleged negligent treatment of a patient who attempts or commits suicide (Bongar et al. 1998). Legal liability risk exists if the psychiatrist fails to involuntarily hospitalize a patient assessed at high risk for suicide who refuses voluntary hospitalization and attempts or completes suicide.

Partial hospitalization programs and intensive outpatient programs treat patients who are at heightened risk for suicide. Partial hospitalization programs ordinarily treat patients who have recently been discharged from inpatient treatment but continue to require transitional care to maintain stability, to maintain safety, and to prevent rehospitalization. Some patients at high risk for suicide who do not adhere to follow-up treatment programs pose significant liability risk for therapists.

Managed care has facilitated the popularity of partial hospitalization programs and intensive outpatient programs as variations of outpatient psychotherapy. Patients' level of suicide risk and severity of mental illnesses are usually greater in partial hospitalization programs and intensive outpatient programs than in outpatient office settings. Worsening of a patient's condition requires the careful assessment of the patient for 1) the risk of suicide and 2) possible rehospitalization. Risk-benefit assessments regarding continued partial hospitalization program or intensive outpatient program treatment versus hospitalization should be carefully documented. If it is determined that the patient in a partial hospitalization program or intensive outpatient program needs to be hospitalized, the patient should be accompanied by a staff member to the emergency department or to the psychiatric unit for admission. Liability exposure exists for failure to hospitalize a patient who is decompensating, who is at high risk for suicide, or whose symptoms that led to the initial hospitalization are recurring.

Coverage should exist for after-hours emergencies. The patient is instructed in how to get help in an emergency and whom to contact. After-hours coverage is usually provided by the patient's outpatient therapist or psychiatrist or is made available through a local hospital emergency department.

Therapeutic Risk Management Strategies for Outpatients

- Conduct an initial screening for suicide risk with new patients. The presence of suicide risk factors alerts the clinician to conduct a systematic risk assessment.
- An accurate diagnosis informs treatment and management of the suicidal patient. Perform and document a differential diagnosis.
- Formulate a comprehensive, rational treatment and management plan before treatment is started. Document the initial treatment plan and any revisions in the patient's record.
- Avoid e-mail communication in the evaluation, treatment, and management of the patient at risk for suicide.
- Suicide risk assessment is an evolving process, not an event. Conduct systematic suicide risk assessments whenever significant changes occur in the condition, treatment, or management of the suicidal patient. Documentation of suicide risk assessments is essential.
- For new patients, obtain records of prior treatments and make direct contact with former treaters, if possible. Records received deserve careful reading.
- Before speaking with family members, obtain the patient's permission. If the patient withholds permission, document the refusal and address it as a treatment issue. Merely listening to family members does not breach confidentiality. To protect the patient at high suicide risk, it is ethical to reveal confidential information (American Psychiatric Association 2001).
- Negative, even hostile, reactions can occur in the treatment of patients at risk for suicide. Identify countertransference reactions and constructively manage them

so as not to interfere with the patient's treatment.

- Limiting the number of suicidal patients in current treatment may help avoid or mitigate exhaustion and negative feelings toward the patient.
- Consider consultation with a colleague regarding assessment, treatment, and management of complex, difficult patients at risk for suicide. Consultation provides a "biopsy" of the standard of care. "Never worry alone."
- Base the decision to hospitalize a patient at risk for suicide on systematic suicide risk assessment combined with a risk-benefit analysis of factors favoring continued outpatient treatment or hospitalization.
- Use involuntary hospitalization as an emergency clinical intervention, not as a way to avoid malpractice liability or to provide a defense against a malpractice suit. Therapeutic risk management places the patient's treatment first. Unfounded fears of lawsuits may interfere with the psychiatrist's clinical judgment.
- Familiarize yourself with the state laws governing involuntary hospitalization. Knowledge of the legal requirements and the availability of community emergency mental health services facilitates involuntary hospitalization, especially in an emergency.
- Standard measures to prevent patients from harming themselves may include enlisting family members and significant others to provide support during the time of a patient's heightened suicide risk (e.g., facilitating removal and safe disarming of guns and other means of suicide, instructing significant others about administering and monitoring the patient's medications).
- When the decision is made to hospitalize a patient, the patient must go directly to the hospital, accompanied by a responsible escort. A detour may provide an opportunity for the patient to attempt/die by suicide.
- Send a certified letter, return receipt requested, to a patient at risk for suicide who unilaterally terminates outpatient therapy, noting unilateral termination, the need for continued treatment, and the offer of assistance in finding another therapist. This procedure also applies to suicidal patients who do not continue treatment after the first appointment.

Collaborative Treatment

Assessment and management of patients at risk for suicide can be especially challenging in collaborative or split-treatment arrangements (see Chapter 15, "Split Treatment," this volume). The hospital length of stay is very short for most psychiatric patients. Consequently, many patients at moderate to high risk for suicide with severe psychiatric conditions receive split treatment.

Patients usually are referred by managed behavioral health organizations or primary care physicians to psychiatrists for medication management and/or to nonphysician therapists for psychotherapy. Managed behavioral health organizations usually authorize patients to see psychotherapists for more frequent and longer sessions than to see psychiatrists who prescribe medication. When the patient's clinical condition deteriorates in therapy, he or she may be referred to a psychiatrist for consultation or medication management. The patient's deterioration is often associated with an increased risk for suicide.

The essence of collaborative treatment is effective communication. "We are in it together" is the operative phrase. Communication in split treatment is essential, whether the psychiatrist and the psychotherapist have low- or high-volume practices. Psychiatrists and psychotherapists with high-volume split treatment practices may not take the time or have the time to collaborate adequately. For example, a psychiatrist who sees 4 patients for medication management every hour, 8 hours per day for 5 days per week, logs 160 patient visits a week. The psychiatrist may have a patient base of more than 500 individuals. Assuming that the psychiatrist receives 20 patient calls a day from this large patient base, the psychiatrist will receive 140 telephone calls a week. Extremely busy, high-volume medication management practices are common. Will the psychiatrist find the time to collaborate? Collaboration takes time and effort. Adequate communication and collaboration between psychiatrist and psychotherapist is standard practice, especially for patients at risk for suicide.

Communication between psychiatrist and psychotherapist is imperative to prevent the patient at risk for suicide from falling between the cracks of split treatment. When the psychiatrist and therapist work together in a clinic or similar arrangement, communication about the patient is more easily accomplished. However, if the psychiatrist's and the therapist's clinical schedules do not overlap, collaboration may fail to occur. When the psychiatrist and psychotherapist are unknown to each other, communication about the suicidal patient may not occur. Moreover, third-party payers do not compensate clinicians for time spent in collaboration.

Split treatment presents unique clinical, ethical, legal, and administrative challenges for each clinician (Meyer and Simon 1999a, 1999b). Sederer et al. (1998) pointed out that collaborative relationships hold the greatest potential ambiguity for clinical duties and responsibilities. Appelbaum (1991) recommended that the responsibilities of the patient, the psychiatrist, and the nonmedical therapist be clearly specified, preferably in a written agreement.

The patient at risk for suicide must be suited for treatment and management in a split-treatment arrangement. The patient's diagnosis, severity of illness, and level of risk for suicide are all essential factors to consider for suitability when the patient is referred for split treatment. Suitability also applies to the relationship between the psychiatrist and the psychotherapist in split treatment. Some psychiatrists will not enter into a split-treatment arrangement unless they know the psychotherapist personally and have a good sense of his or her clinical competence. Some psychiatrists meet quarterly or semiannually with psychotherapists, sometimes over breakfast or lunch.

A psychiatrist and psychotherapist who do not know each other personally or who are unfamiliar with each other's professional competence to conduct treatment should discuss their ability to treat the patient in split treatment. With severely mentally ill patients at moderate to high risk for suicide, the training and clinical experience of the psychiatrist and therapist should be determined before a split-treatment relationship is initiated. Clinicians with limited training and experience may not be appropriate for such suicidal patients.

Each clinician has the right to terminate an unworkable split-treatment relationship. Despite the best efforts to collaborate, teamwork may fail. Problems causing incompatibility may include diagnostic differences, irreconcilable theoretical and practice styles, and interfering transference and countertransference reactions either to the patient or to the other clinician, or both. The clinician in an unworkable collaborative relationship should resign respectfully from treatment and give sufficient notice to allow the patient and the other clinician to make appropriate treatment arrangements. The patient's best interest must guide the explanations that are given about termination. A patient's risk for suicide may be increased by the perception of rejection or actual abandonment (Gutheil and Simon 2003).

Split treatment artificially separates psychotherapy from medication management. Medication management is always accompanied by some psychotherapeutic interaction. The psychiatrist must not only be a drug dispenser. Empathic engagement of the patient as part of medication management encourages the development of a therapeutic alliance and increases the likelihood of medication adherence. The therapeutic alliance is an important protective factor against suicide (Simon 1998a).

Therapeutic Risk Management Strategies for Collaborative Treatment

- Inquire about the psychotherapist's training, clinical experience, licensure, and malpractice insurance coverage. Welcome the same questions from the psychotherapist.
- Unless the psychiatrist intends to supervise a nonmedical therapist, the therapist and the patient must understand that the split-treatment arrangement is not a supervisory relationship. In a supervisory relationship, the psychiatrist is responsible for monitoring and directing *all* aspects of the patient's psychiatric treatment.
- Effective communication and coordination between clinicians are essential in collaborative treatment, minimizing the risk of divergent clinical goals.
- Do not prescribe potentially lethal amounts of medication to patients at moderate to high risk for suicide, despite managed care policies that encourage bulk purchase of medications.
- Obtain consent from the patient for the psychiatrist and psychotherapist to communicate freely.
- Demarcate clinical responsibilities between the psychiatrist and the psychotherapist to prevent harmful role confusion and misalignment between treaters and with the patient, possibly increasing the patient's risk for suicide.
- Document contacts between clinicians.
- Each clinician should provide for routine and emergency availability for patient coverage during nights, weekends, and vacations.
- Tell patients at risk for suicide which clinician to contact for routine calls and emergencies. Provide emergency telephone numbers to patients for each clinician. Instruct the patient to contact the psychotherapist first in an emergency. Questions about medications are referred to the psychiatrist.
- Prescribe medication and sign treatment plans only for patients personally examined or seen in consultation with the treatment team.
- Do not be bound to collaborative treatment that does not conform to the professional standard of care.
- Psychiatrist and psychotherapist have the right and obligation to terminate participation in an unworkable split-treatment arrangement. Provide sufficient notice and treatment alternatives to the patient and to the other clinician.

Inpatients

The inpatient treatment of psychiatric patients has changed dramatically since the advent of managed care. The goal of psychiatric hospitalization is rapid stabilization of severely ill psychiatric patients through crisis intervention and safety management. Most psychiatric units are analogous to intensive care units, providing short-stay, acute care. Psychiatric patients who are suicidal, homicidal, or gravely disabled pass the strict precertification criteria for admission. Many of these patients have comorbid disorders, including substance abuse and substance use disorders (Simon 1998b).

Patients at high risk for suicide may be prematurely discharged because cost-cutting policies have shortened the hospital length of stay. The average length of stay may be as short as 3–4 inpatient days. Close scrutiny by utilization reviewers allows for only brief hospitalization (Wickizer et al. 1996). The hospital administration may push for early discharge to keep patient length-of-stay statistics within predetermined goals.

Premature discharge of severely ill patients at substantial suicide risk is a major clinical and liability problem for inpatient psychiatrists and hospitals. Early discharge planning begins at the patient's admission. Rapid diagnosis and treatment decisions are essential. The psychiatrist must be able to work collaboratively with other mental health professionals on the treatment team to develop and implement a rational treatment plan.

Inpatients come and go quickly. The psychiatrist has little time to develop a working alliance with patients. Some patients are too disturbed to provide a psychiatric history. Information should be obtained from other sources, such as family members or other individuals who know the patient. Current or previous therapists need to be contacted, with the patient's permission. Records of the prior hospitalization should be obtained and read. A faxed copy of the discharge summary is typically the most information the psychiatrist can obtain

quickly. The clinical decision to hospitalize a patient is an indicator of suicide risk (Bostwick and Pankratz 2000).

In this hurly-burly inpatient environment, the systematic assessment of patients at risk for suicide is often neglected or overlooked. In its place, unfounded reliance is often placed on the suicide prevention contract. A suicide prevention contract with a patient places the clinician on notice that suicide is a concern and that an adequate assessment must be done. Systematic suicide risk assessment is essential because it informs and updates treatment planning and safety management.

A suicide-proof psychiatric unit does not exist. Busch et al. (1993) reported that 5%–6% of the estimated 30,000 suicides a year in the United States occur in the hospital. Similar rates of inpatient suicides have been reported in the United Kingdom. Other studies have found that the suicide rate in the psychiatric hospital population is 1% of the total 30,000 admissions a year (Simon 1992). Inpatient suicides tend to occur shortly after admission or discharge and at change of staff (Qin and Nordentoft 2005). Other attempts or completions occur at mealtimes and at resident rotations.

In general, courts hold psychiatrists accountable more often for inpatient than for outpatient suicides. A substantial number of inpatient suicides are litigated. The duty owed inpatients to prevent suicide attempts or suicide is higher than for outpatients (Macbeth et al. 1994). Courts reason that the opportunities to evaluate, observe, monitor, control, and anticipate a patient's risk for suicide are greater on the psychiatric unit than in the therapist's office.

With the length of stay for patients in psychiatric hospitals drastically reduced, a greater percentage of suicides occur within a few days or months after discharge (Morgan and Stanton 1997). Meehan et al. (2006) found that suicide often occurs on the first day after discharge. A malpractice suit filed against the psychiatrist, claiming premature and negligent discharge of the patient, is a distressingly common occurrence. Negligence in diagnostic evaluation, suicide risk assessment, and treatment, and failure to institute protective measures are other common claims in lawsuits filed against inpatient psychiatrists.

The Joint Commission on Accreditation of Healthcare Organizations (2002) analyzed hospital-based suicides between 1996 and 2001 and identified the following environmental and practice deficiencies: nonbreakaway bars, rods, or safety rails; inadequate security; incomplete or inadequate suicide assessment methods; incomplete reassessment; incomplete orientation and training of staff or inadequate staffing levels; incomplete or infrequent patient observations; incomplete communication among caregivers or unavailable information; and inadequate care planning.

Therapeutic Risk Management Strategies for Inpatients

- Fully commit time and effort to the assessment, treatment, and management of the suicidal patient.
- Perform a timely, complete psychiatric examination, including a careful mental status evaluation.
- Formulate, document, and implement a comprehensive, rational treatment plan on admission, to be reviewed and updated as needed.
- Conduct systematic suicide risk assessments at the patient's admission and discharge and at other important clinical decision junctures.
- Monitor and aggressively treat the patient's acute suicide risk factors.

- Mobilize protective factors.
- When patients have threatened or attempted suicide, do not accept their denial of suicidal ideation, intent, or plan without further suicide risk assessment. Be alert for other clinical correlates of suicide risk.
- Adjust the patient's safety precautions according to ongoing systematic suicide risk assessment.
- Obtain prior records of treatment and/ or speak with current or prior treaters.
- Early discharge planning begins at the time of the patient's admission.
- Interview family members or significant others with the patient's permission. If the patient refuses permission, the clinician may listen but not disclose patient information.
- Work closely with the multidisciplinary team in assessing suicide risk, in conducting treatment, and in providing safety management. The team is present 24 hours a day, 7 days a week.
- Designate a responsible family member or other person to remove and safely disarm guns, which could be used by the patient to die by suicide. Ask the responsible individual to call the clinician within a specified time to confirm that guns and ammunition have been removed from the home and are safely secured elsewhere. Feedback is essential because effective compliance with gun removal tends to be low.
- Secure other lethal means for attempting or committing suicide. These may include knives, poisons, over-the-counter and prescription medications (e.g., analgesics), and car keys. A family member may need to dispense and monitor the patient's medication.
- Abide by hospital and psychiatric unit policy and procedures regarding the management of patients at risk for sui-

cide. The standard of care is often reflected in official policies and procedures.

- Contemporaneously document assessment, treatment, and safety management decisions. All documentation should legibly document all times and dates. If the patient attempts or commits suicide and litigation ensues, the plaintiff's attorney may argue to the court that what was not documented was not done.
- Provide patient autonomy and freedom of movement consistent with the patient's treatment and safety needs.
- At the time of contemplated discharge, carefully assess and document the risks and benefits of continued hospitalization compared with the risks and benefits of discharge. What remains unchanged or is different from the time of admission to the time of discharge regarding the patient's mental condition and life situation? Can the patient be managed as an outpatient?
- Structure aftercare planning for maximal compliance by the patient.
- Do not discharge patients who are still on individualized suicide safety precautions. Observe the patient while off safety precautions before discharge.
- Determine whether family members or significant others are supportive or destabilizing to the patient. Especially in the latter instance, determine whether psychosocial interventions are available that could make a difference.
- Exaggerating the severity of the patient's condition to qualify for managed care organization approval exposes the psychiatrist to increased liability risk when the patient is discharged early or prematurely.
- Educate patients and, if feasible, their families about mental disorders.
- Do not discharge patients from the hospital solely for financial reasons. Although the delivery of medical care has changed dramatically under managed care, provide competent care within the system.
- Prior to discharge, discuss with the patient whom to contact or where to go if an emergency arises after discharge. Provide telephone numbers.
- Attend inpatients each day of their hospitalization, including the day of discharge. A patient's clinical condition can deteriorate rapidly as discharge approaches.

Emergency Psychiatric Services

Patients at risk for suicide are frequently assessed and managed in emergency psychiatric services. Wingerson et al. (2001), in a study of 2,319 consecutive patients who visited a crisis triage unit, found that 30% had unipolar depression, 26% had psychosis, 20% had substance use disorder, 14% had bipolar disorder, 4% had adjustment disorder, 3% had anxiety disorder, and 2% had dementia. Dhossche (2000) found that 38% of psychiatric emergencies involved suicidal ideation or behavior. Postdischarge psychiatric patients are frequently evaluated in emergency departments. Ostamo and Lönnqvist (2001), in a 50-year follow-up study of patients treated in hospitals after suicide attempts, found an increase in mortality from suicide, homicide, and other causes. In the follow-up period, 16% of suicide attempters died, 40% by suicide.

Many psychiatric patients who are evaluated in the emergency department of a hospital have more than one psychiatric disorder, substantially increasing the risk for suicide (Kessler et al. 1999). Standardized mortality ratios establish that virtually all psychiatric disorders have an associated risk for suicide (Harris and Barraclough 1997).

Patients evaluated in emergency psychiatric services not only have an increased risk for suicide associated with their psychiatric disorders (necessary factors) but also experience stressful life circumstances (sufficient factors) that impart additional risk. The importance of stress factors in precipitating suicides has been noted in several studies (Heikkinen et al. 1994; Maltsberger et al. 2003). Suicide attempts or completed suicides are invariably caused by the confluence of necessary and sufficient factors.

Important goals of emergency psychiatric services include provision of rapid assessments to determine the appropriate setting for treatment and to provide stabilization and safety for patients. The basic types of emergency psychiatric services are the consultation model and the specialized psychiatric emergency services (Breslow 2002). In the consultation model, the psychiatrist consults with the emergency department staff. A number of emergency departments have crisis counselors who initially evaluate psychiatric patients after they have been "medically cleared" by emergency department physicians. The on-call psychiatrist is usually consulted when an inpatient admission is contemplated or for other emergent matters. The proposed disposition of the patient is discussed with the psychiatrist. The psychiatrist may agree, disagree, or request additional information before making a final decision. When the emergency department physician, crisis counselor, or psychiatrist disagrees with the evaluation or disposition, the psychiatrist is usually required to come to the emergency department and examine the patient. The same situation applies when the emergency department physician calls the on-call psychiatrist in the absence of a crisis counselor arrangement.

Emergency Medical Treatment and Active Labor Act (EMTALA) regulations were enacted to protect patients from dangerous transfers by requiring that they be stabilized first (Quinn et al. 2002). A suicidal patient would likely be considered stable for discharge or transfer when he or she is no longer assessed to be a threat to self or others. Emergency department clinicians (including psychiatrists and crisis counselors) should be familiar with EMTALA requirements for appropriate transfer of patients generally, but especially for patients at risk for suicide.

Therapeutic Risk Management Strategies for Emergency Psychiatric Services

- Perform systematic suicide risk assessment on all psychiatric patients evaluated in the emergency department.
- Remember that suicide prevention contracts have little or no utility in emergency settings.
- Observe and assess other clinical correlates of suicide risk that do not rely on patient reporting. Individuals who come to the emergency department because of suspected suicidal behaviors may deny suicidal ideation, intent, or plan.
- Obtain patient information from collateral sources (e.g., family, significant others, police, emergency department records of previous visits, current and former treaters). The individual may tell significant others the full extent of suicidal intent or a plan. Obtaining collateral information is an important part of the suicide risk assessment process.
- Routinely screen for drug and alcohol use in patients at risk for suicide.
- Some patients at moderate or even high risk for suicide may be managed as out-

patients if sufficient protective factors against suicide are present. Construct a reasonable follow-up plan with the patient, including contact with treaters, if possible.

- Assess the risks and benefits of hospitalization compared with the risks and benefits of discharge as part of the dispositional decision-making process.
- Avoid reflexive or "gut" inpatient admissions or discharges from the emergency department. Careful evaluation and systematic assessment of the patient at risk for suicide inform clinical decision making, especially for patients with "special agendas" (e.g., admission seekers or high-risk suicide deniers).
- In emergencies, when treatment is necessary to save a life or to prevent serious harm, the law "presumes" that consent would have been granted by the patient.
- Secure the patient's safety throughout the assessment process. Patients at high risk for suicide may injure themselves in the emergency department or may elope. Anticipate and institute preventive safety measures when indicated.
- Know what mental health resources are available in the community. It is necessary for psychiatrists who work in or consult with the emergency department to be knowledgeable about the mental health resources available in the community. Patients discharged from the emergency department require followup instructions; when possible, schedule appointments for early evaluation and treatment.
- Thoroughly document evaluations, clinical interventions, suicide risk assessments, risk-benefit determinations, and the decision-making process.
- Carefully assess all patients at risk for suicide without exception. There is no such thing as a "VIP patient."

- Follow EMTALA mandates requiring appropriate screening examination, stabilization, and transfer or discharge of individuals seeking emergency services.

Suicide Aftermath

After a patient's death, the duty to maintain confidentiality of the patient's record continues, unless a court decision or statute provides otherwise. Careful documentation and maintenance of confidentiality of the patient's records provide a sound defense in malpractice litigation as well as in administrative and ethics proceedings. Suicide aftermath presents the clinician with conflicting tensions between maintaining patient confidentiality, providing support to the suicide survivors, and implementing risk management principles that limit liability exposure.

Thomas Gutheil (personal communication, October 1989) recommends postsuicide family outreach by the clinician as crucial for the devastated family members following a suicide. This recommendation, which is based primarily on humanitarian concerns for survivors, has important risk management implications. Gutheil points out that "bad feelings" combined with a bad outcome often lead to litigation. The persons who lived with the patient before the suicide not only currently experience intense emotional pain but also shared it with the patient before death. Some lawsuits are filed because of the clinician's refusal to express, in some way, feelings of condolence, sympathy, and regret for the patient's death.

In Massachusetts, an "apology statute" exists that renders various benevolent human expressions, such as condolences, regrets, and apologies, "inadmissible as evidence of an admission of liability in a civil action" (Mass. Gen. Laws 1986). Slovenko (2002) noted that Texas and California enacted legislation similar to that in Massachusetts. The highest courts of Georgia and Vermont provided apology protection by judicial opinions in 1992. However, as Regehr and Gutheil (2002) noted, "The current empirical evidence is insufficiently solid to support the proposition that apology by oppressors, perpetrators, and a defendant is a panacea leading to healing of trauma under all circumstances" (pp. 429–430).

A fine line exists between a psychiatrist's apology and the perception that fault is being admitted. Admissions of wrongdoing may void insurance coverage (Slovenko 2002). Moreover, another party may be found ultimately at fault in litigation, not the psychiatrist. A skillful lawyer may take feelings of genuine sympathy and turn them against the psychiatrist as an admission of fault. To say "I am sorry" is certainly the appropriate human response, but it may backfire in a litigation context. The psychiatrist must be guided by good judgment, not by guilt-driven feelings.

Attorneys advise psychiatrists in different ways about suicide aftercare. Following a bad outcome, many attorneys recommend that the case be sealed and no communication be established with the family. Some attorneys, however, encourage judicious communication with, consultation with, or even treatment of family members. The treatment of family members by the psychiatrist who treated the patient before his or her suicide is likely doomed from the start by insurmountable transference and countertransference reactions. The family should be referred for treatment. In meeting with family members, the psychiatrist should focus on addressing the feelings of family members rather than the specifics of the patient's care.

Suicide aftercare is similar to any other grief-related therapy or consultation. The value of such consultation in healing grief is important enough for clinicians to consider providing humanitarian support to the survivors of patient suicide. The clinician may justifiably worry that contact with survivors of suicide will increase the risk of a lawsuit. Outreach to survivors of patient suicides should not be undertaken primarily for risk management purposes. No easy answers exist for managing the complex and often conflicting tensions between suicide aftercare and risk management.

Most practicing psychiatrists can expect that a patient suicide will occur during their years of practice. Psychiatrists' reactions to a patient's suicide often include shame, guilt, anger, avoidance behaviors, intrusive thoughts, questioning of competency, and litigation fears (Gitlin 1999; Hendin et al. 2000; see also Chapter 21, "Psychiatrist Reactions to Patient Suicide," this volume). The Clinical Division of the American Association of Suicidology makes several resources available to clinicians whose patients have completed suicide (see www.suicidology.org).

Therapeutic Risk Management Strategies for the Aftermath of Suicide

- The duty to maintain confidentiality of patient records follows the patient in death, unless provided otherwise by a specific court decision or statute.
- The physician-patient privilege that protects confidentiality does not end with the patient's death. It may be claimed by the deceased patient's next of kin or a legal representative.
- Obtain written authorization from the executor or administrator of the deceased patient's estate before a *copy* of the medical record is released.

- If the psychiatrist must disclose confidential information about a deceased patient, legal exposure may be minimized by providing only enough information about the matter at issue.
- Follow standard documentation procedures for correcting errors and misunderstandings. Accurately date postincident written statements.
- Do not tamper with, delete, change, or destroy anything in the patient's record after a suicide.
- Retain patient records at least for the length of time that malpractice claims can be brought according to a state's statute of limitations. Consider keeping patient records indefinitely for administrative, licensure, or ethical proceedings that are not governed by the statute of limitations.
- Consider consulting with an attorney before making any oral or written statements regarding a patient's suicide or suicide attempt or before releasing patient records, unless such actions are to assist in the current clinical care of a patient who has attempted suicide.
- Consider the appropriateness of sending a condolence card or attending the deceased patient's funeral on a case-by-case basis. Discuss with the grieving family their feelings about your attending the patient's funeral. Do not arrive at the funeral unannounced.
- Suicide aftercare is a clinically based outreach effort to survivors of suicide, including clinicians who lose patients to suicide. No easy answers exist for handling the complexity of suicide aftercare and risk management. Case-by-case decisions are required.
- After a patient's suicide, immediately inform the professional liability insurance carrier.

Key Clinical Concepts

- Fully commit the time and effort necessary for the care and treatment of the patient at risk for suicide.

- Perform and contemporaneously document adequate suicide risk assessments.

- Obtain prior treatment records and information from significant others, if possible.

- Consider personal factors that can interfere with care of the suicidal patient.

- Do not allow managed care limitation of payments to interfere with the provision of good clinical care.

References

American Psychiatric Association: Risk management issues in psychiatric practice. Workshop presented at the American Psychiatric Association Psychiatrist's Purchasing Group, Inc., Component Workshop, 155th annual meeting of the American Psychiatric Association, Philadelphia, PA, May 18–23, 2002

American Psychiatric Association: Practice guideline for the assessment and treatment of patients with suicidal behaviors. Am J Psychiatry 160(suppl):1–60, 2003

American Psychiatric Association: Principles of Medical Ethics With Annotations Especially Applicable to Psychiatry, Section 4, Annotation 8. Washington, DC, American Psychiatric Association, 2009

Appelbaum PS: General guidelines for psychiatrists who prescribe medication for patients treated by nonmedical psychotherapists. Hosp Community Psychiatry 42:281–282, 1991

Baldessarini RJ, Tondo L, Hennen J: Lithium treatments and suicide risk in major affective disorders: update and new findings. J Clin Psychiatry 64 (suppl 5):44–52, 2003

Bellah v Greenson, 81 Cal App 3d 614, 146 Cal Rptr 525 (1978)

Black HC: Black's Law Dictionary, 7th Edition. St Paul, MN, West Group, 1999

Bongar B, Maris RW, Berman AL, et al: Outpatient standards of care and the suicidal patient, in Risk Management With Suicide Patients. Edited by Bongar B, Berman AL, Maris FW, et al. New York, Guilford, 1998, pp 4–13

Bostwick JM, Pankratz VS: Affective disorders and suicide risk: a re-examination. Am J Psychiatry 157:1925–1932, 2000

Breslow RE: Structure and function of psychiatric emergency services, in Emergency Psychiatry. Edited by Allen MH. Washington, DC, American Psychiatric Publishing, 2002, pp 35–74

Brown J, Rayne JT: Some ethical considerations in defensive psychiatry: a case study. Am J Orthopsychiatry 59:534–541, 1989

Busch KA, Clark DC, Fawcett J, et al: Clinical features in inpatient suicide. Psychiatr Ann 23:256–262, 1993

Dhossche DM: Suicidal behavior in psychiatric emergency room patients. South Med J 93:310–314, 2000

Egan MP: Contracting for safety: a concept analysis. Crisis 18:17–23, 1997

Federal Tort Claims Act, 28 USCA § § 1346(b), 2674 (1946)

Gitlin MJ: A psychiatrist's reaction to a patient's suicide. Am J Psychiatry 156:1630–1634, 1999

Gutheil TG, Simon RI: Abandonment of patients in split treatment. Harv Rev Psychiatry 11:175–179, 2003

Hairston v Alexander Tank and Equip Co, 310 NC 227, 234, 311 SE2d 559, 565 (1984)

Harris CE, Barraclough B: Suicide as an outcome for mental disorders: a meta analysis. Br J Psychiatry 170:205–228, 1997

Heikkinen M, Aro H, Lönnqvist J: Recent life events, social support and suicide. Acta Psychiatr Scand Suppl 377:65–72, 1994

Hendin H, Lipschitz A, Maltsberger JT, et al: Therapists' reactions to patients' suicides. Am J Psychiatry 157:2022–2027, 2000

Hillard JR: Malpractice: why do we worry so much? (editorial) Curr Psychiatr 3:3, 2004

Jacobs DG, Brewer M, Klein-Benheim M: Suicide assessment: an overview and recommended protocol, in The Harvard Medical School Guide to Suicide Assessment and Intervention. Edited by Jacobs DJ. San Francisco, CA, Jossey-Bass, 1999, pp 3–39

Joint Commission on Accreditation of Healthcare Organizations: Hospital Accreditation Standards. Chicago, IL, Joint Commission on Accreditation of Healthcare Organizations, 2002, PE 1.7.1

Kessler RC, Borges G, Walters EE: Prevalence of and risk factors for lifetime suicide: suicide attempts in the National Comorbidity Survey. Arch Gen Psychiatry 56:617–626, 1999

Kockelman v Segals, 61 Cal App 4th 491, 71 Cal Rptr 2d 552 (1998)

Macbeth JE, Wheeler AM, Sithers J, et al: Legal and Risk Management Issues in the Practice of Psychiatry. Washington, DC, Psychiatrist's Purchasing Group, 1994

Maltsberger JT, Hendin H, Haas AP, et al: Determination of precipitating events in the suicide of psychiatric patients. Suicide Life Threat Behav 33:111–119, 2003

Mass Gen Laws ch. 233, §23D (1986)

Meehan J, Kapur N, Hunt I, et al: Suicide in mental health in-patients and within 3 months of discharge. Br J Psychiatry 188:129–134, 2006

Meyer DJ, Simon RI: Split treatment: clarity between psychiatrists and psychotherapists, part I. Psychiatr Ann 29:241–245, 1999a

Meyer DJ, Simon RI: Split treatment: clarity between psychiatrists and psychotherapists, part II. Psychiatr Ann 29:327–332, 1999b

Miller MC, Jacobs DG, Gutheil TG: Talisman or taboo: the controversy of the suicide prevention contract. Harv Rev Psychiatry 6:78–87, 1998

Morgan HG, Stanton R: Suicide among psychiatric in-patients in a changing clinical scene. Br J Psychiatry 171:561–563, 1997

National Institute of Mental Health: Suicide in the U.S.: Statistics and Prevention. September 27, 2010. Available at: http://www.nimh.nih.gov/health/publications/suicide-in-the-us-statistics-and-prevention/index.shtml. Accessed June 28, 2011.

Ostamo A, Lönnqvist J: Excess mortality in suicide attempters. Soc Psychiatry Psychiatr Epidemiol 36:29–35, 2001

Paddock v Chacko, 522 So2d 410 (Fla Dist Ct App 1988), review denied, 553 So2d 168 (Fla 1989)

Peters PG: The quiet demise of deference to custom: malpractice law at the millennium. Wash Lee Law Rev 57:163–205, 2000

Pokorny AD: Predictions of suicide in psychiatric patients: report of a prospective study. Arch Gen Psychiatry 40:249–257, 1983

Qin P, Nordentoft M: Suicide risk in relation to psychiatric hospitalization: evidence based on longitudinal registers. Arch Gen Psychiatry 62:427–432, 2005

Quinn DK, Geppert CMA, Maggiore WA: The Emergency Medical Treatment and Active Labor Act of 1985 and the practice of psychiatry. Psychiatr Serv 53:1301–1307, 2002

Regehr C, Gutheil TG: Apology, justice and trauma recovery. J Am Acad Psychiatry Law 30:425–429, 2002

Scheiber SC, Kramer TS, Adamowski SE: Core Competencies for Psychiatric Practice: What Clinicians Need to Know (A Report of the American Board of Psychiatry and Neurology). Washington, DC, American Psychiatric Publishing, 2003

Sederer LI, Ellison J, Keyes C: Guidelines for prescribing psychiatrists in consultative, collaborative and supervisory relationships. Psychiatr Serv 49:1197–1202, 1998

Shekelle PG, Ortiz E, Rhodes S, et al: Validity of the Agency for Healthcare Research and Quality clinical practice guidelines: how quickly do guidelines become outdated? JAMA 286:1461–1467, 2001

Siebert v Fink, 280 AD2d 661, 720 NYS2d 564 (2d Dep't 2001)

Simon RI: Coping strategies for the "unduly" defensive psychiatrist. Int J Med Law 4:551–561, 1985

Simon RI: Clinical Psychiatry and the Law, 2nd Edition. Washington, DC, American Psychiatric Press, 1992

Simon RI: Discharging sicker, potentially violent psychiatric inpatients in the managed care era: standard of care and risk management. Psychiatr Ann 27:726–733, 1997

Simon RI: Psychiatrists awake! Suicide risk assessments are all about a good night's sleep. Psychiatr Ann 38:479–485, 1998a

Simon RI: Psychiatrists' duties in discharging sicker and potentially violent inpatients in the managed care era. Psychiatr Serv 49:62–67, 1998b

Simon RI: The suicide prevention contract: clinical, legal and risk management issues. J Am Acad Psychiatry Law 27:445–450, 1999

Simon RI: Concise Guide to Psychiatry and Law for Clinicians, 3rd Edition. Washington, DC, American Psychiatric Publishing, 2001

Simon RI: Suicide risk assessment: what is the standard of care? J Am Acad Psychiatry Law 30:340–344, 2002

Simon RI: Best practices or reasonable care? J Am Acad Psychiatry Law 33:8–11, 2005

Simon RI: Imminent suicide: the illusion of short-term prediction. Suicide Life Threat Behav 36:296–301, 2006

Simon RI: Preventing Patient Suicide: Clinical Assessment and Management. Washington, DC, American Psychiatric Publishing, 2011

Simon RI, Gutheil TG: Abandonment of patients in split treatment. Harv Rev Psychiatry 11:175–179, 2003

Simon RI, Shuman DW: Clinical Manual of Psychiatry and Law. Washington, DC, American Psychiatric Publishing, 2007a

Simon RI, Shuman DE: Therapeutic risk management of clinical-legal dilemmas: should it be a core competency? J Am Acad Psychiatry Law 37:155–161, 2007b

Simon RI, Shuman DW: Clinical-legal issues in psychiatry, in Kaplan & Sadock's Comprehensive Textbook of Psychiatry, 9th Edition. Edited by Sadock BJ, Sadock VA. Philadelphia, PA, Lippincott Williams & Williams, 2009, pp 4427–4438

Slovenko R: Psychiatry in Law/Law in Psychiatry. New York, Brunner-Routledge, 2002

Speer v United States, 512 F Supp 670 (ND Tex 1981), aff'd, 675 F2d 100 (5th Cir 1982)

Stanford EJ, Goetz RR, Bloom JD: The no harm contract in the emergency assessment of suicide risk. J Clin Psychiatry 55:344–348, 1994

Stepakoff v Kantar, 473 N.E.2d 1131, 1134 (Mass 1985)

Wexler DB, Winick BJ: Essays in Therapeutic Jurisprudence. Durham, NC, Carolina Academic Press, 1991

Wexler DB, Winick BJ: Law in a Therapeutic Key: Developments in Therapeutic Jurisprudence. Durham, NC, Carolina Academic Press, 1996

Wickizer TM, Lessler D, Travis KM: Controlling inpatient psychiatric utilization through managed care. Am J Psychiatry 153:339–345, 1996

Wingerson D, Russo J, Ries R, et al: Use of psychiatric emergency services and enrollment status in a public managed mental health plan. Psychiatr Serv 52:1494–1501, 2001

PART VII

Prevention

C H A P T E R 3 0

Suicide Prevention by Lethal Means Restrictions

David Lester, Ph.D.

A universal technique for preventing suicide is the restriction of access to the means (or methods) for committing suicide.[1] If the means for committing suicide were less readily available, then suicidal individuals would be less able to make lethal impulsive suicide attempts. Many scholars have argued for this strategy for preventing suicide, but the notion is usually attributed to Stengel (1964), who discussed the role that the detoxification of domestic gas played in reducing national suicide rates. Seiden and Spence (1983–1984) also drew attention to this strategy, noting, for example, that the Golden Gate Bridge in San Francisco is a much more popular locale for suicide than the Bay Bridge. Erecting fences on Golden Gate Bridge would prevent suicides from that locale.

The first convincing demonstration of the possible effectiveness of this strategy was by Kreitman (1976), who showed that the drop in the English suicide rate was the result of the detoxification of coal gas. The percentage of toxic carbon monoxide in coal gas declined from 13% in 1955 to 0% in 1975 as the country switched to less toxic natural gas for domestic use. The suicide rate by carbon monoxide declined in all age groups and for both sexes. The suicide rate by other methods rose over the same period, but not sufficiently to prevent a decline in the overall suicide rate. This early study illustrated the two questions involved in this strategy: 1) Does the restriction of access to a method for suicide lower the overall suicide rate by that method? 2) What proportion of people would switch to other methods for suicide if their preferred method was not easily available? In this chapter I briefly review the research on these questions and examine the implications of the results of the research for theory and prevention.

---

[1]In earlier terminology, this is a secondary prevention strategy.

A Survey of Research

Research has been conducted on the availability of a number of methods for committing suicide: domestic gas, car exhaust, jumping, medications and poisons, firearms, and charcoal burning.

Domestic Gas

Domestic gas was for many years coal gas, which has a high concentration of carbon monoxide, resulting in a reasonably certain and quick death if inhaled without ventilation. As reserves of natural gas were discovered, many nations switched to natural gas for domestic use. Natural gas is much less toxic, and the suicidal person has to die from suffocation rather than carbon monoxide poisoning. This change was introduced for economic reasons; the prevention of suicide was an unexpected side effect.

Improving on Kreitman's (1976) data analysis, Clarke and Mayhew (1988) documented precisely the gradual detoxification of domestic gas in England and Wales and the declining rate of suicide by means of domestic gas. They showed that the two curves followed each other extremely closely. In 1958, 2,637 suicides out of 5,298 suicides involved domestic gas, or 49.8% of the total number of suicides. By 1977, 8 suicides of 3,944 suicides involved domestic gas, or only 0.2% of the suicides. As can be seen, the total number of suicides also dropped over this period.

Studies of the impact of this change on suicide rates have been carried out in many countries, and always the use of domestic gas for suicide declined. Lester (1995) studied whether the detoxification of domestic gas leads to a reduction in the overall suicide rate. He compared the changes in suicide rates by domestic gas, by all other methods, and overall in six nations: Japan, the Netherlands, Northern Ireland, Scotland, Switzerland, and the United States. In three nations (Northern Ireland, Scotland, and Switzerland), the suicide rate using domestic gas was high initially, and the overall suicide rate declined as domestic gas was detoxified. In three nations (Japan, the Netherlands, and the United States), the suicide rate using domestic gas was low initially, and in all of them the overall suicide rate increased as domestic gas was detoxified. Thus, the total suicide rate appears to have been reduced by making toxic domestic gas less available only in those nations where it was a common method for suicide.

One problem associated with the detoxification of domestic gas is that suicide using car exhaust is a similar method. Clarke and Lester (1989) showed that during the period when domestic gas was detoxified in England and the suicide rate using domestic gas declined, the use of car exhaust for suicide rose. Apparently, the rise in the use of car exhaust was not large enough to offset the decline in the use of domestic gas, but it does look as if switching methods (also known as substitution of methods) did occur to some extent.

Car Exhaust

In 1968, the United States began to impose emission controls for motor vehicles in order to improve air quality. The result was that the carbon monoxide content in car exhaust dropped from 8.5% to 0.05% by 1980. This has made suicide more difficult to commit using car exhaust. Poisoning from carbon monoxide takes some time, thereby increasing the chance of intervention by others and a change of mind by the suicidal person. However, in car exhaust from which the carbon monoxide has been removed, death occurs by suffocation from displacement of the air from the car's cabin. Death from simple suffocation takes much longer than poisoning by carbon monoxide and therefore increases the chances of individuals changing their minds about dying and of intervention by others.

Clarke and Lester (1987) found that the use of car exhaust for suicide in the United States leveled off after 1968 and then declined slightly. (It must be remembered that older, more toxic cars were still in use and that the emission control system can be disconnected to permit gas richer in carbon monoxide to fill the car or garage.) In contrast, in England and Wales, where emission controls had not been imposed on motor vehicles, the use of car exhaust for suicide rose dramatically after 1970. Skilling et al. (2008) found that the use of car exhaust in Scotland increased regularly each year until catalytic converter legislation was introduced in 1993, after which the rate fell.

However, no decline in the use of car exhaust for suicide was observed initially in Australia after emission controls for cars were mandated there. Routley and Ozanne-Smith (1998) suggested several factors in why car exhaust suicides did not decline: 1) carbon monoxide emissions while a car is idling have not been measured for the new cars and could be higher than the levels measured when driving; 2) carbon monoxide emissions have not been measured inside cars, whose cabins vary in volume, when the car exhaust enters through a hose connected to the exhaust pipe; 3) carbon monoxide content may be higher before the engine warms up; and 4) catalytic converters deteriorate over time. However, later research (e.g., Studdert et al. 2010) found a decline in the suicide rate using car exhaust in Australia after 2001, along with declines in the presence of pre-1999 and pre-1986 cars in use. Regions with relatively fewer old cars had relatively greater declines in the suicide rate using car exhaust.

Despite this disparity in the results of research, simple inexpensive changes in car design could reduce the attractiveness of this method for committing suicide, such as changing the shape of the exhaust pipe from a circle to a flattened slit, so that a tube would no longer fit easily over the pipe, or installing automatic turn-off systems if the car engine idles for more than one minute. However, car exhaust is not a very common method for suicide in most countries, and so reducing the use of car exhaust for suicide might not have a significant impact on the overall suicide rate.

Jumping

There are several venues for using jumping as a method for suicide. First, individuals who intend to die by suicide jump from high buildings. In Singapore, Lester (1994) found that the suicide rate by leaping from high-rise apartment buildings was positively associated with their increased availability (as the construction of such buildings increased) and that whereas the suicide rate by all other methods declined, the total suicide rate increased during the period studied. Suicide by jumping is also popular in Hong Kong, another high-density city with many high-rise buildings. Restricting access to the roof and fencing in areas from which people can jump (as has been done for the Empire State Building in New York City) are simple ways to restrict access to this method of suicide.

People also jump in front of trains, especially subway trains. It has been shown that this is especially common for psychiatric patients who have less access to other methods for suicide. In the London subway, the suicide rate is higher in those stations close to psychiatric hospitals. The provision of a pit in the floor beneath the tracks (often called a *suicide pit*) results in some jumpers falling into the pit, thereby not being hit and killed by the train.

Law et al. (2009) used a natural quasi-experiment in the subways of Hong Kong, where one system, the Mass Transit Railway (MTR), installed platform screen doors (in order to reduce air-conditioning costs) in 2002–2005, whereas the other system, the Kowloon-Canton Railway (KCR), did not. On the MTR system, there were 38 suicides in the 5-year period from 1997 through 2001 but only 7 in the 5-year period from 2003 through 2007. In contrast, the corresponding numbers for the KCR system were 13 and 15, respectively. The reduction in suicides on the MTR system seemed to be present for both those with a psychiatric history and those without such a history. Suicide on the railway did not constitute a large proportion of the suicides in Hong Kong, and so the installation of platform doors did not have an impact on the total Hong Kong suicide rate.

Suicidal individuals also jump from bridges. Seiden and Spence (1983–1984) showed that people drove over the Bay Bridge between Oakland and San Francisco in California in order to jump off the Golden Gate Bridge, but rarely, if ever, did people drive over the Golden Gate Bridge in order to jump off the Bay Bridge. No out-of-state suicidal individuals jumped from the Bay Bridge. Thus, fencing in common suicide venues might prevent suicides by those trying to end their lives by jumping. Lester (1993) found that fencing in a bridge that was a common suicide venue in Washington, D.C., not only reduced the number of suicides from that bridge but appeared to lower the total number of bridge suicides in the city as a whole. Glasgow (2011) examined 3,116 American counties and found that those with a landmark bridge had a significantly higher suicide rate by jumping.

Beautrais (2001) took advantage of a decision by a town council in Australia or New Zealand (Beautrais did not want to name the town) to remove safety barriers from a bridge on the grounds that 1) they were unsightly, 2) they impeded rescue efforts, and 3) they did not prevent suicide. In the 4-year periods before and after the removal of the barriers, the number of suicides increased from 3 to 15, with an estimated rate of 0.29 per 100,000 per year before removal of the barriers and a rate of 1.29 afterward.

Beautrais also looked at the evidence for switching. Did more suicides occur by jumping elsewhere in the city? Focusing on the 2-year periods before and after removal of the barriers, the author found that the number of suicides by jumping remained constant (14 in each 2-year period), but the location did switch to the newly unfenced bridge, a change that was statistically significant. These data suggest that switching did occur to the bridge where the barriers had been removed.

Beautrais noted that the majority of the individuals who died by suicide from the bridge were men, persons with schizophrenia, inpatients, or those in residential care at the time. Those jumping from other sites included more women, were somewhat older, and were somewhat less likely to be schizophrenic individuals or psychiatric inpatients, but the numbers were too small for reliable conclusions to be drawn about the differences in the two groups. If the groups did differ in characteristics, then this would argue against switching having occurred. Instead, the removal of the safety barriers may have increased the rate of suicide only among some groups of the population (in this case, schizophrenic individuals).

It is interesting to note that bridge barriers are often erected after strong pressure has been applied from groups representing psychiatric patients. A fence (a "luminous veil") was installed at the Bloor Street Viaduct in Toronto, Canada, after years of pressure from the Schizophrenia Society of Ontario, beginning in 1997 (Lester 2009). The barrier was erected in 2002, after more than 400 people had jumped from the bridge since its opening in 1918. After the barrier was erected, no suicides occurred from the bridge, but suicides from other bridges in Toronto increased (Sinyor and Levitt 2010).

However, suicide by jumping is not a common method. Fencing in bridges, therefore, does not typically have a major impact on the overall suicide rate.

Medications

The restriction of access to medications that can be used for suicide has long been known to reduce their use for suicide. For example, Clark (1985) showed that when prescriptions were required for opiates in England in the early 1900s, the use of opiates for suicide declined. Oliver and Hetzel (1972) presented data that indicated that when sedatives were restricted in Australia in the 1960s, their use for suicide declined, without there being an increase in the use of other methods.

Many medications, including some of those used for treating psychiatrically disturbed individuals who may be suicidal, can be used to die by suicide. Restricting access to a particular medication, such as barbiturates, typically results in a reduction in the use of that medication for suicide, but switching to alternative medications is easily accomplished by individuals who intend to die by suicide.

Prior to 1961, barbiturates were available in Japan as over-the-counter medications. In February 1, 1961, Pharmacy Act S.49 required prescriptions for both barbiturates and meprobamate. Lester and Abe (1989) examined the use of sedatives and hypnotics for suicide prior to and after the implementation of the Pharmacy Act of 1961. The suicide rate using sedatives and hypnotics peaked at 7.05 per 100,000 per year in 1958. Thereafter the suicide rate by sedatives and hypnotics declined consistently. Thus, at the time when the Pharmacy Act was implemented in 1961, the suicide rate using sedatives and hypnotics was already declining. The slope of the declining regression line did increase a little after the implementation of the Pharmacy Act. The suicide rate by all other methods was examined for the same time period. The suicide rate by all other methods began declining even earlier, after 1955 in fact, and continued to decline until 1965. Thus, there is no evidence that people switched methods for suicide once prescriptions were required for sedatives and hypnotics.

Many years ago, Barraclough et al. (1971) suggested the following:

1. Reducing the number of prescriptions for medications that are potentially lethal in overdose
2. Reducing the size of the prescriptions
3. Wrapping tablets individually in tin foil or plastic blisters
4. Using nonbarbiturates (and other less lethal medications) when such medications exist for the same problems
5. Having family physicians recall unused tablets when the treatment is changed or stopped
6. Writing prescriptions in a way that would prevent forgery
7. Having pharmacists monitor large and excessive prescriptions
8. Not prescribing medications or refilling prescriptions without seeing the patient

In Europe, the use of paracetamol (acetaminophen) for suicide results in a fair number of deaths and in kidney damage in many who attempt suicide but survive. A great deal of research has been conducted on restricting access to paracetamol, the results of which are not altogether consistent.

Bateman et al. (2006) examined the impact of restricting sales of paracetamol in Scotland in 1998 on suicide and found that the legislation did *not* have a preventive impact on deaths. In fact, the number of deaths each quarter from paracetamol products increased for both men and women. However, most of the deaths were from ingestion of co-proxamol (a combination of paracetamol and dextropropoxyphene, an opioid), for which the prescription rate declined only from 1.42 million in 1995 to 1.26 million in 2003. The legislation affected only over-the-counter sales for simple paracetamol, not for prescribed paracetamol products.

Sandilands and Bateman (2008) noted that after co-proxamol was withdrawn from the market beginning in 2005, the number of deaths in Scotland from co-proxamol overdose dropped (from 41 in 2004 to 10 in 2006). Interestingly, deaths from all poisons also declined (from 173 in 2004 to 128 in 2006). After the withdrawal of co-proxamol, prescriptions for other analgesics (such as co-codamol [a combination of paracetamol and codeine] and paracetamol) increased, but this was not accompanied by an increase in deaths from these medications, which remained roughly the same as before. Thus, switching of medications for suicide does not appear to have occurred, but Sandilands and Bateman did not examine changes in other methods for suicide or the overall suicide rate.

Gunnell et al. (2000) reviewed many suggestions for reducing the role of paracetamol in overdoses, including 1) adding methionine to the tablets to reduce the toxic effects (but which may lead to side effects for some people), 2) undertaking public education about paracetamol's dangers (which may instead highlight its possibilities for suicide), 3) including warning notices on packets (which may also highlight its possibilities for suicide), 4) using blister packs, 5) restricting sales to only pharmacies (and not permitting sales in supermarkets and other outlets), 6) making paracetamol available only by prescription, and 7) restricting the quantity that may be purchased at one time. Some of these suggestions lead to inconvenience to those who wish to use paracetamol legitimately. However, if the frequency of attempted suicides with paracetamol could be reduced, and if the severity of the medical consequences of the suicide attempts with paracetamol could be reduced, then at least the harm to those individuals could be lessened.

Pesticides

The problem of pesticides as a method for suicide is of current concern because the method is very common in developing nations. Efforts are being made to encourage farmers to store their pesticides safely, but many fail to follow guidelines for this and, furthermore, the farmers and their families know where the pesticides are stored and usually have access to them. Other solutions have focused on making pesticides less toxic.

Kong and Zhang (2010) compared 370 completed suicides of subjects ages 15–34 years in a region of rural China (of whom 66.2% used pesticides for their suicidal act) with 370 living control subjects matched for age and sex. After controlling for education, living situation, marital status, family income, and psychiatric disorder, the adjusted odds ratio for suicide associated with the presence of a pesticide in the home was

3.28 for those ages 24–34 (95% confidence interval=1.62–6.64).[2]

Gunnell and Eddleston (2003) suggested several tactics for reducing the use of pesticides for suicide:

1. Restricting the availability of pesticides directly by restricting their import or use or indirectly by storing them in secure facilities in communities:

   a. Introducing a "minimum" pesticides list and restricting use to a few, less toxic pesticides.
   b. Prohibiting sales of the most toxic pesticides.
   c. Subsidizing the cost of less toxic pesticides.
   d. Keeping all pesticides locked up, with the keys held by licensed users.
   e. Reducing the use of pesticides in farming by implementing other methods of pest control.
   f. Returning unused pesticides to the vendor.

2. Improving public education about the dangers of pesticide ingestion and improving labeling of pesticides.

3. Reducing the toxicity of pesticides.

   a. Adding emetics or antidotes to pesticides.[3]
   b. Making pesticides unpleasant to smell and taste.
   c. Producing less toxic pesticides.

4. Improving the medical management of pesticide poisoning.

The impact of restrictions on the sale of one or more pesticides has been studied, and this approach seems consistently to result in suicidal individuals switching to alternative pesticides. Furthermore, efforts to encourage farmers to store pesticides safely do not always succeed. In a study in Sri Lanka, only 55% of farmers were storing pesticides in locked containers 2 years after the distribution of the lockable devices (Weerasinghe et al. 2008). Weerasinghe et al. (2008) noted that it was difficult to keep the key hidden from children and that, of course, the person with the key had access to the pesticides.

Firearms

In a few countries, including the United States, the most popular method for suicide is a firearm. There are many studies on whether restricting access to firearms has an impact on the use of firearms for suicide (and also for murder). For example, Killias (1993) and Lester (1996) both found that estimates of the percentage of households with guns in nations were positively associated with the suicide rate using firearms but not with the suicide rate by all other methods.

Methodologically sound research on this issue is difficult to accomplish. For example, examining changes over time as firearm regulations are changed allows for the impact of a variety of socioeconomic changes to confound any cause-and-effect conclusions. Furthermore, the passage of legislation does not always ensure strict enforcement of the new laws.

Political realities prevent the imposition of uniform, strict firearm legislation in many countries, including the United States,

---

[2]The adjusted odds ratio for those ages 15–23 was 1.26 and not significantly different from 1.

[3]A less drastic additive (a bittering agent) did not reduce the use of antifreeze for suicide in California and Oregon (White et al. 2008). Making the liquid bitter is, however, a less powerful deterrent than adding a substance to make people nauseous and vomit.

where regions are able to pass their own laws. Lester (2009) reviewed the research on this issue in Canada, a nation where federal laws overrule regional laws, but even in Canada the author was unable to draw firm conclusions about the effectiveness of stricter firearm laws on the use of firearms for suicide. The conflicting results from the many research studies were often a result of different methodologies, and the role of confounding socioeconomic variables could never be ruled out.[4]

Even when uniform laws can be passed nationwide, political realities and public opinions may prevent passage of strict firearm control legislation. There has been some study of politically feasible projects, such as buyback programs. An analysis of the Australian buyback program in 1996–1997, which resulted in the destruction of over 600,000 guns within a few months, has produced conflicting evidence of its impact. Lee and Suardi (2010) found no impact on gun deaths, whereas Leigh and Neill (2010) found a reduction in firearm suicide rates of 80%. The crude suicide rates by firearm and by all other methods indicate a reduction in the firearm suicide rate, but the non-firearm suicide rate also declined, suggesting the role of other socioeconomic variables in these declines.

Because most suicidal individuals use guns owned by them or by a member of their nuclear family (Brent et al. 1991; Johnson et al. 2010), much emphasis has been focused on training individual gun owners in the safe use of firearms and, in particular, safe storage (Coverdale et al. 2010). Guns should not be kept loaded, the ammunition and the gun should be stored in different places, and guns should be kept locked up.

Charcoal Burning

An interesting example of restricting access to a lethal method of suicide occurred in Hong Kong. Suicides by burning of charcoal in a closed space rose from 2% of all suicides in 1998 to over 26% in 2003 (Yip et al. 2010). Publicity of suicides using this method clearly contributed to its rise in popularity, and the use of charcoal spread to other Asian countries. Yip and colleagues noted that those using charcoal to die by suicide differed from those using other methods. For example, they were less likely to have a history of psychiatric illness or substance abuse.

Yip and colleagues chose two districts in Hong Kong, and in one the charcoal was removed from the open shelves of major retail stores. To purchase charcoal in these stores, customers had to ask for the charcoal, which the salesperson would retrieve from a locked container. This change was not publicized, and the public was not informed. Frontline staff were told it was solely an administrative change. In this district, the suicide rate using charcoal dropped from 4.3 per 100,000 per year pre-intervention to 2.0 after intervention. In the control district, the rate increased from 3.0 to 4.3. The overall suicide rate in the targeted district fell from 17.9 to 12.2, whereas in the control district the suicide rate remained steady (12.7 and 12.5).

Charcoal in Hong Kong is not an essential commodity. It is used primarily for recreational purposes. It is impressive that charcoal was not removed from the market completely, but rather a small barrier was imposed on customers. This suggests that a reasonably large proportion of sui-

---

[4]Most of the studies have been correlational, and so cause-and-effect conclusions cannot be drawn.

cides may be impulsive, and so removal of easy, instant access to a method for suicide can prevent these suicides.

Conclusion

In this chapter I have reviewed research on the effects on suicide rates of reducing the availability of firearms, medications, toxic car exhaust, toxic domestic gas, and other methods. Although the studies do not lead to a definitive conclusion, the results do indicate that reducing the availability of a method for suicide reduces its use for suicide and may also reduce the overall suicide rate if the method restricted is commonly used and a lethal method. People who switch methods for suicide are forced to switch to a less lethal method for which survival is more likely. Studies on the likelihood of people switching methods for suicide are needed, and at the present time only preliminary studies have appeared (Lester et al. 1989). It is likely that more research on this important topic will appear in the next few years, hopefully permitting us to evaluate this method of suicide prevention more precisely. Nonetheless, at this point in time, it is possible to suggest a variety of tactics that may be used to restrict access to lethal methods for suicide (see Table 30–1). Some have already been implemented by governments, and others, such as modifying the tailpipes of cars, could be imposed easily with minimal expense.

Lester (1988) has argued that a failure to make lethal methods and venues for suicide less available may render people legally liable for civil damages. For example, all house owners in the United States must fence in swimming pools in their backyards or face civil liability should someone drown in their pool. Lester argued that the municipal government in the Bay Area in California might be held similarly liable by those whose relatives jump from the Golden Gate Bridge, a common suicide venue that has not been fenced in.

The research presented in this chapter has implications for a theory of suicide. It is common to think of suicide as a desperate measure, chosen by seriously dysfunctional people who are at their wits' end. It seems unlikely that such people would be deterred by the effort needed to overcome the restrictions placed upon obtaining a lethal amount of their preferred method for suicide.

However, the research presented here suggests that suicide may often be a logical decision made by people based on rational issues such as the availability of different methods for suicide and one's preferred method for suicide (Clarke and Lester 1989; Yang and Lester 2006). Many people, when asked, say that they would consider one and only one method for suicide. If access to this method were restricted, then suicide might well be averted in these people. The necessity of switching to a less preferred method might introduce costs that were not originally present. For example, those who fear the pain of a bullet and the disfigurement of the wound would in all probability not switch to firearms if medication were no longer available.

Furthermore, these results suggest that it may be heuristic to consider suicide by different methods as distinctly different acts, perhaps with different motivations and determinants. Lester (1991) has shown, for example, that the social correlates of suicide rates by different methods over the American states are quite different from one another and so may be differently determined.

Will people switch methods for suicide if their preferred method is made less easily available? Although this is the critical question for this method of preventing suicide,

---

TABLE 30–1. Ways to limit access to lethal methods for suicide

---

Cars

Emission controls (to reduce carbon monoxide content)

Change shape of tailpipe to end in a narrow slit (to make attachment of hose difficult)

Have automatic ignition turn off once engine has idled for five minutes

Domestic gas

Switch to less toxic natural gas

Automatic gas turn-off if gas not lit within 30 seconds

Make oven doors hinged at base (to make it difficult to put one's head in)

Jumping

Fence in bridges

Fence in tops of high buildings

Restrict access to the tops of buildings

Fence in parking garages

Poisons

Put the common household poisons in childproof containers

Firearms

Pass and enforce strict gun control laws

Require members of gun clubs to store guns at the club in secure rooms

Encourage safe storage of guns by home owners, especially those with children and adolescents

Medications

Limit size of prescriptions

Eliminate automatic refills of prescriptions

Do not prescribe without seeing and evaluating patient

Enclose pills in plastic blisters

Prescribe as suppositories rather than as oral tablets

Set up monitoring system to catch multiple prescribing of patient by several doctors/pharmacists

Prescribe less toxic medications

Set up systems to prevent forging/changing prescriptions by patients
(e.g., by having physicians directly input prescriptions into pharmacies
by computer)

Attempted suicides

Collect lethal agents/implements before releasing attempters to their homes

---

very few studies are relevant to the issue. It remains a matter of opinion. However, for those who would switch methods for suicide, if the new method is less lethal than the former method, then there is a greater likelihood that suicide attempters will survive and, therefore, that some completed suicides will have been prevented.

Key Clinical Concepts

- Always ask potentially suicidal patients about their preferred method for suicide (their suicidal plans) and their access to lethal methods for committing suicide.

- Monitor patients who show signs of impulsiveness and encourage them to remove (or have significant others remove) lethal methods for committing suicide from their homes.

- If patients have made suicide attempts or gestures in the past, inquire about the choice of method and note whether the patient persisted with one method or switched methods.[5]

- Pay attention to the method used in a patient's previous suicide attempt. There is recent, tentative evidence that choice of method for a suicide attempt predicts the future risk of completed suicide, with those who use more violent methods at higher risk (Runeson et al. 2010).

References

Barraclough BM, Nelson B, Bunch J, et al: Suicide and barbiturate poisoning. J R Coll Gen Pract 21:645–653, 1971

Bateman DN, Gorman DR, Bain M, et al: Legislation restricting paracetamol sales and patterns of self-harm and death from paracetamol-containing preparations in Scotland. Br J Clin Pharmacol 62:573–581, 2006

Beautrais AL: Effectiveness of barriers at suicide jumping sites. Aust N Z J Psychiatry 35:557–562, 2001

Brent DA, Perper JA, Allman CJ, et al: The presence and accessibility of firearms in the homes of adolescent suicides. JAMA 266:2989–2995, 1991

Clark MJ: Suicides by opium and its derivatives in England and Wales. Psychol Med 15:237–242, 1985

Clarke RV, Lester D: Toxicity of car exhausts and opportunity for suicide. J Epidemiol Community Health 41:114–120, 1987

Clarke RV, Lester D: Suicide: Closing the Exits. New York, Springer-Verlag, 1989

Clarke RV, Mayhew P: The British gas suicide story and its criminological implications. Crime and Justice 10:79–116, 1988

Coverdale JH, Roberts LW, Balon R: The public health priority to address the accessibility and safety of firearms. Acad Psychiatry 34:405–408, 2010

Glasgow G: Do local landmark bridges increase the suicide rate? Soc Sci Med 72:884–889, 2011

Gunnell D, Eddleston M: Suicide by intentional ingestion of pesticides. Int J Epidemiol 32:902–909, 2003

---

[5]For example, the present author had contact with a woman who preferred overdoses, but who was saved on several occasions. She tried cutting her wrists while in the bathtub, but again was saved. She was then hospitalized after another overdose and hung herself in the hospital after being removed from suicide watch. She had indicated that she was afraid of hanging as a method of suicide, but her willingness to change methods once increased the risk that she would switch to a more lethal method, especially one that she had previously considered.

Gunnell D, Murray V, Hawton K: Use of paracetamol (acetaminophen) for suicide and nonfatal poisoning. Suicide Life Threat Behav 30:313–326, 2000

Johnson RM, Barber C, Azrael D, et al: Who are the owners of firearms used in adolescent suicides? Suicide Life Threat Behav 40:609–611, 2010

Killias M: International correlations between gun ownership and rates of homicide and suicide. CMAJ 148:1721–1725, 1993

Kong Y, Zhang J: Access to farming pesticides and risk for suicide in Chinese rural young people. Psychiatry Res 179:217–221, 2010

Kreitman N: The coal gas story. Br J Prev Soc Med 30:86–93, 1976

Law CK, Yip PS, Chan WS, et al: Evaluating the effectiveness of barrier installation for preventing railway suicides in Hong Kong. J Affect Disord 114:254–262, 2009

Lee WS, Suardi S: The Australian firearms buyback and its effect on gun deaths. Contemporary Economic Policy 28:65–79, 2010

Leigh A, Neill C: Do gun buybacks save lives? Evidence from panel data. American Law and Economics Review 12:462–508, 2010

Lester D: The AAS and political activism. AAS Newslink 14:8, 1988

Lester D: Are the societal correlates of suicide and homicide rates the same for each lethal weapon? European Journal of Psychiatry 5:5–8, 1991

Lester D: Suicide from bridges in Washington, DC. Percept Mot Skills 77:534, 1993

Lester D: Suicide by jumping in Singapore as a function of high-rise apartment availability. Percept Mot Skills 79:74, 1994

Lester D: Effects of the detoxification of domestic gas on suicide rates in six nations. Psychol Rep 77:294, 1995

Lester D: Gun ownership and rates of homicide and suicide. European Journal of Psychiatry 10:83–85, 1996

Lester D: Preventing Suicide: Closing the Exits Revisited. Hauppauge, NY, Nova Science, 2009

Lester D, Abe K: The effect of controls on sedatives and hypnotics and their use for suicide. J Toxicol Clin Toxicol 27:299–303, 1989

Lester D, Fong CA, D'Angelo AA: Chronic suicide attempters who switch methods and those who do not. Percept Mot Skills 69:1390, 1989

Oliver RG, Hetzel BS: Rise and fall of suicide rates in Australia. Med J Aust 2:919–923, 1972

Routley VH, Ozanne-Smith J: The impact of catalytic converters on motor vehicle exhaust gas suicides. Med J Aust 168:65–67, 1998

Runeson B, Tidemalm D, Dahlin M, et al: Method of attempted suicide as predictor of subsequent successful suicide. BMJ 341:c3222, 2010

Sandilands EA, Bateman DN: Co-proxamol withdrawal has reduced suicide from drugs in Scotland. Br J Clin Pharmacol 66:290–293, 2008

Seiden RH, Spence M: A tale of two bridges. Omega (Westport) 14:201–209, 1983–1984

Sinyor M, Levitt AJ: Effect of a barrier at Bloor Street Viaduct on suicide rates in Toronto. BMJ 341:c2884, 2010

Skilling GD, Sclare PD, Watt SJ, et al: The effect of catalytic converter legislation on suicide rates in Grampian and Scotland 1980–2003. Scott Med J 53:3–6, 2008

Stengel E: Suicide and Attempted Suicide. Baltimore, MD, Penguin, 1964

Studdert DM, Gurrin LC, Jatkar U, et al: Relationship between vehicle emissions laws and incidence of suicide by motor vehicle exhaust gas in Australia, 2001–06. PLoS Med 7:e1000210, 2010

Weerasinghe M, Pieris R, Eddleston M, et al: Safe storage of pesticides in Sri Lanka: identifying important design features influencing community acceptance and use of safe storage devices. BMC Public Health 8:276, 2008

White NC, Litovitz T, White MK, et al: The impact of bittering agents on suicidal ingestions of antifreeze. Clin Toxicol (Phila) 46:507–514, 2008

Yang B, Lester D: A prolegomenon to behavioral economic studies of suicide, in Handbook of Contemporary Behavioral Economics. Edited by Altman M. Armonk, NY, ME Sharpe, 2006, pp 543–559

Yip PS, Law CK, Fu KW, et al: Restricting the means of suicide by charcoal burning. Br J Psychiatry 196:241–242, 2010

C H A P T E R 3 1

Suicide Prevention Programs

Maurizio Pompili, M.D., Ph.D.

Marco Innamorati, Psy.D.

David Lester, Ph.D.

Suicide prevention is a relatively young endeavor. The first attempts to develop crisis services and suicide prevention programs date back to 1893, but the major breakthrough in suicide prevention was the establishment of the Los Angeles Suicide Prevention Center by Edwin Shneidman, Norman Farberow, and Robert Litman in the mid-1950s.

Suicide prevention has become a world imperative (see Table 31–1). Resources have been invested in order to reduce the tragic loss of human lives due to suicide and thousands of scholarly papers have been published, yet the reduction of suicide rates does not parallel this ever-increasing investment both in economic and in human resources. O'Carroll et al. (1994) noted that the scientific information about the efficacy of suicide prevention strategies was insufficient, citing as an example that the National Center for Injury Prevention and Control (1992), in its summary of research *Youth Suicide Prevention Programs:*

A Resource Guide, published by the Centers for Disease Control and Prevention (CDC), was not able to recommend one strategy over another.

One of the most important obstacles in the prevention of suicide is the absence of evidence-based practices for delivering meaningful intervention (Pompili 2010). However, evidence-based practice in suicide prevention may be limited by specific features of this behavior (Goldney 2005). For example, suicide is rare, and so we need extremely large sample sizes in order to demonstrate the effectiveness of a suicide prevention program. The aim of this chapter is to review strategies for suicide prevention at the population, at-risk group, and individual level. Notably, the prevailing prevention model in the prevention of suicide focuses on universal, selective, and indicated prevention (see Table 31–2). Approaches reported in this chapter refer to populations as categorized according to this model.

TABLE 31–1.	World Health Organization six-step approach to the prevention of suicidal behavior

Psychiatric treatment

Firearm possession control

Gas detoxification

Control of toxic substances and medicine

Responsible media reporting

Use of physical barriers to deter jumping from high places

Source. World Health Organization 1998.

School-Based Suicide Prevention Programs

In many countries and regions, most adolescents attend school, and this appears to provide an excellent place to develop and provide programs for suicide prevention. However, to improve the likelihood that a school suicide prevention program will be effectively implemented and maintained, it is necessary to establish policies and procedures before implementing programs that are focused on such issues as how to respond effectively to a student who may be indicating suicidal ideation or making suicidal threats, how to respond to the aftermath of a suicidal attempt or a death by suicide, and the various roles school personnel may play in preventing, intervening, and coping with a student who may be suicidal (Lazear et al. 2003).

Curriculum-Based Programs for Education and Awareness About Suicide

Programs of education about suicide are generally focused on dispelling myths and increasing correct knowledge about adolescent suicide and encouraging seeking help when necessary.

Results on the effectiveness of curriculum-based programs to promote awareness

TABLE 31–2.	Strategies in suicide prevention programs

Universal strategies
Those addressing an entire population (the nation, state, local county or community, school, or neighborhood). Universal interventions include programs such as public education campaigns, school-based suicide awareness programs, means restriction, education programs for the media on reporting practices related to suicide, and school-based crisis response plans and teams.

Selective strategies
Those addressing at-risk groups that have a greater probability of becoming suicidal. This level of prevention includes screening programs, gatekeeper training for frontline adult caregivers and peer "natural helpers," support and skill-building programs for at-risk groups in the population, and enhanced accessible crisis services and referral sources.

Indicated strategies
Those addressing high-risk individuals within the population. Programs include skill-building support groups in high schools and colleges, parent support training programs, case management for high-risk adolescents at school, and referral sources for crisis intervention and treatment.

are mixed, with some studies reporting no benefits at all or potentially dangerous results. Thus, Beautrais et al. (1997) recommended that school-based programs aimed at increasing the awareness of young people about youth suicide not be undertaken. Lazear et al. (2003) suggested that a curriculum approach focused on reducing the stigma associated with suicide, which presents suicide as a reaction to the common stressors of adolescence, may be harmful because it normalizes the behavior and reduces protective taboos, especially when the intervention is extremely brief (often only one session of 2–4 hours). The authors recommended using a model that identifies suicide as a complicated, abnormal reaction to a number of overwhelming factors. Programs should also emphasize the association between suicide and mental illness, and "one-shot" approaches with students must be avoided. Furthermore, schools that wish to use a suicide curriculum as a preventive method should use this approach in conjunction with other preventive strategies, such as gatekeeper training, screening, establishing community links, and skills training. The authors pointed out that schools should not avoid using this approach due to a fear that talking about suicide and teaching students about suicide will only provide students with ideas and methods for suicidal behaviors, because this is simply not true.

School programs that have used education and awareness about suicide include Signs of Suicide (SOS; Aseltine and DeMartino 2004). This is a 2-day secondary school–based intervention. Students are screened for depression and suicide risk and referred for professional help as indicated. Students also view a video that teaches them to recognize warning signs of depression and suicide in others. They are taught that the appropriate response to these warning signs is to acknowledge them, let the person know you care, and tell a responsible adult (either with the person or on that person's behalf). Students also participate in guided classroom discussions about suicide and depression.

In an attempt to provide a reference for evidence-based practice in the prevention of suicide in general, and among youth in particular, the Best Practices Registry for Suicide Prevention, a collaboration between the Suicide Prevention Resource Center and the American Foundation for Suicide Prevention (AFSP), has been established. The registry looked at the strength and limitations of the SOS program and assessed its readiness for dissemination using a criterion of 2.5 on a 0–4 scale. In two studies involving more than 10,000 students, SOS program participants were 40% less likely than comparable students who did not participate in the intervention to report attempting suicide in the past 3 months (Aseltine et al. 2007).

Skills-Based School Programs

Skills-based school programs focus on appropriate social skills, problem-solving strategies, coping skills, and help-seeking skills (for examples, see Table 31–3). The rationale behind such programs is that adolescents with deficits in such skills are more prone to suicide. Social skills, problem-solving strategies, and coping skills can be taught directly through lessons or indirectly by incorporating these skills into existing classes. There has been some evidence that skills-based school programs can reduce suicidal behavior and improve the students' attitudes, emotions, and coping skills (Klingman and Hochdorf 1993; Orbach and Bar-Joseph 1993; Zenere and Lazarus 1997).

Some studies have focused specifically on skills training and social support programs for students at high risk for school failure or dropout (Eggert et al. 1995; Randell et al. 2001; Thompson et al. 2000, 2001) and have demonstrated enhanced protective factors and reduced risk factors following the "active" interventions, compared with "intervention as usual," which did not increase protective factors (Gould et al. 2003) (for example, see Coping and Support Training and Reconnecting Youth, Table 31–3). Randell et al. (2001) noted the superiority of skills-based interventions in reducing depression and enhancing perceived family support, but the decrease in suicidal behaviors did not differ from "intervention as usual." The improvement in self-efficacy, personal control, and problem-solving was

TABLE 31–3. Examples of skills-based school programs

The Good Behavior Game (GBG) (Barrish et al. 1969)
- The goal of the GBG is to create an integrated classroom social system that is supportive of all children being able to learn with little aggressive, disruptive behavior.
- GBG promotes good behavior by rewarding teams that do not exceed maladaptive behavior standards as set by the teacher.
- The methods involve helping teachers to define unacceptable behaviors clearly and to socialize children with regulation of a teammate's behavior through a process of team contingent reinforcement and mutual self-interest.
- The results supported the hypothesis that first graders assigned to GBG classrooms experienced lower incidences of suicidality throughout childhood and adolescence and into young adulthood compared with control subjects, with half the reported lifetime rates of ideation and attempts of their matched control subjects.

Coping and Support Training (CAST) (Eggert et al. 2002; Randell et al. 2001; Thompson et al. 2001) and CARE (Care, Assess, Respond, Empower) (formerly Counselors CARE)
- CAST is intended to decrease suicidal behavior, depression, and drug involvement in high-risk 14- to 19-year-old youth who screen positive for suicidal risk.
- The CAST program is used in conjunction with C-CARE.
- Students potentially at risk for suicidal behavior are included in a small-group (6–8 students per group) intervention delivered two times per week (1-hour session) for a 6-week period.
- 10 skill-training sessions targeting three overall goals: increased mood management (depression and anger), improved school performance, and decreased drug involvement.
- Self-recognition of progress is provided through the program.
- Every session ends with "lifework" assignments that call for the youth to practice the session's skills with a specific person in their school, home, or peer-group environment.
- The sessions are administered by trained, master's-level high school teachers, counselors, or nurses with considerable school-based experience.
- When used together, C-CARE and CAST have been shown to be effective at decreasing suicidal risk, depression, hopelessness, stress, and anger, and in increasing self-esteem and the ability to use social support.
- Readiness for dissemination=3.5 on a 0–4 scale (Best Practices Registry for Suicide Prevention).
- In a clinical randomized controlled trial that compared CAST participants with usual care for youth at suicide risk (a 30-minute, one-on-one session with a school counselor or nurse), CAST participants showed significantly greater declines relative to usual-care youth in two of the four suicide risk factors: positive attitudes toward suicide and suicidal ideation. For suicidal ideation, the initial declines were maintained throughout the 9 months of follow-up.

Reconnecting Youth (Eggert and Nicholas 2004; Eggert et al. 1995, 2001; Thompson et al. 2000).
- This program targets young people in grades 9–12 who show signs of poor school achievement, potential for school dropout, and suicide risk.
- Skills are taught to build resiliency with respect to risk factors and to moderate early signs of substance abuse and depression/aggression.
- The program is one semester in duration.
- The program is divided into five modules: 1) getting started, 2) self-esteem enhancement, 3) decision making, 4) personal control, and 5) interpersonal communication.
- Small-group work and life-skills training models are used to enhance personal and social protective factors for high-risk youth.

specific to the skills-training component (Randell et al. 2001).

In another study, group leader support was found to be critical for building a positive peer group culture. Higher levels of depression at baseline predicted lower levels of personal control at follow-up, suggesting that strategies to address existing depression are important for enhancing the adolescent's personal control (Thompson et al. 2000). Interventions in which suicide education is incorporated within a life-skills approach show more consistent evidence of an effect, but the effect on the suicide-specific behavior remains uncertain (Burns and Patton 2000).

Gatekeeper Training Programs

Gatekeeper training is an essential component for any suicide prevention program. The United Nations (United Nations Department for Policy Coordination and Sustainable Development 1996), along with numerous review articles on general methods of suicide prevention, have recommended that gatekeeper training be considered in implementing an effective strategy to prevent suicide (Beautrais et al. 2007; Gould and Kramer 2001; Mann et al. 2005). Gatekeeper training teaches specific groups of people to identify people at high risk for suicide and then to refer those people for treatment (see Table 31–4). In general, gatekeepers are people who have primary contact with those at risk for suicide and can identify them by recognizing suicidal risk factors. The function of gatekeeping is seen as an attempt to make informal channels of help more effective rather than to build or superimpose formal channels through social engineering.

Historically, these gatekeepers have been divided into two main groups, defined as

TABLE 31–4. Example of a gatekeeper training program

Question, Persuade, Refer (QPR) (Wyman et al. 2008)

- QPR consists of 1.5 hours of training covering the following themes: rates of youth suicide, warning signs and risk factors for suicide, procedures for asking a student about suicide, persuading a student to get help, and referring a student for help.
- The training is conducted by staff who receive QPR instructor training and triage training (12–16 hours).
- The training is co-led by a counselor in each school who receives instructor training (6–8 hours) and who serves as the primary source for referrals in the school.
- The adolescents who participated in the study were in 8th- and 10th-grade health classes.
- The authors found a consistent positive impact on staff knowledge and appraisals.
- The training had a medium-size effect on increasing participants' accuracy in identifying warning signs and risk factors for youth suicide and in recommending intervention behaviors.

either *designated* or *emergent* (Isaac et al. 2009; Ramsay et al. 1990). The designated group consists of people who are trained and designated as helping professionals (e.g., those who work in the fields of medicine, social work, nursing, and psychology). The emergent group consists of community members who may not have been formally trained to intervene with someone who is at risk for suicide but who emerge as potential gatekeepers as recognized by those with suicidal intent. Because schools provide a valuable window of observation through which young people at risk can be identified, school staff should be encouraged to share this responsibility by taking part in regular and ongoing training that includes increasing knowledge of the symptoms of distress and risk of suicide, increasing staff members' confidence and competence to refer and support distressed young people, increasing staff members' willingness to do this, and increasing competence to work in these situations (Beautrais et al. 1997).

Gatekeeper training usually consists of training any adult who interacts with or observes students in order for him or her to be able to identify any students who may be at risk for suicide, determine the level of risk, know where to refer a potentially at-risk student, know how to contact these referral sources, and know what school policies are in place that relate to suicidal crisis situations. Although teachers are expected to act as gatekeepers and know how to identify a student potentially at risk for suicidal actions, they should be informed that they are not meant to take on an additional role as a mental health counselor but are simply meant to act as a watchful eye and "sound the alarm" (Lazear et al. 2003). However, teachers usually do not feel confident about being able to recognize an adolescent at risk (K.A. King et al. 1999).

Isaac et al. (2009) performed a systematic review of gatekeeper training as a preventive intervention for suicide. The authors found that the highest level of evidence for gatekeeper training programs was level 1B (i.e., randomized controlled trials). The authors examined two main outcomes when reporting the use of gatekeeper training: 1) the impact of the training on increasing knowledge, changing attitudes, and imparting skills to the trainee; and 2) the effect on the suicide rate. Gatekeeper training programs have been studied in school counselors, educators, and peer helpers, with positive effects on knowledge, skills, and attitudes (Garland and Zigler 1993; Gould and Kramer 2001; K.A. King and

Smith 2000; National Center for Injury Prevention and Control 1992; Wyman et al. 2008).

Isaac et al. (2009) noted that despite numerous studies showing an increase in skills, attitudes, and knowledge generally, there is a dearth of studies on the effectiveness of school-based gatekeeper training programs in decreasing rates of suicidal ideation, suicide attempts, or deaths by suicide. The authors concluded that gatekeeper training holds promise as part of a multifaceted strategy to combat suicide. It has been proven to positively affect the skills, attitudes, and knowledge of people who undertake the training in many settings. Although research is limited in demonstrating an effect on suicide rates and ideation, gatekeeper training is seen in many circles as an extremely promising initiative to prevent suicide.

Peer Support Groups

Research suggests that peer gatekeeper training may be useful in preventing adolescent suicide because up to 40% of male peers and 60% of female peers know someone who has attempted suicide, but only 25% have confided in an adult (Kalafat and Elias 1995). Peers may help youth at risk to develop more appropriate coping skills, reduce feelings of isolation, and ameliorate substance abuse and other early risk factors while enhancing important protective factors (White and Jodoin 1998). Some of the existing programs that use peers focus on having peers listen for and report any possible warning signs, whereas others involve the peers in counseling responsibilities (Gould et al. 2003).

Gatekeeper training has been examined in a peer gatekeeper program, with similar effects on skills, attitudes, and knowledge as in studies of educators (Stuart et al. 2003). However, negative side effects have not been adequately examined (Gould et al. 2003), and there is some concern about peers being involved in counseling suicidal youth because of the potential risks posed to the nonsuicidal peer (Steele and Doey 2007).

Lazear et al. (2003) suggest that schools have to use these programs in conjunction with screening programs in order to identify students at risk. In addition, schools should not use peer support programs as a substitute for professional counseling or therapy.

Educating Parents and Community Members

Gatekeeper programs can also be directed to parents and community members. The approach is based on the hypothesis that parental psychiatric disorder and dysfunction are more prevalent in suicidal adolescents' families and that connectedness with adults may minimize the impact of environmental risk factors.

C.A. King et al. (2006) investigated the efficacy of the Youth-Nominated Support Team—Version 1 (YST-1), a psychoeducational social network intervention, with 289 suicidal, psychiatrically hospitalized adolescents. Adolescents were randomly assigned to treatment as usual plus YST-1 or treatment as usual only. Assessments were completed pre- and postintervention (6 months). YST-1 was designed to supplement routine care for suicidal adolescents following psychiatric hospitalization, provide psychoeducation for support persons whom youth nominate from within and outside their family, and facilitate the supportive weekly contact of these support persons with the suicidal adolescent. However, the hypothesis that the program would be effective in reducing suicidality was not supported, although gender effects were evident, with adolescent girls reporting greater effects from the program.

Although it may not be the responsibility of schools to train community members, schools should make sure that there are established agreements between the school and crisis services. Only when these links are in place can a perceptive and educated staff member make an effective referral for a student potentially at risk. These links also increase the likelihood that students will receive clear, consistent messages about suicide, which research has shown increase a student's feeling of competence. Schools should also provide information to parents about warning signs, risk factors, protective factors, community resources, and what to do following a suicidal crisis. Research has found that when schools communicate with parents and involve them in school activities and programs, parents are more likely to cooperate with the school and help the school maintain these programs (Carlyon et al. 1998; Marx and Northrop 1995).

The Australian Institute of Family Studies conducted an evaluation of the National Youth Suicide Prevention Strategy (Mitchell 2000), which has funded seven parenting projects, which together formed the National Parenting Initiative (Table 31–5). Results from the meta-analysis of parenting projects fell into four major themes: 1) effective strategies for recruiting and engaging parents; 2) interventions that are effective in enhancing parenting skills, knowledge, and confidence; 3) increasing well-being and reducing risk factors for young people; and 4) sustaining and disseminating effective parenting programs. Some crucial aspects of these projects are reported in Table 31–5.

Local or community-based support structures are vital to the maintenance of these programs. Community-based support

---

TABLE 31–5. National Parenting Initiative results

Recruiting parents—universal strategies

Resourceful Adolescent Program for Parents (RAP-P; Shochet and Ham 2004)

- A program developed for the urban setting that focused mainly on the school setting for recruitment efforts.
- The program targets parents with children facing the transition to high school.
- School-based staff are trained to deliver the program as part of the school's usual services.
- Parent group-based modes of program delivery are only partially successful in engaging parents.
- RAP-P uses two different strategies to recruit parents to the program: recruitment through the general community using mass media, including radio, television, and newspapers, and a strategy that involved targeting whole schools.
- Community recruitment strategy may be more effective in targeting socioeconomically disadvantaged parents.

Recruiting parents—selective strategies

- These programs targeted families that were experiencing difficulties with their children.
- These projects mainly focused on Australian minorities such as Aboriginal people.
- The programs emphasize the importance of addressing the historical and political factors that continue to impact family well-being.

Enhancing parenting skills, knowledge, and confidence

Program for Parents is effective in increasing parents' confidence and satisfaction and decreasing parental depression compared to a control group (Program for Parents Project 1999).

- Almost all of the parenting programs placed central importance on building parents' self-esteem by encouraging awareness of and building on their strengths.
- Meeting parents' needs for friendship, support, and positive regard is critical to parents' ability to parent effectively.
- A group-based approach to parenting skills training is used.
- The program curriculum encourages parents to move from negatively interpretating adolescent behavior toward seeing many adolescent behaviors as normative.
- Home visiting is a primary prevention tactic and early intervention program that provides flexible support to socially isolated new mothers.
- There is advantage in including parents with a range of abilities in the parent groups.

Increasing well-being and reducing risk factors for young people

- Only one of the group of parenting projects included evaluation of outcomes for young people.
- Improvements were believed to be mediated through changes in the parents' perceptions of their adolescents.
- The results support the view that when programs are implemented within a school system, positive effects may extend beyond the minority of families who participate directly in the program.
- The cognitive reframing approach is designed to move parents away from authoritarian and permissive parenting styles toward authoritative styles.

TABLE 31–5. National Parenting Initiative results *(continued)*

Disseminating effective parenting programs

- The main strategy employed in the dissemination of the parenting programs was to provide training to professionals for delivering the programs.
- The features of the programs involved in their effectiveness and diffusion included a systematic documentation of program curricula in manuals (the projects relied on a wide variety of media to promote the programs to both parents and to service providers), ongoing support, and coordination provided to program workers or staff who delivered the programs.
- The roles of local/regional coordinators included marketing the program to appropriate agencies; coordinating referrals to the program; organizing programs; supporting group leaders; liaising with other local/regional and national/state level coordinators regarding support needs in training, consultation, and evaluation; and writing funding submissions.
- The roles of state/territory or national coordinators included liaising with and providing support for local/regional coordinators; providing consultation for leaders involved in running their own programs; providing ongoing training and support for program leaders; and performing ongoing evaluation and program development.

Source. Mitchell 2000.

structures appear to be particularly critical to the uptake and maintenance of programs targeting rural-remote and indigenous communities. Involvement of schools is particularly helpful in recruiting parents to programs. Parenting programs may also be more effective in engaging parents and achieving outcomes if they are run in parallel with programs for adolescents and children. Ongoing funding also is essential to the maintenance and dissemination of programs of this nature. Significant cost inefficiencies result from dependence on short-term project funding to sustain parenting programs.

Parent education programs may be combined with preventive programs directed to restrict access to potentially lethal weapons (Lazear et al. 2003). The Adolescent Health Committee of the Canadian Paediatric Society (2005) published guidelines about youth and firearms. The committee recommended the following:

1. Physicians should routinely inquire about the presence of a firearm in the home and inform parents of the risks of gun ownership if one is present.

2. Physicians have an obligation to share this information with parents until such time that an effective approach to anticipatory guidance relating to the prevention of firearm injuries is established.

3. Physicians should recommend removal of the firearm from the home in cases where there are risk factors for adolescent suicide.

4. Firearm safety interventions that include education and environmental interventions—such as the provision of trigger locks and gun safes—would likely be more effective than an education-only program.

5. Childhood firearm safety education cannot be recommended at present because currently available programs have not been shown to result in behavior change in children, and such education may have unintended negative effects, such as reduced parental vigilance.

However, research that has investigated parents' attitudes about physician counseling on firearm dangers has had mixed results (Brent et al. 2000; Grossman et al. 2000; Oatis et al. 1999). Family physicians play key roles in the community and may have a major role in assessing and treating suicidal youth because most of these youth report that they are most likely to consult their family physician when distressed (Davidson and Manion 1993). However, suicidal adolescents are underdiagnosed by their primary care physician. Thus, it is necessary to train primary care physicians in the recognition and management of suicidal youth. A study conducted in Sweden indicated that a 2-day training course for primary practitioners on how to evaluate mood disorders and suicidality was followed by a reduction in the number of suicides and suicide attempts (among female patients) (Rutz et al. 1992). However, ongoing repetition of educational programs was needed to maintain gains (Steele and Doey 2007).

Screening

Screening is a prevention strategy that is intended to identify students who are potentially at risk for suicide through interviews and self-report questionnaires. Screening tools typically consist of asking students directly about whether they are experiencing symptoms associated with depression or are currently having or have previously had suicidal ideation or have attempted suicide, and assessing the presence of risk factors for suicide.

Screening can be done in two ways (Lazear et al. 2003). The first way is a broad approach, which seeks to identify students potentially at risk for suicide by screening all students in the school. However, surveys of both high school principals and school psychologists reveal that they view schoolwide student screening programs as less acceptable than curriculum-based, inservice programs for staff (Eckert et al. 2003; Miller et al. 1999). Insufficient staffing and budgets, scheduling issues, legal concerns,

and potential negative responses of administrators, parents, and students are potential real-world barriers to program adoption and implementation (Hayden and Lauer 2000).

Focused screening, on the other hand, uses screening in combination with other methods for identifying students at risk for suicidal actions, such as using gatekeepers or peers. Once identified and referred by gatekeepers or peers, those students potentially at risk are screened and subsequently evaluated by a mental health professional. The underlying rationale behind these programs is that, given that suicide is a low-incidence event, prevention may be more effective and efficient if only those students who are potentially at risk for suicide are identified and referred.

Lazear et al. (2003) noted that because suicidality fluctuates in adolescents, repeated screening must be done to measure the changes in suicidality and to avoid missing a student who is not suicidal at one time but becomes suicidal subsequently. Also, screening may identify as many as 10% of the adolescents at school as being at risk for suicide, creating a costly need to follow up those identified as such. Lastly, in order for schools to initiate a screening session, they must have cooperation and consent from parents. However, research has found that parental consent runs close to only 50%, which means that schools may only be able to screen half of the at-risk students, thereby possibly missing students potentially at risk before screening even begins. In the last decade, several randomized trials assessed the efficacy of screening programs in school students. Some examples of these programs are reported on in Table 31–6.

It is important that schools use screening tools that have been evaluated as effective methods for identifying students po-

TABLE 31–6. Examples of screening programs

Reconnecting Youth (Hallfors et al. 2006)

- Students are administered an audio-computer-assisted, self-interviewing format of the High School Questionnaire (Eggert et al. 1994a, 1994b), a questionnaire assessing school deviance and school connectedness; peer bonding; family support; emotional issues such as self-esteem, stress, anxiety, hopelessness and personal control; high-risk behaviors; substance use; suicide; and several demographic variables.
- Items assessing suicide are part of the Suicide Risk Screen (Thompson and Eggert 1999), a screening instrument focusing on sets of rank-ordered criteria based on confirmed suicide risk factors (e.g., suicidal ideation, depression, previous suicide attempts, indirect/direct threats of suicide, and drug misuse).
- A total of 29% of the participants were rated as at risk for suicide. In further analyses, about half of the students identified were deemed at high risk on the basis of high levels of depression, suicidal ideation, or suicidal behavior.
- The authors believe that the low specificity resulted in too many false positives for the instrument to be practical in schools; therefore, they recommend testing a simplified instrument that identifies only students who have attempted suicide in the past year, who have high current levels of suicidal ideation, or who have high current levels of depression and exhibit any degree of suicidal ideation. This instrument identified approximately 11% of urban high school youth for assessment.
- School personnel were reluctant to participate in training.
- Excessive staff turnover and changes in administrative personnel can hamper successful implementation.
- Only a few schools were able to comply with the protocols and act as partners in evaluating the program.

CARE (Care, Assess, Respond, Empower; formerly called Counselors CARE) (Eggert et al. 1995, 2002; Randell et al. 2001; Thompson et al. 2001)

- CARE is a high school–based suicide prevention program targeting high-risk youth.
- It includes a 2-hour, one-on-one computer-assisted suicide assessment interview followed by a 2-hour motivational counseling and social support intervention.
- The counseling session is designed to deliver empathy and support, provide a safe context for sharing personal information, and reinforce positive coping skills and help-seeking behaviors.
- CARE expedites access to help by connecting each high-risk youth to a school-based caseworker or a favorite teacher and establishing contact with a parent or guardian chosen by the youth.
- The program also includes a follow-up reassessment of broad suicide risk and protective factors and a booster motivational counseling session 9 weeks after the initial counseling session.
- The CARE program is typically delivered by school or advanced-practice nurses, counselors, psychologists, or social workers who have completed the CARE implementation training program and certification process.
- In the first study, suicide risk factors decreased by at least 25% from baseline to 5- and 10-month follow-up assessments in more than 85% of the youth exposed to the CARE program ($P<0.001$).
- CARE participants' reduction in suicide risk factors was replicated with a specific decrease in suicidal ideation ($P<0.05$) in a second study that compared CARE participants with a usual-care control group of suicidal youth over a 9-month follow-up period.
- Readiness for dissemination rating=2.2 (Best Practices Registry for Suicide Prevention [BPR]).

TABLE 31–6. Examples of screening programs *(continued)*

Columbia TeenScreen Program (Scott et al. 2009; Shaffer et al. 2004)

- Committed to using screening tools to identify and arrange treatment for youth who are suffering from depression and other undiagnosed mental illnesses and those who are at risk for suicide.
- The measures used include the Voice DISC (Diagnostic Interview Schedule for Children). This computerized diagnostic interview uses DSM-IV-TR criteria to assess for more than 30 different psychiatric disorders found in children and adolescents.
- The TeenScreen, a paper and pencil prescreen, is used before the DISC in order to identify those who require further assessment and those who do not.
- Two studies found that the program efficiently and effectively identified many adolescents who were at high risk for suicidal behaviors (Scott et al. 2009; Shaffer et al. 1996).
- Readiness for dissemination rating=3.8 (BPR).

tentially at risk for suicide. Screening is just one component of a suicide prevention program. Schools should not rely solely on screening in order to effectively address adolescent suicide. An effective program is a comprehensive program.

Pena and Caine (2006), in a comprehensive review of suicide screening programs, proposed seven validated screening instruments with good psychometrics that assess suicidal ideation and attempts: Columbia Suicide Screen, Risk of Suicide Questionnaire, Suicidal Ideation Questionnaire, Suicidal Ideation Questionnaire JR, Diagnostic Predictive Scales, Suicide Risk Screen, and Suicide Probability Scale. In high school settings, the Columbia Suicide Screen, the Suicidal Ideation Questionnaire, and the Suicidal Ideation Questionnaire JR tend to yield a large number of false positives. The two most commonly used instruments are the Suicide Risk Screen and the Suicidal Ideation Questionnaire (Joe and Bryant 2007). The Suicidal Ideation Questionnaire is used as an instrument to assess current suicidal ideation in adolescents. The 30-item version is meant for students in grades 10–12, whereas the Suicidal Ideation Questionnaire JR is a shorter, 15-item questionnaire created for grades 7–9 (Gutierrez et al. 2004). Both versions of the Suicidal Ideation

Questionnaire have good internal consistencies, ranging from 0.93 to 0.97.

Media Campaigns

In recent years, media campaigns promoting suicide prevention awareness have become more frequent. Although media initiatives have most often focused on modifying portrayals of suicide to reduce the likelihood of imitation, there have also been campaigns noting that suicide is a neglected topic and that try to inform the general public about the problem.

The Institute of Medicine (2002, pp. 276–277), in its report on reducing suicide, discussed evidence for suicide imitation:

> Throughout history, people have expressed concern about suicide imitation as evidenced by various anecdotal accounts in the literature of suicide imitation and clustering. For example, Goethe's 1774 novel *The Sorrows of Young Werther*, in which the title character shoots himself after a failed love affair, was banned in Denmark, Saxony, and Milan in order to prevent further suicides that were thought to be a result of young men imitating the behavior of Werther (Phillips 1974, 1985). These events led to the term "the Werther effect" being used to describe imitation of this sort.

Research shows that suicide contagion mediated through the media is real (for reviews, see Gould 2001a, 2001b). Recent meta-analyses report that studies conducted by clinically oriented investigators yield the strongest support for suicide imitation (cited in Schmidtke and Schaller 2000).

The Institute of Medicine (2002, pp. 278–279) went on to summarize guidelines for responsible media coverage of suicide:

Many elements of media presentations influence the likelihood of imitation, and these all provide opportunities for prevention. In efforts to prevent contagion, several countries (including Australia, Austria, Canada, Germany, Japan, New Zealand, and Switzerland) and organizations, including the World Health Organization (United Nations [United Nations Department for Policy Coordination and Sustainable Development] 1996; WHO [World Health Organization] 2000), have formulated guidelines for media coverage of suicide. The National Strategy for Suicide Prevention in the United States includes as one of its major goals improving 'the reporting and portrayals of suicidal behavior, mental illness, and substance abuse in the entertainment and news media' (PHS [Public Health Service] 2001). To advance that goal, guidelines for media coverage of suicide were formulated by the Annenberg Public Policy Center of the University of Pennsylvania, the American Association of Suicidology (AAS), and the American Foundation for Suicide Prevention (AFSP) in collaboration with several government agencies (CDC, NIMH [National Institute of Mental Health], Office of the Surgeon General, Substance Abuse and Mental Health Services Administration [SAMHSA]), the WHO, and other international suicide prevention groups. They were released in August 2001, and the full text of these guidelines can be found on the sites of the partner organizations that developed them, including www.

appcpenn.org and www.afsp.org. The guidelines, titled "Reporting on Suicide: Recommendations for the Media," update those developed in 1989 at a national consensus conference on the topic.

The media guidelines include the stipulation that media accounts of suicide should neither romanticize nor normalize suicide; that is, individuals who kill themselves should not inadvertently be idealized as heroic or romantic. They also urge the inclusion of factual information on suicide contagion and mental illness, provide suggestions for questions to ask of relatives and friends of the victim, and suggest that information on treatment resources be included. The guidelines also address issues of language such as the use of terms like "a successful suicide" and speak to special situations that may arise such as a celebrity death by suicide. Finally, they suggest that media professionals address suicide as an issue in its own right, reporting on stigma, treatments, and trends in suicide rates, rather than only in response to a tragedy (AFSP 2001) [see also National Strategy for Suicide 2002].

Currently, many comprehensive suicide prevention programs include components to improve media response to suicide, including the Finland National Program, [the] Maryland [Suicide Prevention Model], and the Washington State Youth Suicide Prevention Program (Eggert et al. 1997), with the state programs often using the nationally formulated guidelines. The Washington program included a media education component that was designed to impact reporting practices by (1) educating media personnel in ways to report youth suicide stories that prevent potential contagion effects and (2) educating select personnel such as crisis line workers, gatekeepers, and school personnel in how to respond to media requests for information and stories related to youth suicide and suicide prevention. It also focused on ensuring that the youth suicide prevention message was "in the news" by providing information to the media and encouraging ongoing and responsible coverage of suicide and suicide prevention.

Role of the Internet in Suicide Prevention

The Internet is no doubt a useful tool for those who are seeking help (www.suicidology.org; www.befrienders.org).[1] For example, Befrienders, an international organization devoted to suicide prevention (whose centers are typically called Samaritans), introduced crisis intervention for suicidal individuals by e-mail in 1994. In recent years, informal counseling of suicidal individuals has also utilized instant messaging. Organizations such as the National Suicide Prevention Lifeline introduced a Google search mechanism in April 2010. Queries regarding suicide posted to Help.com generate an automatic response with the Lifeline's toll-free number, 800-273-TALK (Boyce 2010). However, the Internet may also be used to seek information about methods for committing suicide (Yang et al. 2011).

The use of the Internet for providing psychological help began in the mid-1990s (Huang and Alessi 1996; Murphy and Mitchell 1998) and has grown in recent years, sometimes focusing on particular groups such as adolescents (Swanton et al. 2007). The services have grown to include psychological advice, support groups, testing and assessment, and counseling and therapy. This may be especially useful for segments of the population such as adolescents, who may not turn to other media for their information (Gould et al. 2002). The Internet can provide information about mental health issues, including suicide, but, as Mandrusiak et al. (2006) have documented in their study of warning signs for suicide posted on various Web sites, the information may not be reliable (Jorm et al. 2010; Szumilas and Kutcher 2009), and the quality standards of the online suicide prevention Web sites may not be the best (van Ballegooijen et al. 2009).

Two published examples of using the Internet for counseling suicidal clients have appeared (SAHAR and the Befrienders), and these are described in the following sections.

SAHAR

SAHAR is the Hebrew acronym for Support and Listening on the Net, which was designed to attract people in crisis and provide listeners, who are trained paraprofessionals, online. SAHAR uses Hebrew but, being online, is accessible to Hebrew speakers anywhere in the world. Barak (2007) noted that an online service provides easy accessibility and greater anonymity because tracing is not possible and because age, sex, and ethnicity are more easily hidden. An online service also provides immediate access to information on a variety of topics. Online services make working with groups easier, and there are other advantages such as saving the dialogue for future reference, permitting a counselor to handle several clients at the same time, and allowing both immediate feedback (instant messaging) and delayed feedback (e-mails).

SAHAR began operation in February 2001, after training the first group of counselors and after other administrative formalities (such as getting insurance coverage and organizing as a nonprofit organization). SAHAR is managed by one paid person and

---

[1]Local programs have also incorporated Web sites into their suicide prevention programs.

supported by volunteers, including counselors and programmers. The Web site (www. sahar.org.il) has several sections: 1) informative articles on various aspects of distress, such as psychiatric disorders, helping a suicidal friend, and myths about suicide; 2) a list of community support services with addresses, telephone numbers, e-mail addresses, and links where available; 3) information on telephone hotlines and emergency services for those needing immediate help; 4) an extensive list of recommended books and other readings; 5) links to other relevant sites for people in distress; and 6) a page about SAHAR and information about volunteering and donating.

For counseling, SAHAR offers individual, personal communication via personal chat software or instant messaging, and counseling via e-mail for those who prefer this medium. In the latter case, clients can use their own e-mail address or use an online forum at the site in order to preserve their anonymity. In addition, SAHAR offers group communication by online forums and chat rooms (protected by passwords and monitored by paraprofessional helpers). There are four forums: youngsters, adults, enlisted soldiers, and creative support (using poetry, stories, and painting). The counselors all remain anonymous to prevent relationships developing between clients and helpers.

SAHAR operates only 3 hours each day. Conversations last on the average 45–60 minutes, and the Web site is accessed more than 10,000 times each month (350 times each day). The data indicate that there have been more than 300,000 visits by 120,000 unique users. Approximately 1,000 personal conversations take place each month, with about 50% from clearly suicidal clients. SAHAR has also intervened, using community services such as the police, in roughly 100 cases in which people were in the process of committing suicide.

Barak (2007) noted problems similar to those reported by telephone counseling services (Lester 2002): imposters presenting as suicides, fake messages in the forums that distress the other participants, emotional stress and burnout in the counselors, difficulty maintaining discipline in the volunteers (so that they act professionally), and software glitches that interrupt the service. The fact that all e-therapy sessions are saved makes supervising the volunteers easier than in telephone hotlines, the majority of which do not automatically record all calls. However, Barak noted that many distressed individuals do not find writing easy, and so this type of service is not for them.

Gilat and Shahar (2007) compared clients using a service that provided a telephone hotline, personal chat over the Internet, and an asynchronous online support group. They found that high-risk suicidal communications were much more common in the asynchronous online support group than in the two other modes (15.3% vs. 1.4% and 0.3%).

The Befrienders: Suicide Prevention by E-Mail

Sustained counseling using e-mail communications is offered by the Befrienders (also known as the Samaritans). In these situations, a client contacts the suicide prevention center by sending an e-mail communication. Within 24 hours, a counselor reads the communication and writes and sends a response. This exchange may continue for a period of time.

For the Samaritans, there is a central address for e-mail messages from clients (Armson 1997; Bale 2001; Baughan 2000; Howlett and Langdon 2004; Morgan 1996).

The central computer then assigns the message to a center. Encryption (scrambling) of the letters is possible if clients desire this.[2] In 1998, this service had 15,309 contacts, of which 51% involved suicidal ideation (Baughan 2000); in 2001, 61 branches online had received 64,000 e-mails, with 50% suicidal in nature (Howlett and Langdon 2004).

E-Therapy

In recent years, Web companies (e.g., MyTherapyNet.com, HelpHorizons.com) have introduced services that link clients with therapists where counseling can be conducted using instant messaging, and some therapists are offering instant messaging as a supplement to office-based counseling (LaVallee 2006).

LaVallee (2006) noted that online providers generally agree that instant messaging is not appropriate for suicidal clients. The e-therapy sites typically urge suicidal people to call 911 and ask them to indicate that they have read this warning before a chat session can begin. However, there is no guarantee that suicidal clients will actually read such a warning or heed it.

Barak, Klein, and Proudfoot (2009) classified Internet-supported interventions into four categories, based on their approach: 1) Web-based interventions, 2) online counseling and therapy, 3) Internet-operated therapeutic software, and 4) other online activities. These interventions are described in further detail in Table 31–7.

Other Suicide Prevention Programs and Modalities

Helplines

There are over 350 Befrienders International Centers, associated with the Samaritans, in over 40 countries (Scott 2001), and there were over 1,000 teen suicide hotlines alone in the United States as of 1992 (National Center for Injury Prevention and Control 1992). Hotlines and crisis intervention services include a broad scope of services, including anonymous or non-anonymous phone counseling for suicidal individuals and/or their family and friends, face-to-face counseling, and referrals by professionals, paraprofessionals, and/or volunteers with various training. These services can intervene during an acute suicidal crisis and connect individuals to additional mental health services that they might not otherwise seek. Certification is available through the American Association of Suicidology for North American phone helplines and from the Samaritans by membership in Befrienders International, based in London. Accreditation or membership, however, does not require formal evaluation of services nor is monitoring of services provided (Mishara and Daigle 2001).

Helplines for suicide prevention are generally part of wider suicide prevention programs. In reviewing data on the role of helplines, Lester (2010) observed that their role in the suicide rate, although small, is encouraging. It is critical that researchers continue to work on this issue using longer time periods, other nations, and more sophisticated research designs so that we can

---

[2]Access is limited to a Web site (www.compulink.co.uk/~careware/samaritans/) and Internet e-mail. E-mails are always answered by real volunteers; there are no "automatic" responses. Other Internet techniques, such as Telnet or anonymous ftp, do not work.

TABLE 31–7. Categories of Internet-supported interventions

Web-based interventions

- Self-guided intervention program that is executed by means of a prescriptive online program operated through a Web site and used by consumers seeking health- and mental health–related assistance.
  - Provision of health-related material and use of interactive Web-based components:
    - Program content
    - Multimedia use/choices
    - Interactive online activities
    - Guidance and supportive feedback

Online counseling and therapy

- Client must have technical and writing skills.
- Client must have mild to moderate pathology.
- Directed to the individual or to groups.
- Invisibility may cause group therapy to be more complicated and limited than individual counseling.
- Therapists should be prepared to make emergency provisions (identifying and locating clients, using external help from a distance) should they identify a dangerous state, such as a client being suicidal.

Internet-operated therapeutic software

- Therapeutic software that uses advanced computer capabilities for robotic simulation of therapists providing dialogue-based therapy with patients, rule-based expert systems, and gaming and three-dimensional virtual environments, such as Second Life.

Other online activities

- Online activities such as the publication of personal blogs; participation in support groups via chat, audio, or Web cam communication channels; the use of online assessments; and accessing health-related information.
- These activities may be used as stand-alone functions by individuals or prescribed by therapists as supplements to the main treatment modality.

Source. Barak et al. 2009.

---

have a more reliable meta-analysis in the future.

The Air Force Suicide Prevention Strategy

The U.S. Air Force has implemented a comprehensive suicide prevention program. A multilayered intervention was targeted at reducing the risk factors and enhancing the factors that are considered protective. The intervention consisted of removing the stigma of seeking help for a mental health or psychosocial problem, enhancing the understanding of mental health, and changing policies and social norms. Relative risk reductions (the prevented fraction) for suicide and other outcomes were hypothesized to be sensitive to broadly based community prevention efforts (family violence, accidental death, and homicide).

Additional outcomes not exclusively associated with suicide were included because of the comprehensiveness of the program. Implementation of the results of the program was associated with a sustained decline in the rate of suicide and other adverse outcomes. A 33% relative risk reduction was observed for suicide after the intervention, whereas reductions for other outcomes ranged from 18% to 54% (Knox et al. 2003). After the implementation of this broadly based, community-level suicide prevention program, there were fewer suicides.

Primary Care Physician Training Program for Recognition and Management of Depression and Suicide Prevention

Most people who die by suicide are found to have contacted their primary care physician within a few weeks prior to death (Luoma et al. 2002; Mesec Rodi et al. 2010). This suggests a need to have primary care physicians become familiar with suicide assessment.

In 2008, the World Health Organization launched the Mental Health Gap Action Programme (mhGAP) to address the lack of care, especially in low- and middle-income countries, for people suffering from mental, neurological, and substance use disorders. The mhGAP Intervention Guide was developed for use in nonspecialized health care settings. It is aimed at health care providers working at first- and second-level facilities. These providers may be working in a health center or as part of the clinical team at a district-level hospital or clinic and include general physicians, family physicians, nurses, and clinical officers. Suicide assessment is part of this program, with flowcharts that help those who are not familiar with suicide prevention to generate decisions.

The Gotland study is the most famous of this type of suicide prevention program. This study on education of primary care practitioners on depression was conducted between 1983 and 1984 on the Swedish island of Gotland. This educational program was offered to all general practitioners of the island during a 2-year period and involved two training sessions. The program was characterized by a combination of oral and written information, group work, videotaped and written case reports, sharing of personal experiences, and an integrative ideology describing the process of becoming depressed and suicidal and recovering from it in a multidimensional way (Rutz 2001).

The training was evaluated starting at baseline prior to the educational intervention and at 5 years after the intervention. The general practitioners reported increased knowledge and capacity to detect patients with depressive conditions, improved capacity for risk assessment concerning suicidality, and improved diagnostic, therapeutic, and monitoring ability to detect and follow-up depressions in a comprehensive way. Two years after the educational intervention, referrals to psychiatry for depressive conditions had decreased by about 50%, and the number of suicides had fallen by 60%. However, 4 years after the educational program ended, inpatient care for depression and the suicide rate returned again to almost baseline values, and the prescription of antidepressants stabilized, indicating that the effects were strictly time related to the educational program. In 1988, 50% of the general practitioners who participated in the educational program had left their positions in Gotland (Rutz 2001).

Furthermore, detailed study on all suicides in Gotland showed that the main decrease in suicides was in female suicidal patients with a diagnosis of major depression. Male violent suicides were unaffected by the educational program, except for older men who were in contact with general practitioners. Those men who were known to the medical system but later died by suicide belonged to a group not diagnosed as depressed and suicidal and often presenting with aggressive behaviors and poor adherence to treatment (Rihmer et al. 1995; Rutz 2001).

Henriksson and Isacsson (2006) evaluated the effects of a continuing medical education program (eight interactive seminars conducted between 1995 and 2002) for general practitioners in Jämtland county in Sweden. The authors found that the mean suicide rate of the county decreased by 36% in the intervention period, compared with the pre-intervention period (1970–1994), whereas the mean suicide rate of Sweden as a whole decreased by 30% during the same time. In the same years, the use of antidepressants in Jämtland county increased from 25% below the Swedish average to the same level. In line with the greater reduction of suicide rate in Jämtland county, the use of antidepressants increased by 161% in this county, whereas the same figure for the whole of Sweden was 108%.

A similar intervention was conducted in Kiskunhalas, Hungary (Kalmár 2008; Szanto et al. 2007). The rate of antidepressant prescriptions and the rate of antidepressant-treated persons increased significantly more in the intervention region than in the control region. Further, the decrease in the annual suicide rate was significantly greater in the intervention region (9.8 per 100,000) compared with the control region (6.9 per 100,000) and with Hungary as a whole (4.5 per 100,000).

More recently, Roskar et al. (2010) evaluated the effects of a training program on the recognition and management of depression and suicide risk for 82 Slovenian primary care physicians from two Slovenian regions (with a neighboring region used as a control). The 4-hour training consisted of two lectures providing theoretical information about depression and suicide (e.g., etiology, prevalence) and practical guidelines about treating depression. The lectures were followed by a longer workshop that included a role-play between a physician and a depressive/suicidal patient. The results indicated a significant increase in the number of antidepressant prescriptions, but the 12% decrease in the number of suicides between the two observation periods in the intervention regions was not significantly larger than the 4% decrease in the control region.

PROSPECT (Prevention of Suicide in Primary Care Elderly: Collaborative Trial) is a program that aims to prevent suicide among older primary care patients by reducing suicidal ideation and depression (http://nrepp.samhsa.gov/ViewIntervention.aspx?id=128). PROSPECT is a multidimensional intervention whose components are 1) recognition of depression and suicidal ideation by primary care physicians, 2) application of a treatment algorithm for geriatric depression in the primary care setting, and 3) treatment management by health specialists (e.g., nurses, social workers, psychologists). The treatment algorithm assists primary care physicians in making appropriate care choices during the acute, continuation, and maintenance phases of treatment.

Bruce et al. (2004) studied the effect of the PROSPECT program. They hypothesized that older patients randomly assigned to receive the intervention and compared with usual care (usual care was enhanced by initially educating physicians about the treatment guidelines and notifying them when a patient met criteria for a diagnosis of depression) would demonstrate 1) a greater reduction in suicidal ideation and 2) a greater reduction in depressive symptoms, increased response rates, and greater remission rates in depressive symptoms. Enrollment included patients with a major depression or clinically significant minor depression as defined by DSM-IV and a random sample of patients who screened negative ($N=598$; 320 intervention, 278 usual care). The study was conducted in 20 primary care practices from greater New York City, Philadelphia, and Pittsburgh.

The results indicated that intervention patients were significantly more likely than usual-care patients to report depression treatment at each follow-up period (4, 8, 12 months). Intervention patients had higher rates of medication-only ($P<0.001$) and psychotherapy-only ($P<0.001$) treatment. The small number of patients receiving combination treatment did not differ between groups ($P=0.23$). Despite the fact that patients in the intervention group were more likely to report suicidal ideation at baseline than patients in the usual-care group, by 4 months and at each subsequent follow-up period, rates of suicidal ideation no longer differed between groups, reflecting a significantly greater decline in suicidal ideation in the intervention group after adjusting for the baseline difference. In the intervention group, raw rates of suicidal ideation declined from 29.4% to 16.5% compared with 20.1% to 17.1% in the usual-care group ($P=0.01$).

Two sets of post hoc analyses examined the effect of the PROSPECT intervention stratified by both depression diagnosis and suicidality. Among patients who reported suicidal ideation at baseline, suicidal ideation had resolved by 4 months in 66.7% of intervention patients compared with 58.7% of patients receiving usual care ($P=0.34$). The difference between groups was more pronounced and statistically significant at 8 months (70.7% vs. 43.9%; $P=0.005$). By 12 months, about two-thirds of both groups no longer expressed suicidal ideation (68.7% vs. 65.8%, $P=0.89$). Consistent with the group difference peaking at 8 months, the omnibus test for change across time was significant ($P=0.03$). The pattern was similar within the major depression and the minor depression subgroups, although the omnibus test did not reach statistical significance in either group (major depression, $P=0.09$; minor depression, $P=0.09$).

The European Alliance Against Depression

The European Alliance Against Depression began with the Nuremberg Alliance Against Depression (NAAD) and later expanded to other European Union countries. The NAAD was carried out as a subproject of the German Research Network on Depression and Suicidality (*Kompetenznetz Depression, Suizidalität*) and was funded by the German Federal Ministry of Education and Research in the city of Nuremberg (500,000 inhabitants) during 2001–2002.

The NAAD intervention used a four-level approach that included education of general practitioners through the use of training sessions and videos (level 1); public relations activities (level 2); training sessions for key figures such as priests, social workers, geriatric caregivers, teachers, and the media (level 3); and help for high-risk groups (such as individuals who had attempted suicide) and their relatives (level 4) (see Figure 31–1). Hegerl et al. (2006) evaluated the effects of a 2-year intervention in Nuremberg with respect to a 1-year baseline and a control region (Würzburg). The results indicated a reduction in the frequency of suicidal acts in Nuremberg during the 2-year intervention (2000–2002: –24%; $P<0.01$) and suicidal attempts (2000–2002: –26.5%; $P<0.001$). The study failed to find evidence for a significant reduction in completed suicides when compared with the control region.

Following these promising results, activities were initiated in Regensburg in 2003 (Hübner-Liebermann et al. 2010). Hübner-Liebermann et al. (2010) compared the rate of suicide in the city of Regensburg with the rates in the control regions of the county districts of Regensburg and Neumarkt, where no activities took place, as well as with the overall suicide rate of Germany. The study revealed significant changes in suicide rates from 1998 to 2007 only for the city of Regensburg, especially in the male population.

The Nuremberg approach was used as a model for OSPI-Europe (optimizing sui-

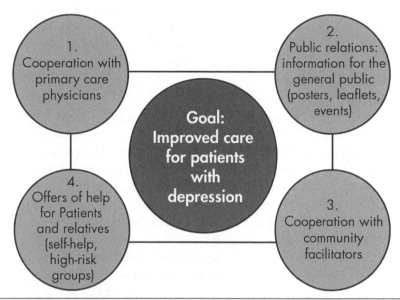

FIGURE 31–1. Four-level approach of Nuremberg Alliance Against Depression interventions.

cide prevention programs and their implementation in Europe) (Hegerl et al. 2009), a collaborative research project funded by the European Commission under the Seventh Framework Programme (http:// www.ospi-europe.com/en/ospi-project-description.php). OSPI-Europe supplemented the Nuremberg intervention approach with a fifth level: restriction of access to lethal means.

Conclusion

It should be clear that suicide prevention programs that attempt to deal with suicide as if it were a unique disorder may be far too narrow in their focus. This may be particularly the case when dealing with populations in which there are significantly heightened levels of other disorders and/or heightened exposure to high levels of multiple risk conditions for such disorders.

Key Clinical Concepts

- Worldwide, the prevention of suicide has not been adequately addressed due to basically a lack of awareness of suicide as a major problem and the taboo in many societies to discuss it openly. In fact, only a few countries have included prevention of suicide among their priorities.

- To some extent, suicide prevention programs have been implemented before appropriate assessments have been completed; gaps may exist in knowledge about the efficacy, effectiveness, safety, or economic impact of specific prevention strategies. Without evaluation of programs, we do not know if the program benefits or harms the people we are trying to help.

- The interest in classifying populations of suicidal patients by their psychiatric diagnoses is being supplemented by an interest in understanding what makes a minority of patients within any given diagnostic category suicidal while the majority are not suicidal. It is clear that suicide prevention requires intervention also from outside the health sector and calls for an innovative, comprehensive multisectorial approach, including both health and nonhealth sectors (e.g., education, labor, police, justice, religion, law, politics, the media).

- Before a suicide prevention program is initiated, it is necessary to establish policies and procedures focused on such issues as how to respond effectively to a student who may be indicating suicidal ideation or threats, how to respond to the aftermath of a suicide attempt or a death by suicide, and the various roles school personnel may play in preventing suicide and intervening and coping with a student who may be suicidal. Such policies increase the likelihood that a school suicide prevention program will be effectively implemented and maintained.

- The conceptualization of developmental pathways as the primary focus of preventive interventions that we have offered here has direct implications for the evaluation of prevention programs. Initial and ongoing assessments of the efficacy of suicide prevention efforts can and should be built, at least in part, on the degree to which they are successful in reducing those risk factors and vulnerabilities and/or increasing those protective factors and competencies that they identify as primary targets. For example, our first assessments of program impact would focus on the degree to which levels of risk have been reduced and levels of enhancing conditions increased. Next, we would assess the degree to which the incidence and prevalence of vulnerabilities and competencies in the population have been changed.

- Prevention efforts should occur within the context of health education programs and cultural development processes that promote a safe and healthy environment, increase self-esteem, and address adolescent difficulties. In general, efforts should be made to address and manage the difficulties faced by young people from adverse childhood backgrounds who have multiple problems of personal adjustment (including disorders such as depression, alcohol and drug abuse, and conduct disorders).

- Governments should seek to integrate suicide prevention into existing health, mental health, substance abuse, education, and human services activities. Settings that provide related services such as schools, workplaces, clinics, medical offices, correctional and detention centers, elder care facilities, faith-based institutions, and community centers are all important venues for seamless suicide prevention activities.

- There should be an emphasis on early interventions to reduce risk factors for suicide and promote protective factors. As important as it is to recognize and help suicidal individuals, progress depends on measures that address problems early and promote strengths so that fewer people become suicidal.

References

Adolescent Health Committee of the Canadian Paediatric Society: Youth and firearms in Canada. Paediatr Child Health 10:473–477, 2005

American Foundation for Suicide Prevention: Reporting on Suicide: Recommendations for the Media. New York, American Foundation for Suicide Prevention, 2001

Armson S: Suicide and cyberspace—befriending by e-mail. Crisis 18:103–105, 1997

Aseltine RH Jr, DeMartino R: An outcome evaluation of the SOS suicide prevention program. Am J Public Health 94:446–451, 2004

Aseltine RH Jr, James A, Schilling EA, et al: Evaluating the SOS suicide prevention program: a replication and extension. BMC Public Health 7:161, 2007

Bale C: Befriending in cyberspace—challenges and opportunities. Crisis 22:10–11, 2001

Barak A: Emotional support and suicide prevention through the Internet: a field project report. Computers in Human Behavior 23:971–984, 2007

Barak A, Klein B, Proudfoot JG: Defining internet-supported therapeutic interventions. Ann Behav Med 38:4–17, 2009

Barrish HH, Saunders M, Wolf MM: Good Behavior Game: effects of individual contingencies for group consequences on disruptive behavior in a classroom. J Appl Behav Anal 2:119–124, 1969

Baughan R: E-listening: the Samaritans' experience. Counselling 11:292–293, 2000

Beautrais AL, Coggan CA, Fergusson DM, et al: The Prevention, Recognition, and Management of Young People at Risk of Suicide: Development of Guidelines for Schools. Wellington, New Zealand, National Advisory Committee on Health and Disability, 1997

Beautrais AL, Fergusson D, Coggan C, et al: Effective strategies for suicide prevention in New Zealand: a review of the evidence. N Z Med J 120:U2459, 2007

Boyce N: Pilots of the future: suicide prevention and the internet. Lancet 376:1889–1890, 2010

Brent DA, Baugher M, Birmaher B, et al: Compliance with recommendations to remove firearms in families participating in a clinical trial for adolescent depression. J Am Acad Child Adolesc Psychiatry 39:1220–1226, 2000

Bruce ML, Ten Have TR, Reynolds CF III, et al: Reducing suicidal ideation and depressive symptoms in depressed older primary care patients: a randomized controlled trial. JAMA 291:1081–1091, 2004

Burns JM, Patton GC: Preventive interventions for youth suicide: a risk factor–based approach. Aust N Z J Psychiatry 34:388–407, 2000

Carlyon P, Carlyon W, McCarthy AR: Family and community involvement in school health, in Health Is Academic: A Guide to Coordinated School Health Programs. Edited by Marx E, Wooley SF, Northrop D. New York, Teachers College Press, 1998, pp 67–95

Davidson S, Manion IG: Canadian Youth Mental Health and Illness Survey: Survey Overview, Interview Schedule, and Demographic Cross Tabulations. Ottawa, ON, Canada, Canadian Psychiatric Association, 1993

Eckert TL, Miller DN, DuPaul GJ, et al: Adolescent suicide prevention: school psychologists' acceptability of school-based programs. School Psychology Review 32:57–76, 2003

Eggert LL, Nicholas LJ: Reconnecting Youth: A Peer Group Approach to Building Life Skills, 2nd Edition. Bloomington, IN, National Educational Service, 2004

Eggert LL, Thompson EA, Herting JR, et al: Preventing adolescent drug abuse and high school dropout through an intensive school-based social network development program. Am J Health Promot 8:202–215, 1994a

Eggert LL, Thompson EA, Herting JR, et al: Prevention research program: reconnecting at-risk youth. Issues Ment Health Nurs 15:107–135, 1994b

Eggert LL, Thompson EA, Herting JR, et al: Reducing suicide potential among high-risk youth: tests of a school-based prevention program. Suicide Life Threat Behav 25:276–296, 1995

Eggert LL, Randell BR, Thompson EA, et al: Washington State Youth Suicide Prevention Program: Report of Activities. Seattle, University of Washington, 1997

Eggert LL, Thompson EA, Herting JR, et al: Reconnecting youth to prevent drug abuse, school dropout, and suicidal behaviors among high-risk youth, in Innovations in Adolescent Substance Abuse Intervention. Edited by Wagner E, Waldron HB. Oxford, UK, Elsevier Science, 2001, pp 51–84

Eggert LL, Thompson EA, Randell BP, et al: Preliminary effects of brief school-based prevention approaches for reducing youth suicide—risk behaviors, depression, and drug involvement. J Child Adolesc Psychiatr Nurs 15:48–64, 2002

Garland AF, Zigler E: Adolescent suicide prevention: current research and social policy implications. Am Psychol 48:169–182, 1993

Gilat I, Shahar G: Emotional first aid for a suicide crisis: comparison between Telephonic hotline and internet. Psychiatry 70:12–18, 2007

Goldney RD: Suicide prevention: a pragmatic review of recent studies. Crisis 26:128–140, 2005

Gould MS: Suicide and the media. Ann N Y Acad Sci 932:200–221; discussion 221–204, 2001a

Gould MS: Suicide contagion: Workshop presentation at the Institute of Medicine's Workshop on Suicide Prevention and Intervention, May 14, 2001. Washington, DC, National Academy Press, 2001b, pp 8–10

Gould MS, Kramer RA: Youth suicide prevention. Suicide Life Threat Behav 31(suppl):6–31, 2001

Gould MS, Munfakh JL, Lubell K, et al: Seeking help from the internet during adolescence. J Am Acad Child Adolesc Psychiatry 41:1182–1189, 2002

Gould MS, Greenberg T, Velting DM, et al: Youth suicide risk and preventive interventions: a review of the past 10 years. J Am Acad Child Adolesc Psychiatry 42:386–405, 2003

Grossman DC, Cummings P, Koepsell TD, et al: Firearm safety counseling in primary care pediatrics: a randomized, controlled trial. Pediatrics 106:22–26, 2000

Gutierrez PM, Watkins R, Collura D: Suicide risk screening in an urban high school. Suicide Life Threat Behav 34:421–428, 2004

Hallfors D, Brodish PH, Khatapoush S, et al: Feasibility of screening adolescents for suicide risk in "real-world" high school settings. Am J Public Health 96:282–287, 2006

Hayden DC, Lauer P: Prevalence of suicide programs in schools and roadblocks to implementation. Suicide Life Threat Behav 30:239–251, 2000

Hegerl U, Althaus D, Schmidtke A, et al: The alliance against depression: 2-year evaluation of a community-based intervention to reduce suicidality. Psychol Med 36:1225–1233, 2006

Hegerl U, Wittenburg L, Arensman E, et al: Optimizing suicide prevention programs and their implementation in Europe (OSPI Europe): an evidence-based multi-level approach. BMC Public Health 9:428, 2009

Henriksson S, Isacsson G: Increased antidepressant use and fewer suicides in Jämtland county, Sweden, after a primary care educational programme on the treatment of depression. Acta Psychiatr Scand 114:159–167, 2006

Howlett S, Langdon R: Messages to Jo, in Writing Cures: An Introductory Handbook of Writing in Counseling and Therapy. Edited by Bolton G, Howlett S, Lago C, et al. New York, Brunner-Routledge, 2004, pp 160–169

Huang MP, Alessi NE: The Internet and the future of psychiatry. Am J Psychiatry 153:861–869, 1996

Hübner-Liebermann B, Neuner T, Hegerl U, et al: Reducing suicides through an alliance against depression? Gen Hosp Psychiatry 32:514–518, 2010

Institute of Medicine: Reducing Suicide: A National Imperative. Edited by Goldsmith SK, Pellmar TC, Kleinman AM, et al. Washington, DC, National Academies Press, 2002

Isaac M, Elias B, Katz LY, et al: Gatekeeper training as a preventative intervention for suicide: a systematic review. Can J Psychiatry 54:260–268, 2009

Joe S, Bryant H: Evidence-based suicide prevention screening in schools. Child Sch 29:219–227, 2007

Jorm AF, Fischer JA, Oh E: Effect of feedback on the quality of suicide prevention websites: randomised controlled trial. Br J Psychiatry 197:73–74, 2010

Kalafat J, Elias MJ: Suicide prevention in an educational context: broad and narrow foci. Suicide Life Threat Behav 25:123–133, 1995

Kalmár S: Programs for prevention of depression and suicide in Kiskunhalas, Hungary [in Hungarian]. Psychiatr Hung 23:244–248; discussion 248, 2008

King CA, Kramer A, Preuss L, et al: Youth-Nominated Support Team for Suicidal Adolescents (Version 1): a randomized controlled trial. J Consult Clin Psychol 74:199–206, 2006

King KA, Smith J: Project SOAR: a training program to increase school counselors' knowledge and confidence regarding suicide prevention and intervention. J Sch Health 70:402–407, 2000

King KA, Price JH, Telljohann SK, et al: High school health teachers' perceived self-efficacy in identifying students at risk for suicide. J Sch Health 69:202–207, 1999

Klingman A, Hochdorf Z: Coping with distress and self harm: the impact of a primary prevention program among adolescents. J Adolesc 16:121–140, 1993

Knox KL, Litts DA, Talcott GW, et al: Risk of suicide and related adverse outcomes after exposure to a suicide prevention programme in the US Air Force: cohort study. BMJ 327:1376, 2003

LaVallee A: Chat therapy. The Wall Street Journal, March 28, 2006, p D1

Lazear K, Roggenbaum S, Blase K: Youth Suicide Prevention School-Based Guide—Overview. Tampa, FL, Department of Child and Family Studies, Division of State and Local Support, Louis de la Parte Florida Mental Health Institute, University of South Florida, 2003

Lester D: Crisis Intervention and Counseling by Telephone. Springfield, IL, Charles C Thomas, 2002

Lester D: Evidence-based suicide prevention by helplines: a meta-analysis, in Evidence-Based Practice in Suicidology: A Source Book. Edited by Pompili M, Tatarelli R. Cambridge, MA, Hogrefe Publishing, 2010, pp 139–151

Luoma JB, Martin CE, Pearson JL: Contact with mental health and primary care providers before suicide: a review of the evidence. Am J Psychiatry 159:909–916, 2002

Mandrusiak M, Rudd MD, Joiner TE Jr, et al: Warning signs for suicide on the Internet: a descriptive study. Suicide Life Threat Behav 36:263–271, 2006

Mann JJ, Apter A, Bertolote J, et al: Suicide prevention strategies: a systematic review. JAMA 294:2064–2074, 2005

Marx E, Northrop D: Educating for Health: A Guide for Implementing a Comprehensive Approach to School Health Education. Newton, MA, Education Development Center, 1995

Mesec Rodi P, Roskar S, Marusic A: Suicide victims' last contact with the primary care physician: report from Slovenia. Int J Soc Psychiatry 56:280–287, 2010

Miller DN, Eckert TL, DuPaul GJ, et al: Adolescent suicide prevention: acceptability of school-based programs among secondary school principals. Suicide Life Threat Behav 29:72–85, 1999

Mishara BL, Daigle M: Helplines and crisis intervention services: challenges for the future, in Suicide Prevention: Resources for the Millennium. Edited by Lester D. Philadelphia, PA, Brunner-Routledge, 2001, pp 153–171

Mitchell P: Primary Prevention and Early Intervention: Evaluation of the National Youth Suicide Prevention Strategy. Melbourne, Australia, Australian Institute of Family Studies, 2000

Morgan C: Befriending by e-mail. Befriending Worldwide 49:11, 1996

Murphy LJ, Mitchell DL: When writing helps to heal: e-mail as therapy. Br J Guid Counc 26:21–32, 1998

National Center for Injury Prevention and Control: Youth Suicide Prevention Programs: A Resource Guide. Atlanta, GA, Centers for Disease Control and Prevention, 1992

National Strategy for Suicide: Reporting on suicide: recommendations for the media. Suicide Life Threat Behav 32:viii–xiii, 2002

Oatis PJ, Fenn Buderer NM, Cummings P, et al: Pediatric practice based evaluation of the Steps to Prevent Firearm Injury program. Inj Prev 5:48–52, 1999

O'Carroll PW, Potter LB, Mercy JA: Programs for the prevention of suicide among adolescents and young adults. MMWR Recomm Rep 43:1–7, 1994

Orbach I, Bar-Joseph H: The impact of a suicide prevention program for adolescents on suicidal tendencies, hopelessness, ego identity, and coping. Suicide Life Threat Behav 23:120–129, 1993

Pena JB, Caine ED: Screening as an approach for adolescent suicide prevention. Suicide Life Threat Behav 36:614–637, 2006

Phillips DP: The influence of suggestion on suicide: substantive and theroretical implications of the Werther effect. Am Sociol Rev 39:340–354, 1974

Phillips DP: The Werther effect: suicide, and other forms of violence, are contagious. Sciences (New York) 25:32–39, 1985

Pompili M: Evidence-based practice in suicidology what we need and what we need to know, in Evidence-Based Practice in Suicidology: A Source Book. Edited by Pompili M, Tatarelli R. Cambridge, MA, Hogrefe, 2010, pp 3–25

Program for Parents Project: Program for Parents: a program of Parenting Australia, Part B: summary report of evaluation by the Centre for Adolescent Health (executive summary). 1999. Available at: http://www.jss.org.au/files/Docs/policy-and-advocacy/publications/program_for_parenting.pdf. Accessed August 13, 2011.

Public Health Service: National Strategy for Suicide Prevention: Goals and Objectives for Action. Rockville, MD, U.S. Department of Health and Human Services, 2001

Ramsay RF, Cooke MA, Lang WA: Alberta's suicide prevention training programs: a retrospective comparison with Rothman's developmental research model. Suicide Life Threat Behav 20:335–351, 1990

Randell BP, Eggert LL, Pike KC: Immediate post intervention effects of two brief youth suicide prevention interventions. Suicide Life Threat Behav 31:41–61, 2001

Rihmer Z, Rutz W, Pihlgren H: Depression and suicide on Gotland: an intensive study of all suicides before and after a depression-training programme for general practitioners. J Affect Disord 35:147–152, 1995

Roskar S, Podlesek A, Zorko M, et al: Effects of training program on recognition and management of depression and suicide risk evaluation for Slovenian primary-care physicians: follow-up study. Croat Med J 51:237–242, 2010

Rutz W: Preventing suicide and premature death by education and treatment. J Affect Disord 62:123–129, 2001

Rutz W, von Knorring L, Walinder J: Long-term effects of an educational program for general practitioners given by the Swedish Committee for the Prevention and Treatment of Depression. Acta Psychiatr Scand 85:83–88, 1992

Schmidtke A, Schaller S: The role of mass media in suicide prevention, in The International Handbook of Suicide and Attempted Suicide. Edited by Hawton K, Van Heeringen K. Chichester, UK, Wiley, 2000, pp 675–697

Scott MA, Wilcox HC, Schonfeld IS, et al: School-based screening to identify at-risk students not already known to school professionals: the Columbia Suicide Screen. Am J Public Health 99:334–339, 2009

Scott V: Crisis services: Befrienders International: volunteer action in preventing suicide, in Suicide Prevention: Resources for the Millenium. Edited by Lester D. Philadelphia, PA, Brunner-Routledge, 2001, pp 265–273

Shaffer D, Gould MS, Fisher P, et al: Psychiatric diagnosis in child and adolescent suicide. Arch Gen Psychiatry 53:339–348, 1996

Shaffer D, Scott M, Wilcox H, et al: The Columbia Suicide Screen: validity and reliability of a screen for youth suicide and depression. J Am Acad Child Adolesc Psychiatry 43:71–79, 2004

Shochet I, Ham D: Universal school-based approaches to preventing adolescent depression: past findings and future directions of the Resourceful Adolescent Program. International Journal of Mental Health Promotion 6:17–25, 2004

Steele MM, Doey T: Suicidal behaviour in children and adolescents, Part 2: treatment and prevention. Can J Psychiatry 52 (suppl 1):35S–45S, 2007

Stuart C, Waalen JK, Haelstromm E: Many helping hearts: an evaluation of peer gate-keeper training in suicide risk assessment. Death Stud 27:321–333, 2003

Swanton R, Collin P, Burns J, et al: Engaging, understanding and including young people in the provision of mental health services. Int J Adolesc Med Health 19:325–332, 2007

Szanto K, Kalmár S, Hendin H, et al: A suicide prevention program in a region with a very high suicide rate. Arch Gen Psychiatry 64:914–920, 2007

Szumilas M, Kutcher S: Teen suicide information on the internet: a systematic analysis of quality. Can J Psychiatry 54:596–604, 2009

Thompson EA, Eggert LL: Using the suicide risk screen to identify suicidal adolescents among potential high school dropouts. J Am Acad Child Adolesc Psychiatry 38:1506–1514, 1999

Thompson EA, Eggert LL, Herting JR: Mediating effects of an indicated prevention program for reducing youth depression and suicide risk behaviors. Suicide Life Threat Behav 30:252–271, 2000

Thompson EA, Eggert LL, Randell BP, et al: Evaluation of indicated suicide risk prevention approaches for potential high school dropouts. Am J Public Health 91:742–752, 2001

United Nations Department for Policy Coordination and Sustainable Development: Prevention of Suicide: Guidelines for the Formulation and Implementation of National Strategies. New York, United Nations, 1996

van Ballegooijen W, van Spijker BA, Kerkhof AJ: The quality of online suicide prevention in the Netherlands and Flanders in 2007 [in Dutch]. Tijdschr Psychiatr 51:117–122, 2009

White J, Jodoin N: Before-the-Fact Interventions: A Manual of Best Practices in Youth Suicide Prevention. Vancouver, BC, Canada, University of British Columbia, 1998

World Health Organization: Guidelines for the Primary Prevention of Mental, Neurological, and Psychosocial Disorders. Geneva, World Health Organization, 1998

World Health Organization: Preventing Suicide: A Resource for Media Professionals. Geneva, World Health Organization, 2000

Wyman PA, Brown CH, Inman J, et al: Randomized trial of a gatekeeper program for suicide prevention: 1-year impact on secondary school staff. J Consult Clin Psychol 76:104–115, 2008

Yang AC, Tsai SJ, Huang NE, et al: Association of Internet search trends with suicide death in Taipei City, Taiwan, 2004–2009. J Affect Disord 132:179–184, 2011

Zenere FJ III, Lazarus PJ: The decline of youth suicidal behavior in an urban, multicultural public school system following the introduction of a suicide prevention and intervention program. Suicide Life Threat Behav 27:387–402, 1997

C H A P T E R   3 2

Suicide Research

Knowledge Gaps and Opportunities

Alan L. Berman, Ph.D., A.B.P.P.

The scientific study of suicide (suicidology) arguably began with the work of Émile Durkheim, the French sociologist, and was indelibly marked by the publication of his book *Suicide: A Study in Sociology* (1897/1951). In truth, suicidal behavior had been studied before Durkheim, notably by Morselli, in Italy (see Goldney and Schioldann 2000), but Durkheim's efforts were clearly the first major theory-driven investigations of the effect of social forces (independent variables) on suicide rates (dependent variables).

Official statistics on deaths by suicide, Durkheim's dependent variables, remain "fraught with inaccuracies" (Goldsmith et al. 2002) to this day. For this reason, and because of the low base rate for deaths by suicide upon which hypothesized impacts of interventions must rely to demonstrate significant effect, more modern research studies have relied heavily on samples of nonfatal attempters, a heterogeneous group of persons who have engaged in a range of self-injurious behaviors across a range of potential lethality with varying degrees of

stated or unstated intent. Notably, because of the lack of specificity in subject selection in most research investigations, a great deal of effort has gone into the development of a standardized nomenclature to help define and guide selection of more homogeneous groups for study (see later in this chapter).

Suicide investigations have evolved from an early focus on epidemiology and demographics to much more sophisticated research designs and statistical analyses that have provided a wealth of significant data regarding populations and individuals at risk. However, perhaps because suicide and suicidal behaviors are considered worst-case outcomes of complex interactions across a multifaceted spectrum of domains (e.g., psychiatric, biological, psychological, sociological, philosophical), there remain a great number of gaps in our understanding of those at risk and of the pathways they travel that end in suicidal deaths or nonfatal attempts. One unfortunate result is that we have yet to develop effective interventions. As a consequence, the annual incidence of suicides and suicidal behaviors in the United States has not changed significantly across the last century. Another result is that there remains a great need to further refine our understanding sufficiently to train clinicians better in assessing suicidal risk, reasonably formulating levels of risk, and developing effective interventions to reduce that level of risk or strengthening protections against risk from ever developing in the first place.

This chapter is designed to highlight selectively and briefly describe areas of clinical research that remain significantly unfocused and demanding of better attention to provide consequent findings of value to clinical work with patients who are at risk for suicide.

The Past as Prologue

The National Institute of Mental Health (NIMH) established, in 1965, the Center for Studies of Suicide Prevention (CSSP) to coordinate and direct national research activities to further basic knowledge and practical wisdom about the problems of suicide and the techniques for aiding the suicidal individual (Yolles 1967). The CSSP, unfortunately, was the victim of shifting political will and was ended in the early 1970s. During its brief tenure, the CSSP was able to fund and appoint a task force of some 50 leaders and students in the field of suicide prevention, self-destructive behaviors, and dying and bereavement, charging them with establishing directions and priorities for the field for the decade ahead. The task force assembled in Phoenix in January 1970 and published its reports and recommendations 3 years later (Resnik and Hathorne 1973).

The task force forged five breakout committees, one of which focused on research. The research committee argued for the need for greater rigor in research designs and the use of more sophisticated statistical analyses, the promotion of cross-fertilization among scientific disciplines studying suicide, and the development of a national data bank that would allow for the computer-accessible retrieval for study of a large number of individual cases. Most profoundly, the committee saw the need for longitudinal and in-depth investigations that would elucidate the course of suicidal behavior (pathway analyses) and inform the nature of its development and amelioration, as well as refining of criteria for the assessment of risk among subgroups at highest risk. The fields that defined the historical tradition in suicidology, epidemiology and demography, were deemed of lowest priority in the advancement of research-based knowledge in the coming years.

In 2000, the Institute of Medicine of the National Academy of Sciences was asked to assess the science of suicidology and to comment on gaps in knowledge and research opportunities. Their findings and recommendations were presented in a report (Goldsmith et al. 2002), more than 400 pages in length, that, in a number of respects, repeated many of the same calls to action voiced in the NIMH task force report three decades earlier (e.g., the need for longitudinal, prospective studies and interdisciplinary research labs).

In spite of considerable growth and evidence of much greater research sophistication in the field of suicidology, it is painfully apparent that there remain significant gaps in the state of our knowledge and, consequently, in our efforts to translate that knowledge into practical clinical applications. To this day, we have few significant longitudinal studies (of presuicidal pathways) in the literature, we lack a national data bank of in-depth studies of deaths by suicide, the number of cases that have received (psychological autopsy) investigations remains quite small (Fleischmann et al. 2005), and interdisciplinary research studies conducted by teams are few and far between—hence there is a preponderance of guild-driven, potentially biased research foci—and high-risk subgroup-specific risk profiles remain elusive.

Two recent reviews of current research efforts and funded studies have been conducted, one in Australia (Robinson et al. 2008), the other in the United States (Brown and Pearson 2011). In spite of the 1970 Phoenix task force's perspective that epidemiological studies are of the lowest priority, each review reported a continuing trend in both countries to significantly fund and publish epidemiologic studies. Robinson et al. (2008) examined all Australian peer-reviewed journal articles published between 1999 and 2006 ($N=263$) in which suicide or suicidal behavior was the primary focus of the research and found that 57% of the articles were epidemiological studies. Published research studies, the authors argued, represent varied sources of funding, ranging from federal grants to local health departments. Brown and Pearson (2011) more narrowly examined the 2008–2009 research portfolio (federally funded grants) of the U.S. National Institutes of Health in which suicide, attempted suicide or suicidal behavior, or suicidal ideation was examined as part of the study (102 unique grants; 81% funded by NIMH) and, similarly, found that epidemiological surveys predominated as a research method (37.3% of funded grants). The amount of funding for research on psychological and/or pharmacological interventions combined to only three-fourths that provided for epidemiological research.

The authors of the Australian review concluded that more intervention studies were both warranted and identified by stakeholders as of highest priority for future suicide prevention research. The review of the national suicide research agenda in the United States was conducted, in part, to inform research opportunities in both the short and long term. As of this writing, these opportunities are being examined by a federally appointed task force working to make recommendations to the U.S. National Action Alliance for Suicide Prevention.

It is therefore apparent that a great deal more effort needs to be made to use science to inform clinical practice to prevent suicide. Clinicians are faced with a near impossible task to assess and treat those at risk for suicide at a point in time where an insufficient knowledge base remains to reasonably inform how to do this. The following sections selectively define a number of gaps and opportunities, suggesting a range of potential landmark research studies that should move us toward accomplishing scientifically sound understandings and even, perhaps, an evidence-based clinical practice in working with individuals at risk for suicide.

Toward the Future

Risk Identification

A great deal is known about factors that perpetuate and predispose to lifetime risk for suicide and suicidal behaviors. Examples of perpetuating risk factors (permanent and nonmodifiable) include family history of suicide and major psychiatric disorders, and early childhood trauma or abuse. Examples of predisposing and potentially modifiable risk factors include current Axis I, II, and/or III diagnoses; a lack of acceptance of LGBTQQI (lesbian, gay, bisexual, transgender, questioning, queer, intersex) sexual orientation; media exposure to another's suicide; and genetic abnormalities (see also Willour et al. 2011). However, whereas elevated lifetime risk is significant in informing a clinician's index of suspicion for potential suicide risk (and selective prevention programs that focus on high-risk groups), the essential focus for the clinician must be on knowing and identifying variables that define acute (near-term) risk for suicide and suicidal behaviors. Notably, as clinicians are deemed to be negligent if and when a patient's suicide or suicidal behavior can be retrospectively identified as imminent (but was not so identified prospectively), the crucial focus for clinicians must be on identifying imminent risk factors for suicide. We are light-years away from achieving that knowledge competency.

Current definitions of acute risk, at best, have attempted to distinguish risk factors specific to the *last 12 months of a patient's life* (Rudd et al. 2006), an operational definition of acute that is something far short of any reasonable definition of acute. As suicide and suicidal behaviors are relatively rare events, and as even the more acute risk factors thus far identified are comparatively quite common (e.g., insomnia, suicidal ideation), the clinical task of discriminating true- from false-positive cases remains daunting. Remarkably, we have no studies that have exclusively focused on the last 30 or 7 days of life of those who have died by suicide. Case-controlled psychological autopsy studies with this temporal focus are needed and should be high priorities on public and private research agendas.

In a similar vein, we lack studies that have developed a clearer understanding of the pathways or trajectories describing how an individual at chronic risk moves to a level of more acute or imminent risk, and of the complex interplay among risk and protective factors that ultimately leverages suicidal action versus successful resistance to the urge for suicidal action. Research data teach us that protective factors—for example, religiosity or marriage with children—lead to lowered suicide rates, but anecdotal cases offer exceptions to the rule—the religiously devout have died by suicide, filicide-suicides have occurred—when factors of acute risk overwhelm coping skills. A better understanding of how protective factors break down or are otherwise insufficient to prevent suicidal behavior would go a long way to better informing clinical judgment (see later in this chapter)—for example, when patients state, as they commonly do, they would never act on suicidal urges because of their children or because their religion prohibits such behavior.

Lifetime suicide risk has been clearly tied to the presence of one or more mental disorders, with an average of 90% of psychological autopsied cases having retrospectively diagnosed mental and/or substance use disorders. Tanney (1992) appropriately cautioned and reminded us that although mental disorders have clearly been found to be associated with suicide, association does not equate to causation. He proposed a number of direct, indirect, interactive, and co-occurring mechanisms to explain the observed association. There remains a compelling need to better understand and explore these underlying mechanisms and, in particular, the multiple driving forces that lead one severely pathological person to suicide and an equally pathological person to a sustained life in spite of the impact of his or her mental disorder. Although we have isolated a few disorder-specific risk factors (Oquendo et al. 2004), we lack similar data across a wide range of disorders associated with heightened lifetime risk for suicide. One-third of all suicides in the United States involve alcohol or drug use disorders, yet less than 10% of federally funded suicide studies involve even a mention of interest in these disorders (Berman 2006b).

In the same vein, we have insufficient knowledge to differentiate what turns one person's psychological despair into suicidal ideation, another's into suicidal impulse, and yet a third's into suicidal behavior, much less to describe the pathway from despair to ideation to impulse to behavior within the same individual. That said, we know practically nothing of significance about "the other 10%" (Berman 2006a). As mental disorders impair resilience and coping skills, amplify distress, and erode protections, it makes intuitive sense to understand the association between mental disorders and, notably, comorbidity and suicidal behavior. But what about subsyndromal factors? What symptoms and/or psychological processes are powerful enough to promote suicidal behavior when a diagnosable mental illness is not present? One such factor that has potential for independent effect might be impulsive aggression, but current research has not yet assessed its contribution to suicide risk independent of diagnoses in which it is a diagnostic criterion (e.g., borderline personality disorder) (Chesin et al. 2010).

Lastly, there is great need to go beyond the medical model to explore and explicate the impact and role of specific affects and cognitions common to suicide—the role of shame and humiliation, for example, as they interact with particular aspects of character and coping ability.

Risk Formulation

Reasonably formulating a patient's risk for suicide in the near term requires an understanding of research-based risk factors, an integration and prioritization of all information available, the application of critical thinking, and an articulated rationale for making a judgment about that patient's level of risk. The American Psychiatric Association's (2003) *Practice Guideline for the As-*

sessment and Treatment of Patients With Suicidal Behaviors calls "the estimation of suicide risk, at the culmination of the suicide assessment, the quintessential clinical judgment" (p. 12). Remarkably, however, there has been no documented attempt to assess whether this "quintessential clinical judgment" can be trained.

Knowing what to look for (risk factors) is not the same as knowing how to apply a reasonable rationale to evaluating a patient's level of risk. Practice guidelines (American Psychiatric Association 2003; Magellan Health Services 2002) offer one such principle, stating that risk factors may be additive, risk increasing with the number of risk factors. In fact, there is some evidence for this, although it is only for a subsequent nonfatal attempt (within 5 years of an index attempt) (Beautrais 2004). However, no actuarial or mathematical approach has yet been offered or evaluated to address improved clinical judgment in making a suicide risk formulation.

Two models for doing this are currently being implemented but remain untested. The National Suicide Prevention Lifeline, the managers of the United States' 800-SUICIDE 24/7 national hotline, has presented a model of formulating a caller's level of risk based on a synergy between an evaluation of the caller's desire, capability, and intent for suicide and the presence or absence of buffers (Joiner et al. 2007). The model is built on a wide range of empirically defined risk factors, but their interrelations and proposed synergy in defining levels of risk remain untested. In contrast, the American Association of Suicidology has developed an intensive clinical training program, Recognizing and Responding to Suicide Risk, that has been shown to change clinicians' attitudes and behavior (Jacobson and Berman 2010). In this training, a model based on separate evaluations of chronic risk (vulnerability to suicide) and the presence of one or more acute risk factors is presented and applied across a number of practice cases to train clinical judgment. This model also awaits rigorous evaluation.

Whether we can train to good clinical judgment, especially judgment validated by known outcomes among actual cases, hence with some application to future judgment, remains to be seen, but a more worthwhile endeavor is hardly imaginable. By analogy, would anyone want to board an airplane piloted by someone who has not been maximally taught to make good judgments about whether to take off or to land based on myriad interacting variables (e.g., visibility, snow or ice, thunderstorms, fatigue, the one glass of alcohol consumed 3 hours before flight time) of consequence to passenger safety? Should we expect less of clinical professionals? Principles and corollaries (see also Smith and Paauw 2000), at the least, should be offered and tested, then taught.

The most consequential level of formulated risk (i.e., imminent risk) is, at once, the least well articulated and the least evidence based. Hirschfeld (1998) asserted that the risk of suicide is imminent "if the patient has expressed the intent to die, has a plan in mind, and has lethal means available" (pp. 127–128), and framed imminent risk as spanning a period of 48 hours or less. This perspective has widespread clinical acceptance and defines the essence of most directives toward clinical inquiry (i.e., first, ask about the presence of suicidal thoughts; then, if present, whether they entail intent, involve associated plans, and are accompanied by the accessibility of means to carry out those plans). The American Psychiatric Association's (2003) practice guideline for the treatment of patients with suicidal behaviors, as but one example, asserts that "the more detailed and specific the suicide

plan, the greater will be the level of risk" (p. 26), an assertion repeated by some managed care company guides for assessing suicidal behaviors (e.g., www.ubhonline. com/html/regionalInformation/newsletters/IOPLetter.pdf?).

Simon (2006) has appropriately noted that the notion of *imminent* risk is illusory, a construction of our attorney friends, without any tie to empirical validity or reliability. Imminent risk is best defined by the concept of *foreseeability*. Foreseeability is the reasonable anticipation of the possibility of suicide or suicidal behavior in the very near future. The foreseeability of an individual's future suicidal behavior is a prediction, yet suicidologists are unanimous in the belief that the prediction of suicide is impossible. Even persons at very high risk—for example, depressed people admitted to a hospital because of suicidal ideation or suicide attempt—have been found to have only a 6% lifetime risk of suicide (Bostwick and Pankratz 2000). Even in the presence of research-defined "powerful predictors of future suicidal acts," among patients with a major depressive or bipolar disorder and the current presentation of a depressive episode, the risk of suicide in the next 2 years may be only slightly greater than 1% (Oquendo et al. 2004). That said, mental health clinicians are expected to make judgments regarding a patient's level of risk and to develop treatment plans on the basis of that judgment.

The foreseeability of an individual's future suicidal behavior must be considered within a time frame, yet even Hirschfeld's (1998) suggested 48-hour window for defining imminent risk is well beyond any clinician's level or reasonable competency. Eggleston (2008) tested the validity of television weather forecasts of precipitation in the Kansas City area and found that predictions of rain beyond the next 24 hours were no better than those achieved by flipping a coin, and accurate only slightly better than 50% of the time over the next 48 hours. Weather forecasting involves sophisticated technology (e.g., Doppler radar) but is no better than chance over a 24-hour period of time, yet clinicians have a responsibility to be correct in predicting human behavior in the next 48 hours?

As noted previously, we have yet to define sensitive markers to describe acute risk for suicide or suicidal behaviors in any time frame more proximate to the suicide than 12 months (Rudd et al. 2006). The clinical demand is to better observe and judge risk in the very short term (i.e., hours to days), because this judgment must inform triage and the need for close monitoring or hospitalization. Thus, there is a siren call to intensively study a large number of completed suicides and suicide attempts of various lethalities relative to both observed and observable signs and symptoms in the very near term (e.g., last 24 hours or last week of life) through psychological autopsies or standardized chart review studies and, then, to validate any derived acute risk factors through case-control research with high-risk subjects. Further, the potential to link near-term clinical manifestations of heightened risk to a biologic marker to predict these, no less to pharmacologic interventions to inhibit these, presents an exciting collaborative opportunity bridging the psychosocial and neurobiological research communities.

One principle associated with near-term and/or imminent risk formulation implications that has been offered by practice guidelines (American Psychiatric Association 2003) is that the more detailed and specific the suicide plan, the greater will be the level of risk. Although this makes good intuitive sense, there is published research neither to defend it nor to support its corollary—that risk is lessened if suicidal ideation is not active and planned.

The standard protocol for assessing suicide risk begins with queries about the presence of suicidal thoughts. Absent any communicated thoughts, or when suicidal thoughts are denied by the patient, the average practitioner generally does little more to formulate a patient's risk for suicide. A number of studies have reported that as many as 80% of those who died by suicide had communicated suicidal thoughts, but a closer reading of many of these and more recent reports finds that the majority of patients had communicated their intent through verbal communications or *behavior* (e.g., Portzky et al. 2005; Shneidman and Farberow 1957).

Remarkably, in this regard, it may well be that the majority of patients who die by suicide actually deny having suicidal thoughts when asked immediately prior to their death or communicate their risk in more behavioral versus verbal messaging (Appleby et al. 1999; Barraclough et al. 1974; Busch et al. 2003; Chavan et al. 2008; Delong and Robins 1961; Hall et al. 1999; Hjelmeland 1996; Isometsä et al. 1995). In fact, one recent study (Wenzel et al. 2011) found that an important predictor of eventual suicide was taking active precautions against discovery of an index suicide attempt. Therefore, the denial of suicidal ideation or intent, rather than the communication of ideation or intent, may be the more important variable associated with heightened suicide risk. On the other hand, ideation with a plan may be most significant in leading to a risk formulation among adolescents with no clearly diagnosed psychopathology (Brent et al. 1993). As noted previously, research addressing last-week communications (verbal and nonverbal) by those who die by suicide is sorely needed.

Risk Reduction

The purpose of assessing and formulating suicide risk is to define a treatment plan (and setting) best designed to reduce imminent and/or acute risk (i.e., suicidal behavior in the immediate future) and thereby allow time to focus on that which makes the individual vulnerable and predisposed to engage in suicidal behavior.

The relative scarcity of randomized clinical trials has been well documented elsewhere (Comtois and Linehan 2006; Hawton et al. 1999; Linehan 1997; Rudd 2000). Research in this area remains hampered by 1) the relative exclusion from study of high-risk patients; 2) relatively short follow-up durations, necessarily limited by available funding but therefore maximizing focus on brief cognitive-behavioral and other structured interventions and relatively short-term outcomes (long-term treatment follow-up studies appear to be bounded at only 24 months); 3) a lack of differentiation among those studied into groups judged to be at acute versus chronic risk; 4) a lack of precision, consequent to our continuing muddled nomenclature (see below) in defining homogeneous groups (e.g., ideators, attempters, repetitive attempters) for research study; 5) a lack of differentiation, thereby, among patient-subjects with regard to their relative lethality and intent; and 6) our reliance, consequent to the relatively short-term duration of studies, on indirect markers (e.g., symptom reduction or one-time measures of suicidal ideation) for treatment outcomes versus direct markers (e.g., no suicidal behavior sustained over longer periods of follow-up). Moreover, reviews of clinical trials focused on reducing suicide risk per se have been limited with regard to statistical power to detect possible positive treatment effects.

Similarly, the available research on psychopharmacological interventions is plagued by problems of classification and a lack of standardized data collection by pharmaceutical houses during clinical trials; relatively brief durations of study; overreliance on single-question markers of treatment response (e.g., responses to a single scale [e.g., Hamilton Rating Scale for Depression] or even one item of that scale [e.g., item 3]) on a rating scale to measure suicide risk; the lack of dechallenge-rechallenge studies; a better understanding of why nonresponders are nonresponders; and, with regard to selective serotonin reuptake inhibitors (SSRIs) in particular, an understandable lack of interest in exploring the relatively high rate of placebo response, which may account for as much as 80% of observed benefit from active medications.

Although an association has been found between SSRIs and suicidal ideation and nonfatal suicide attempts in children, adolescents, and young adults, leading to the U.S. Food and Drug Administration–mandated black box warning in the United States, this association does not equate to a statement of causality. Preexisting suicidality was neither examined nor controlled for as a potential confounding variable in studies of reported adverse events. Moreover, pharmaceutical company–identified adverse event descriptions were highly variable in their specificity and not systematically ascertained (Posner et al. 2007). More sophisticated study of those suffering adverse events such as increased suicide risk has yet to be reported and is sorely needed.

Lastly, given the observed odds ratios for suicide consequent to discharge from psychiatric hospitalization (Qin and Nordentoft 2005), the effectiveness of hospitalization as a treatment intervention and questions regarding discharge planning and continuity of care procedures and implementation (Beautrais 2006; Knesper et al. 2010) all call for investigation and answers.

Moreover, there is no evidence supporting hospitalization as a treatment intervention for suicidal patients diagnosed with Axis II disorders; therefore, there remains a need to ascertain what treatment setting is best suited to the care of such a patient when in the throes of an acute suicidal crisis.

Compliance

Crucial to effective treatment interventions is a compliant patient, yet this construct remains more theoretical than empirically studied. We have reason to presume that noncompliant patients are compromised by a number of factors, ranging from gender role socialization (males are more noncompliant than females) to influences stemming from their psychopathology and character that compromise trust, willingness to be in a dependent position to a caregiver, and so on. It is noteworthy, for example, that two studies (Leon et al. 2006; Moskos et al. 2005) of adolescent suicides found that only one patient out of 72 (combined samples) who had been prescribed an antidepressant had evidence of that medication in his or her blood upon toxicological analysis at the time of autopsy. In this regard, studies of help seeking and help receiving, particularly among males at risk for suicide (Motto et al. 1985), are crucial to better develop methods to enhance these behaviors and thus engagement in caregiving and compliance with recommended treatments (Berman 2005; Stanley 2006). With that being said, the association between enhanced compliance and a reduction in suicidal behavior remains to be demonstrated (Heard 2000).

Ethical Issues in Suicide Research

Fisher et al. (2002) summarized discussions and issues raised from an NIMH-sponsored workshop on ethical issues related to inclusion of suicidal individuals in clinical research. Among the many issues posed were the following:

- Individuals perceived to be at risk for suicide are excluded from clinical trials.
- Perceived liability burdens to individual researchers and their institutions mean that few researchers are willing to conduct trials with suicidal individuals.
- Valid risk assessment criteria and rescue procedures with long-term effectiveness have yet to be established.
- No study has assessed the competency to consent to research of individuals assumed to be at risk for suicide.
- Ethical concerns have been raised about the use of placebo or nontreatment control groups for suicide research.

A decade has passed since this workshop, and there remains much yet to be accomplished in resolving these issues (Pearson, personal communication, May 20, 2011). NIMH grant reviewers have been increasingly involved in shaping proposals to include more persons at risk in submitted studies, but high-risk individuals (indicated populations) still are not in evidence. The pool of funded researchers testing interventions remains small, and institutional review boards at their institutions remain wary of potential liability issues. Although we have some evidence that participating in a suicide research protocol does not induce suicidal ideation or attempts (Cukrowicz et al. 2010), this evidence is based on a small sample of persons at increased chronic risk for suicide (depressed ideators and depressed persons with a history of suicide attempt) and not on patients at elevated acute risk for suicide. Competency questions remain unaddressed.

Funded treatment interventions typically have no more than an 18- to 24-month duration for follow-up; therefore, long-term outcome data are limited. Although we know that there are effective interventions (see Brown et al. 2005), the holy grail of demonstrating long-term effectiveness has yet to be established. The one area in which there has been some clear shift is in the use of nontreatment control groups. More typically these are now defined as enhanced treatment-as-usual groups, with periodic monitoring and crisis referrals available if deemed necessary.

Other Issues

Building Resiliency and Strengthening Protective Factors

An alternative and necessarily secondary treatment intervention (or primary prevention) approach to working with individuals at risk for suicide is to strengthen protective factors. However, little is known about how to enhance protective factors in individuals already at risk (Felner et al. 2000).

Nomenclature

As noted in the introduction to this chapter, the most frequently researched population among suicidal individuals is those identified as ideators or as attempters, because both groups remain alive and available for study. However, too frequently samples of ideators and attempters are admixed, as if they are one and the same. Moreover, even when the study population includes only nonfatal attempters, this population, too, is a highly heterogeneous group of individuals with a range of lethalities and intentions describing their suicidal behaviors. No uniform set of definitions for suicidal behaviors exists to guide research and clinical communication. There is a great need to foster studies that use universally accepted op-

erational definitions and homogeneous subject populations. Considerable effort has gone into creating a consensually accepted nomenclature (Brenner et al. 2011; DeLeo et al. 2006; Silverman et al. 2007a, 2007b), but adoption by clinicians and researchers remains a challenge.

Cultural Issues

Suicidal behaviors are subject to considerable cultural variation in their expression, in their demography, and in the degree to which they may be related to psychiatric disorders—and thus in the way they may be treated within or outside of a mental health system, in treatment methods used, in sociocultural stigmatization, and so on. Cultural issues affect different minority groups and/or immigrant groups in the same country as much as they differentially affect native born citizens in different countries. Risk factors are not the same across cultures, age and gender groups, or developed, low-income, and middle-income countries. There is a great need to validate universal versus culturally specific profiles of persons at acute and chronic risk across different cultures; this area of research is but in its infancy.

Conclusion

In the history of science, there is ample evidence that it may take centuries of intensive empirical study to understand a clinical phenomenon well enough to establish effective interventions and, yet again, centuries to widely implement effective treatments to eradicate the disease entity. Take, for example, smallpox, which had existed for millennia before Edward Jenner demonstrated in 1798 that an inoculation could control the disease. The World Health Organization certified in 1978 that smallpox had been eradicated. That is, it took almost 200 years to sufficiently prevent the disease caused by but a single organism (variola virus).

In contrast, suicide is caused by a complex and dynamic interplay of both internal and external causes, and as noted in the introduction to this chapter, the study of suicide must be considered a very young science. We have enough as yet unaddressed and unanswered questions to drive researchers for centuries to come.

One of the best books on the subject describes suicide assessment as an art (Shea 1999; see also Chapter 2, "The Interpersonal Art of Suicide Assessment," in this volume). Our challenge lies in translating science into practice and in improving through science our understandings of what works and how to best implement what works—in short, in providing a more scientific foundation to the art of working with suicidal patients. Interventions that have been shown to be effective are slow to translate into everyday clinical practice. It may well be that randomized clinical trials, with tightly controlled, often manualized interventions, simply do not translate well into everyday clinical practice, where the work of treatment is highly individualized (this is yet another example of the "art" of working with persons at risk for suicide). Moreover, suicidal patients are often difficult to engage and difficult to treat, frequently evoking strong countertransference reactions, ranging from anger to aversion and from helplessness to contagious hopelessness. These may well be those patients who never enter into or who drop out of clinical trials. Therefore, we remain challenged by questions of how best to form therapeutic alliances with patients who lack the skill sets needed to benefit from collaborative therapeutic work, who are ambivalent in their motivation toward receiving help, and who are driven by a countertherapeutic urge to end life.

Perhaps there is no more compelling patient problem in the mental health arena than that of the suicidal patient, with whom our gaps in understanding are so great and our opportunities for making a difference are so profound.

Key Clinical Concepts

- Clinical practice must be informed by empirical study of suicidal individuals.
- There is a pressing need to study final pathways, hence acute risk factors, displayed by those who die by suicide to inform the assessment and formulation of near-term and imminent risk for suicide.
- Both the communication and denial of current suicidal ideation should trigger further evaluation of near-term risk for suicidal behavior.
- There is an urgent need to develop research-based models for the formulation of level of suicide risk based on an assessment of that risk.
- Studies are urgently needed that address long-term outcomes of clinical interventions and models to increase adherence to prescribed interventions among those at risk for suicide.

References

American Psychiatric Association: Practice guideline for the assessment and treatment of patients with suicidal behaviors. 2003. Available at: http://www.psychiatryonline.com/pracGuide/pracGuideTopic_14. aspx. Accessed August 15, 2011.

Appleby L, Shaw J, Amos T: Suicide within 12 months of contact with mental health services: national clinical survey. BMJ 318:1235–1239, 1999

Barraclough BM, Bunch J, Nelson B, et al: A hundred cases of suicide: clinical aspects. Br J Psychiatry 125:355–373, 1974

Beautrais AL: Further suicidal behavior among medically serious suicide attempters. Suicide Life Threat Behav 34:1–11, 2004

Beautrais AL: Is suicidal behavior a chronic condition? Presented at the 39th annual conference of the American Association of Suicidology, Seattle, WA, April 2006

Berman AL: Help-seeking among men: implications for suicide prevention. Acta Suicidologica Slovenica 3:36–51, 2005

Berman AL: The Other Ten Percent. Washington, DC, American Association of Suicidology, 2006a

Berman AL: "The Time Has Come," the Walrus Said, "to Talk of Many Things…" Dublin Award presentation at the 39th annual conference of the American Association of Suicidology, Seattle, WA, April 2006b

Bostwick JM, Pankratz VS: Affective disorders and suicide risk: a reexamination. Am J Psychiatry 157:1925–1932, 2000

Brenner LA, Breshears RE, Betthauser LM, et al: Implementation of a suicide nomenclature within two VA healthcare settings. J Clin Psychol Med Settings 18:116–128, 2011

Brent D, Perper J, Moritz J, et al: Suicide in adolescents with no apparent psychopathology. J Am Acad Child Adolesc Psychiatry 32:494–500, 1993

Brown GK, Pearson JL: National suicide research agenda: what is being funded and what isn't. Paper presented at the 44th annual conference of the American Association of Suicidology, Portland, OR, April 2011

Brown GK, Ten Have T, Henriques GR, et al: Cognitive therapy for the prevention of suicide attempts: a randomized controlled trial. JAMA 294:563–570, 2005

Busch KA, Fawcett J, Jacobs DG: Clinical correlates of inpatient suicide. J Clin Psychiatry 64:14–19, 2003

Chavan BS, Singh GP, Kaur J, et al: Psychological autopsy of 101 suicide cases from northwest region of India. Indian J Psychiatry 50:34–38, 2008

Chesin MS, Jeglic EL, Stanley B: Pathways to high-lethality suicide attempts in individuals with borderline personality disorder. Arch Suicide Res 14:342–362, 2010

Comtois KA, Linehan MM: Psychosocial treatments of suicidal behaviors: a practice-friendly review. J Clin Psychol 62:161–170, 2006

Cukrowicz K, Smith P, Poindexter E: The effect of participating in suicide research: does participating in a research protocol on suicide and psychiatric symptoms increase suicide ideation and attempts? Suicide Life Threat Behav 40:535–543, 2010

DeLeo D, Burgis S, Bertolote JM, et al: Definitions of suicidal behavior: lessons learned from the WHO/EURO Multicentre Study. Crisis 27:4–15, 2006

Delong WB, Robins E: The communication of suicidal intent prior to psychiatric hospitalization: a study of 87 patients. Am J Psychiatry 117:695–705, 1961

Durkheim E: Suicide: A Study in Sociology (1897). Translated by Spaulding JA, Simpson G. New York, Free Press, 1951

Eggleston JD: How valid are T.V. weather forecasts? 2008. Available at: http://www.freakonomics.com/2008/04/21/how-valid-are-tv-weather-forecasts/. Accessed August 15, 2011.

Felner RD, Felner TY, Silverman MM: Prevention in mental health and social intervention, in Handbook of Community Psychology. Edited by Rappaport J, Seidman E. New York, Kluwer Academic/Plenum, 2000, pp 9–42

Fisher CB, Pearson JL, Kim S, et al: Ethical issues in including suicidal individuals in suicide research. IRB 24:9–14, 2002

Fleischmann A, Bertolote JM, Belfer M, et al: Completed suicide and psychiatric diagnoses in young people: a critical examination of the evidence. Am J Orthopsychiatry 75:676–683, 2005

Goldney RD, Schioldann JA: Pre-Durkheim suicidology. Crisis 21:181–186, 2000

Goldsmith SK, Pellmar TC, Kleinman AM, et al (eds): Reducing Suicide: A National Imperative. Washington, DC, National Academies Press, 2002

Hall RCW, Platt DE, Hall RC: Suicide risk assessment: a review of risk factors in 100 patients who made severe suicide attempts: evaluation of suicide risk in a time of managed care. Psychosomatics 40:18–27, 1999

Hawton K, Townsend E, Arensman E, et al: Psychosocial versus pharmacological treatments for deliberate self harm. Cochrane Database of Systematic Reviews 1999, Issue 4. Art. No.: CD001764. DOI: 10.1002/14651858.CD001764.

Heard HL: Psychotherapeutic approaches to suicidal ideation and behavior, in The International Handbook of Suicide and Attempted Suicide. Edited by Hawton K, van Heeringen K. Chichester, UK, Wiley, 2000, pp 503–518

Hjelmeland H: Verbally expressed intentions of parasuicide, II: prediction of fatal and nonfatal repetition. Crisis 17:10–14, 1996

Hirschfeld RM: The suicidal patient. Hosp Pract (Minneap) 33:119–123, 127–128, 131–133, 1998

Isometsä ET, Heikkinen ME, Marttunen MJ, et al: The last appointment before suicide: is intent communicated? Am J Psychiatry 152:919–922, 1995

Jacobson J, Berman AL: Outcomes from behavioral outcomes evaluations of the RRSR training (Recognizing and Responding to Suicide Risk): an advanced training program for the clinical practitioner. Paper presented at the 43rd annual conference of the American Association of Suicidology, Orlando, FL, April 2010

Joiner T, Kalafat J, Draper J, et al: Establishing standards for the assessment of suicide risk among callers to the National Suicide Prevention Lifeline. Suicide Life Threat Behav 37:353–365, 2007

Knesper DJ, American Association of Suicidology, Suicide Prevention Resource Center: Continuity of Care for Suicide Prevention and Research: Suicide Attempts and Suicide Deaths Subsequent to Discharge From the Emergency Department or Psychiatry Inpatient Unit. Newton, MA, Education Development Center, 2010

Leon AC, Marzuk PM, Tardiff AK, et al: Antidepressants and youth suicide in New York City, 1999–2002. J Am Acad Child Adolesc Psychiatry 45:1054–1058, 2006

Linehan MM: Behavioral treatments of suicidal behaviors: definitional obfuscation and treatment outcomes. Ann N Y Acad Sci 836:302–328, 1997

Magellan Health Services: Magellan Clinical Practice Guideline for Assessing and Managing the Suicidal Patient. 2002. Available at: http://www.magellanprovider.com/MHS/MGL/providing_care/clinical_guidelines/clin_prac_guidelines/suicide.pdf. Accessed August 15, 2011.

Moskos M, Olson L, Halbern S, et al: Utah youth suicide study: psychological autopsy. Suicide Life Threat Behav 35:536–546, 2005

Motto JA, Heilbron DC, Juster RP: Development of a clinical instrument to estimate suicide risk. Am J Psychiatry 142:680–686, 1985

Oquendo MA, Galfalvy H, Russo S, et al: Prospective study of clinical predictors of suicidal acts after a major depressive episode in patients with major depressive disorder or bipolar disorder. Am J Psychiatry 161:1433–1441, 2004

Portzky G, Audenaert K, Van Heeringen K: Suicide among adolescents: a psychological autopsy study of psychiatric, psychosocial, and personality-related risk factors. Soc Psychiatry Psychiatr Epidemiol 40:922–930, 2005

Posner K, Oquendo MA, Gould M, et al: Columbia Classification Algorithm of Suicide Assessment (C-CASA): classification of suicidal events in the FDA's pediatric suicidal risk analysis of antidepressants. Am J Psychiatry 164:1035–1043, 2007

Qin P, Nordentoft M: Suicide risk in relation to psychiatric hospitalization: evidence based on longitudinal registers. Arch Gen Psychiatry 62:427–432, 2005

Resnik HLP, Hathorne BC (eds): Suicide Prevention in the 70s (CHEW Publ No HSM-72-9054). Washington, DC, U.S. Government Printing Office, 1973

Robinson J, Pirkis J, Krysinska K, et al: Research priorities in suicide prevention in Australia. Crisis 29:180–190, 2008

Rudd MD: Integrating science into the practice of clinical suicidology: a review of the psychotherapy literature and a research agenda for the future, in Review of Suicidology, 2000. Edited by Maris RW, Canetto SS, McIntosh JL, et al. New York, Guilford, 2000, pp 47–83

Rudd MD, Berman L, Joiner T, et al: Warning signs for suicide: theory, research, and clinical application. Suicide Life Threat Behav 36:255–262, 2006

Shea S: The Practical Art of Suicide Assessment. New York, Wiley, 1999

Shneidman ES, Farberow NL: Clues to Suicide. New York, McGraw-Hill, 1957

Silverman MM, Berman AL, Sandall ND, et al: Rebuilding the tower of Babel: a revised nomenclature for the study of suicide and suicidal behaviors. Part I: background, rationale, and methodology. Suicide Life Threat Behav 37:248–263, 2007a

Silverman MM, Berman AL, Sandall ND, et al: Rebuilding the tower of Babel: a revised nomenclature for the study of suicide and suicidal behaviors, Part II: suicide-related ideations, communications, and behaviors. Suicide Life Threat Behav 37: 264–267, 2007b

Simon RI: Imminent suicide: the illusion of short-term prediction. Suicide Life Threat Behav 36:296–301, 2006

Smith CS, Paauw DS: When you hear hoof beats: four principles for separating zebras from horses. J Am Board Fam Pract 13:424–429, 2000

Stanley B: Psychological interventions for people at risk for suicide: what works and what does not? Presented at the 11th European Symposium on Suicide and Suicidal Behaviours, Potoroz, Slovenia, September 2006

Tanney BL: Mental disorders, psychiatric patients, and suicide, in Assessment and Prediction of Suicide. Edited by Maris RW, Berman AL, Maltsberger JT, et al. New York, Guilford, 1992, pp 277–320

Wenzel A, Berchick ER, Tenhave T, et al: Predictors of suicide relative to other deaths in patients with suicide attempts and suicide ideation: a 30 year prospective study. J Affect Disord 132:375–382, 2011

Willour VL, Seifuddin F, Mahon PB, et al: A genome-wide association study of attempted suicide. Mol Psychiatry March 22, 2011 [Epub ahead of print]

Yolles S: Foreword, in Bulletin of Suicidology. Washington, DC, National Institutes of Mental Health, July 1967

PART VIII

Aftermath of Suicide and the Psychiatrist

CHAPTER 33

Psychiatrist Reactions to Patient Suicide

Michael Gitlin, M.D.

The suicide of a patient in ongoing treatment has been and continues to be among the most traumatic events in the professional life of a psychiatrist. Despite the occasional article urging more attention to this area, systematic examinations of the prevalence of psychiatrists' reactions to patient suicide, the specific reactions that are typically seen, and predictors of these responses, as well as recommendations for optimal coping mechanisms in these situations, continue to be remarkably sparse in the psychiatric literature. This is especially noteworthy given that in the last year reported (2009), more than 36,000 individuals in the United States died by suicide (Kochanek et al. 2011), and over half of these individuals had received care for their psychiatric problems in the year before their suicide (although nonpsychiatrists may have provided a substantial proportion of this care) (Jamison and Baldessarini 1999).

A number of potential reasons have been proposed for our field's relative silence in considering what are frequently traumatic events for psychiatrists. It has been sug-

gested that some individuals become psychiatrists to avoid dealing with death (Sacks 1989). Consistent with this, an early study noted greater anxiety about death in medical students planning on specializing in psychiatry (Livingston and Zimet 1965). Additionally, even though a substantial percentage of psychiatrists will experience a patient's suicide, it remains a relatively very-low-frequency event. As an example, in a study from Scotland that surveyed psychiatrists about patient suicide, 87% had experienced six or fewer patient suicides over an average career of 17.5 years, yielding an average of less than one suicide every 3 years (Alexander et al. 2000). In another study of private practitioners and hospital-based psychiatrists and psychologists, no private practitioners had experienced more than one patient suicide in the previous 5 years (Wurst et al. 2010). In contrast, those working in institutional settings were more likely to experience multiple patient suicides, with two-thirds having had more than one patient suicide during the same time frame. Overall, with relatively few suicides per psychiatrist, the topic never becomes one that demands an agreed-upon set of coping skills that has been shaped and taught over the generations. Finally, with death a more common outcome in most of the other medical specialties, medical schools treat it as a natural outcome of disorders that physicians treat and generally do not focus on suicide as playing a unique role as stress-generator in treating physicians.

Nonetheless, a substantial proportion, estimated to range from 15% to 68%, of psychiatrists have experienced at least one patient suicide (Alexander et al. 2000; Chemtob et al. 1988b; Wurst et al. 2010). Among trainees, even with their relatively brief experience in the field, one-third to two-thirds have had a patient die by suicide (Brown 1987a, 1987b; Ruskin et al. 2004; Wurst et al. 2010). In the largest survey of its type, 31% of psychiatrists (74/239) recalled the suicide of a patient while in training, with over half of these suicides having occurred during the first year of residency (Ruskin et al. 2004). Between 5% and 20% of psychiatrists report having had more than one patient suicide during training. Thus, despite the relative infrequency of patient suicide over a psychiatrist's professional lifetime, patient suicide occurs with regularity, especially with psychiatric residents. It behooves us, then, to better understand our own reactions and potential coping mechanisms.

General Reactions to Patient Suicide

The few surveys that have examined psychiatrists' reactions to patient suicides consistently show that in general, a significant proportion of those affected show strong negative reactions, affecting professional and personal lives at levels of distress that are frequently comparable with those seen in clinical populations. In one survey of 88 psychotherapists, the most common cause of professional anxiety was patient suicide (Menninger 1991). Chemtob et al. (1988b), using the Impact of Event Scale, found that scores of both intrusive thoughts related to the event and avoidance of reminders were similar to those seen in patients seeking therapy after a parent's death in more than half of the surveyed psychiatrists. In a parallel study surveying psychologists, in which the Impact of Event Scale was used, half the clinicians had intrusion scores similar to a clinical population's, but only 27% had comparable avoidance scores (Chemtob et al. 1988a). On an ordinal scale, 38% of psychiatrists rated their distress after patient suicide as 7 out of 10 or higher, classified as severe by Hendin et al. (2004). Similarly, one-third of psychiatrists and psychologists rated their distress as severe (visual analogue scale score >70) (Wurst et al. 2010).

Consideration of discontinuing practicing psychiatry would be a clear and rather dramatic expression of distress. In one survey of psychiatrists in Great Britain, one-third described patient suicide as having affected their personal lives; they became more irritable at home and coped less well with family problems. Fifteen percent of these psychiatrists considered taking early retirement; however, only 3% considered it seriously (Alexander et al. 2000).[1] Another fantasy of "having to leave town,

---

[1]The consideration of retirement is similar to the plan of a young psychiatrist in a single case report to change the city in which he practiced if a second patient died by suicide in his practice, reasoning that his professional community would never tolerate a psychiatrist who had had two patient suicides (Gitlin 1999).

shunned like a leper for the terrible act I had committed" has also been recorded (Perr 1968, p. 177). Finally, in a qualitative study of psychoanalytic clinicians who experienced patient suicide, one clinician reported that she "longed for a job with the least amount of interpersonal contact and responsibility...and laughed about her fantasy of working as a forest ranger" (Tillman 2006, p. 166).

After patient suicides, many psychiatrists develop rather classic symptoms of anxiety, depression, or acute or posttraumatic stress symptoms. These include sleep difficulties, suicidal thoughts, accident proneness, intrusive thoughts, and exaggerated startle responses (Alexander et al. 2000; Chemtob et al. 1988b; Gitlin 1999; Ruskin et al. 2004; Sacks 1989; Tillman 2006). At least three papers (Gitlin 1999; Hendin et al. 2004; Sacks 1989) note that for up to 1 year or more afterward, some psychiatrists show an exaggerated startle response to late-night telephone calls or pages, with the reflexive assumption that news about another patient suicide is impending.

Finally, a few surveys have noted the remarkable vividness of feelings, specific memories, and dreams/fantasies surrounding a patient's suicide, even years or decades later (Brown 1987b; Gitlin 1999; Hendin et al. 2000; Tillman 2006), indicating that despite the general healing that occurs over time, the experience often remains deeply etched in clinicians' psyches. In a descriptive study, half the interviewed clinicians cried during the research interview when recalling their experience of a patient's suicide, often years after the event (Tillman 2006).

For the majority of clinicians, however, distress levels diminish over time. As an example, in one study, distress scores declined over time such that by 6 months after the suicide, most psychiatrists' scores had decreased to nonclinical levels (Chemtob et al. 1988a). In a more recent study, the high levels of distress seen immediately after a patient suicide had decreased significantly by 2 weeks later, and after 6 months had decreased even more (Wurst et al. 2010).

Specific Reactions to Patient Suicide

Beyond the general intensity of psychiatrists' reactions to patients' suicides, a characteristic set of psychological responses, shown in Table 33–1, can be identified (Brown 1987b; Gitlin 1999; Hendin et al. 2000; Litman 1965; Sacks 1989; Sacks et al. 1987; Tillman 2006; Wurst et al. 2010).

Of course, not every psychiatrist exhibits each of the typical reactions, nor is the evolution or order of the responses invariant. In general, these responses reflect universal responses to the death of another with whom we have deep emotional ties, altered by the special role of psychiatric physicians in our society (Litman 1965). Compared with other physicians, psychiatrists generally have deeper ties with their patients, reflecting a more emotionally intimate knowledge of them, given that the medium of discussion is psychological feelings or symptoms rather than the more distanced physical symptoms. This may be true even with patients seen only in psychopharmacological treatment, with whom discussions of mood or cognitions may still be experienced as intimate. This is especially relevant because psychiatrists, who identify themselves as biologically oriented, are more likely to experience patient suicide, either because they see higher volumes of patients or because they treat more ill patients (Ruskin et al. 2004).

TABLE 33–1. Reactions to patient suicide

Initial reactions
   Shock
   Disbelief
   Denial
   Depersonalization
Second-phase reactions
   Grief
   Shame
   Guilt
   Fear of blame
   Anger
   Relief
   Finding of omens and subsequent
     behavioral changes
   Conflicting feelings of specialness

Initial Responses: Shock, Disbelief, Denial, and Depersonalization

Typically, initial responses revolve around the difficulties in assimilating the new information about the patient's suicide, the intense affective arousal that the suicide engenders, and the internal mechanisms used to diminish that intensity. Initial responses include comments such as "I could hardly believe it" (Litman 1965) and convictions such as "There must be a mistake" (Sacks et al. 1987). Depersonalization feelings—numbness, a sense of unreality, or spaciness—frequently accompany or follow the initial shock. These descriptors are entirely consistent with the symptoms described in DSM-IV-TR as acute stress disorder (American Psychiatric Association 2000).

Second-Phase Responses: Grief, Shame, Guilt, and Fear of Blame

Typically following, but often intermingling with, the initial disbelief responses are reactions related to grief, shame, and guilt commonly associated with fear of blame. In one study, grief was the most commonly observed reaction in psychiatrists after patient suicide (Perr 1968). The experience has been described as consistent with an acute grief reaction (Tillman 2006). Grief can be related to a number of different simultaneous losses. First, of course, is that of losing a patient with whom the psychiatrist has often had a deep, meaningful relationship. This type of grief encompasses both the loss of the person and the loss of the possibility of the patient achieving the hoped-for positive goals of treatment. Another type of grief, however, reflects a different type of loss— that of the psychiatrist's own fantasies of power, influence, and the ability to make a difference in patients' lives (Gitlin 1999; Sacks 1989). One psychiatrist acknowledged his own primitive fantasy that "with his skill, empathy, and good training, he would make a positive difference in all his patients' lives. That [his patient] could kill himself despite [the psychiatrist's] best efforts and judgments made the practice and outcome of psychiatric treatment far less certain" (Gitlin 1999, p. 1631). Another psychiatrist expressed almost identical thoughts and feelings: "I really thought if you were good enough you could help almost everybody. That these things only happen to clinicians who miss something and I learned that this is not true....This was a turning point, a reorienting point" (Tillman 2006, p. 164). The loss of this youthful grandiosity is, in the long run, appropriate and necessary for optimal professional development. It is presumed (but not studied) that this second type of grief is more likely to occur when the treating psychiatrist is young and has been practicing for a relatively short period of time. Thus, although traumatic, this type of grief ultimately serves a larger, necessary purpose. The mourning of unrealistic youthful fantasies is analogous to the effect of other losses in one's personal life, leading to a deeper appreciation of the finiteness of life. Of course, as with other losses, timing is critical, and it can be postulated that losses at a too-early stage of development can be deeply scarring.

Shame and guilt are also very common reactions to patient suicide, with at least one observer suggesting these as the most universal responses (Sacks 1989). Questions and responses arise such as "Did I listen to him?" "How did I miss it?" (Litman 1965), and ""I'm wracking my brain for what I missed" (Tillman 2006). Among the four factors identified in one study as the most common sources of severe distress, two related to technical decisions made regarding the patient's care with subsequent feelings of (presumably) guilt (Hendin et al. 2004). The aforementioned fantasies of moving to another city or retiring are linked to the deep shame and guilt that some psychiatrists experience after patient suicide. At times, severe guilt has led to false confessions of wrongdoing. In one example, a psychiatrist gave an incorrectly low dosage of the antidepressant he had been prescribing, with the (incorrect) implication of his having treated the patient inadequately (Sacks 1989). Another psychiatrist admitted prescribing the sleeping pills with which a patient died by suicide, even though another physician had prescribed them (Litman 1965).

The shame and guilt reactions are inextricably linked to fear of blame or reprisal. Foremost among these is the fear of a potential malpractice suit (Gitlin 1999; Hendin et al. 2000, 2004; Tillman 2006; Wurst et al. 2010). Even in Germany and Switzerland, two countries generally considered to be less litigious than the United States, overall distress levels after patient suicide correlated significantly with fear of lawsuits (Wurst et al. 2010). A corollary of this is the fear that

even without a malpractice suit, colleagues will be deeply critical of a psychiatrist who has had a patient die by suicide and will stop referring patients, and one's reputation and career will be ruined. Implied in these concerns is the common fantasy that a patient suicide, with or without subsequent litigation, is a very public event to colleagues, potential patients, and the community. Concerns about public exposure and humiliation are common and very powerful despite the fact that public discussions of these issues are rare. In one survey, only 9% of patient suicides eventuated in a lawsuit and only 2% (2/120) went to trial. Consistent with these themes, one study found that after a patient suicide, 79% of psychiatrists felt professionally devalued and were concerned that they would no longer be respected professionally (Ruskin et al. 2004).

Anger

Although not as universal as grief, guilt, and shame, anger is a common and, in many ways, a more difficult psychological response for psychiatrists after a patient suicide. What differs among individuals is the object of the anger and the rationale for the anger. Among those treating outpatients, the likely objects of anger are the patient and his or her family. If an inpatient commits suicide, however, the list of potential objects lengthens to include nurses and administrators. If the treating psychiatrist is a trainee, others to be angry at might include supervisors and residency directors or the institution itself.

Rationales for anger are similarly diffuse. Feelings of betrayal toward the patient who did not, for example, honor a therapeutic contract, such as calling the psychiatrist if intense suicidal feelings erupt, may emerge (Hendin et al. 2000). Some psychiatrists feel angry at the waste of the previous therapeutic work. Others feel angry at the patient for engendering such painful feelings in the psychiatrist as guilt and shame or for making the therapist look stupid in his or her own eyes. In one detailed case report, a young psychiatrist focused his anger on the patient's having died by suicide by overdose of the antidepressant medications prescribed. It felt unfair to the psychiatrist that the patient had killed himself and caused great psychological pain to the psychiatrist using the "personal healing ministrations of the doctor, the actual means of his healing" (Gitlin 1999, p. 1632).

When the suicide occurs in an institutional setting with the trainee as the treating psychiatrist, the theme of the anger is that of receiving inadequate support, help, or guidance or of being pressured to discharge a patient from a more protected setting such as an inpatient unit. (Of course, the supervisors may also be angry at the treating trainee.) As in so many other situations in which anger is a dominant affect, the anger often serves to protect the individual against excessive guilt or blame ("It's their fault, not mine").

Relief

Less common, yet still conflictual when they arise, are feelings of relief. Relief is likely to be experienced after the suicide of a chronically suicidal patient who has exhausted those around him or her by endless threats or attempts. These feelings may also arise in the family members of chronically suicidal individuals, who, like the treating psychiatrists, have often lived in dread of the late-night phone calls surrounding either suicidal threats or self-destructive behavior. In these cases, the mixture of the more classic feelings—sadness, grief, guilt, and self-blame—with feelings of anger and relief can make for a very difficult internally conflicted brew.

Finding of Omens and Behavioral Changes

Among the more interesting psychological sequelae of patient suicide is the finding of omens (Sacks 1989), in which the psychiatrist retroactively considers signs signaling the coming suicide that were, of course, missed. These typically include rather trivial differences in nuance, such as an ending greeting of "good-bye" instead of "so long" or a different look at the end of the last session. The purpose of finding these omens is to provide an illusory sense of control over an event that makes the psychiatrist feel helpless. If signs exist, even if they were missed, then suicide is predictable and therefore preventable in the future.

The finding of omens—or, more broadly, the examination of potentially missed signals of impending suicide and identification of high-risk situations based on a completed suicide—typically leads to behavioral changes. On the surface, as with the finding of omens, the purpose of these behavioral changes is to learn from the suicide and to prevent future suicides. In fact, more frequently these behavioral changes simply serve as rituals, repetitive behaviors that bind the caregivers' anxiety and reduce the feelings of helplessness that accompany patient suicide. As an example, after a patient suicide, inpatient units may decrease the threshold for the intensive observation of suicide watch (e.g., 15-minute observation intervals) and require it for many more patients. After a patient suicide, one outpatient psychiatrist began to ritualistically ask all patients (even those who had never had suicidal ideation) at every visit about the presence of suicidal thoughts. Because his patient had died by suicide via an overdose of prescribed antidepressants, he also became excessively anxious about all his other patients and began ritualistically quizzing them about the exact amounts of medications at home and their thoughts of overdosing (even with those patients with whom overdosing had never been raised or considered), until a patient confronted him on his anxious questioning (Gitlin 1999). After a patient suicide, one psychiatrist demanded that some of her suicidal patients be hospitalized far more quickly than was typical for her, whereas another psychiatrist acknowledged attempting to have a suicidal patient terminate with him because he could not bear to lose another patient (Tillman 2006).

Conflicting Feelings of Specialness

In some situations, especially in institutional settings where there is frequent contact with other professionals, a psychiatrist experiencing a patient suicide develops feelings of isolation and specialness (Gitlin 1999; Sacks 1989; Tillman 2006). The isolation feelings reflect the irrational conviction that no one else has had the same experience—that one is "branded" as different by the suicide. If the suicide is not discussed openly, the treating psychiatrist may feel shunned. In association with these feelings, however, is also a sense of specialness, of having gone through a rite of passage, of becoming a member of a very special club, in which only those who have had a similar experience really understand, similar to that described by war veterans; "to survive it is testimony to one's hardiness, endurance, and being a 'real' physician" (Sacks 1989, p. 568). Although overall the feelings of specialness generate isolation and shame, it is important to acknowledge the positive and adaptive, albeit defensive, nature of these feelings.

Predictors of Distress

Among the predictors of increased distress among psychiatrists who experience a patient suicide, shown in Table 33–2, the most consistent are age and experience (which are, of course, highly correlated), with older age and more years of experience predicting somewhat less distress.

This finding can be seen in most, but not all, of the few data-based papers examining the topic (Chemtob et al. 1988b; Hendin et al. 2004; Ruskin et al. 2004; Wurst et al. 2010) as well as in most impressionistic papers. That age and experience are the most important factors in predicting distress is deeply intuitive. No differently than when coping with other losses or tragedies, psychiatrists develop perspectives over time that buffer them from greater pain after the loss of a patient. A number of papers have highlighted the greater vulnerability of trainees who experience a patient suicide. Trainees, the youngest and least experienced of our field, are uniquely vulnerable because they typically have not yet been able to internalize a self-image as a competent professional who can successfully treat some patients despite the tragedy of a patient suicide (Brown 1987a, 1987b; Goldstein and Buongiorno 1984; Sacks 1989).

Another factor commonly assumed to predict greater distress after patient suicide is the intensity of involvement between the professional and the patient. Surprisingly, no data exist to support this assumption. (In the one study that examined this issue systematically, a patient's length of time in treatment did not contribute to ratings of therapist distress [Hendin et al. 2004].) Nonetheless, greater emotional involvement with the patient is likely to be associated with greater distress. The involvement may not always be measurable by simply establishing the length of treatment. Related fac-

TABLE 33–2. Potential predictors of distress after patient suicide

Age (negative predictor)

Experience (negative predictor)

Intensity of involvement with patient

Treatment setting

Gender of psychiatrist

Clinician's personality

Clinician's history of depression and anxiety

tors might also be the sheer volume of time spent with the patient, with the possibility that the suicide of a therapy patient may have a deeper effect than that of a patient seen in medication management. At the same time, however, remarkably deep ties often develop between patients and psychiatrists whose role is purely as psychopharmacologists.

Work setting (inpatient vs. outpatient, private practice vs. institutional setting) has also not been shown to be related to distress after patient suicide. However, treatment setting will certainly dictate the reaction of others to the suicide and will therefore have an impact on the treating psychiatrist. As noted earlier, in a private practice setting, only the psychiatrist and the patient's family are ordinarily involved in the aftermath of the suicide. In an institutional setting, especially if the patient was either an inpatient or a partial hospital (day treatment) patient, other professionals and administrators become involved. If the treating physician is a trainee, supervisors and other faculty may be added to the list. In these situations, either greater support and cohesion or projected anger and blame could emerge. In one study, negative reaction by the therapist's institution was one of four factors identified as sources of severe distress (Hendin et al. 2004). The different ways in which institutions respond to the suicide may play a role in the incon-

sistent relationship between treatment setting and individual clinicians' responses to patient suicide.

In the three studies examining the issue, female psychiatrists were almost twice as likely to experience severe distress as their male counterparts after patient suicide (Hendin et al. 2004), more likely to experience more severe distress (Wurst et al. 2010), and exhibited higher rates of shame, guilt, and self-doubt (Grad et al. 1997). This may reflect the observation that women experience bereavement in general more deeply (Cleiren et al. 1994). Of course, greater distress should not always be considered as a negative finding. Emotional denial and excessive repression may interfere with optimal learning from experience.

Finally, among the most important factors in predicting reactions to patient suicide is the individual clinician's personality and own psychiatric history. In one study, psychiatrists who were less distressed after a patient suicide were more likely to identify changes in treatment they might consider in the future, a possible marker for flexible thinking and the ability to learn from the suicide as opposed to feeling dominated by guilt and self-blame (Hendin et al. 2004). Although never studied, overall resilience—with its roots in both temperament/biology and prior experience—might be the single most important factor in predicting response to suicide. Other psychological factors, such as tendencies for introjection versus projection, are also likely to be important. Finally, the individual psychiatrist's potential past history of depression and anxiety might also play a role in predicting individual vulnerability to greater distress. Although speculative, the finding of greater distress among female psychiatrists could reflect the greater likelihood of depressive disorders and most anxiety disorders among women versus men in general (Robins and Regier 1991). In one study, a past personal experience with suicide in a close friend or family member did not predict greater distress after patient suicide (Ruskin et al. 2004).

Coping With Patient Suicide

A number of methods for optimal coping with suicide have been suggested. These methods may be broadly divided into four categories (Table 33–3): decreasing isolation, using philosophical and cognitive approaches, effecting temporary behavioral changes, and instituting reparative, constructive behaviors (Gitlin 1999).

Decreasing Isolation

Despite a lack of data, reducing the feelings of isolation is the most commonly recommended method of combating the negative effects of a patient's suicide (Alexander et al. 2000; Brown 1987b; Chemtob et al. 1988a; Gitlin 1999; Goldstein and Buongiorno 1984; Hendin et al. 2000, 2004; Sacks 1989; Sacks et al. 1987). This coping method, which can be accomplished in a broad variety of ways, is perfectly analogous to the suggestions we make to our patients after tragedies in their own lives. Talking to others one trusts and respects, whether lovers, friends, family, or colleagues, is likely to be helpful. Discussion with former or current supervisors (assuming they know something about this area) can be exceedingly helpful. It is surprising how few papers comment on the use of the psychiatrist's own individual psychotherapy as a useful method of decreasing isolation (see Tillman 2006 for an exception). Colleagues sharing their own experiences with the suicide of a patient may be more helpful than the soothing comments about the inevitability of the death or reflexive reassurance ("You did

TABLE 33–3. Optimal coping methods after patient suicide

Decreasing isolation
Using philosophical and cognitive approaches
Effecting temporary behavioral changes
Instituting reparative, constructive behaviors

nothing wrong") (Hendin et al. 2004; Tillman 2006).

A specific method of decreasing isolation is meeting with the significant others of the person who died by suicide and/or going to the person's funeral or memorial service. In two case series, 60%–66% of psychiatrists saw their patients' relatives after the suicides (Hendin et al. 2004; Ruskin et al. 2004). Although meeting with family members is typically described as positive, this is not always the case. Fear of relatives' reactions correlated with greater degrees of distress in one study (Wurst et al. 2010). The psychiatrist must be aware of the possibility that relatives will be angry because of the feeling that they do not know enough about the specifics of their relative's psychopathology, because of projected anger, or because of well-meaning decisions by the psychiatrist that may indeed have not prevented or may have even contributed to the suicide. Therefore, a psychiatrist meeting with the relatives of a patient who died by suicide must be prepared for anger and must be able to respond in a nondefensive manner while not being too quick to accept blame caused by guilt feelings. Care must also be taken in these meetings with regard to patient confidentiality, which extends beyond the death of a patient. It is possible, although delicate, to provide sufficient feedback and discussion with family members without violating the core of the patient's privileged information.

As noted earlier, suicides within institutional settings provide unique opportunities for decreasing isolation or engaging in blaming behaviors. In many situations, the group setting provides greater support. As Litman (1965) noted in one of the earliest papers on the topic, the helpfulness of an institution "is especially true if there was a spirit of mutual support, shared responsibility, and cooperative teamwork among the staff" (p. 574). A psychological autopsy often occurs as a mandated suicide review in certain psychiatric hospitals. Its goal is to review the suicide, understand its causes, and learn so as to treat patients better in the future. When done properly, it should be a supportive, constructive learning experience. However, it is too easy for the psychological autopsy to become a public shaming by blaming the treating professional (Sacks 1989). In today's environment, in which the concern/threat of lawsuits psychologically dominates many situations, it is particularly important that the perceived institutional response not be dominated by projecting blame away from the institution and toward one or more treating professionals.

Using Philosophical and Cognitive Approaches

Understanding a patient's suicide using philosophical and cognitive approaches is a second useful strategy. These approaches may sound trite when written but may be powerful when presented in interactive discussion. In many ways, they may be most helpful if they are inculcated during psychiatric training and *before* a suicide instead of after one.

The first of these approaches acknowledges that psychiatrists who treat patients with serious psychiatric disorders—depression, bipolar disorder, drug and alcohol abuse, schizophrenia, borderline personality disorder—must embrace the expectation that some of their patients will die because of the natural course of their disorder. It must be understood that we cannot prevent the worst outcome of every case any more than can our colleagues in cardiology or oncology. Additionally, it must be understood that although there are clear demographic and clinical predictors of suicide among groups of patients, the field is unable to accurately predict suicidal risk for any individual patient (Porkorny 1983). These statements must not be used to foster a passivity, fatalism, or therapeutic nihilism in our therapeutic work; rather, they should be used to understand the inherent inconsistent effect of our best efforts (implied in the earlier discussion of the loss of omnipotence or grandiosity in young psychiatrists after a patient suicide).

Effecting Temporary Behavioral Changes

Because of the frequency with which patient suicide adversely affects psychiatrists, a number of relatively simple, temporary behavioral changes can be effected to help diminish distress and to ensure that the psychiatrist continues to practice optimal care. In the immediate aftermath of a patient suicide, most psychiatrists, especially younger ones, feel distinctly less trusting of their own judgment. This typically leads to an overly conservative set of decisions and behaviors, such as more aggressively querying patients about suicide (in ways that are neither appropriate nor therapeutic) or too quickly hospitalizing other suicidal patients (Tillman 2006). If possible, therefore, after a patient suicide, it is often helpful to not accept patients who are euphemistically described as "challenging" or "interesting," and certainly not those described as "difficult," until one has regained enough balance to utilize judgment based on the current case and not the suicide that occurred previously.

Instituting Reparative, Constructive Behaviors

Although rarely utilized in the immediate aftermath of a patient suicide, helping others cope with similar incidents may be a remarkably effective and constructive long-term behavior. Such help would include being available to other, younger colleagues who have had a first patient die by suicide, presenting about the topics at conferences, and writing about the experience (Biermann 2003; Gitlin 1999). Because this type of activity requires some distance from the traumatic event itself, it usually becomes a viable option only months or even years later and typically in those who have achieved some maturity and experience in the field. Of course, being more open about personal experiences with patient suicide decreases isolation both in the presenter and in the audience, thereby effectively using two of the most important techniques of coping.

Impact of Patient Suicide on Trainees

As previously noted, trainees are more likely (one-third to two-thirds) to experience patient suicides than are more experienced psychiatrists (Brown 1987a, 1987b; Ruskin et al. 2004; Wurst et al. 2010). Although issues of competence and experience may play some role in this disparity, the more likely factor is the inherently more psychiatrically ill patients that trainees see in their hospital-based training compared with office-based clinicians. This is consistent with a previously cited study that found that 85% of hospital-based psychiatrists and psychologists experienced a patient suicide within 5 years, compared with 17% of office-based practitioners (Wurst et al. 2010). In one study, 20% of psychiatric trainees experienced more than one suicide (Ruskin et al. 2004).

In most ways, residents describe feelings after patient suicide that are similar to those of older psychiatrists, but, as previously noted, they are at higher risk of being more traumatized by the experience. Soon after the suicide, 25% of trainees met criteria for acute stress disorder and, later, 20% met criteria for posttraumatic stress disorder (Ruskin et al. 2004).

As previously noted, one of the potential tasks after a patient suicide is to deal with the family of the patient, and with the myriad potential responses that may be seen. Partly because of a lack of experience and partly because they may have seen the patient for a briefer period of time, residents are particularly uncomfortable in this arena and frequently avoid the family.

Strategies for helping trainees after a patient suicide are the same for trainees as they are for more experienced psychiatrists. However, given the less well-formed professional self-image of trainees, the psychological stress may be greater, and it may also be more difficult for the trainee to ask for the help needed. As an example, in one study, one-quarter of trainees found themselves unable to ask for help even though they knew that others were available to them (Ruskin et al. 2004).

The experience of the psychological autopsy as destructive, as previously noted, seems to be perceived frequently when the treating psychiatrist is a trainee. As an example, in one of the earlier surveys, 12 of 20 trainees stated that chart reviews and psychological autopsies compounded doubt rather than aided recovery, especially when performed very soon after the patient suicide (Goldstein and Buongiorno 1984). In another study, the two therapists who felt that their institution's response to the suicide of their patients contributed greatly to their distress were both trainees (Hendin et al. 2004). Trainees often find both their colleagues and their supervisors to be helpful after a patient suicide (Ruskin et al. 2004). In psychiatric training programs, trainee groups (if they exist) may be useful in diminishing isolation in a nonblaming atmosphere (Kolodny et al. 1979).

In working with trainees, the critical point must be to help them understand that clinical failures do not make them personal failures (Brown 1987a). (Hopefully, as psychiatrists mature in their careers, this lesson is learned, at least to some degree.) Unfortunately, few training programs have integrated psychological preparation for patient suicides. Anticipating the possibility of a patient suicide during their careers, or even their training years, should be made explicit. This can and should be introduced and discussed early in the first or second postgraduate year (Brown 1987b). Discussing the likely reactions that a resident might feel after a patient suicide as delineated in this chapter would help block the potential shock if and when these feelings arise. Faculty who have had the experience of a patient suicide can provide experience, reduce feelings of isolation, and model a successful future after the event. Additionally, if a tradition arises in which more senior residents are available to more junior ones in these situations, a closer peer-oriented modeling would enhance buffering of the experience.

Conclusion

A substantial proportion of psychiatrists will experience the suicide of a patient at some point in their careers. Trainees are at higher risk of having a patient die by suicide because they treat the patients with the greatest psychopathology. Responses to the suicide are similar to those seen in others who have lost an important person in their life, exacerbated by the shame, guilt, and fear of reprisal given the current climate of blame and malpractice threats in our country. In the immediate aftermath of a patient suicide, many psychiatrists will exhibit psychiatric distress and symptoms comparable to those in clinical populations. Typically, these symptoms diminish over the next few months. The most important predictor of greater distress after a patient suicide is the psychiatrist's age and experience, with younger clinicians exhibiting greater difficulty.

Optimal coping with a patient's suicide involves a number of different interactions and techniques. First and foremost is to decrease the (irrational) feelings of isolation. This can be accomplished in a number of ways, no one of which is superior to the others. In institutional settings such as hospitals with training programs, group discussions should be handled in a constructive, supportive manner while still attempting to help members learn from the suicide. In these situations, care must be taken not to use the group discussions to establish blame for the event (typically directed toward the youngest, least experienced clinician involved).

Anticipating suicides during one's career, especially during training, would help psychiatrists prepare psychologically. Given how frequently residents experience patient suicide and how vulnerable they are to negative effects from these suicides, more attention needs to be paid to formal instruction in this area in training programs. It would also be helpful if senior psychiatrists were more open about their experiences in this area, modeling for younger psychiatrists and decreasing the sense of isolation common after patient suicides.

Key Clinical Concepts

- A substantial proportion of psychiatrists will experience the suicide of a patient at some point in their careers.

- Responses to patient suicide resemble reactions to other meaningful losses, including denial, grief, and anger exacerbated by shame, guilt, and fear of blame.

- The most important predictors of distress after a patient suicide are younger age and lesser experience of the treating psychiatrist.

- The most important coping technique after patient suicide is decreasing isolation of the treating psychiatrist.

- Training programs should institute formal instruction for trainees in anticipating and coping with patient suicide.

References

Alexander DA, Klein S, Gray NM, et al: Suicide by patients: questionnaire study of its effect on consultant psychiatrists. BMJ 320:1571–1574, 2000

American Psychiatric Association: Diagnostic and Statistical Manual of Mental Disorders, 4th Edition, Text Revision. Washington, DC, American Psychiatric Association, 2000

Biermann B: When depression becomes terminal: the impact of patient suicide during residency. J Am Acad Psychoanal Dyn Psychiatry 31:443–457, 2003

Brown HN: The impact of suicide on therapists in training. Compr Psychiatry 28:101–112, 1987a

Brown HN: Patient suicide during residency training, I: incidence, implications, and program response. J Psychiatr Educ 11:201–216, 1987b

Chemtob CM, Hamada RS, Bauer G, et al: Patient suicide: frequency and impact on psychologists. Prof Psychol Res Pr 19:416–420, 1988a

Chemtob CM, Hamada RS, Bauer G, et al: Patients' suicides: frequency and impact on psychiatrists. Am J Psychiatry 145:224–228, 1988b

Cleiren MP, Diekstra RF, Kierkof AJ, et al: Mode of death and kinship in bereavement: focusing on "who" rather than "how." Crisis 15:22–36, 1994

Gitlin MJ: Clinical case conference: a psychiatrist's reaction to a patient's suicide. Am J Psychiatry 156:1630–1634, 1999

Goldstein LS, Buongiorno PA: Psychotherapists as suicide survivors. Am J Psychother 38:392–398, 1984

Grad OT, Zavasnik A, Groleger U: Suicide of a patient: gender differences in bereavement reactions of therapists. Suicide Life Threat Behav 27:379–386, 1997

Hendin H, Lipschitz A, Maltsberger JT, et al: Therapists' reactions to patients' suicides. Am J Psychiatry 157:2022–2027, 2000

Hendin H, Haas AP, Maltsberger JT, et al: Factors contributing to therapists' distress after the suicide of a patient. Am J Psychiatry 161:1442–1446, 2004

Jamison KR, Baldessarini RJ: Effects of medical interventions on suicidal behaviors. J Clin Psychiatry 60:4–6, 1999

Kochanek KD, Xu J, Murphy SL, et al: Deaths: preliminary data for 2009. National Vital Statistics Reports, March 16, 2011. Available at: http://www.cdc.gov/nchs/data/nvsr/nvsr59/nvsr59_04.pdf. Accessed June 22, 2011.

Kolodny S, Binder RL, Bronstein AA, et al: The working through of patients' suicides by four therapists. Suicide Life Threat Behav 9:33–46, 1979

Litman RE: When patients commit suicide. Am J Psychother 19:570–576, 1965

Livingston P, Zimet CN: Death anxiety, authoritarianism and choice of specialty in medical students. J Nerv Ment Dis 140:222–230, 1965

Menninger WW: Patient suicide and its impact on the psychotherapist. Bull Menninger Clin 55:216–227, 1991

Perr HM: Suicide and the doctor-patient relationship. Am J Psychoanal 18:177–188, 1968

Porkorny AD: Prediction of suicide in psychiatric patients. Arch Gen Psychiatry 40:249–257, 1983

Robins LN, Regier DA: Psychiatric Disorders in America. New York, Free Press, 1991

Ruskin R, Sakinofsky I, Bagby RM, et al: Impact of patient suicide on psychiatrists and psychiatric trainees. Acad Psychiatry 28:104–110, 2004

Sacks MH: When patients kill themselves, in American Psychiatric Press Review of Psychiatry, Vol 8. Edited by Tasman A, Hales RE, Frances AJ. Washington, DC, American Psychiatric Press, 1989, pp 563–579

Sacks MH, Kibel HD, Cohen AM, et al: Resident response to patient suicide. J Psychiatr Educ 11:217–226, 1987

Tillman JG: When a patient commits suicide: an empirical study of psychoanalytic clinicians. Int J Psychoanal 87:1159–1177, 2006

Wurst FH, Mueller S, Petitjean S, et al: Patient suicide: a survey of therapists' reactions. Suicide Life Threat Behav 40:328–336, 2010

CHAPTER 34

Aftermath of Suicide

The Clinician's Role

Frank R. Campbell, Ph.D., L.C.S.W., C.T.

After a death by suicide there are individuals who, because of their relationships to the deceased, will be affected. That group is collectively known as *survivors of suicide*. Historically, only the immediate family members of the deceased have been assigned the title "survivor." This assignment happens most commonly through the obituary, which reports the name of the deceased and then states, "survived by..." By this notification to the public, a parameter of impact is drawn that somewhat artificially restricts who is considered a survivor; however, there are many others in any community who, by the nature of their relationships to the deceased, will be affected by the suicide. In the United States, suicidologists have estimated that between 6 (Shneidman 1969) and 45 (Campbell 2001, 2011; Linn-Gust and Cerel 2011) survivors are affected by each suicide; however, clinicians are not included in these estimates. It is realistic to note that any person engaged in providing treatment to the deceased will be affected, and these individuals should not be excluded from consideration when resources to assist survivors are being developed and provided.

An estimated 12 clinicians lose a patient to suicide each week in the United States, necessitating interaction with survivors (Peterson et al. 2002). In the course of their practices, at least half of psychiatrists can expect that a patient will die from suicide (American Psychiatric Association 2003). A variety of factors influence the clinician's role in the aftermath of suicide, including barriers that may be both external and internal. An example of an internal barrier is the incorporation of specific gender responses to suicide that are products of the socialization process (Grad et al. 1997). External barriers include but are not limited to institutional policy and protocol, peer pressure, legal opinion, malpractice insurance constraints, and professional association recommendations. Therefore, the clinician has to overcome pressures that are both internal and external in order to contact the survivors and/or seek support for his or her own role as a survivor.

It is well documented that survivors are at increased risk for suicide (Cain 1972) as well as other maladaptive coping behaviors. When a clinician has experienced the loss of a patient to suicide, what is considered appropriate among psychiatrists and other clinicians varies greatly by the setting in which they practice. For example, psychiatrists in the United States report a reluctance to contact survivors of the deceased for fear of being held responsible for failing to prevent the death. In other countries, however, treatment of the survivors by the attending psychiatrist following suicide is an accepted and often expected practice. Regardless of the range of efforts to assist the survivors, a poverty of care for clinicians is consistent. Herein lies the paradox for the clinician. Survivors have expressed desires to discuss their particular concerns and ask questions of the clinician. Clinicians, often conflicted by the need for self-care, care for survivors, and other internal and external constraints, are unsure how to proceed.

In reviewing the role of the clinician after the suicide of a patient, it is important to point out the barriers that may be real or assumed by the professionals. Institutional barriers are very real, and when imposed by hospitals or practice settings, they often prevent clinicians from providing services desired by survivors. Institutional barriers to caring for survivors stem from many factors, including ever-changing restraints concerning confidentiality, fear of retribution or blame, malpractice insurance limitations, and governmental guidelines, and result in policies and protocols that may hinder clinicians' ability to respond to survivors.

Some of the same realities that influence institutional response also affect clinicians' personal beliefs about their roles following

suicide. Governmental laws and guidelines, including licensure, malpractice insurance, and peer review, all contribute to clinicians' interpretations about what constitutes appropriate care. Financial considerations and fear of damage to reputation also affect each clinician's determination of how to practice his or her profession. Wrongful death suits after a suicide are the most predictable legal entanglements that psychiatrists will face during their careers. Training, mentors, peers, prior experience and practice, and personal and religious beliefs all contribute to the value system internalized by clinicians and must be examined as factors that also influence responses to survivors. Ironically, many of the things that influence a clinician's response after a suicide create the barriers that are cited by survivors as the major factors in their decision to bring legal action against both institutions and clinicians.

Because research is lacking regarding the efficacy of services for survivors, it remains unclear what is appropriate and what is needed for survivors, including clinicians. In the absence of rigorous research into efficacy of treatments for survivors, clinicians remain dependent on the anecdotal reports by survivors of what they want and need from the treatment provider after a suicide.

Active Postvention Model

Having worked with survivors for more than 25 years and having developed an active postvention model (APM; Campbell 1997), I have accumulated an in-depth understanding of survivor needs. Since 1998, the APM has provided the opportunity for survivor-sensitive mental health professionals and paraprofessional survivor volunteers to respond to more than 100 suicide scenes in order to deliver care and information about services to the new survivors. This environment, while the body is still present, allows the wants and needs of the newly bereaved to be expressed and recorded.

APM is a volunteer service affiliated with the local coroner's office and a free program of the Baton Rouge Crisis Intervention Center. It is staffed primarily by survivors, facilitating immediate acceptance at the scenes of suicides and a level of trust by the newly bereaved that might not otherwise be achieved if provided by clinicians alone. This service provided at the scenes of suicides is known as Local Outreach to Suicide Survivors, more commonly referred to as the LOSS Team. It is particularly noteworthy that the survivor team members have an instant rapport with the newly bereaved because they share a traumatic loss experience. This bonds the new survivors to the LOSS Team members and has resulted in a reduction of the elapsed time between the loss and seeking support services (Campbell et al. 2004).

Prior to the LOSS Team program, survivors in one study waited an average of 4.5 years before seeking treatment (Campbell 1997). Six years into providing LOSS Team support, the mean elapsed time between death and seeking help for the newly bereaved who received the APM was 43 days. The anecdotal information is gathered from survivors, both at the scene and in individual intakes for services, in a more timely manner, thus increasing the validity and reliability of reporting.

Because of the APM and the unique opportunity it presents for reporting the wants and needs of the newly bereaved, certain themes have surfaced regarding the clinician's role in the aftermath of suicide. Individuals who are in treatment, individuals who have received treatment in the past, and individuals who have never received

treatment die by suicide. Although survivors of those who have never received treatment could contribute their insights on services, the discussion in this chapter is limited to deaths by suicide of individuals recently in treatment with a clinician.

The insights derived from the APM study are in the category of postvention services and are specific to the field of suicidology. Shneidman (1972) defined *postvention* as "appropriate and helpful acts that come after a dire event" for the purpose of "alleviation of the effects of stress in the survivor-victims of suicidal deaths, whose lives are ever after benighted by that event" (p. x). Along with this definition in 1972, Shneidman stated that "postvention is prevention for the next generation." If his statement is correct, then clinicians might justifiably seek to provide such "appropriate and helpful acts" to the survivors who seek counsel after a suicide as an effort to prevent future suicides. Until robust research into postvention is completed, Shneidman's theories about helping survivors remain the only reasonable approach for clinicians to adopt after the suicide of a patient. In addition, clinicians must be diligent about caring for themselves during their treatment of and follow-up with suicidal patients and survivors of suicide. Survivors who received APM services at the scene of a suicide informed the recommendations in Table 34–1 by members of the LOSS Team of the Baton Rouge Crisis Intervention Center.

Firsthand accounts are included in this chapter to illustrate, from the survivors' perspectives, the importance of adopting these recommendations in the clinician's practice whenever possible. Each story is a case example representing a survivor's answer to the question "What would you have wished that the clinician who was treating your loved one provided to you following the suicide?" These responses have not been altered in content and should be read in the context of e-mail correspondence. The first case example comes from a mental health professional who lost her sister (a therapist herself as well) and then, years later, her mother to suicide. Both of her family members were in treatment at the time of their death.

> When considering what I would have wished for from the clinicians who treated both my mother and sister at the times of their suicides, it would be these two specific things:
>
> 1. Show up at the visitation or funeral (my sister's clinician did and my mother's did not).
> 2. Offer to meet with me to discuss my concerns, and answer questions.
>
> Note: my sister's therapist did offer to meet with me and I decided to honor my sister's confidence with her therapist and not seek any information regarding her treatment…, but my appreciation of the offer can't be underestimated. Had my mother's psychiatrist made the offer, I would not have taken him up on it, either. Had I pursued a meeting with either therapist, the top two questions would have simply been.
>
> 1. What was she most fearful of in life?
> 2. What was she most angry about/resentful of in life?

It is important to note that this survivor assigned value to the attendance by one therapist and noted the absence of the other. Regardless of the clinician's personal comfort or beliefs regarding attending the visitation or funeral of the patient, this survivor's account represents the wishes of hundreds of survivors with whom I have had personal contact. LOSS Team members attend many of the visitations and funerals and corroborate the importance of the clinician making contact during visitation. The clinician's attendance at the visitation or funeral pro-

TABLE 34–1. Recommendations to clinicians for reaching out to survivors of suicide at the time of death

Be assertive in contacting the survivors.

Attend the funeral or visitation.

Support ongoing help for survivors.

Offer referrals or treatment if appropriate.

Provide information about psychological autopsy.

Be knowledgeable about survivor resources in your community.

vides another opportunity to encourage survivors to seek support or treatment by reassuring them about the availability and importance of postvention.

Outreach to Survivors After the Initial Period Following Loss

After the initial visitation period, it is a valid consideration for the clinician to follow up on any referrals made to the survivors. A sincere inquiry into the survivors' ability to cope with the activities of daily living (eating, sleeping, exercise, and concentration) is helpful in determining other referrals that might be needed. If a survivor reports compromised activities of daily living, then medication and/or individual treatment may be indicated. A survivor who is functioning in a depressed state may begin to overidentify with the deceased and experience suicidal ideation, therefore requiring thorough assessment. Follow-up reinforces not only the need for ongoing support for the survivor but also the clinician's willingness to be a resource. Mental health centers throughout the United States may be a referral resource for the clinician to consider for survivors who are suicidal and lack other mental health resources (private insurance or ability to pay).

For many survivors, *psychological autopsy* is a method of review that can answer specific questions regarding the deceased's behavior, compliance to treatment, and complications in his or her successful treatment. The next case example demonstrates how an interview with the clinician of the deceased might have provided some insight for the survivor into the deceased's ability to mask his symptoms. The following e-mail is from a survivor who lost her adult son to suicide. He had been in treatment for bipolar disorder prior to his death.

Pete had seen a counselor about a week before he died, at our urging. We had tried to get him to see the psychiatrist that he had seen in the past or to go to the mental health center, but he chose to see the counselor to just talk about the problem (he admitted to feeling depressed to us). He had promised us that he would go to the mental health center but changed his mind. He told us he had talked to the counselor and that all had gone well and that they felt he didn't need medicine but would talk again the following week. (The next week was too late.) He had seen this counselor about a year ago for about 6 months when he was feeling stressed, to talk about the problems he was having. I wish I knew what occurred or how Pete hid his manic state so well from a professional. He was very good at hiding his true feelings so much of the time.

Had this parent been afforded the opportunity for psychological autopsy of her son, she might have gained answers into the stressors that precipitated his death and how he was able to disguise what to her appeared to be a manic state. Her son was considered high functioning and resourceful by other counselors who had assisted him over the years. The following e-mail came from his counselor, who had worked with him for more than 2 years at a vocational rehabilitation program: "I was shocked by the news of his passing. He was one of my favorite clients, and one of my most successful. I remember the last time I saw him we had a good talk. He was showing me his new tattoo and talking about his new girlfriend. I will miss him."

The rehabilitation counselor clearly acknowledges confusion over Pete's ability to appear life oriented in a counseling session and yet later take his own life. This acknowledgment of the deceased's ability to mask his thoughts of suicide validates the mother's confusion over the same issue. One of the many benefits of psychological autopsy is providing an environment in which such questions can be explored.

Providing other resources of which the survivor may not be aware is another benefit of follow-up. Reading lists of survivor-focused materials create opportunities for bibliotherapy, which many survivors report as helpful. Because so much of the literature is relationship specific (e.g., loss of child, spouse, sibling), clinicians' recommendations could be more effective and should be founded on their firsthand knowledge of the material and their assessments of the needs of the survivor. Some survivor literature features information directed to survivors regardless of their relationship to the deceased. Carla Fine's (1997) book *No Time to Say Goodbye* contains both her personal journey as a survivor of her physician husband's suicide and the stories of persons surviving the deaths of loved ones of other relationships. The opportunity to read (see "Suggested Readings" at the end of this chapter) about what helped so many survivors could help normalize the complicated process that follows suicide for the newly bereaved.

Another possible outcome of reading survivor literature is a reduction in resistance to participating in survivors of suicide (SOS) support groups. Although SOS groups do not exist in every community, they are more common today and have provided a low- or no-cost local environment where many survivors gain support. Contact information about many of the SOS groups can be found in survivor literature. Should the survivor be interested in attending an SOS group, the clinician should be well informed about making referrals to the group and other services for survivors that may be provided.

Another referral resource that might be considered by clinicians treating survivors is a local crisis line. These lines often provide support for suicidal callers and survivors of suicide experiencing compromised activities of daily living and other issues related to the suicide. Because it is available 24 hours a day, 7 days a week, the crisis line becomes a resource during off-hours for clinicians and other services. Many crisis lines also provide up-to-date information and referral to resources in the community.

Since September 11, 2001, many communities have begun providing telephone access to current information and referral resources by a three-digit phone number known simply as 211. Like other three-digit resources (411 for directory assistance, 911 for emergency services), it is gaining in recognition and usage over time. Just as 911 is not available in all communities in the United States, 211 is presently limited, and clinicians can determine whether it is available in their communities by dialing 211 (cellular services are currently not mandated to provide access to this resource).

Through the use of the Internet, Web sites hosted by survivors and agencies and programs that provide information specific to survivors are readily identified and are usually more current. Clinicians should include the Internet in their referrals to survivors because it provides an environment in which support, via e-mail and online chat rooms, is available. Such electronic support can reduce the isolation that many survivors, especially in rural settings, report due to their distance from the limited resources that may be available.

Survivors have indicated their appreciation of clinicians who identify important dates and difficult times (i.e., holidays and the deceased's dates of birth and death) and use that information in tandem with a contact management program to follow up with ongoing support. This contact, although only a small gesture, may be a key to helping the survivor through a very complicated bereavement process. This personalized contact on key dates (for the survivors) helps mitigate the grief experienced during seasonal spikes that time alone cannot erase. The value to the survivor is incalculable. A spouse who lost her husband just prior to their anniversary noted the following example of such a follow-up approach:

> Each year on the anniversary of his death and during the holidays I get a simple card from the doctor who was treating my husband. He writes in his own hand something like "I know this can be a difficult time of year and I hope you are taking care of yourself." He then signs at the bottom. I have kept them all, and it means so much to me that he remembers. I realize it may be just a function of a mail-out system that he has for his office but that really does not matter. What is important is that someone remembers my loss besides me.

Clinicians must be vigilant to ensure that any correspondence is appropriate and comforting. The following example illustrates how routine correspondence, such as billing for services, might cause pain and create animosity for survivors after the suicide of a patient. The mother of an adult son who took his life while in treatment after 4 years with the same physician stated:

About 2 weeks after the funeral I went to his apartment to pick up the last of the mail the landlord was keeping for me. There in the mail was a letter from his doctor. I assumed it was going to be some sort of acknowledgment about his death and offer to help; was I wrong! It was a note reminding him that he had "missed an appointment" (we had notified the office, on the same day he died, that he had killed himself) and that "the office policy requires payment if you do not cancel more than 48 hours before the appointment day." Well, I was furious! I called and gave them a piece of my mind. I told the office manager that to get something like this in the mail was criminal. I also told her that if they wanted to "report his debt for collection" as they threatened in the letter, then they might want to know where he is buried so they can take it up with him in person. She was sorry and apologized, and when I hung up all I could do was cry. The poor landlord saw me in the parking lot and came out to see if he could help. If only the doctor's office would have been more efficient, I would not have had to go through such a difficult and embarrassing experience.

Clinicians must be diligent in reviewing their accounts and marketing procedures and instructing their staff members to avoid being part of unintended harassment of survivors dealing with the financial and legal considerations after an unexpected death. Caring professionals who take the time to explain the processes and offer assistance can mitigate those taxing and painful concerns. The following case example tells how the spouse of the deceased dealt with the frustrations of such details:

It seemed that daily I would get a call from some bank or insurance company to verify something with him, sell him something, or just want to talk to him. Each time I would have to explain that

he was dead, and then they would want to know how he died, and I would just hang up. I called to cancel his cell phone, and they told me that I could not cancel it for him and I had to bring in a death certificate to prove he was dead. I just kept paying the bill for almost a year because the death certificate made it real and paying the bill let me pretend he was just away on a trip. I know that was crazy, but I could not get up the courage to go and face some cell phone person and show them his death certificate. A part of me wanted to ask them if he had called anyone in the past year!

Clinicians should take particular care to recommend hospital or institutional treatment for a patient where the clinician him- or herself will be available for consultation with the patient and supervision of the patient's treatment plan while in the facility. Because family members and significant others of a suicidal patient become exhausted from hypervigilance over the suicidal patient, they can experience cognitive impairments, difficulty processing complex information, and caregiver ambivalence. They place immense trust in the clinician's treatment recommendations and assume that all treatment will be safe and effective and that the admitting clinician will be present during admission and for their loved one's treatment. When a suicide is completed in a hospital or institutional setting, loss of trust occurs for clinicians and the survivors. When a clinician recommends hospitalization and is then unable to see the patient for days following admission, the impact is confusing to the survivors. The following e-mail describes such a loss of trust by a surviving spouse:

The doctor reassured me that hospitalization would be the best thing for him. My husband begged me not to sign the papers and have him committed. I had to trust the doctor; after he killed himself I found out they put him in a lockdown ward and left him there for the weekend. He was not given any medication to help him sleep or calm down. The doctor (I found out later) went away for the weekend and was not even available to be called if a consultation could have been arranged. My husband was put in a unit with several actively psychotic patients who would just walk in his room and wake him up (if he did manage to fall asleep). The following Monday the doctor returned and saw him for 10 minutes that morning and gave him a shot to "calm him down"; the next day he hanged himself with a belt left by another patient. How can I ever trust anyone again?

Clinicians must also disclose the limitations of any treatment recommendations. Defining limitations of treatment may not change the ultimate outcome of the treatment; however, it might eliminate the loss of trust that occurs when expectations are overestimated. When a suicide occurs in a hospital—a safe place as perceived by caregivers—their loss of trust is outweighed only by an elevated fear that something else bad will happen. That fear may remain elevated for years past the survivors' renewed ability to trust. Clinicians could use the following example of a script that might have been a better alternative for handling the prior case:

> You are both exhausted! Your wife is exhausted from standing guard day and night, protecting you from yourself, and you are exhausted from the apparent suicidal depression you are fighting. By going into the hospital you might both get some rest; however, it will be difficult for both of you to cope with being away from each other, having been so close during this battle with suicide. The limitations I have in treating you include not being in town this weekend,

and this means I will not be able to begin your treatment until Monday. The depression can get much worse before it gets better. Can you commit to beginning treatment under these limitations?

This approach allows the patient and family to be aware of the clinician's limitations to begin treatment due to other prior responsibilities as well as acknowledging the need for everyone to share in the commitment to get help and rest. Treatment expectations may come from media, books, firsthand accounts, or survivors' own experiences in hospitals for physical complications. Loved ones may have unrealistic expectations of treatment options in inpatient settings. Expectations of patients, loved ones, and clinicians may be varied, making it necessary to prepare all parties for realistic goals and treatment outcomes.

The following case example is from a spouse whose physician husband was admitted to a private psychiatric hospital, where he hanged himself within 48 hours of admission. Clinicians might discern from this example how to avoid long-term trauma for survivors stemming from the method and content of the notification of the suicide and the identification of the deceased:

> He has been dead 20 years, but I can remember that day as if it was yesterday. I remember very clearly his psychiatrist taking me to see his body and pulling back the sheet to show me the ligature marks. He then stated, "They weren't too bad," as if that would give me some comfort.

Viewing the body can produce many intrusive images. The LOSS Team has discovered that whether the survivors choose to view the body or not, being given the *choice* is paramount in importance. Clinicians should make every effort to prepare the survivors by informing them about the condition of the body and how it will be presented (e.g., on a gurney, in a body bag, as it was found). Such preparation can reduce the negative consequences of viewing. Viewing only a small portion of the body may achieve what survivors desire (a mother said she just needed to see his hand, and then she would know this was her son). The case example continues with what the survivor wanted at the time of her physician husband's inpatient suicide:

> The first thing I wanted from any ONE of them was an explanation of how this happened; he was in a private psychiatric hospital on "arm's length" suicide watch, being checked every 30 minutes. Of course, now I realize this can be a legal question and very tricky, because I later brought a lawsuit against the hospital, et al. BUT I thought that putting him in a private, small, specialty hospital on suicide watch would lessen by far the chance of him carrying out his plans. And I am intelligent enough to realize that where there is a will, there is a way, and when he made up his mind to die, nothing was going to hold him back; but this is after the fact. The hospital was very unclear on the circumstances of his death. I just wanted to talk, talk, talk, and THE PROFESSIONALS DID NOT WANT TO LISTEN. There was no SOS group in our city and in general the whole medical community was closed to me after his death, perhaps because he was a physician, and they did not want to admit that one of their own had done this.

Her desires to get answers and to "talk, talk, talk" about her feelings and fears were her immediate needs and could have been accomplished with the support of caring and competent clinicians. However, the lack of survivor-sensitive postvention care, the exposure to a traumatic sight (viewing the body), the limited availability to provide treatment by the clinician, and the lack of comprehension over how this could have happened in an inpatient setting were all factors in her decision to file a lawsuit:

> I brought a wrongful death lawsuit a year after he died because there was a 45-minute gap in the nurses' notes about checking him, and that's exactly when he took the opportunity to kill himself. The psychiatrist had pulled him off all his medications and was doing tests (mental and physical) to try to determine if it was a chemical imbalance in his brain that was causing the depression. We never got the chance to find out. I sued the hospital, the psychiatrist who was treating him, and the two nurses who were his main caregivers. I was in a courtroom for 12 awful days, on the stand myself for a day and a half, and lost the lawsuit. The hospital's slick lawyer came up with a surprise defense only 24 hours before the trial started. He said that he died of autoerotic asphyxiation, and a jury of my peers believed him. His family testified for the defense. I think I would still have brought the lawsuit against them [the hospital, the psychiatrist who was treating him, and the two nurses involved in his care] because they were not doing their duty in checking him every 30 minutes. They treated him like a physician instead of a patient (asking him if he had suicidal ideations instead of doing their job and physically checking him). The fact that he had been pulled off all his medications didn't help. Also, the chemical dependency unit (CDU) downstairs from him filled up, and on his second night there he was given a roommate. His own belts and sharps had been taken, but his second-night roommate had his belt because he was from the CDU and not on suicide watch. So during the 45-minute gap in the nurses' notes, he took his roommate's belt, went all the way down to the end of the hall to a bathroom, locked the door, hooked the belt to a hook on the wall, and hung himself.

Thirty minutes later someone reported to the nurses' station that a shower had been running for a long time down the hall.

Her continued efforts to get answers and the ensuing lawsuit resulted in more trauma and distancing from supports.

The legal implications of an apology to the survivors by the treating clinician make it a complex and difficult decision. The potential for the apology to be used against the clinician varies in the United States on a state-by-state basis. The following memorandum from a legal researcher (Adam Haney) to an attorney (Allen Posey) is an example of the paradigm shift that is ongoing in the United States on the issue of apology:

> Oregon and Colorado have statutory privileges regarding apologies in medical malpractice cases. The statutes state that apologies by or on behalf of medical professionals are inadmissible not only in court but also in arbitration and other alternative forums.
>
> The Vermont Supreme Court has also ruled that an apology by a physician for an "inadequate" operation is not an admission of liability (*Phinney v. Vinson* [1992] 605 A.2d 849). The court similarly held that an apology for a serious mistake made during surgery does not establish an element of a malpractice claim (*Senesac v. Associates in Obstetrics and Gynecology* [1982] 449 A.2d 900).
>
> California also has a similar but less expansive statute. That state's law is that general apologies or statements of regret are inadmissible to prove liabil-

ity. However, if a person makes a statement outright admitting liability, that statement may be admissible.

> (Memorandum from Adam Haney, Capital Clerks, to Attorney Allen Posey, April 25, 2005)[1]

Many other states have bills in their legislatures or in committees that are attempting to address this issue. Thus, the clinician is caught in an ongoing transition that will affect his or her practice outcomes as well as redefine malpractice coverage. Until such legal issues are resolved, clinicians not only must know their particular jurisdictional limitations but also must be knowledgeable about the policies of their workplace and the restrictions set forth by their malpractice carrier. The following correspondence from Professor Ralph Slovenko, author of *Law in Psychiatry* and *Psychiatry in Law*, illustrates these very complex areas of apology:

> May 5, 2005
>
> A number of states have enacted legislation, and a number of others are considering it, that excludes an expression of sorrow as an admission, but this legislation only ensures freedom to say one is sorry, but not of other types of admission. Thus, if someone says, "I'm sorry, this is all my fault, I was yelling at my wife on my cell phone and wasn't looking," everything after "I'm sorry" is admissible in evidence as an admission.
>
> It is also to be noted that an admission obviates the requirement of expert testimony that is ordinarily required to prove a case of malpractice.

---

[1]Important insights into how apology laws impact settlement issues can be found using a LEXSEE search for Citation 59 DePaul L. Rev. 489 by Jennifer K. Robbennoit, Professor of Law and Psychology, University of Illinois (2010). LEXSEE search for Citation 46 San Diego L. Rev. 137 by Michael B. Runnels, Assistant Professor of Law and Social Responsibility Department, Sellinger School of Business and Management, Loyola College in Maryland. Louisiana Revised Statutes Title 13. Courts and Judicial Procedure, Chapter 17 Witnesses an Evidence Part 2. Evidence in General, La. R.S. 13:3715.5 (2011).

Moreover, liability insurance companies consider an admission by the insured party that he has done something wrong is failure of cooperation, voiding insurance coverage.

Lawyers understand the importance of never admitting to anything—it's the lawyer's commandment. It is most important, at least from a legal perspective, to say nothing and particularly to admit no responsibility whatsoever. It's typical lawyer advice: "If you start explaining or apologizing, you will be providing crucial evidence for a lawsuit."

The Japanese, who by culture apologize profusely, learn not to apologize when working in the United States.

Regards,
Ralph Slovenko

Because several states have begun to address the need for an "apology law" that allows clinicians to say they are sorry, it is imperative that clinicians know the statutes and policies that apply in the jurisdictions where they practice. This effort to facilitate an environment in which apology cannot be used to punish the clinician may be the result of all parties agreeing that both the clinician and the family benefit from such a condolence. Attorney George Anding, partner in the Baton Rouge law firm of Rainer, Anding, and McLindon, states:

> While some defense counsel or professional groups may advise against it, in my experience a physician's sympathetic and concerned communication with a grieving family generally goes a lot farther toward avoiding a claim than inciting one. When a physician either fails or refuses to communicate with the family of the deceased, whether or not on advice of counsel, their frequent (and natural) assumption is that he or she may have something to hide, and that it's probably inculpatory. Even in a situation where the physician may be at fault, caring communication with the family may prevent a claim that a lack of such contact may significantly promote. Louisiana legislation passed in 2005 actually encourages such expressions of caring, by providing that any communication by a health care provider "expressing or conveying apology, regret, grief, sympathy, commiseration, condolence, compassion, or a general sense of benevolence made to a patient, a relative of the patient, or an agent or representative of the patient, shall not constitute an admission against interest...and shall not be admissible in evidence to establish liability...." (G.K. Anding, personal communication, March 2011, quoting from La. R.S. 13:3715.5)

Mr. Anding's 35-year practice has included both the defense and prosecution of medical malpractice claims. His insight may be the basis of legislative reform regarding the use of apology in legal cases in the United States.

Survivors who file lawsuits may have a variety of reasons to pursue such "remedies," including a desire to fix a mental health system that has failed to keep promises made (or assumed) regarding the safety and treatment of the deceased. They also hope to determine the responsible parties and perhaps prevent future suicides. The efforts to do so, whether successful or not, often result in significant financial and emotional tolls for survivors and clinicians.

Perhaps the most deficient response to the aftermath of a patient suicide is in the clinician's self-care. How the death of his or her patient affects the clinician's own psychological well-being is often ignored and/or routinely dismissed. Clinicians are trained in techniques to ameliorate the negative effects of exposure to a sudden and traumatic death. However, when it relates to oneself or to a colleague, the resolve to seek support and/or treatment seems lacking. This implies a paradoxical understanding of the importance of treatment. Clinicians must be diligent to ensure their own self-care following the suicide of a patient by considering the recommendations in Table 34–2.

Informed studies focusing on the needs of survivors and clinicians following suicide are needed and would certainly assist professionals in determining how to reduce the negative effects. Until such appropriate research is completed, clinicians must depend on anecdotal evidence to determine best practices in assessment of suicide and the ensuing follow-up.

TABLE 34–2. Recommendations for clinicians for self-care after the suicide of a patient

Seek survivor-sensitive peer support and/or consultation.

Be knowledgeable about survivor symptoms that are role specific to caregivers.

Monitor your personal activities of daily living as well as any increased hypervigilance, cognitive confusion, or levels of dissociation.

Be aware of any change in the incidence of hospitalization and/or referral of patients who present with issues or problems similar to those of the deceased patient (could be a projection issue).

Be aware of any increased use of gallows humor, paranoia, or inappropriate affect and content.

Avoid distancing, withdrawal, or isolation from supports.

Note any increased use of maladaptive behaviors (e.g., drinking, poor eating, drug use).

Key Clinical Concepts

- After a death by suicide, individuals with relationships to the deceased, collectively known as *survivors of suicide*, are at increased risk for suicide as well as other maladaptive coping behaviors.

- Persons engaged in providing treatment to the deceased will be affected and should not be excluded from consideration when resources to assist survivors are being developed and provided.

- The active postvention model (APM) is a volunteer service affiliated with the local coroner's office and a free program of the Baton Rouge Crisis Intervention Center. Staffed primarily by survivors, it facilitates immediate acceptance at the scenes of suicides and a level of trust by the newly bereaved that might not otherwise be achieved if provided by clinicians alone.

- It is recommended that clinicians who are reaching out to survivors of suicide at the time of death 1) be assertive in contacting the survivors, 2) attend the funeral or visitation, 3) support ongoing help for survivors, 4) offer referrals or treatment if appropriate, 5) provide information about psychological autopsy, and 6) be knowledgeable about survivor resources in your community.

- After the initial visitation period, it is a valid consideration for the clinician to follow up on any referrals made to the survivors. A sincere inquiry into the survivors' ability to cope with the activities of daily living is helpful in determining other referrals that might be needed. For many survivors, psychological autopsy is a method of review that can answer specific questions regarding the deceased's behavior, compliance to treatment, and complications in his or her successful treatment. Follow-up also allows the clinician to refer survivors to other resources about which they may not be aware, such as reading lists, survivors support groups, local crisis lines, and Web sites.

- Clinicians must be vigilant to ensure that any correspondence with survivors is appropriate and comforting. Clinicians must be diligent in reviewing their accounts and marketing procedures and instructing their staff members to avoid being part of unintended harassment of survivors dealing with the financial and legal considerations after an unexpected death. Caring professionals who take the time to explain the processes and offer assistance can mitigate those taxing and painful concerns.

- Clinicians should take particular care to recommend hospital or institutional treatment for a patient where the clinicians themselves will be available for consultation with the patient and supervision of the patient's treatment plan while in the facility. Family members and significant others of a suicidal patient place immense trust in the clinician's treatment recommendations and assume that all treatment will be safe and effective and that the admitting clinician will be present during admission and for their loved one's treatment. When a suicide is completed in a hospital or institutional setting, loss of trust occurs for clinicians and the survivors. When a clinician recommends hospitalization and is then unable to see the patient for days following admission, the impact is confusing to the survivors. Clinicians must also disclose the limitations of any treatment recommendations, in part to mitigate the loss of trust that occurs when expectations are overestimated.

- The legal implications of an apology to the survivors by the treating clinician make it a complex and difficult decision. The potential for the apology to be used against the clinician varies in the United States on a state-by-state basis. Clinicians not only must know their particular jurisdictional statutes and policies, including whether there is a so-called apology law, but also must be knowledgeable about the policies of their workplace and the restrictions set forth by their malpractice carrier. Effort to facilitate an environment in which apology cannot be used to punish the clinician may be the result of all parties agreeing that both the clinician and the family benefit from such a condolence.

- Perhaps the most deficient response to the aftermath of a patient suicide is in the clinician's self-care. The effect of the death on the clinician's own psychological well-being is often ignored and/or routinely dismissed. It is recommended that clinicians 1) seek survivor-sensitive peer support and/or consultation, 2) be knowledgeable about survivor symptoms that are role specific to caregivers, 3) monitor their personal activities of daily living as well as any increased hypervigilance, cognitive confusion, or levels of dissociation, 4) be aware of any change in the incidence of hospitalization and/or referral of patients who present with issues or problems similar to those of the deceased patient (could be a projection issue), 5) be aware of any increased use of gallows humor, paranoia, or inappropriate affect and content, and 6) avoid distancing, withdrawal, or isolation from supports.

Suggested Readings

Allen BG, Calhoun LG, Cann A, et al: The effect of cause of death on responses to the bereaved: suicide compared to accident and natural causes. Omega (Westport) 28:39–48, 1993

Bailley SE, Kral MJ, Dunham K: Survivors of suicide do grieve differently: empirical support for a common sense proposition. Suicide Life Threat Behav 29:256–271, 1999

Barrett TW, Scott TB: Suicide bereavement and recovery patterns compared with non-suicide bereavement patterns. Suicide Life Threat Behav 20:1–15, 1990

Bengesser G, Sokoloff S: After suicide-postvention. Eur J Psychiatry 3:116–118, 1989

Brent DA, Perper J, Moritz G, et al: Bereavement or depression? The impact of the loss of a friend to suicide. J Am Acad Child Adolesc Psychiatry 32:1189–1197, 1993

Brent DA, Perper JA, Moritz G, et al: Psychiatric risk factors for adolescent suicide victims: a case-control study. J Am Acad Child Adolesc Psychiatry 32:521–529, 1993

Brent DA, Moritz G, Bridge J, et al: The impact of adolescent suicide on siblings and parents: a longitudinal follow-up. Suicide Life Threat Behav 26:253–259, 1996

Callaghan J: Predictors and correlates of bereavement in suicide support group participants. Suicide Life Threat Behavior 30:104–124, 2000

Campbell FR: Suicide: an American form of family abuse. New Global Development 16:88–93, 2000

Campbell FR: Changing the legacy of suicide through an active model of postvention. Proceedings of the Irish Association of Suicidology 6:26–29, 2001

Campbell FR: Living and working in the canyon of why. Proceedings of Irish Association of Suicidology 6:96–97, 2001

Campbell FR, Cataldie L: Survivor support teams. Paper presented at the Survivors of Suicide Research Workshop Program, National Institute of Mental Health/National Institutes of Health Office of Rare Diseases and the American Foundation for Suicide Prevention, Bethesda, MD, May 2003

Dunne EJ, McIntosh JL, Dunne-Maxim K (eds): Suicide and Its Aftermath: Understanding and Counseling the Survivors. New York, WW Norton, 1987

Dyregrov K: Assistance from local authorities versus survivors' needs for support after suicide. Death Stud 26:647–668, 2002

Farberow NL, Gallagher-Thompson D, Gilewski M, et al: The role of social supports in the bereavement process of surviving spouses of suicide and natural deaths. Suicide Life Threat Behav 22:107–124, 1992

Goldsmith SK, Pellmar TC, Kleinman AM, et al (eds): Reducing Suicide: A National Imperative. Washington, DC, National Academies Press, 2002

Hendin H: Suicide in America, New and Expanded Edition. New York, WW Norton, 1995

Jordan JR: Is suicide bereavement different? A reassessment of the literature. Suicide Life Threat Behav 31:91–102, 2001

Jordan JR, McMenamy J: Interventions for suicide survivors: a review of the literature. Suicide Life Threat Behav 34:337–349, 2004

Knight KH, Elfenbein MH, Messina-Soares JA: College students' perceptions of helpful responses to bereaved persons: effects of sex of bereaved persons and cause of death. Psychol Rep 83:627–636, 1998

Leenaars AA, Wenckstern S: Principles of postvention: applications to suicide and trauma in schools. Death Stud 22:357–391, 1998

Maltsberger JT, Hendin H, Haas A, et al: Determination of precipitating events in the suicide of psychiatric patients. Suicide Life Threat Behav 33:111–119, 2003

Maris RW, Berman AL, Silverman MM: Comprehensive Textbook of Suicidology. New York, Guilford, 2000

Myers MF, Fine C: Touched by Suicide: Hope and Healing After Loss. New York, Gotham Books, 2006

Ness DE, Pfeffer CR: Sequelae of bereavement resulting from suicide. Am J Psychiatry 147:279–285, 1990

Pfeffer CR, Karus D, Siegel K, et al: Child survivors of parental death from cancer or suicide: depressive and behavioral outcomes. Psychooncology 9:1–10, 2000

Prigerson HG: Suicidal ideation among survivors of suicide. Paper presented at the Survivors of Suicide Research Workshop Program, National Institute of Mental Health/National Institutes of Health Office of Rare Diseases and the American Foundation for Suicide Prevention, Bethesda, MD, May 2003

Prigerson H, Jacobs S: Traumatic grief as a distinct disorder: a rationale, consensus, criteria, and a preliminary empirical test, in Handbook of Bereavement Research: Consequences, Coping and Care. Edited by Stroebe MS, Hansson RO, Stroebe W, et al. Washington, DC, American Psychological Association, 2001, pp 613–647

Provini C, Everett JR, Pfeffer C: Adults mourning suicide: self-reported concerns about bereavement, needs for assistance, and help-seeking behavior. Death Stud 24:1–20, 2000

Range LM: When a loss is due to suicide: unique aspects of bereavement, in Perspectives on Loss: A Sourcebook. Edited by Harvey JH. Philadelphia, PA, Brunner/Mazel, 1998, pp 213–220

Runeson B, Åsberg M: Family history of suicide among suicide victims. Am J Psychiatry 160:1525–1526, 2003

Saarinen P, Irmeli H, Hintikka J, et al: Psychological symptoms of close relatives of suicide victims. Eur J Psychiatry 13:33–39, 1999

Shneidman ES (ed): On the Nature of Suicide. San Francisco, CA, Jossey-Bass, 1969

Shneidman ES: Deaths of Man. New York, Quadrangle Books, 1981

Shneidman ES: The Suicidal Mind. New York, Oxford University Press, 1996

Stephens BJ: Suicidal women and their relationships with husbands, boyfriends, and lovers. Suicide Life Threat Behav 15:77–89, 1985

Suicide Prevention Resource Center: Featured resources: prevention support. Available at: http://www.sprc.org/featured_resources/ps/index.asp. Accessed June 22, 2011.

U.S. Department of Health and Human Services: The Surgeon General's call to action to prevent suicide, 1999. Available at: http://www.surgeongeneral.gov/library/calltoaction/. Accessed June 22, 2011.

U.S. Department of Health and Human Services: National Strategy for Suicide Prevention, 2001. Available at: http://www.sprc.org/library/nssp.pdf. Accessed June 22, 2011.

World Health Organization: The World Health Report 2001. Mental Health: New Understanding, New Hope. Geneva, Switzerland, World Health Organization, 2001

Zisook S, Chentsova-Dutton Y, Shuchter SR: PTSD following bereavement. Ann Clin Psychiatry 10:157–163, 1998

References

American Psychiatric Association: Practice guideline for the assessment and treatment of patients with suicidal behaviors. Am J Psychiatry 160(suppl):1–60, 2003

Cain AC (ed): Survivors of Suicide. Springfield, IL, Charles C Thomas, 1972

Campbell FR: Changing the legacy of suicide. Suicide Life Threat Behav 27:329–338, 1997

Campbell FR: Changing the legacy of suicide through an active model of postvention. Proceedings of the Irish Association of Suicidology 6:26–29, 2001

Campbell FR: Baton Rouge Crisis Intervention Center's LOSS Team Active Postvention Model approach, in Grief After Suicide: Understanding the Consequences and Caring for the Survivors. Edited by Jordan JR, McIntosh JL. New York, Routledge, 2011, pp 327–332

Campbell FR, Cataldie L, McIntosh J, et al: An active postvention program. Crisis 25:30–32, 2004

Fine C: No Time to Say Goodbye: Surviving the Suicide of a Loved One. New York, Doubleday, 1997

Grad OT, Zavasnik A, Groleger U: Suicide of a patient: gender differences in bereavement reactions of therapists. Suicide Life Threat Behav 27:379–386, 1997

Linn-Gust M, Cerel J: Seeking Hope: Stories of the Suicide Bereaved. Albuquerque, NM, Chellehead Works, 2011

Peterson EM, Luoma JB, Dunne ED: Suicide survivors' perceptions of the treating clinician. Suicide Life Threat Behav 32:158–166, 2002

Shneidman ES: On the Nature of Suicide. San Francisco, CA, Jossey-Bass, 1969

Shneidman ES: Foreword, in Survivors of Suicide. Edited by Cain AC. Springfield, IL, Charles C Thomas, 1972, pp ix–xi

APPENDIX 1

Case Scenario Questions for Self-Study

Robert I. Simon, M.D.

The assessment, management, and treatment of the patient at risk for suicide is a core competency requirement for clinicians. This case-based multiple-choice self-test is a teaching instrument designed to enhance the clinician's suicide assessment and management of patients at risk for suicide. The 15 questions and accompanying commentaries in the Answer Guide are derived from the referenced sources.

Suicide risk assessment and management are complex, difficult, and challenging tasks, raising clinical issues that do not have clear-cut or easy answers. Thus, the test taker is asked to choose the "best response" for each question, rather than the customary but more restrictive "correct answer." Scoring is by and for the test taker.

Question 1

A psychiatrist is conducting an initial outpatient psychiatric evaluation of a 34-year-old professional basketball player who complains of weight loss, early-morning awakening, and dysphoric mood of 1 month's duration. The patient's performance on the basketball court has declined. His wife is seeking a separation. The patient describes "fleeting" suicidal thoughts. There is no history of suicide attempts or depression. The patient does not abuse alcohol or drugs. The initial assessment approach would be to

A. Obtain a suicide prevention contract.
B. Assess suicide risk and protective factors.
C. Determine the cause of the depression.
D. Have the patient complete a self-report suicide risk assessment form.
E. Contact the patient's wife for additional history.

References

American Psychiatric Association: Practice guideline for the assessment and treatment of patients with suicidal behaviors. Am J Psychiatry 160 (suppl 11):1–60, 2003

Resnick PJ: Recognizing that the suicidal patient views you as an adversary. Curr Psychiatr 1:8, 2002

Simon RI: Suicide risk assessment forms: form over substance? J Am Acad Psychiatry Law 37:290–293, 2009

Simon RI: Preventing Patient Suicide: Clinical Assessment and Management. Washington, DC, American Psychiatric Publishing, 2011

Stanford EJ, Goetz RR, Bloom JD: The No Harm Contract in the emergency assessment of suicidal risk. J Clin Psychiatry 55:344–348, 1994

Question 2

A 56-year-old single schoolteacher is admitted to a psychiatric unit for severe depression and suicidal ideation without a plan. She attends church regularly and is devoutly religious, stating, "I won't kill myself; I don't want to go to Hell." The patient has a history of chronic recurrent depression with suicidal ideation. There is no history of suicide attempts. A diagnosis of bipolar II disorder is suspected. In assessing religious affiliation as a protective factor against suicide, the psychiatrist should consider which of the following?

A. Nature of patient's religious conviction.
B. Espoused religion's position on suicide.
C. Severity of patient's illness.
D. Presence of delusional religious beliefs.
E. All of the above.

Reference

Dervic K, Oquendo MA, Grunebaum MF, et al: Religious affiliation and suicide attempt. Am J Psychiatry 161:2303–2308, 2004

Question 3

An 18-year-old male is admitted to an inpatient psychiatric unit with severe agitation, thought disorder, disorganized speech, and auditory hallucinations. The patient was threatening to jump from a nearby building. There is no history of substance abuse. The psychiatrist conducts a comprehensive suicide risk assessment that includes the patient's psychiatric diagnosis as a risk factor. Which of the following psychiatric diagnoses is associated with the highest suicide mortality rate?

A. Schizophrenia.
B. Eating disorders.
C. Bipolar disorder.
D. Major depressive disorder.
E. Borderline personality disorder.

Reference

Harris CE, Barraclough B: Suicide as an outcome for mental disorders. A meta-analysis. Br J Psychiatry 170:205–228, 1997

Question 4

A 64-year-old recently divorced lawyer is admitted to the psychiatric unit from the emergency room. Colleagues brought the patient to the emergency room because he had made suicide threats. On the unit, the patient denies suicidal ideation, planning, or intent. Agitation and suspiciousness are prominent. He refuses authorization for staff to contact his colleagues, his ex-wife, or other family members, including phone contact for the psychiatrist to just listen. The patient also forbids contact with his outpatient therapist. The patient demands immediate discharge. As a conditional voluntary admission, he is placed on 72-hour hold. The psychiatrist should

A. Contact family members, as an emergency exception to confidentiality.
B. E-mail family members with questions.
C. Contact the patient's therapist, as permitted by the Health Insurance Porta-

bility and Accountability Act of 1996 (HIPAA).

D. Try to develop a therapeutic alliance with the patient.

E. None of the above.

References

American Psychiatric Association: The Principles of Medical Ethics With Annotations Especially Applicable to Psychiatry. Section 4, Annotation 8. Washington, DC, American Psychiatric Association, 2009

Health Insurance Portability and Accountability Act of 1996 (HIPAA). Pub. L. 104-191, 110 Stat. 1936; enacted August 21, 1996

Simon RI, Shuman DW: Clinical Manual of Psychiatry and Law. Washington, DC, American Psychiatric Publishing, 2007

Question 5

A 42-year-old engineer is rehospitalized after a failed attempt to hang himself. Initially, the patient is profoundly depressed, but he improves suddenly and requests discharge. The psychiatrist and clinical staff are perplexed. Is the sudden improvement real or feigned? Useful options for the treatment team to consider in evaluating this question include all of the following except

A. Obtain records of prior hospitalizations.

B. Check collateral sources of information.

C. Assess the patient's compliance with treatment.

D. Obtain psychological testing to determine the patient's veracity.

E. Determine whether behavioral indications of depression are present.

Reference

Simon RI, Gutheil TG: Sudden improvement in high-risk suicidal patients: should it be trusted? Psychiatr Serv 60:387–389, 2009

Question 6

In midwinter, a 46-year-old homeless woman presents to the emergency room of a general hospital reporting depression and auditory hallucinations commanding suicide. She has had five previous admissions to the psychiatry unit with similar complaints. The psychiatrist conducts a comprehensive suicide risk assessment in which acute and chronic risk factors for suicide are identified and protective factors are considered. The psychiatrist analyzes (weighs) and synthesizes the risk and protective factors into an overall assessment of suicide risk. The main purpose of suicide risk assessment is to

A. Predict the likelihood of suicide.

B. Determine imminence of suicide.

C. Inform patient treatment and safety management.

D. Identify malingered suicide.

E. Provide a legal defense against a malpractice claim.

References

American Psychiatric Association: Practice guideline for the assessment and treatment of patients with suicidal behaviors. Am J Psychiatry 160 (suppl 11):1–60, 2003

Pokorny AD: Predictions of suicide in psychiatric patients: report of a prospective study. Arch Gen Psychiatry 4:249–257, 1983

Simon RI: Imminent suicide: the illusion of short-term prediction. Suicide Life Threat Behav 36:296–301, 2006

Simon RI, Shuman DW: Therapeutic risk management of clinical-legal dilemmas: should it be a core competency? J Am Acad Psychiatry Law 37:155–161, 2009

Question 7

A 40-year-old computer analyst is being treated by a psychiatrist in once-a-week psychotherapy with medication management for the recent onset of panic and depression symptoms that began after the breakup of a romantic relationship. A therapeutic alliance develops with the psychiatrist. The psychiatrist performs a systematic suicide risk assessment to evaluate the level of suicide risk and the possibility that hospitalization may be necessary. Overall suicide risk is determined by the assessment of individual risk and protective factors. The patient admits using alcohol to sleep. He reports occasional suicidal ideation but no plan. He states that he finds the idea of suicide to be morally repugnant. The patient has continued to pursue his interests and to participate in civil causes. Evidence-based factors considered protective against suicide include all of the following except

A. Presence of a therapeutic alliance.
B. Strong survival and coping beliefs.
C. Responsibility to family.
D. Fear of suicide.
E. Moral objections to suicide.

References

Linehan MM, Goodstein JL, Nielsen SL, et al: Reasons for staying alive when you are thinking of killing yourself: the Reasons for Living Inventory. J Consult Clin Psychol 51:276–286, 1983

Malone KM, Oquendo MA, Haas GL, et al: Protective factors against suicidal acts in major depression. Am J Psychiatry 157:1084–1088, 2000

Question 8

A 28-year-old mother of a newborn child is admitted to the psychiatric unit after expressing suicidal thoughts to her husband. Although there is no history of suicide attempts, the patient previously was hospitalized following a hypomanic episode and severe depression. A diagnosis of bipolar II disorder (recurrent major depressive episodes with hypomanic episodes) is made. The patient's maternal aunt has bipolar disorder, and her paternal grandfather died by suicide. The psychiatrist conducts a systematic suicide risk assessment and determines the patient to be at high suicide risk. He prescribes a psychotropic drug that has been shown to reduce suicide and suicide attempts in bipolar II patients. This drug is

A. Clozapine.
B. Clonazepam.
C. Lorazepam.
D. Lithium.
E. Quetiapine.

Reference

Baldessarini RJ, Pompili M, Tondo L: Bipolar disorder, in The American Psychiatric Publishing Textbook of Suicide Assessment and Management. Edited by Simon RI, Hales RE. Washington, DC, American Psychiatric Publishing, 2006, pp 277–299

Question 9

A 60-year-old patient is admitted to a psychiatric unit after an overdose suicide attempt. The patient became depressed after the loss of his business and was "treating" his depression and anxiety with alcohol. In the unit, the patient is successfully withdrawn from alcohol and responds to medication and support. The patient is much improved and eager to go home. However, during a family meeting with staff, the patient's wife states that he keeps a gun by his bedside. Before discharging the patient, the psychiatrist or staff should

A. Instruct the patient to remove the gun from the house.

B. Instruct the wife to remove the gun from the home.

C. Instruct the wife to search the house in case there is more than one gun.

D. Instruct the wife to call the staff once guns and ammunition are safely removed according to a prearranged safety plan.

E. Instruct the wife to lock up the gun in a place unknown to the patient.

Reference

Simon RI: Gun safety management with patients at risk for suicide. Suicide Life Threat Behav 37:518–526, 2007

Question 10

A recently admitted 58-year-old inpatient is discovered wrapping a towel around her neck. The psychiatrist is notified. The patient denies suicidal intent; however, the treatment team views the incident as a suicide rehearsal. The patient is placed on one-to-one close observation. Inpatient suicides most frequently occur

A. Shortly after admission.

B. During staff shift changes.

C. At mealtimes.

D. Shortly after discharge.

E. All of the above.

References

Appleby L, Shaw J, Amos T, et al: Suicide within 12 months of contact with mental health services: national clinical survey. BMJ 318:1235–1239, 1999

Meehan J, Kapur N, Hunt I, et al: Suicide in mental health in-patients and within 3 months of discharge: national clinical survey. Br J Psychiatry 188:129–134, 2006

Qin P, Nordentoft M: Suicide risk in relation to psychiatric hospitalization: evidence based on longitudinal registers. Arch Gen Psychiatry 62:427–432, 2005

Question 11

A 44-year-old single woman in acute suicidal crisis is admitted to the psychiatric unit of a general hospital. She is diagnosed with bipolar I disorder, most recent episode depressed, and borderline personality disorder. The patient has a history of multiple psychiatric hospitalizations, all precipitated by a suicidal crisis. The average length of stay on the psychiatric unit is 6.3 days. After 7 days of intensive treatment, the patient is stabilized. Suicide risk is reduced, and the treatment team prepares for the patient's discharge. The patient's suicide risk at discharge is most likely

A. Indeterminate.

B. Low.

C. Moderate.

D. Chronic high.

E. Acute high.

Reference

Qin P, Nordentoft M: Suicide risk in relation to psychiatric hospitalization: evidence based on longitudinal registers. Arch Gen Psychiatry 62:427–432, 2005

Simon RI: Preventing Patient Suicide: Clinical Assessment and Management. Washington, DC, American Psychiatric Publishing, 2011

Question 12

A 20-year-old college student is hospitalized following an overdose suicide attempt. Failing grades, panic attacks, and depression precipitated the suicide attempt. After 8 days of hospitalization, the young woman is much improved and ready for discharge. The patient is assessed as being at low to moderate risk for suicide. A family meeting is convened by the treating psychiatrist and the social worker. Both of the patient's parents and her older brother are present. The role of the family following discharge is discussed. Helpful family roles after the patient's discharge include all of the following except

A. Provide continuous 24-hour family supervision.
B. Provide emotional support.
C. Observe and report symptoms and behaviors of concern.
D. Encourage adherence to treatment.
E. Provide helpful feedback about the patient's thoughts and behavior.

Reference

Simon RI: Preventing Patient Suicide: Clinical Assessment and Management. Washington, DC, American Psychiatric Publishing, 2011

Question 13

During the initial evaluation of patients, psychiatrists routinely inquire about current and past suicidal ideation. An affirmative answer prompts a systematic suicide risk assessment. Even in the absence of current risk, a psychiatrist should conduct a systematic suicide risk assessment if exploration of a patient's history reveals the presence of chronic suicide risk factors. Which of the following chronic risk factors has the highest association with suicide?

A. Family history of mental illness or suicide.
B. Childhood abuse.
C. Prior suicide attempt.
D. Impulsivity/aggression.
E. Prior psychiatric hospitalization.

References

Harris CE, Barraclough B: Suicide as an outcome for mental disorders: a meta-analysis. Br J Psychiatry 170:205–228, 1997
Simon RI: Preventing Patient Suicide: Clinical Assessment and Management. Washington, DC, American Psychiatric Publishing, 2011

Question 14

A psychiatrist is treating a 38-year-old physician for anxiety and depression. The psychiatrist sees the patient twice a week for psychotherapy and medication management. A recent lawsuit filed against the physician has severely exacerbated her symptoms. The patient is able to sleep only a few hours each night. Suicidal ideation has emerged, alarming the patient and her family. The psychiatrist performs a systematic suicide risk assessment and determines that the patient is at acute high risk for suicide. The psychiatrist recommends immediate hospitalization. The patient adamantly refuses. The psychiatrist decides not to involuntarily hospitalize the patient because she does not meet the substantive criteria of the state's involuntary commitment statute (e.g., overt suicidal behaviors). Instead, he chooses to continue outpatient treatment. Which of the following clinical interventions can help reduce the patient's suicide risk?

A. See the patient more frequently.
B. Adjust medications.
C. Obtain a psychiatric consultation.
D. Refer the patient to an adjunctive, intensive outpatient program.
E. All of the above.

References

Simon RI: Preventing Patient Suicide: Clinical Assessment and Management. Washington, DC, American Psychiatric Publishing, 2011

Simon RI, Shuman DW: Clinical Manual of Psychiatry and Law. Washington, DC, American Psychiatric Publishing, 2007

Question 15

A 52-year-old married CEO is admitted to an inpatient unit because of acute alcohol intoxication and suicidal threats. The patient has had two similar episodes within the past year. After the patient undergoes successful detoxification, the psychiatrist and treatment team conduct a risk-benefit analysis for both discharge and continued hospitalization. A psychiatric consultation is also obtained. Which of the following factors should carry the most weight in the discharge decision?

A. Presence of family support.

B. Compliance with follow-up care.

C. Availability of dual-diagnosis programs.

D. Results of a systematic suicide risk assessment.

E. Psychiatric consultation.

References

Appleby L, Dennehy JA, Thomas CS, et al: Aftercare and clinical characteristics of people with mental illness who commit suicide: a case-control study. Lancet 353:1397–1400, 1999

Meehan J, Kapur N, Hunt I, et al: Suicide in mental health in-patients and within 3 months of discharge: national clinical survey. Br J Psychiatry 188:129–134, 2006

A P P E N D I X   2

Answer Guide to Case Scenario Questions for Self-Study

Robert I. Simon, M.D.

Question 1

A psychiatrist is conducting an initial outpatient psychiatric evaluation of a 34-year-old professional basketball player who complains of weight loss, early-morning awakening, and dysphoric mood of 1 month's duration. The patient's performance on the basketball court has declined. His wife is seeking a separation. The patient describes "fleeting" suicidal thoughts. There is no history of suicide attempts or depression. The patient does not abuse alcohol or drugs. The initial assessment approach would be to

A. Obtain a suicide prevention contract.
B. Assess suicide risk and protective factors.
C. Determine the cause of the depression.
D. Have the patient complete a self-report suicide risk assessment form.
E. Contact the patient's wife for additional history.

Best response is B. Suicide prevention contracts do not prevent suicide (Stanford

et al. 1994). Contacting the patient's wife may be an option at a later stage of the evaluation or treatment, if the patient grants permission. Determining the cause of the depression will likely require ongoing assessment. Assessing suicide risk factors without also assessing protective factors is a common error. A comprehensive suicide risk assessment requires that both risk and protective factors be examined (American Psychiatric Association 2003; Simon 2011). Suicide risk assessment forms frequently omit assessment of protective factors (Simon 2009). Self-report suicide risk assessment forms should not be used because of their reliance on the patient's truthfulness. Patients who are determined to die by suicide regard the psychiatrist as the enemy (Resnick 2002).

References

American Psychiatric Association: Practice guideline for the assessment and treatment of patients with suicidal behaviors. Am J Psychiatry 160 (suppl 11):1–60, 2003

Resnick PJ: Recognizing that the suicidal patient views you as an adversary. Curr Psychiatr 1:8, 2002

Simon RI: Suicide risk assessment forms: form over substance? J Am Acad Psychiatry Law 37:290–293, 2009

Simon RI: Preventing Patient Suicide: Clinical Assessment and Management. Washington, DC, American Psychiatric Publishing, 2011

Stanford EJ, Goetz RR, Bloom JD: The No Harm Contract in the emergency assessment of suicidal risk. J Clin Psychiatry 55:344–348, 1994

Question 2

A 56-year-old single schoolteacher is admitted to a psychiatric unit for severe depression and suicidal ideation without a plan. She attends church regularly and is devoutly religious, stating, "I won't kill myself; I don't want to go to Hell." The patient has a history of chronic recurrent depression with suicidal ideation. There is no history of suicide attempts. A diagnosis of bipolar II disorder is suspected. In assessing religious affiliation as a protective factor against suicide, the psychiatrist should consider which of the following?

A. Nature of patient's religious conviction.
B. Espoused religion's position on suicide.
C. Severity of patient's illness.
D. Presence of delusional religious beliefs.
E. All of the above.

Best response is E. Dervic et al. (2004) evaluated 371 depressed inpatients according to their religious or nonreligious affiliation. Patients who had no religious affiliation made significantly more suicide attempts, had more first-degree relatives who had died by suicide, were younger, were less frequently married, less often had children, and had fewer contacts with family members.

Religious affiliation is a general protective factor but may not be a protective factor in an individual patient. Religious affiliation, like other presumed general protective factors, requires further scrutiny. Assumptions must be avoided. For example, a depressed, devoutly religious patient cursed God for abandoning her. A bipolar patient believed that God would forgive her for committing suicide. A presumed protective factor may not be protective or might even be a risk factor. Psychotic patients with religious delusions are an example.

The Abrahamic religions (i.e., Judaism, Christianity, and Islam) prohibit suicide. Severe mental illness, however, can overcome the strongest religious forbiddance against suicide, including the fear of eternal damnation. For many psychiatric patients, religious affiliations and beliefs are protective factors against suicide, but only relatively. No protective factor against suicide, however strong, provides absolute protection against suicide. Moreover, other risk and protective factors must also be comprehensively assessed.

Reference

Dervic K, Oquendo MA, Grunebaum MF, et al: Religious affiliation and suicide attempt. Am J Psychiatry 161:2303–2308, 2004

Question 3

An 18-year-old male is admitted to an inpatient psychiatric unit with severe agitation, thought disorder, disorganized speech, and auditory hallucinations. The patient was threatening to jump from a nearby building. There is no history of substance abuse. The psychiatrist conducts a comprehensive suicide risk assessment that includes the patient's psychiatric diagnosis as a risk factor. Which of the following psychiatric diagnoses is associated with the highest suicide mortality rate?

A. Schizophrenia.
B. Eating disorders.
C. Bipolar disorder.
D. Major depressive disorder.
E. Borderline personality disorder.

Best response is B. The patient's psychiatric diagnosis is an important risk factor that should be considered in a comprehensive suicide risk assessment. Harris and Barraclough (1997) conducted a meta-analysis of 249 separate studies, from which they estimated the standardized mortality ratios (SMRs) for death by suicide associated with common mental disorders. (SMRs are calculated by dividing observed mortality by expected mortality in the general population.) Although nearly all of the disorders (exceptions were mental retardation and dementia) were associated with an increased degree of suicide risk, the highest SMRs were found for eating disorders. Depression and demoralization frequently accompany this group of disorders.

Reference

Harris CE, Barraclough B: Suicide as an outcome for mental disorders: a meta-analysis. Br J Psychiatry 170:205–228, 1997

Question 4

A 64-year-old recently divorced lawyer is admitted to the psychiatric unit from the emergency room. Colleagues brought the patient to the emergency room because he had made suicide threats. On the unit, the patient denies suicidal ideation, planning, or intent. Agitation and suspiciousness are prominent. He refuses authorization for staff to contact his colleagues, his ex-wife, or other family members, including phone contact for the psychiatrist to just listen. The patient also forbids contact with his outpatient therapist. The patient demands immediate discharge. As a conditional voluntary admission, he is placed on 72-hour hold. The psychiatrist should

A. Contact family members, as an emergency exception to confidentiality.
B. E-mail family members with questions.
C. Contact the patient's therapist, as permitted by the Health Insurance Portability and Accountability Act of 1996 (HIPAA).
D. Try to develop a therapeutic alliance with the patient.
E. None of the above.

Best response is C. The Health Insurance Portability and Accountability Act of 1996 (HIPAA) permits a psychiatrist and other "health care providers" who are treating the same patient to communicate without the expressed permission of the patient (45 Code of Federal Regulations § 164.502). This is the most expeditious and productive way of obtaining essential clinical information.

E-mail merely changes the mode of unauthorized communication with significant others. The patient is agitated and suspicious; developing a therapeutic alliance with such a patient would require time. It is necessary to gather information about the patient's psychiatric status as soon as possible. An emergency exception to maintaining confidentiality is another option (Simon and Shuman 2007). The definition of emergency varies among jurisdictions. Consultation with a knowledgeable attorney may be necessary, but such advisement usually takes time. Ethically, it is permissible to breach confidentiality to protect the suicidal patient (American Psychiatric Association 2001).

References

American Psychiatric Association: The Principles of Medical Ethics With Annotations Especially Applicable to Psychiatry. Section 4, Annotation 8. Arlington, VA, American Psychiatric Association, 2009

Health Insurance Portability and Accountability Act of 1996 (HIPAA). Pub. L. 104-191, 110 Stat. 1936; enacted August 21, 1996

Simon RI, Shuman DW: Clinical Manual of Psychiatry and Law. Washington, DC, American Psychiatric Publishing, 2007

Question 5

A 42-year-old engineer is rehospitalized after a failed attempt to hang himself. Initially, the patient is profoundly depressed, but he improves suddenly and requests discharge. The psychiatrist and clinical staff are perplexed. Is the sudden improvement real or feigned? Useful options for the treatment team to consider in evaluating this question include all of the following except

A. Obtain records of prior hospitalizations.
B. Check collateral sources of information.
C. Assess the patient's compliance with treatment.
D. Obtain psychological testing to determine the patient's veracity.
E. Determine whether behavioral indications of depression are present.

Best response is D.   Short lengths of hospital stay and expectations of progress make it difficult to assess sudden patient improvement (Simon and Gutheil 2009).

Real improvement of a high-risk suicidal patient is a *process,* even when it occurs quickly. Feigned improvement is an *event.* Obtaining patient information from collateral sources is crucial. Sudden improvement can be the result of the patient's resolve to complete suicide. Identifying a mosaic of clinical factors and patient behaviors is necessary. A single factor, such as treatment adherence, can indicate either real patient improvement or an attempt to gain rapid discharge. Behavioral risk factors associated with psychiatric disorders inform the clinician's systematic suicide risk assessment of the guarded or dissimulating patient. Psychological testing will take time and should not be a substitute for careful clinical assessment.

Reference

Simon RI, Gutheil TG: Sudden improvement in high-risk suicidal patients: should it be trusted? Psychiatr Serv 60:387–389, 2009

Question 6

In midwinter, a 46-year-old homeless woman presents to the emergency room of a general hospital reporting depression and auditory hallucinations commanding suicide. She has had five previous admissions to the psychiatry unit with similar complaints. The psychiatrist conducts a comprehensive suicide risk assessment in which acute and chronic risk factors for suicide are identified and protective factors are considered. The psychiatrist analyzes (weighs) and synthesizes the risk and protective factors into an overall assessment of suicide risk. The main purpose of suicide risk assessment is to

A. Predict the likelihood of suicide.
B. Determine imminence of suicide.

C. Inform patient treatment and safety management.
D. Identify malingered suicide.
E. Provide a legal defense against a malpractice claim.

Best response is C. Suicide cannot be predicted (Pokorny 1983). The idea that suicide imminence can be determined implies the foreseeability of an inherently unpredictable act (Simon 2006). The process of comprehensive or systematic suicide risk assessment encompasses identification, analysis, and synthesis of risk and protective factors that inform the treatment and safety management of the patient (American Psychiatric Association 2003). The overall suicide assessment is an exercise in clinical judgment that estimates risk along a continuum of low to high. In the above case example, a comprehensive suicide risk assessment will assist the clinician in determining the patient's overall level of suicide risk and making an appropriate disposition. Without the guidance provided by a systematic suicide risk assessment methodology, the clinician has little choice but to robotically admit every patient who presents with self-reported suicidal symptoms, including the pejoratively labeled "frequent flyer" who is seeking sustenance and lodging.

Although protection from clinician liability is not the main purpose of the suicide risk assessment, a systematic and comprehensive assessment can help provide a sound legal defense if a suicide malpractice claim alleging negligent assessment is filed against the clinician (Simon and Shuman 2009).

References

American Psychiatric Association: Practice guideline for the assessment and treatment of patients with suicidal behaviors. Am J Psychiatry 160 (suppl 11):1–60, 2003

Pokorny AD: Predictions of suicide in psychiatric patients: report of a prospective study. Arch Gen Psychiatry 4:249–257, 1983

Simon RI: Imminent suicide: the illusion of short-term prediction. Suicide Life Threat Behav 36:296–301, 2006

Simon RI, Shuman DW: Therapeutic risk management of clinical-legal dilemmas: should it be a core competency? J Am Acad Psychiatry Law 37:155–161, 2009

Question 7

A 40-year-old computer analyst is being treated by a psychiatrist in once-a-week psychotherapy with medication management for the recent onset of panic and depression symptoms that began after the breakup of a romantic relationship. A therapeutic alliance develops with the psychiatrist. The psychiatrist performs a systematic suicide risk assessment to evaluate the level of suicide risk and the possibility that hospitalization may be necessary. Overall suicide risk is determined by the assessment of individual risk and protective factors . The patient admits using alcohol to sleep. He reports occasional suicidal ideation but no plan. He states that he finds the idea of suicide to be morally repugnant. The patient has continued to pursue his interests and to participate in civil causes. Evidence-based factors considered protective against suicide include all of the following except

A. Presence of a therapeutic alliance.
B. Strong survival and coping beliefs.
C. Responsibility to family.
D. Fear of suicide.
E. Moral objections to suicide.

Best response is A. Although clinical consensus holds that the therapeutic alliance is an important protective factor against suicide, no evidence-based research supports or refutes this widely held belief among clinicians.

Linehan et al. (1983) developed the Reasons for Living Inventory, a self-report instrument that evaluates six facets of life-affirming values: 1) survival and coping beliefs, 2) responsibility to family, 3) child-related concerns, 4) fear of suicide, 5) fear of social disapproval, and 6) moral objections to suicide. They found that survival and coping beliefs, responsibility to family, and child-related concerns were the most useful factors in differentiating between suicidal and nonsuicidal groups.

Malone et al. (2000) administered the Reasons for Living Inventory to 84 inpatients with major depression, 45 of whom had attempted suicide. The depressed patients who had not attempted suicide demonstrated a stronger sense of responsibility toward family, greater fear of social disapproval, stronger moral objections to suicide, greater survival and coping skills, and greater fear of suicide than did the patients who attempted suicide. Malone and colleagues recommended that the Reasons for Living Inventory be included as part of the standard assessment of patients at risk for suicide.

References

Linehan MM, Goodstein JL, Nielsen SL, et al: Reasons for staying alive when you are thinking of killing yourself: the Reasons for Living Inventory. J Consult Clin Psychol 51:276–286, 1983

Malone KM, Oquendo MA, Haas GL, et al: Protective factors against suicidal acts in major depression. Am J Psychiatry 157:1084–1088, 2000

Question 8

A 28-year-old mother of a newborn child is admitted to the psychiatric unit after expressing suicidal thoughts to her husband. Although there is no history of suicide attempts, the patient previously was hospitalized following a hypomanic episode and severe depression. A diagnosis of bipolar II disorder (recurrent major depressive episodes with hypomanic episodes) is made. The patient's maternal aunt has bipolar disorder, and her paternal grandfather died by suicide. The psychiatrist conducts a systematic suicide risk assessment and determines the patient to be at high suicide risk. He prescribes a psychotropic drug that has been shown to reduce suicide and suicide attempts in bipolar II patients. This drug is

A. Clozapine.
B. Clonazepam.
C. Lorazepam.
D. Lithium.
E. Quetiapine.

Best response is D. Prospective, randomized controlled trials consistently have found lower rates of suicide and suicide attempts during lithium maintenance treatment among patients with bipolar disorder and other major affective disorders (Baldessarini et al. 2006).

Reference

Baldessarini RJ, Pompili M, Tondo L: Bipolar disorder, in The American Psychiatric Publishing Textbook of Suicide Assessment and Management, 2nd Edition. Edited by Simon RI, Hales RE. Washington, DC, American Psychiatric Publishing, 2012, pp 159–176

Question 9

A 60-year-old patient is admitted to a psychiatric unit after an overdose suicide attempt. The patient became depressed after the loss of his business and was "treating" his depression and anxiety with alcohol. In the unit, the patient is successfully withdrawn from alcohol and responds to medication and support. The patient is much improved and eager to go home. However, during a family meeting with staff, the patient's wife states that he keeps a gun by his bedside. Before discharging the patient, the psychiatrist or staff should

A. Instruct the patient to remove the gun from the house.
B. Instruct the wife to remove the gun from the home.
C. Instruct the wife to search the house in case there is more than one gun.
D. Instruct the wife to call the staff once guns and ammunition are safely removed according to a prearranged safety plan.
E. Instruct the wife to lock up the gun in a place unknown to the patient.

Best response is D. Guns in the home are associated with a significant increase in suicide. All patients at risk for suicide must be asked whether guns are available at home or easily accessible elsewhere, or whether they intend to purchase a gun (Simon 2007). Gun safety management requires a collaborative team approach that includes the clinician, the patient, and a designated person responsible for removing guns from the home or elsewhere. A callback to the clinician from the designated person is required, confirming that the gun or guns have been removed and secured according to plan. These principles of gun safety management

apply to outpatients, inpatients, and emergency patients, although their implementation varies according to the clinical setting.

Asking a patient to remove guns from the home is too risky. Guns must be safely secured before the patient is discharged. Enlisting the help of a spouse, another family member, or a partner is necessary. The person designated to help must be willing to remove the guns and ammunition according to a prearranged plan requiring a callback upon completion. A callback is essential because denial may lead to doing nothing to remove the gun(s) or to merely locking up or "hiding" them in the house where they can be found by a determined suicidal patient. Guns also may be available outside the home (e.g., car, office) or may be purchased.

The essence of gun safety management is verification. Trust but verify—or, better yet, verify, then trust.

Reference

Simon RI: Gun safety management with patients at risk for suicide. Suicide Life Threat Behav 37:518–526, 2007

Question 10

A recently admitted 58-year-old inpatient is discovered wrapping a towel around her neck. The psychiatrist is notified. The patient denies suicidal intent; however, the treatment team views the incident as a suicide rehearsal. The patient is placed on one-to-one close observation. Inpatient suicides most frequently occur

A. Shortly after admission.
B. During staff shift changes.
C. At mealtimes.
D. Shortly after discharge.
E. All of the above.

Best response is E. Inpatient suicides also occur at increased frequency at times of staff rotation (especially of psychiatric residents) and in understaffed psychiatric units (Qin and Nordentoft 2005). Undue delay in the evaluation of a newly admitted patient who is at acute high risk may allow that patient an opportunity to die by suicide.

By far the greatest number of patient suicides occur shortly after hospital discharge (a few hours, days, or weeks later). Appleby et al. (1999) found that the highest number of suicides occurred during the first week after discharge. Meehan et al. (2006) found that suicide most frequently occurred during the first 2 weeks postdischarge. The highest number of suicides occurred on the first day after discharge.

References

Appleby L, Shaw J, Amos T, et al: Suicide within 12 months of contact with mental health services: national clinical survey. BMJ 318:1235–1239, 1999

Meehan J, Kapur N, Hunt I, et al: Suicide in mental health in-patients and within 3 months of discharge: national clinical survey. Br J Psychiatry 188:129–134, 2006

Qin P, Nordentoft M: Suicide risk in relation to psychiatric hospitalization: evidence based on longitudinal registers. Arch Gen Psychiatry 62:427–432, 2005

Question 11

A 44-year-old single woman in acute suicidal crisis is admitted to the psychiatric unit of a general hospital. She is diagnosed with bipolar I disorder, most recent episode depressed, and borderline personality disorder. The patient has a history of multiple psychiatric hospitalizations, all precipitated by a suicidal crisis. The average length of stay on the psychiatric unit is 6.3 days. After 7 days of intensive treatment, the patient is stabilized. Suicide risk is reduced, and the treatment team prepares for the patient's discharge. The patient's suicide risk at discharge is most likely

A. Indeterminate.
B. Low.
C. Moderate.
D. Chronic high.
E. Acute high.

Best response is D. The length of stay in many acute-care psychiatric facilities is less than 7 days. The goal of hospitalization is stabilization of the patient and discharge to appropriate community mental health resources. Current brief length of hospital stays may not allow sufficient time to stabilize some suicidal patients, thus increasing their suicide risk (Qin and Nordentoft 2005). Discharge planning begins at the time of admission.

Reducing this patient's suicide risk to low or moderate is unlikely, given her diagnoses, frequent hospitalizations, and acute high risk for suicide on admission. After patients at acute high risk of suicide are treated, many remain at chronic high risk for suicide.

Patients at chronic high risk for suicide frequently are treated as outpatients, except when an acute suicidal crisis requires hospitalization (Simon 2011). At discharge from the hospital, the goal is to return the patient to outpatient treatment.

A discharge note identifies the acute suicide risk factors that have abated and the chronic (long-term) suicide risk factors that remain. The discharge note also addresses the patient's chronic vulnerability to suicide. For example, the patient can become acutely suicidal again, depending on a number of factors, including nature and cause of the psychiatric illness, adequacy of future treatment, adherence to treatment recommendations, and unforeseeable life vicissitudes.

Reference

Qin P, Nordentoft M: Suicide risk in relation to psychiatric hospitalization: evidence based on longitudinal registers. Arch Gen Psychiatry 62:427–432, 2005

Simon RI: Preventing Patient Suicide: Clinical Assessment and Management. Washington, DC, American Psychiatric Publishing, 2011

Question 12

A 20-year-old college student is hospitalized following an overdose suicide attempt. Failing grades, panic attacks, and depression precipitated the suicide attempt. After 8 days of hospitalization, the young woman is much improved and ready for discharge. The patient is assessed as being at low to moderate risk for suicide. A family meeting is convened by the treating psychiatrist and the social worker. Both of the patient's parents and her older brother are present. The role of the family following discharge is discussed. Helpful family roles after the patient's discharge include all of the following except

A. Provide continuous 24-hour family supervision.
B. Provide emotional support.
C. Observe and report symptoms and behaviors of concern.
D. Encourage adherence to treatment.
E. Provide helpful feedback about the patient's thoughts and behavior.

Best response is A. There is an important role for the family of the discharged inpatient, but it is not as a substitute for the round-the-clock safety management provided by trained mental health professionals on an inpatient psychiatric unit (Simon 2011). Early discharge of an inpatient on the basis of reliance on family supervision can be precarious. Most patients are discharged at some level of suicide risk, given the short lengths of hospital stay. If an outpatient at suicide risk requires continuous 24-hour family supervision, then psychiatric hospitalization is indicated.

Patients who are intent on killing themselves often find ingenious ways to attempt or die by suicide. Asking family members to keep a continuous watch on such patients usually fails. Most family members will not follow the patient into the bathroom or be able to stay up all night to observe the patient. Moreover, family members find reasons to make exceptions to the requirement for constant surveillance, whether out of denial, fatigue, or the need to attend to other pressing matters.

Reference

Simon RI: Preventing Patient Suicide: Clinical Assessment and Management. Washington, DC, American Psychiatric Publishing, 2011

Question 13

During the initial evaluation of patients, psychiatrists routinely inquire about current and past suicidal ideation. An affirmative answer prompts a systematic suicide risk assessment. Even in the absence of current risk, a psychiatrist should conduct a systematic suicide risk assessment if exploration of a patient's history reveals the presence of chronic suicide risk factors. Which of the following chronic risk factors has the highest association with suicide?

A. Family history of mental illness or suicide.

B. Childhood abuse.
C. Prior suicide attempt.
D. Impulsivity/aggression.
E. Prior psychiatric hospitalization.

Best response is C.   A comprehensive suicide risk assessment may not be required at the initial outpatient evaluation if there is no evidence of acute suicide risk factors. However, chronic suicide risk factors may be present, and, if revealed, should prompt a full assessment.

Harris and Barraclough (1997) conducted a meta-analysis in which they estimated the standardized mortality ratios (SMRs) for death by suicide associated with common mental disorders. (The SMR is a measure of the relative risk of death compared with the expected rate in the general population [i.e., SMR of 1.00].) In this study, the SMR for prior suicide attempts by any method was 38.61. Suicide risk was highest in the 2 years following the first attempt.

Some chronic suicide risk factors are static (e.g., a family history of mental illness, a prior suicide attempt). Other chronic risk factors, usually representing trait characteristics, can become acute (e.g., impulsivity/ aggression, deliberate self-harm). Assessment of chronic suicide risk factors is an essential component of a comprehensive assessment (Simon 2011).

References

Harris CE, Barraclough B: Suicide as an outcome for mental disorders: a meta-analysis. Br J Psychiatry 170:205–228, 1997
Simon RI: Preventing Patient Suicide: Clinical Assessment and Management. Washington, DC, American Psychiatric Publishing, 2011

Question 14

A psychiatrist is treating a 38-year-old physician for anxiety and depression. The psychiatrist sees the patient twice a week for psychotherapy and medication management. A recent lawsuit filed against the physician has severely exacerbated her symptoms. The patient is able to sleep only a few hours each night. Suicidal ideation has emerged, alarming the patient and her family. The psychiatrist performs a systematic suicide risk assessment and determines that the patient is at acute high risk for suicide. The psychiatrist recommends immediate hospitalization. The patient adamantly refuses. The psychiatrist decides not to involuntarily hospitalize the patient because she does not meet the substantive criteria of the state's involuntary commitment statute (e.g., overt suicidal behaviors). Instead, he chooses to continue outpatient treatment. Which of the following clinical interventions can help reduce the patient's suicide risk?

A. See the patient more frequently.
B. Adjust medications.
C. Obtain a psychiatric consultation.
D. Refer the patient to an adjunctive, intensive outpatient program.
E. All of the above.

Best response is E.   To hospitalize or not to hospitalize, that is the conundrum that psychiatrists often face with high-risk suicidal patients. The decision is considerably more complicated when the need for hospitalization is clear but the patient refuses the recommendation. The decisions that the psychiatrist makes at this point are crucial for treatment and risk management (Simon 2011).

Consultation and referral are good options for the clinician to consider, if time and the patient's condition allow. The psychiatrist should never worry alone. Sleepless nights benefit neither the psychiatrist nor the patient.

As in the case example, a psychiatrist may decide not to hospitalize a patient who is assessed to be at moderate to high risk of suicide. Protective factors may permit the patient to continue outpatient treatment. A therapeutic alliance may be present when the psychiatrist has worked with the patient for some time. Family support may also be available. The psychiatrist determines whether the patient's suicide risk can be managed by more frequent visits and treatment adjustments. In addition, supportive family members can help by providing observational data.

Nonetheless, a patient assessed as being at only moderate risk for suicide may need hospitalization when protective factors are few or are absent. Furthermore, protective factors can be overwhelmed by a severe mental illness.

A psychiatrist may determine that a patient at high risk for suicide who refuses hospitalization does not meet the substantive criteria for involuntary hospitalization. States have provisions in their commitment statutes granting immunity from liability for the clinician who certifies a patient for involuntary hospitalization, provided that the clinician uses reasonable clinical judgment and acts in good faith (Simon and Shuman 2007). Civil commitment is a judicial or quasi-judicial determination.

References

Simon RI: Preventing Patient Suicide: Clinical Assessment and Management. Washington, DC, American Psychiatric Publishing, 2011

Simon RI, Shuman DW: Clinical Manual of Psychiatry and Law. Washington, DC, American Psychiatric Publishing, 2007

Question 15

A 52-year-old married CEO is admitted to an inpatient unit because of acute alcohol intoxication and suicidal threats. The patient has had two similar episodes within the past year. After the patient undergoes successful detoxification, the psychiatrist and treatment team conduct a risk-benefit analysis for both discharge and continued hospitalization. A psychiatric consultation is also obtained. Which of the following factors should carry the most weight in the discharge decision?

A. Presence of family support.
B. Compliance with follow-up care.
C. Availability of dual-diagnosis programs.
D. Results of a systematic suicide risk assessment.
E. Psychiatric consultation.

Best response is D. All of the factors listed in options A through E are important considerations in the discharge planning of patients at risk for suicide. However, conducting a systematic suicide risk assessment to inform discharge planning is the most critical. The patient in the case example has had two previous psychiatric admissions for alcohol abuse and suicidal ideation. The patient is at chronic suicide risk but escalates to acute high risk when intoxicated.

Discharge planning begins at admission and is refined during the inpatient stay. Before the patient is discharged, a final post-discharge treatment and aftercare plan is necessary. Following discharge, suicide risk increases when the intensity of treatment is decreased (Appleby et al. 1999).

The patient's willingness to cooperate with discharge and aftercare planning is a critical determinant in establishing contact with follow-up treaters. The psychiatrist and treatment team structure the follow-up plan so as to encourage compliance. For example, psychotic patients at risk for suicide who have a history of stopping their medications after discharge can be given a long-acting intramuscular neuroleptic that will last until they reach aftercare. Patients with comorbid drug and alcohol abuse disorders can be referred to agencies equipped to manage dual-diagnosis patients.

Beyond stabilization of the patient, the psychiatrist's options in bringing about positive changes may be limited or nonexistent. Also, the patient's failure to adhere to postdischarge plans and treatment often results in rehospitalization, hopelessness, and greater suicide risk.

Psychiatric patients at moderate or moderate to high risk for suicide are increasingly treated in outpatient settings. It is the responsibility of the psychiatrist and the treatment team to competently hand off the patient to appropriate aftercare. With the patient's permission, the psychiatrist or social worker should call the follow-up agency or therapist before discharge to provide information about the patient's diagnosis, treatment, and hospital course. Follow-up appointments should be scheduled as close to the time of discharge as possible, given that suicide often occurs on the first day after discharge (Meehan et al. 2006).

References

Appleby L, Dennehy JA, Thomas CS, et al: Aftercare and clinical characteristics of people with mental illness who commit suicide: case-control study. Lancet 353:1397–1400, 1999

Meehan J, Kapur N, Hunt I, et al: Suicide in mental health in-patients and within 3 months of discharge: national clinical survey. Br J Psychiatry 188:129–134, 2006

Index

*Page numbers printed in **boldface** type refer to figures and tables. Those followed by "n" refer to footnotes.*